Man to Man

A Journal of Discovery for the Conscious Man

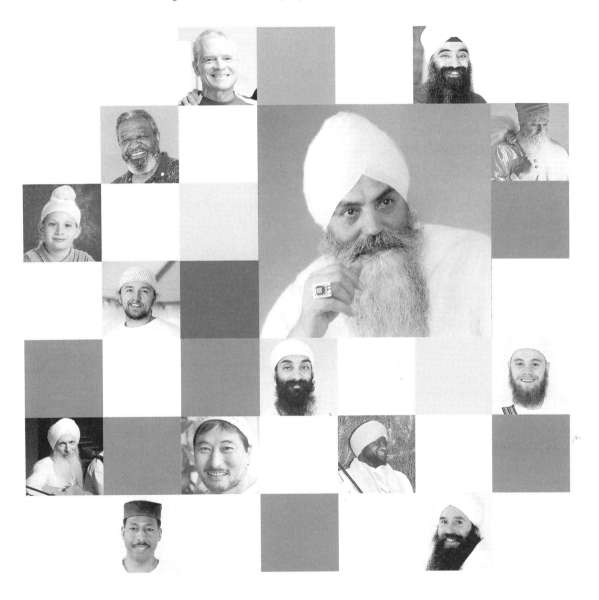

The Men's Teachings of **Yogi Bhajan**, PhD
Master of Kundalini Yoga

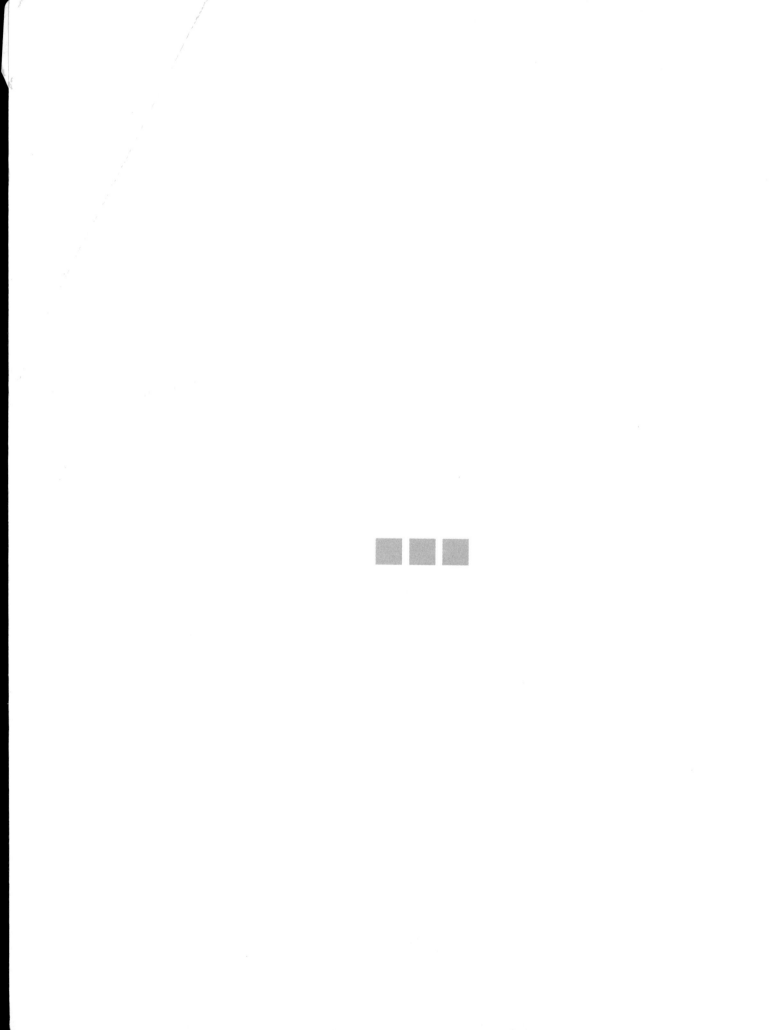

Man to Man
A Journal of Discovery for the Conscious Man

With special thanks to:
Siri Dharma Kaur Khalsa, Tej Kaur Khalsa, Vikram Kaur Khalsa, Gurubanda Singh Khalsa,
Pritpal Kaur Khalsa, Seva Simran Siri Kaur Khalsa, Gurushabd Singh Khalsa,
Gurumander Singh Khalsa and Awtar Kaur Khalsa without whose original work on
these manuals, this volume could not have been completed.

All illustrations were made from photographs taken at the course by Siri Dharma Singh Khalsa.
Illustrations by: Dharm Darshan Kaur Khalsa

Managing Editor: Sat Purkh Kaur Khalsa
Book Design and Production: Ravitej Singh Khalsa & Tara Kemp
Cover Design: Ravitej Singh Khalsa
Contributing Editors: Gurucharan Singh Khalsa, Nirvair Singh Khalsa
Other Contributors: Satya Kaur Khalsa, Kirpal Singh Khalsa, Siri Neel Kaur Khalsa,
Sewa Singh Khalsa, Hari Jiwan Singh Khalsa, Dharm Singh Khalsa
Original Recordings: Siri Ved Singh Khalsa
Photography: Jaime Kowal, Ravitej Singh Khalsa, Convivial Design, Gurudarshan Kaur Khalsa
Models: Sarbjit Singh, Tom Khu, Himat Singh Khalsa, Roger Woods,
Har Rai Singh Khalsa, Dyal Singh Khalsa, Har Pal Singh Khalsa, Lakhmi Chand Singh Khalsa,
Nirmal Singh Khalsa, Sat Purkha Singh Khalsa, Ravitej Singh Khalsa, Gurprakash Singh Khalsa.

13-Digit ISBN 978-1-934532-05-8 Man to Man: A Journal of Discovery for the Conscious Man.
10-Digit ISBN 1-934532-05-3 Man to Man: A Journal of Discovery for the Conscious Man.

Copyright 2008 Kundalini Research Institute. All teachings, yoga sets, techniques, kriyas and meditations courtesy of The Teachings of Yogi Bhajan. Reprinted with permission. Unauthorized duplication is a violation of applicable laws. ALL RIGHTS RESERVED. No part of these Teachings may be reproduced or transmitted in any form by any means, electronic or mechanical, including photocopying and recording, or by any information storage and retrieval system, except as may be expressly permitted in writing by the Kundalini Research Institute.
To request permission, please write to KRI at PO Box 1819, Santa Cruz, NM 87567 or see www.kriteachings.org.

Rev 5.16

Kundalini Research Institute
PO Box 1819 Santa Cruz, NM 87567
www.kriteachings.org

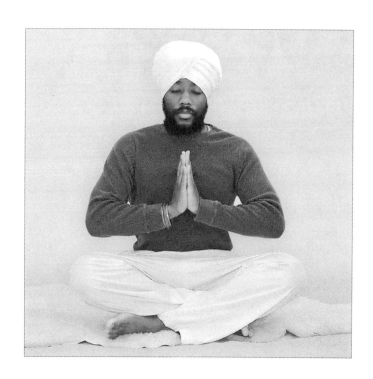

You are the men of God. May you recognize it.
You are the men of the universe. May you deal with it in the light of God.
You are men to be men. May you feel the pride of it and be in grace.
You are the men of success. May you accomplish it.
You are the men of self, light and respect. May you understand it.
You are the men of merits. May your virtues be known.
You are the men of knowledge. May your compassion be known.
You are the men of absolute determination. May your kindness be known.
May you be men whom the world, the Earth, the Universe, may be proud of.
Sat Nam.

—Yogi Bhajan

A Few Words from a Few Good Men

Yogiji[1] communicated a magnificent description of the Aquarian male, the new age man: a man who is conscious of his word, a man who is kind, generous, successful and full of love. We had never heard these words used to describe what we could be. Gracious, respectful, contained, aware, sensitive and potent, learned, beautiful and wise. This vision of man's true Self was nowhere in the mainstream media, it was certainly not in American culture.

Sitting among the men at Yogiji's Men's Courses was completely enthralling. No one moved while he spoke. There was electricity in the air. The moments between his sentences were pregnant with concentration, every one of us waiting for the next sentence, wondering what was coming next. An entire room full of men, each one unique, with completely diverse backgrounds, sitting in awestruck silence, with eyes on him. There was incredible intensity but deep trust. There was softness of the divine behind the surface. We watched his hands and his eyes. His entire being was a living mudra.

Then he would give us a kriya. Sweat would pour and tears would drop, potential would be achieved, the infinite light would become your best friend, songs would resound in your cellular structure, and I don't think we were ever the same again.

But the most valuable thing he gave us was the yoga, which let us achieve this vision of our potential. It was not just a vision–there was a way to get there. Because this yogic methodology is available, it means that every man has the tools to achieve this vision of the Aquarian man. I don't think the men's courses were ever fully understood by us at the time. We tried to comprehend. Yet he always said that we would understand more in the future. After years of practice I still feel his teachings are as alive as ever and continue to sink in and touch me at greater and greater depths.

This volume from KRI, which compiles the courses under one cover, is a remarkable achievement. It strings the series of men's courses, which spanned decades, onto one coherent thread, linking them into a continuum of teachings, making them accessible and understandable as a life work.

Blessings,
Dharm Singh Khalsa

Studying with Yogi Bhajan in the Men's Courses was an unforgettable experience. Yogiji always knew how to communicate with his audience. He knew how to really reach the students and his language and approach reflected that mastery.

These courses were attended by young men. We wanted the information straight and we did not have the time or the patience for anything less than an avalanche of earthy practical knowledge about relationships, health, sex and spirituality. Yogiji delivered—period.

The courses themselves were very fun. I remember the very first course I attended. I was a little hesitant because I really did not know what to expect and was accustomed to the style he used in his other public lectures. I was amazed that he communicated and taught us more like he would in a private audience. He worked us hard, too. The kriyas were really challenging and being with other men really inspired us—read, competition—to do our best.

I am so glad I took these courses. Reading them again recently, I was once again shocked, confronted, uplifted, amused and inspired by the information and awed by the magnificent Teacher Yogi Bhajan was and is to this day. I am doubly grateful that my son studied these timeless courses when he was in school in India. What a wonderful thing to be exposed to this information as a teenager! He knows what it means to be a real man in the truest sense of the word.

Blessings,
Nirvair Singh Khalsa
The Kundalini Research Institute

---

[1] Yogiji was a nickname or familiar name for Yogi Bhajan, used by some of his students.

Yogi Bhajan rarely taught classes exclusively for men; I had the great good fortune of attending most of those precious events. I am ever grateful to him, because even the most minor application of his teachings in my life has yielded immense and wonderful outcomes.

At the time, I had to stretch very hard to grasp the meaning of his words. Our culture had rejected traditional boundaries and the search for a new model of behavior for people in love was basically a free for all. What he offered in the midst of this sea of experimentation was truly ancient wisdom with its roots in the core physical, mental, emotional and spiritual nature of the human being.

It is amazing that this man had the courage and audacity to give a message of restraint in the midst of a sexual revolution. One could only imagine which was less palatable, this or his message to reject drugs and alcohol. Considering the number of people who took his message to heart and restricted their previously unfettered sexual activity, the outcome had vast consequences. His timing was precise; at the very least, hundreds, if not thousands of people were likely spared death by AIDS/HIV, not to mention the suffering brought on by other STDs and unwanted pregnancies. And this was just the background to a much subtler body of teachings.

To my knowledge, Yogi Bhajan never made any claim or reference to this outcome. In hindsight, like with so many of his actions, we see an incredible and selfless vision spanning time and space; touching humanity in ways never imagined by the casual observer.

It is my prayer that through the application of the wisdom in this book, the reader, like many before them, may find their life's destiny changed in profoundly positive ways.

Blessings,
Sewa Singh Khalsa

■ ■ ■

Where do we go from here? What do I do? Who am I, really? Why is there a Ladies' Camp and not a men's course? In 1978 Yogi Bhajan addressed these questions by beginning an annual course for men. Believe me—these courses were for men only. He would blow in and teach with all the testosterone only a master Yogi can conjure; and, we'd wonder why we had asked for these classes.

After many, very strenuous yoga sets (as if he were saying, 'you asked for it, now take it'), our energy would rise to a level at which we could begin to match his. This quasi-balance in the aura would call for his lecture to begin. And, begin it did; for it has never ended. I still carry teachings from these courses with me today. Many times, at innocuous moments, some mundane thought or action will remind me of what he taught at one of these courses. They have grown deeper and been understood at different levels at the appropriate times in my life. For this, I am forever grateful. These teachings are sacred, blessed and infinite.

If there was one word I'd use to describe Yogi Bhajan it would be: intuition. *Man to Man* reflects the progression toward becoming a man of intuition. To quote Yogi Bhajan in all his humility, "In this world, all you need to be is just to be a man." A "man" possessing all the qualities of an elevated being, and of course, all the qualities attributed to reality are included in this concept. For the blessed practitioner, these teachings progress from understanding to acceptance; from memorization to coalescence; from integration to intuition.

Man to Man offers great insight into the relationship men have with themselves, their partners and others. Our habits are a product of our subconscious mind. The result is a continuum that our memory has created. Developing an awareness and understanding of this history, this circle of memory and action, leads to change. To have the courage and discipline to move out of this limiting cycle creates a new, elevating reality. These notes lead one to face the truth so that relationships and life itself change in a positive manner.

These Men's notes are offered here for your perusal, enjoyment and elevation. Yogi Bhajan's distinct style of candor and humor offer the reader infinite understanding and also entertainment. Take them for what they are; be who you are; and receive them for who and what they will lead you to be. I can only express my personal experience: these teachings are the essence of totality, Godliness brought to the Earth. They have blessed my life. They are offered to you in the prayer that you, too, will be blessed in the same way.

Blessings,
Hari Jiwan Singh Khalsa

Just Be a **Man**!

In a rapidly changing world, full of turbulence and crises, how do we experience fulfillment as a Man? How do we define our identity, our sense of belonging, our meaning and purpose, and our social roles and gender? Our minds don't help: we are filled with ideas and impulses that often cloud our direct perception and understanding of what it means biologically, mythically and functionally to be a man. Add to this our constant fascination with our polarity—the feminine—and you can see that there's lots of room for guidance.

The dance of men and women has gone on from the beginning. So we can call on the wisdom of the ages, but of course, that wisdom is overlaid with just as much fantasy, fear, desire, culture and phobias as well. In tribal cultures, there is ritual—rites of passage—where elders help the younger men sift out the wisdom from the whimsical and prepare the boy to be a man, to handle himself and his duties rightly, along with this "other creature," the woman, who holds such a central place in his subconscious. We have largely lost this place by the fire; this sincere appreciation of our masculine nature and this clarity in relation to the feminine. In our globalized networked environment and the fluid interaction of cultures, it feels like we have lost our compass, our common ground, our North Star—what does it really mean to be a man? Instead, it all seems to be cultural history or religious narratives, not relevant to contemporary life and lifestyles.

Yogi Bhajan gathered men together and challenged them with straight talk and hard exercise. He shined a strong light on our individual nature, our shared natures and our universal nature. He discussed being a man from so many different facets. How do we think about being a man? What is our fundamental nature as man and woman? How do we communicate and acknowledge our basic tendencies? How do we learn to express our unique attitudes and personalities? What are the pitfalls in male–female relationships? What are our common distractions? What are the fundamental tendencies and differences in the masculine and feminine experience? How can they work well together?

In these discussions he engaged and embraced us—just as men. He was not a professor. He did not proceed along a careful linear path of points and propositions. Instead, we traversed a long and twisting mountain path, fraught with dangers but leading to unexpected vistas. He did not hold our hands like children. He walked with us side by side as men. He leapt ahead and challenged us to prove ourselves to our Self—our own potential and grit. He asked each of us to pause on our path, to break our hypnotic march through life and resist the steady beat of impulse and defensiveness. He woke us up and asked us to understand the nature of being a man and what it takes to walk on the path as a man.

Yogi Bhajan said that if we would just be who we are as a man there would be no problem. Love your design as a man. You are built to defend. You are designed to be steady. You are crafted by nature and time to be direct and think in terms of action and strategy. Sure you tend to act with half a brain—that's called cutting to the chase! What would it look like if you could stand with dignity? If your word was your law? If you understood the polarity of the feminine? If you recognized that she read your subconscious not just your conscious projection, with all its spectral flashes of bluster?

He filled his talks with simple classical metaphors—man is the sun, woman is the moon, and earth is the realm of action, material things and money. The masculine–feminine dance is as orchestrated and polar as the approach of the spermatozoa to the ovum. It is driven by cellular rituals and attended to by the handmaidens of smell, vision and touch. On top of this infrastructure of simple metaphors, he layered practical knowledge: herbs and food for health and potency, techniques for self-discipline to give us strength and awareness as men, and nuanced wisdom to see beyond surface judgments and primal impulses.

There is a historical context to this universal wisdom. When he came to teach in the United States, it was in the midst of a "sexual revolution" that was part political and part radical, questioning the norms and strictures of sexual choice. It was also a time that pushed the proposition that men and women were not different, as the Women's Movement fought for equal rights under the law and equitable economic practices. Yogi Bhajan did two things. He started a small women's movement to raise the consciousness and the dignity of women so that they would recognize their powerful creative energy. As many women challenged the status quo and dressed provocatively, he asked these women to dress themselves in a royal manner that communicated self-contentment, self-esteem and self-respect. As part of this effort he began the women's camp experience to get women together to learn the technology of the feminine and to discuss and bond with each other. Second, he elaborated the differences between men and women and taught men to be men. This flew directly in the face of the times.

Over the years, his teachings have spread and become more accepted, incorporated by other authors and vindicated in their practical usefulness. Science has also moved ahead. We now know that 2% of our genes are linked to gender differences that affect the metabolism of 40% of our body's tissues and organs. This has profound implications, from the cellular level to the individual personality. Yogi Bhajan explained that men are 40% feminine; and we all start from an egg, that is, a woman. Although that difference may seem small, it is profound and Yogiji[1] said that the best way to perfect the essence of being a man was to be in a male body. His concept contains two primary thoughts: First, sexuality exists in men and women on a spectrum that is determined by the hormonal actions of the pituitary, androgens and other glands. He taught that the balance of these hormones was both genetic and influenced by experience and the environment of the womb. So he was open to the individuality of gendered experience and sexual choice. Second, he understood that as the sexual "temperature" increases it goes through a phase shift. Think of the temperature of water increasing from -2C to +2 C. The water suddenly shifts from ice to liquid. A small change in temperature changes the form, function and possibilities of the water. So he would say if you are 1% more man, then be 100% man. Cultivate and excel in the character and accomplishments of being a man.

Yogi Bhajan's perception was nuanced. We are both individually crafted in our proportion of masculine and feminine energy—our gender expression—and we get the best out of our self when we recognize the impersonal patterns of our masculine energy and consciously optimize them. To continue with the metaphor, we get the best experience of ice if we recognize it is different from water. We can walk on ice across the lake, skate at high speeds, keep our drinks cold or sculpt ice castles. So as a man, if we recognize and cultivate the shift in form and phase that attends it, we can realize and optimize our innate potential. This conversation is important. And to have it from a spiritual perspective laced with the practical technology of exercise, nutrition, relationships and meditation is unusual. You will find in the many dialogues with his students that the men ask direct and frequently blunt questions; and he answers in kind. Yogi Bhajan invites us to explore our self as a human and as a man.

I had the blessing to go through these courses with him. I recommend that you read it once through from beginning to end. Get the whole vista he described. Don't stop at a point of interest or contention; don't pause at what attracts you, or stop at what challenges you. Take it all in like a gift. Recognize the conversation as a living document—the legacy of interaction and communication between a Master, Yogi Bhajan, and a community of men—then go back and pick through the points of interest. Try the meditations. Explore the impact of the diets. Explore what disciplines and perspectives serve you as an individual to experience and deliver your excellence as a man. Forge from this raw steel a tempered sword of clarity about how to be a man.

Gurucharan Singh Khalsa, PhD
Director of Training
Kundalini Research Institute

Table of Contents

A Few Words from a Few Good **Men** V

Just Be a **Man**! *by Gurucharan Singh Khalsa, PhD*
Director of Training for The Kundalini Research Institute VII

Table of **Contents** IX

Man to **Man** 1: *Talks with Yogi Bhajan* 1
"If man is man, there cannot be any problem. . . . Woman has to be woman and man has to be man. If man is not man it starts a chain reaction."

- If Man Is **Man** 2
- The Secret to Sexual **Satisfaction** 14
- Phobias and **the Man** 20

Man to **Man** 2: *Inside the Real Man* 27
"We are talking about the inside man—the real man. . . . in the past, there was nothing more beautiful before a man than a man himself."

- Potency and **Potentiality** 28
- The Downfall of **the Man** 31
- Potent Potential of the **Inner Being** 36
- Exercises for Potency and **Potentiality** 38
- Creativity of **Consciousness** 45

Man to **Man** 3: *Incentive and Invocation of Polarities* 49
"Each male and female relationship is not physical at all. The physical relationship is the culmination of the relationship. It is initiated by invocation through the auric body."

- Incentive and Invocation of **Polarities** 50
- Invoke, Don't **Provoke** 58
- Magnetic **Preference** 64
- If You Can Fake It, You Can **Make It** 70

Man to **Man** 4: *Growing as a Man* 73
"After a man presents himself, he must communicate. . . . When you communicate, the only friend you have is the art of creative dialogue. That is what establishes you as a man."

- The Multiple **Man** 74
- The Growing **Man** 86

Man to **Man** 5: *The Real Strength of Man* 99
"Your ultimate desire is a desire that uplifts you, your spirit, and your consciousness. It is always positive to you and your surroundings and your framework. . . . It is a love of self and grace. It is a consciousness, which has nothing but radiance about it.

- Your **Arcline** 100
- Developing Your **Arcline** 102
- Creative **Relevance** 107
- Woman and **Wisdom** 112
- The Ultimate **Desire** 119

Man to **Man** 6: *Sex, Success and Prosperity* 123
"You must understand, thoroughly understand, one thing: this energy, this psyche, this creative energy, this sexual energy is totally yours and nobody can share it."

- Creative **Sexuality** 124
- Creative Sensitivity: **The Fundamental You** 129

- Sex and Your **Life Span** 132
- Sex Is a Natural **Thing** 139
- The Origins of Sexual **Neuroses**: *An Interview with Michael Ebner, PhD* 143

Man to **Man** 7: *The Successful Man* 149
"In the garden of God, you are His one and only rose. Carry your own smell with your own deeds."

- Aspects of **Success** 150
- Physical **Aspects** 151
- Mental **Aspects** 160

Man to **Man** 8: *The Invincible Man* 171
"You must realize that the strength in you is you. The material world around you is to supplement your strength or to complement your strength; it is not your strength."

- Evergreen **Exercises** 172
- The Flow of **Life** 180
- Communication Is **Personality**: 186
- Health Is **Flexibility** 192
- **Who** Are You Subject To? 198

Man to **Man** 9: *The Blocks Men Can't Talk About* 203
"There are blocks that men can't talk about. These blocks are keeping you from achieving your potential as men. If we are not willing to talk about something, how can we get rid of it?"

- Growing **Up** 204
- Living the You Within **You** 213

Man to **Man** 10: *Being a Man* 223
"The greatest tragedy that mankind was given to understand or believe was that you have to find God. You can never, ever find God. You are God—part of God. And the whole God is with you, behind you and within you."

- Realize the Reality of Being a **Man** 224
- Realizing **Success** 241

Man to **Man** 11: *The Qualities of a Successful Man* 255
"Nothing in the world can destroy you. Nothing in the world can build you. It is only the art of communication."

- Communicating **Successfully** 256
- Claim Your **Virtues** 266
- Communicate **Prosperity** 276

Man to **Man** 12: *Excel as a Man* 283
"What is a man? Man is a living experience, which can confront every temptation and still resurrect itself. . . . It is an endless seed; it lives to seed. Its faculty, its quality, its generality, its temperament, its achievement is not mortal."

- The Faculty of **Man** 284
- Three Kriyas to Become a **Man** 287

Man to **Man** 13: *On Being a Spiritual Man* 291
"If you can nurse, nurture, love, take care, make a person grow, and from the heart, the person says "thank you," there is no more blessing than that, there is no more prayer than that, there is no more goodwill than that."

- The Technology of Being a **Man** 292
- Wake Up Like a **Man** 309
- Life in **Balance** 324

Appendix **A**: *Additional Recommended Kriyas* 329

- Hidden Self **Kriyas** 1 & 2 330
- Sat **Kriya** 332

- Sodarshan Chakra **Kriya** 333
- Kirtan **Kriya** 334

Appendix **B**: *Healing and Healthy Foods for Men* 337
- A-Z Foods and Supplements for **Potency** 339
- Fasts, Recipes, and **Remedies** 343
- Rejuvenating Foods from Around the **World** - *Presented by Soram Singh Khalsa, M.D.* 352

Index 361

Man to **Man**: *Exercises, Kriyas, and Meditations*
- Exercises for Potency and **Potentiality** 42
- Narayan **Kriya** 96
- 8-Stroke Breath **Meditation** 116
- Dancing Ardas Bhaee **Meditation** 121
- Peacock Pose 126
- Kriya to Create **Balance** 128
- Special Exercises for **Men** 131
- Breath of **Fire** 133
- Kirtan **Kriya** 134
- Meditation for Mental Control of **Metabolism** 161
- Meditation for **Success** 166
- Pratyahar/Pranayam Sank Chalnee **Kriya** 168
- Evergreen **Exercises** 173
- Guru Gobind Singh's **Jaap Sahib** 179
- Kriya for the Evening **Star** 184
- Kriya to Communicate and Create **Companionship** 189
- Chitra Kriya: **Mirror Exercises** 194
- Invincible Man **Exercises** 200
- Meditation to Realize the Reality of a **Man** 226
- Meditation to Turn Yourself into **Water** 230
- Palate and Tongue **Kriya** 233
- Yoga Therapy for **Anger** 235
- Kriya to Free Yourself from **Karma** 239
- Kriya to Unfold Your **Virtues** 243
- Kriya to Realize **Success** 245
- Kriya to Awaken the Vibrant **Self** 247
- Kriya to Develop the Art of Selling Your **Self** 250
- Meditation to Move through the **Ethers** 253
- Kriya for Infinite Strength and **Communication** 259
- Kriya to Communicate as **You** 265
- Lingam **Kriya** 266
- Kriya to Claim Your **Virtues** 274
- Drib Drishti Kriya to Show You the **Future** 280
- Becoming **Divine** 287
- Balancing the Apana **Energy** 288
- How to Overcome **Crisis** 289
- Charan **Japa** 298
- Kriya to Create a **Saint** 302
- The Faculty of a **Man** 307
- Wake Up **Exercises** 309
- Exercise for **Clarity** 313
- Relaxation **Exercise** 314
- Kriya to Invoke the Internal Power of a **Man** 315
- Kriya to Prevent **Impotence** 317
- Kriya to Be a **Man** 321
- Meditation: Tantric Yantra to Receive All **Knowledge** 327

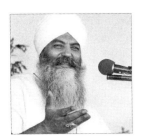

Man to **Man** 1

Talks with Yogi Bhajan

Circa 1978

If man is man, there cannot be any problem. . . .
Woman has to be woman and man has to be man.
If man is not man it starts a chain reaction.

- If Man Is **Man**
- The Secret to Sexual **Satisfaction**
- Phobias and the **Man**

If Man Is Man

In particular relationships in life there are simple facts you have to study from the law of nature.

Lose everything on this planet but hope. Hope is the last thing one should lose. If you want to build up what you need to build up, there's no magic which can help you except sadhana. I know the majority of you are lazy in relation to sadhana for one reason or another, but that is not what I call laziness. Nor do I call it negativity or self-depression. It is self-denial. Men do suffer with one thing, self-denial. While woman is very involved in recognizing herself and making herself to be recognized, man is equally good at self-denial and escapism. Have you seen men talking with this flowery talk? God, it is worthwhile listening. They want to represent themselves for what they are not.

Today we'll talk on a man to man basis. If man is man, there cannot be any problem. Any problem you face in life indicates how much minus-man you are. I'll help you understand why this is so in a very harmonious and rhythmical way. All you seem to understand about a man is that he is a guy who has something between his two legs. Some believe that's what makes them a man. This is not true. Fundamentally and scientifically, this does not make you a man at all. The urinary function of the penis is exactly the same as a female's. You must recognize one fact: by nature, in your normal day to day life, your penis remains relaxed. It is only when the thought wave stimulates a particular part of the brain that the master gland, the pituitary, sends a signal and the male organ becomes stiff. Then you feel that you are different from the female.

Today we are at the crossroads of the greatest human trauma. The circumstances are very heavy. Females are becoming berserk and man is not trained to be a man. For example, consider this: A successful doctor makes about $250,000 each year. He has three children and a beautiful blonde wife. He has a car for her and one for himself, and so on. One day he comes home and finds a note on the door. It says, "Your entry has been prohibited under the advice of my attorney. Please have your attorney contact my attorney, if you wish. Any other effort on your part will be considered an interference with my life." In the morning she kissed him, she hugged him and she wished him goodbye for the day. In the evening, he gets a note posted on the outside of the door and he finds that the lock has already been changed. If he wants to enter, he will be considered a trespasser. Can you compute that life? Can you understand it?

Woman has to be woman and man has to be man. If man is not man it starts a chain reaction. Initially, your thoughts which arise through the intellect create an emotional state. Next your desires become commotional, disturbed and destructive. From this you have neuroses and deepening problems. The intellect releases 1,000 thoughts per 1/10th of a second. Each thought can become an emotion; there's that possibility. This is very important. Each emotion can become a desire. When you come to the point of desire, there is a point of diversion: that desire can become a commotional desire or a devotional desire. When it becomes commotional, it creates neurosis. Neurosis can bring patterns and these patterns can bring you constant and continuous unhappiness. Or, a desire can become devotion. Devotion can become compassion, and compassion can become sacrifice. Sacrifice can bring you happiness within your Self. There is no way to find happiness outside of you. All these efforts: "if I do this, I'll be happy, or if I do that, I'll be happy" are totally escapism. This is what is facing you. It is trying to confront you as a man.

In particular relationships in life there are simple facts you have to study from the law of nature. Most men have trouble with their neurosis because they don't understand that the male and the female are two different situations. The female has the mechanism to sprout the seed. When she gets your spermatozoa with her egg, she gives you a baby. If you give her a thought, she will give you a whole scheme. If you know how to use a woman—it is such an essential, natural asset, you cannot even believe it. Give her something, give her anything and tell her to build it up into a program, from a thought, and she will do it perfectly. For you it is a hassle.

Now there are fundamental problems in which we get involved and I'm going to list those problems one by one. First of all, we have an image of a woman. Each male has an image of a female and he continuously searches to meet that female. This image can be either exactly like his mother or contrary to that [image]. It depends on how he establishes himself within the first five years. Now this is a most important thing to remember: When you meet a woman, you don't just meet a woman. You are looking for your female image within that woman. When you become an adult, you become almost insane, forgetting the creature and trying to find the image. So the woman you look at is not a woman at all. What you are looking at is a statue of a woman. If you want to relate to a statue, you are not relating to a woman. For example, men say, "Oh, I married her because she was beautiful. I married her because she was a blonde. I married her because she was pretty." Now that is a statue. Why don't you get a marble slab and have a statue made and look at it all the time? Woman is not a statue; she is a living organic thing.

No woman in her lifestyle is complete. In the scriptures, woman is described as the moon. Just as the moon goes full and then wanes and is constantly fluctuating, so the woman fluctuates mentally, physically and spiritually. The flow of her spiritual strength also goes in that variance. One day she is very bright and charming; after a couple of days she is totally dumb and non-communicative. This is called the normal woman mood. The normal flow of a woman's moods is a rhythmic cycle. Woman has her own natal chart in which there is a moon. Her mind is in a certain zodiac sign and that is her momentary mood. Also, physically the moon moves through her, and all the three make a combination in time and space called the menstruation cycle. She is very much influenced by that cycle.

Using a woman, in a normal rhythmic sense, just for sexual and sensual purposes is just like taking a biscuit and eating it when you are very hungry. Normally, most sexual intercourse between a man and a woman is this: the man has the gratification and satisfaction of having conquered. You have done it. You have achieved it. Ejaculation is nothing but a satisfaction to the very ego of the male. It is not what

The Do's and **Don'ts**

I'll explain more of the process now—the do's and don'ts. You must not have relations with a woman if you have eaten within two or three hours. If you have food in your stomach—if you have eaten—the game of love is out and the game of food is in. Food is in, love is out. Remember this. Otherwise, you will invite so many diseases. There are two things you must not do: You must not meditate when you have eaten and you must not have sexual relationships when you have eaten. Otherwise, it will not make a saint out of you, but a piglet—and I'm serious! It's a very damaging thing. If you meditate with a full stomach, instead of all of the blood going to the stomach to take care of the body's whole system, it starts turning itself into serum and going to the brain. You are then causing an unnecessary diversion and an unnecessary problem. Simply, when you have taken food, everything should concentrate towards the stomach. If you are ejaculating downstairs, you are just creating a problem.

Now, when you are tired, one thing as a man you must declare, "I am tired. And I need a truce." A man who's shy to declare he's tired is asking for trouble. "Come, trouble, come," that is the mantra. It is ridiculous; if you are tired, you need rest. If you need rest and you are not getting rest, you are going to rust. You can get a lot of sympathy, a lot of feeling from the other side if you say, "I am very tired, I need rest and you will be a great help to me, to let me rest."

Q: *You're just talking about sex; you're not talking about when you're tired in other cases are you?*
Yogi Bhajan: *No, I'm saying that sometimes when people are tired, they become very sensual, sexual, and they engage in intercourse. That is very sickening because that causes a lot of serious diseases—to the extent that you can cause blood diseases, or intestinal diseases, which come only when you are tired and indulge in sex and don't take a rest. That's what we are talking about, the don'ts. These are the don'ts. We are trying to give out precautions, to make you aware of the cautious situations.*

Q: *If we cut back on our sleep a little for sadhana, does that mean we will be tired at other times?*
Yogi Bhajan: *No, because when you sleep you are not sleeping. If you take eight hours of sleep, actually you sleep deeply for half an hour. The rest of the time either you dream, or you go into scupid.[1] Peaceful sleep that you call sleep is actually napping. Let us put it in a Western term. If you can take a half an hour nap, you can survive the rest of the time in absolute glory. Nap means switch off and switch on–sleep. [If you have slept deeply and you're still tired during the day, nap.]*

Q: *What is the best time to nap?*
Yogi Bhajan: *Nap? Anytime. But the most wonderful time is when you have eaten food. During the daytime, at what is called lunchtime, you can nap for **10 to 15 Minutes**.*

Q: *What if you switch it on and it won't switch off?*
Yogi Bhajan: *I understand. When you can switch off and you cannot switch on, either your digestive system is wrong or your lower back is wrong.*

[1] Scupid: A particular state of consciousness reached during sleep.

you think it is. After all, an ejaculation is not a small thing. It takes 80 drops of blood to produce 1 drop of semen. Also, it is a very great release. It is not beneficial in any way or form—except one. You must understand the play before the ejaculation.

The most sensitive system which you have is touch. Both parties must touch each other. It is called a system of body blend. Sometimes you do it wrong. You start with the membrane systems. You start kissing or trying to stimulate other membranes which are very touchy and sensitive. You just want a short cut and that is definitely just a defeatist male policy. Such marriages and such relationships will always end up very unhappy. First off, you must understand that there is no female, whosoever she may be, however ugly she is or however clean and beautiful she is, who doesn't want her body to be appreciated. Even if she tells you she is fat or ugly, tell her she is beautiful; because she doesn't care whether she's beautiful or ugly, she just wants you to care. You are the target. If she knows she's fat and ugly, she should have taken care of it. If she is not taking care of it, then she's very happy about what she is. Some men ruin their marriages or their relationships at that moment when she is without clothes. It's called the strip-off method: "Just take off your clothes; come on, let's go, let's do it; O.K., done; thank you; get out." You are in trouble. Because when you do that, you have a terrible fear calling on you. It is called mother phobia. Under the sensitivity of the sexual pressure, you can have intercourse; but in basic reality, you are still acting under a clear phobia. You feel like there is a sword hanging over you. You feel you have to hurry up. This is not how to do it.

Let me explain to you how nature sees the relationship between male and female. There is the sun. There is the moon. There is the earth. When the moon comes between the sun and the earth, a solar eclipse occurs. The male is considered to be the sun. If you prefer the earth and earthly possessions over your female, the moon, you will be eclipsed. Period. Let me put it in simple language: You can either love your dollar or you can love your woman. Choose either of the two, but you can't love both. Do you understand? It's a law of nature. Don't just think that I am saying it. I didn't say that you will be eliminated; I said you will be eclipsed. If woman comes between you and your ego, and she is in the center of it, you shall be eclipsed. That is the law of nature. Understand? All relationships which break, break because of this. You must change the situation, under normal and abnormal circumstances. Don't let your woman come between you and your earth.

Now, what happens otherwise? There is a situation where the earth comes between the sun and the moon. What is it? This is a lunar eclipse. Who is eliminated? Woman. So actually, in any relationship which you have or which you build, the problem is the earth. When earth comes in-between, one shall be eliminated. For the male, it is the sun. For the female, it is the moon. They say a man who does not know the earth *shastra* (how to manage property, how to manage wealth, how to manage your earthly relationship) is not going to be a happy man.

I remember once a woman called her husband, "Darling, my friends have come and I want to show them the city. Can you come away from the office for half a day so that we can do it?" It is a very ordinary request. He said, "No, my work is very important." So she took them herself, and in the evening, she took them to a restaurant. What did she see there? Her husband was sitting with one of the office employees, gossiping and taking tea. She was very intelligent, so she asked the waiter, "Oh, those people sitting at that table, when did they come?" He said, "Three o'clock." And she remembered that she had called at two o'clock.

A female needs constant social security and constant leadership. That is why a female looks to a male: social security and leadership. The female doesn't look to the man for sex—that is a by-product. She likes to bring up her concerns as a proposition. Remember, no woman wants to bring up problems. For a woman, there is no problem. Her problems are propositions. You don't understand that, which is why you get in trouble with women. Woman doesn't believe that what she says is a problem at all. This is one area in which the male and female greatly differ. For a male, it is a problem; for a female, it is a proposition. A woman will give you a proposition, you end up with a problem—and it is your problem, not hers.

Woman wants a constant security. This is to counter her waning and waxing. Just like the moon, she goes up and down; and so she needs a constant security. To test that constant security, it is her nature to continue giving problems in the shape of propositions to the male she loves the most. Sometimes it reaches the point of insanity. If you get involved in her insanity, that's what she wants. In this way, she proves to herself that you are insane, you are not a competent leader, and therefore she has the right to revolt.

First she will establish one thing, then her mind will establish the second, then it will establish the third. First she tries to establish that you are not a competent leader. There is no equal in this game. If you are a failure, you usually do certain things. Number one, you will stop communication. You will become angry and then you will stop communication. Next, out of the lack of communication, you will go outside of her orbit. These are the natural things you do as a man. You show your anger, stop communication, and get out of her orbit, to get out of her aura. These are the three things she needs to begin her proposition to get rid of you. There is a very common saying which I would like to translate to you, "Stop communicating with a woman and start the trouble." It makes the most rotten situation. If you can talk to a woman, you can get away with everything. So remember, the first thing she wants to establish, however, is the leadership. It is good for a man to be an established leader, but leadership has to be established in her eyes not in yours. Don't think you can say, "Oh well, I am a wonderful man." You may be wonderful by your own nature, but her nature must accept it.

Another issue which is very positive for a man to understand is that woman doesn't care whether you are very wise or you are very dumb. Some of you have a very phobic situation and feel that you have to be super intelligent. No, that is not what woman needs. Woman needs to experience whether or not you can communicate with her as a leader. You may be the most intelligent; you may be the most intellectual; you may be the most humorous; you may be the most of everything; but if she cannot accept your talk as a leader, you have lost yourself—with all your money and all your male chauvinism and all the diamond dust you have eaten. It has gone to waste. No sensual, sexual and charming situation can save the relationship if you cannot be accepted as a leader by law.

Whose law is that? It is that of woman. That is called focus. That is what it is all about: a lady and a law. A lady has a law and you are the focus of it. If you are out of focus, you are out of the picture. Don't make yourself a hero; make yourself be in that focus. If the lens is wide, be that wide, so then nothing else will come in. Got it? Do you understand? I know you don't want to understand. I understand that, too. To not try to know what a woman's focus is, is a basic suicide in relationship. That is why they say "know your lady." Understand what she says, what she means, what she thinks, how she thinks, and so on. Analytically these are very important things. If you are married to a woman who is the last child, you have married the most spoiled child in the family. If you are dating a woman who is the first child, you are actually marrying your own ego. Remember the first child is given too much care and too much love; last child is given too much free will and too much love. This is the "fundamental" [nature] of the person. If you do not understand the fundamental [nature] of the person, if you do not understand the woman, you are going to hit against a brick wall. Don't look at her blonde hair. Blonde hair is not what you are going to live with. Those blonde hairs are going to go around your neck! Remember even with beautiful red lips, there are very sharp teeth right behind them. You forget that. You only look at the lips, but what about those 32 big molars and teeth behind it. They can be used on you, too!

The Law of **Approach**

One important law to understand is the Law of Approach. If you want to come into focus, you must establish your approach to any woman. Even now you can do that. To a simple individual who is a man and nothing but a man, there is a simple law: he shall approach everything as a man. I have seen a lot of ladies who have divorced professional people. They always end up saying, "I married the man, not the profession." Though the profession sustains the whole family life and the marriage life, still, it is for her, the man.

In the Law of Approach there are four aspects. First, talk directly to your woman. Some men think that buttering a woman up or by going hodge-podge about things, everything will work out. This will cause you the greatest trouble. Be direct. Be a fact. Don't tell her that you have no money when you have $3,000 in the bank. Dummy! If she finds out, she's never going to forgive you. Woman by nature has a very fact-finding part in her. She is the nosiest creature. Woman is the nosiest creature created by God on this planet. There is a saying, and I am quoting the scriptures now, "A woman is five feet tall, but she has a ten foot long unseen nose. That is how nosy a woman is." Sometimes it sounds like this:

"Oh, where did you go?"
"Oh, I went to the bathroom."
"Which bathroom?"
You must have faced this question. "Oh I went into that bathroom."
"But Ji, you took so much time."
What can you say? "Oh ya, that was a long time."
"What for?"
"Oh, I don't know, there were a lot of people, lot of passengers, you know, there was no urinal."
"Oh, I see. Poor Ji, you really had trouble. But did you—everything is all right now?"

What can you do? This is a common state of mind for a normal woman. Exactly her height—double that is her nosy nature. You can't escape it; there's no way. Try to know what you are dealing with before you even begin dealing. Be direct, be a fact. Don't get caught by your woman so she can prove to you with facts and figures that you are wrong. Plead the Fifth Amendment. Actually, you will always see that in most conversations, women say, "I don't know." It is much better that you should say, "I cannot say exactly now." Don't say, "I don't know," then you look like a dummy, then you are no leader. You have to keep your leadership, so you have to say, "I do not exactly know now." If she says, "When are you going to know it?", you say, "Soon."

Never get beaten by time in direct or indirect relationships with a woman. Say, "We have got a lot of problems, let us discuss them. Let's talk it out." She replies, "Oh, when are we going to get it out?" You say, "I am going to lay it out. Don't you understand? As fast as time will permit me?" The speed may be two miles an hour, what do you care? Never in your conversation get tied by the time. Don't give woman time and space. If you give her time and space then only do it when you can be exact. So be direct, be a fact and be exact. First preference is don't give her time and space. You understand? If you do this blunder, out of your compassionate or your idiotic nature, I don't care whatever it is, then be exact. Tell her 4:30 p.m. and be there at exactly one minute to 4:30. That means 4:29.

You forget one law, the sun is alive. The moon reflects. She shall reflect you. Woman shall reflect you. She can never be you. It is a law of nature. What she reflects of you is your subconscious. She will never reflect your conscious. The worst you can do is expect that whatever you are consciously, that is what your woman should represent. No. She is a polarity. Woman shall represent your subconscious. I know practically in my own case my subconscious is very compassionate. If you deal with me either directly or indirectly, you will find it. All the women on my staff say, "All he knows is mercy." Men won't say that. They say, "Be afraid of him. Don't get under his claw, he'll tear you apart." This is because subconsciously woman can see you more. She may not see you as the aura, but subconsciously woman can see you. It is her automatic intuition. You can never hide your subconscious intuition from a woman.

I will give you an example: "Oh darling, congratulations are in order. I got all my back salary, ha ha ha. I thought I should bring a present for you. I bought you a diamond ring." She will say, "Wait a minute. Thank you very much. It looks pretty, but how much salary did you get?" You will have to come out with the exact amount. The moment you bring her a present, she will intuitively feel that there is some extra amount which you have spent which you don't want to tell her about and you are covering it up with a present. You think that if you bring a woman a present she'll be happy, forget it. If you bring her a present, you are starting a whole commission of inquiry. Originally, presents were to make a woman inquisitive. A present means communication starts, if communication is not happening. You think that if you bring a present to her then you have established a relationship. No, no, no. It is not true in the case of woman. When you take a present to her, she will want to know why you brought red roses today and white yesterday; and why you brought four roses yesterday and seven today. That's basic.

I said be direct, be a fact. Don't give her time and space. Be exact. That is the law of approach. Now you can ask me why do we have to hassle about this? You have to hassle about it because a woman is your opposite polarity. If you are the north pole, she is your south pole. You can either live with a woman, or you can love a woman, or you can totally hate a woman. You can hate her. You can love her. You can live with her. Beyond that, no state of mind exists. Do you understand? Now I will tell you what you can do. If you love her, L-O-V-E, she'll be a dove to you. You know what a dove is? It is known as a symbol of peace. If you love a woman, no matter how neurotic, how obnoxious, or how idiotic she is, somehow she will bring peace to your life, directly or indirectly. If you live with her, then she will only let you think of time and space. You will live a life of curiosity. If you hate her, then you live the life of your destruction. Rejection of your own polarity is a rejection of you.

There is a worse hatred: you indulge in a woman and then she has children. You love the child, the boy or the girl, more than her. It is called hatred at a distance. The moment a woman knows that she loves you and you love the children, she's going to play those children against your ego and mess up your life. This can happen even with your own wife. That is the worst thing you can have in your life. But a woman will only do certain things in a certain state of mind, when she's insecure. When a woman is insecure—do you know that proverb which says, "You have a snake in your armpit"? Well, if you have a snake in your armpit, neither can you move nor can you not move. You understand what I mean? If you move, you are in danger; it will bite you. And if you don't move, you're stranded and you don't know what to do. An insecure woman is a snake in the armpit. So spend some time and make her secure.

Now there is a problem in the Western world which doesn't exist in the Oriental world. Here woman can earn her own money. What can you do? You as a man are a pivot. Your balance of ego is based on the personality of the female's ego. Despite the fact that you have that balance, still you want to make a move, because you must move in order to establish your leadership. How do you do that? You do it through intercourse, or you do it through fighting, or you give her time and space, you run away. You must move! One is a physical indulgence. The other is the mental indulgence and the third is that you can move in time and space.

You do not understand your problem as a male. You are born of a woman. The basic elemental ingredients of you come from her earth. Therefore in your own chemistry, you carry the woman in you. The only area where you fall in your life is when you match up the moon with the earth. Now question is what to do instead? Match up the moon with the ether. It is the law of continuity. You cannot give guidance to a woman based on earthly law. She knows better than you. Therefore, you have one option. If you can be divine, you can keep the balance. You must establish a divine approach. Is that clear? That satisfies for now the Law of Approach.

Question and **Answer**

Q: You said the two things to establish are social security and your own leadership. What are the basic techniques of establishing social security?

Yogi Bhajan: Be direct, don't give her time and space, and be exact. That is what I laid down in the Law of Approach. It is a law which you cannot afford to forget. If you think woman is a sexual and sensual object for you, then for her you are only the one who exploits her. She will not bother to exploit you sexually, but her appearance of respect toward you is just to blind you. She's going to put blinders on you. Be direct in approach, effectual, don't give her time and space, and be exact.

Q: *Can you explain mother phobia? Its cause, its manifestation and its cure?*
Yogi Bhajan: Yes. Mother phobia: I'm going to take it as a second subject. I'm going to completely explain it.

Q: *What about using the silent treatment that you have mentioned before in your lectures?*
Yogi Bhajan: The silent treatment is a communication. You can only use the silent treatment to freak-out a woman—it is a 25 millimeter gun. Just become silently happy. If you are silently sad, then she thinks you are cursing yourself, then it is O.K. for her. But when you become silent toward her and you are happy, you can kill her in minutes. There is no woman yet born on this planet, including Goddesses, who can stand the silence of a man with a smiling face. Because her nature is to inquire, she wants to know why you are happy but you are silent. That's the death.

You know that is the treatment I have learned and that is the treatment I can give to anybody. It's just very calm and very quiet and simple and absolutely divine. Be a yogi and that's it.

Q: *What about how you feel underneath?*
Yogi Bhajan: Don't worry about your underneath. You have got two pounds of stool in your stomach, but do you show everybody? Underneath there are a lot of problems—and that's one of the problems. But the factual problem is your Law of Approach. You should be direct with her. You are smiling and you are just silent. That is what she cannot stand.

Q: *Are there any special things to know when living with a woman who was adopted and who doesn't know who her parents are?*
Yogi Bhajan: Oh, I'm going to cover that—bring that question up when I am discussing mother phobia. That is my next lecture.

Q: *I don't understand why giving a woman a gift causes her to inquire about it? That makes her unhappy. It seems like she could be happy.*
Yogi Bhajan: You think by giving a gift to a woman you are conquering a woman. Actually giving a gift is triggering the inquiry in her. The moment you bring a gift to a woman you are getting into her focus. The moment you get into focus, there is an endless inquiry. That is within her nature; she wants to know. If you become tired and lie down on the bed and forget about yourself, she understands you are tired. She will take off your shoes, take off your socks, take cold water and wash your feet, give you a good drink or whatever you need to recuperate. She will put a blanket over you and she will sympathize with you. That is her mother nature, the nursing nature will come out. If you stopped on the way and brought flowers and then came in and went to bed, she will think that you took flowers to somebody else and that she was not in and now you are sad. She can go 180° opposite. Woman doesn't think like a man. Her mechanism of thinking is much shrewder and much sharper because she can have a child. She has a super-sensitive nature to feel, and she fills in the feelings. Woman is never satisfied with the feeling, no way. She will fill in the feeling and when she starts filling in the feeling and you do not know how to be straight, you are getting into a mess. So don't trigger it.

Q: *In the silent treatment, wouldn't she be sensitive to what was underneath?*
Yogi Bhajan: Oh, yes. She knows that she cannot budge you. Woman never likes to confront a man and the silent treatment forces her to confront you. The moment she confronts you, she has to look into your eyes and she knows there is something wrong. The only way she can get out of this is to correct herself, and if you can make her do that, you are a very good man. In her nature, you are the perfect leader and that's all a woman needs.

Q: *How do you find out a woman's focus?*
Yogi Bhajan: Oh, that is one thing a woman can never hide. Out of the eight chakras, one chakra is her focus. Either she likes intelligent people, fabulous people, or sensuous people. Her focus is very elementary. There's no way she can hide it. If you do not know the focus of the woman, you do not know the woman. Do not try to be there. You understand what I mean? If you don't know her focus, you are putting yourself on the hot plate by involving yourself with her. But this is a common mistake we make as commotional people. We get into a proposition without knowing what the proposition is. You've got to know her focus and the lens she uses and whether it is a wide-range lens or a narrow lens, etc. You have to know that.

Q: *What do you mean by the width of the lens?*
Yogi Bhajan: Woman loves to talk. If you love to listen, then she can tell you everything about herself. Unfortunately, the majority of you do not even take the time to know who she is. That causes the problem.

Q: *There's the law that you have to communicate with a woman, and also there's the silent treatment. How do you reconcile those two?*

Yogi Bhajan: The law of silence is a law of communication. You must be there within her aura. You can always communicate. Your silence is not your true nature. You're doing it as a communication. You are not uttering a word because in the game of words she's sharper than you. She will cut you left and right. Have you seen any man who can win an argument with a woman? He usually gets angry and breaks the walls or a head or a plate. Forget it. Argument is her basic nature. She can argue and make you totally frustrated. When you start arguing with a woman, you are asking to become angry and leave the room in a couple of minutes. It can be 15 minutes for you, 10 minutes for somebody else and 20 minutes in most cases. But there is a decent and divine way; just be silent.

Q: I don't think I understood the pivot point. Is it the balance between the ego of the man and the woman?
Yogi Bhajan: Yes. The ego between the man and the woman is based on a pinpoint called personality, but you also have to act.

Q: Can you explain what you mean by not giving a woman time and space?
Yogi Bhajan: Not giving her time and space means either don't accept her and direct her, or accept her and become silent. Next, don't move. The majority of the people say, "I love you, but…" There's no such thing as "I love you but…" If you love her then it is very positive for you; just stay where you are.

Here is a typical case to study: There was a woman who was having problems. In the evening she would ask, "How was your day?" The man would say, "My day was fine. Your day was also wonderful, but you did this, this, and this, and even though I know you should not have done it, I won't say anything because I love you." This freaks her out. After months, she fell apart. She wanted to go to a professional person to get out of this problem. She wanted to understand her behavior. During this inquiry, I came into the play. I gave her a character analysis. She then could understand why she was behaving as she did and she got out of it. But the man had used a very positive approach. If you give her time and space, and be dignified about it, the strongest arm you have is your nobility. Be a noble man. There's no more powerful virtue in you as a man. You can be an established leader and a noble person. If she is sure that you are a noble person, you have no problem.

Q: You say either accept her the way she is and give her the time and space or…..?
Yogi Bhajan: No I didn't say that. You are reversing it. If you have given her time and space, then don't start an argument. That's called the law of forgiveness. Once you have established this with her that is it. You have done it. That's it, then forget it.

Q: I didn't quite understand about the bringing of gifts.
Yogi Bhajan: I'm just saying that if you bring a gift to a woman, don't bring a gift thinking it will conquer her. When you bring a gift you must understand you are triggering in her the inquiry. When you bring a gift to a woman, then you are triggering the inquisitive nature in her. Normally, men falter. They feel that by bringing a gift to a woman everything is taken care of. I have seen people buying a bunch of flowers and romantically thinking that she's already hugging them. All they know is that after 3 minutes, they are sitting in their car driving 80 miles an hour to get out of the house. Don't presume that if you give a gift to a woman you have already established everything you want to establish. No, you have started a situation and then you must end it properly. Got it?

Q: What about a woman who is apparently very attached to the earth and is afraid of the divine?
Yogi Bhajan: Woman is very attached to the earth in one way only—when she is very insecure about her husband. A woman who is attached to the earth is totally detached from you because you are the ether. You have got to act to correct that situation from the very beginning, before it is too late.

Q: What would be the approach?
Yogi Bhajan: The approach is to sit and negotiate. Don't leave it until tomorrow. You must understand if she's talking earth, earth, all the time and you are the polarity of earth as ether, it means she is telling you to go to the dogs, go to hell, etc. It's a very indirect language she is using. You understand? At that moment it is important for you to sit down and just establish contact. For example, "Well, wait a minute, this earth business concerns me and you. Let us now talk about ourselves."

Pull her over. She knows then that when she talks earth, you feel rejected, and she's not going to do it. She reflects the subconscious, not the conscious, not the physical love you make to her. No woman will ever reflect that. It is very important for you to know this. For example, some women want children right away. They are not secure with their husbands; a minus-husband is there. They either want a child or the house in their name. These behaviors and situations reflect the intolerance that she has been living with and they must be confronted and talked about. A clear understanding must be reached.

Q: Consider a hypothetical situation where a man imagines that he is the leader. Yet in reality he is totally dominated by the woman. The woman knows this and thus not only dominates, but manipulates the man to her whims and fancies.
Yogi Bhajan: Oh, that is a "banana man." That situation definitely exists. It will be covered. I must tell you I am trying to teach this course chapter by chapter, as I learned

it, to establish within you a scientific knowledge that has been achieved by the sages over thousands of years. It is important to complete this fundamental knowledge of the nature of man and woman. You must know what man is and how you can tackle him. If you do not know the outline, how can you know how you are supposed to act and what you are supposed to do? You can end up in a lot of trouble. In the beginning, when I said, "if you are a man you have no trouble," I didn't mean to give you a boost. Facts are facts and it took me four years to learn this aspect of knowledge; and I needed seven years to see its implementation in my life; and I have by my experience found it to be true. I believe that if you try to understand what we are discussing today and you implement that in your life, you will be very happy. You may have your experience; you may have your doubts; you may have your fears; and you may not be able to say directly what you want to know; but if those issues are discussed, they can throw light on all of us.

It is a combination of life. What is knowledge? Knowledge is a practical combination of life that is lived. That's all it is. Nothing comes from heaven; it's all created here. Earth is what earth is—in experience.

Q: When a man is not the leadership, the sun, that the woman wants him to be, then she resents the fact that he is a banana man.

Yogi Bhajan: When you are not the leader, she is not satisfied. That is her nature; that is her fundamental nature. The relationship between a man and a woman is based on this fundamental law. She wants to have leadership, otherwise she doesn't need a man for any reason. In matriarchal tribes, where woman has every right, she still needs a man for leadership.

Q: When do you compromise?

Yogi Bhajan: You compromise toward mutual righteousness. You should never compromise to your mutual benefit. It must be right for both. It must be right and divine. Your consciousness must agree it is right. When you compromise for mutual benefit—like two thieves, for example the husband is committing a theft and the wife does not want to tell the police—ultimately you run into trouble. As a man, you are not superior to your consciousness; instead you are subject to your consciousness. Therefore, you must answer to your consciousness. Because the woman is looking into your subconscious, she is the polarity of your consciousness. Ultimately, the relationship will be established when you establish a relationship with your own consciousness. If your woman doesn't know that you're a man of consciousness, your leadership can never be established. As long as the woman knows she can manipulate you, you are just a chess game. She will love to play it again and again. You'll not get peace of mind at all. This is why I say: if she loves you, she'll bring peace to you; but if she lives with you, you better forget it. Thinking that woman is just a subject of sensuality and sexuality is not real. That has no meaning if you truly want to look into the life of a man.

Q: If it's never right for a woman to publicly criticize a man, I don't understand how it's all right for a man to criticize a woman.

Yogi Bhajan: Man will criticize a woman out of sheer ego, and woman will criticize a man for sheer insecurity. If communication is established, then they use sign language in public. Between an established relationship of a male and a female, there is always a sign language which is never known from one pair to another. For example, if you do something wrong, your wife looks for her purse or touches your arm and this means, shut up idiot, you are lying. You know consciously what she is saying, and she knows what she is saying to you; but she will never say it in a way that everybody else may understand. I know a woman who becomes silent when you speak the truth very directly to her. She says she has nothing to say, which means she would like to live it, but she can't. She doesn't want to accept it. This is called father phobia. This is one of the qualities of the father phobia: Woman can be goaded to truth, but she will not accept it because she is not willing to accept anything from a man. When I discuss mother phobia and father phobia you will be surprised how much of life is messed up by these two things. That is why I say openly, clearly, give your children the values, not the life.

Q: You said you can't give a woman advice on earthly laws and that you must have the divine approach. Can you give an example of what you mean by this law and how it is used?

Yogi Bhajan: Earthly law is when in the time and space you want to escape from a situation, at that moment, if there is a problem, confront it, face it, establish it and clear it out. Don't put it off and ignore it. Once an inquiry starts in the mind of a woman it must be totally ended, completely satisfied. Escape is not the way. Divine is when you approach a problem from a totality.

Q: When you establish social security and leadership in a relationship and the woman, through past experiences, doesn't want to trust you because you're a man, what techniques can you use to overcome that?

Yogi Bhajan: Be constant in your own Self. Once she has been with Henry, Jack, Smith, Grant and Bob, there's a very clear auric expression. As her earth, she who can take your seed and sprout it, it's very difficult to get around the past. But on a long-term basis, if she finds the leadership and continuity in you, and comes to trust in you and your leadership, she will totally try to forget those earlier experiences. That will ease the past. Past can be erased in a woman if you are constant, or your continuity is constant.

If you fluctuate and are up and down like an idiot, forget it. You are another Henry, Smith, Jack, whatever it is. Then for her it is another time-to-time relationship. It is temporary. Don't establish a relationship with anybody on a time-to-time basis. It is going to be totally insane as far as you as a male are concerned.

Q: How do you know when you're leading a woman and when you're manipulating a woman?

Yogi Bhajan: Well, manipulation is when you treat her as an object. That is when you are manipulating a woman. The moment she knows that you are manipulating her, then you are being manipulated and the woman will never trust you. Remember, I told you about woman as a snake in the armpit. Once a woman is convinced of an idea in the depth of her mind, the subconscious, it is very difficult to change. She is a polarity. If she feels you are a cheat, you'll have to become a saint—200%. I can give you my own example. When I got married, I was an administrator. I was an officer in the government of India, wearing a lot of brass on my shoulders. My life was, "Yes. No. This. That." Do you understand? Part of my life I was still a yogi, but it was a side. Now the main part of my life is as a yogi, but my wife still feels that I am this man who is an executive. This morning when I telephoned her, I asked her about her health. She said, "I know I should have talked to you and asked you to pray for me. I would have been healthier." Now it is a constant for her. After 9 years, she has started to understand that I am more a divine man than an executive man.

I'm saying a life can totally happen, and when you are constant, when you are continuous, when you are very direct, when you are very honest, then everything is cool. It takes time and you must use that time. Don't try to hurry things. I'm sorry, but there is no other way.

Q: A couple of nights ago, in a discussion you were having, you said that you're not a man. What does that mean? You said, "They don't understand I'm not a man.

Yogi Bhajan: This is because my compassionate nature doesn't make me a man. When you treat me like a man, you are treating your own reflection, your own ego. I have nothing to lose, nothing to gain. I have no ego. What does it matter to me if I go out and I am killed? It doesn't matter to me at all. Simply, I'll be free. I'll be free today. My job is to complete a mission, right? It is not my job to live. To me, life and death no longer matter. My consciousness doesn't relate to it. But to an ordinary man, to live and to die is a big deal.

So when you treat me like a man, then you treat me as though I have advantages and disadvantages. I have no advantage and I have no disadvantage. I don't care. And I shall never care. It doesn't matter to me who's the President of the United States. What do I lose, who is who? Does it matter? It doesn't matter. I cannot focus my security in a man, in a government. I have to focus my security in God. Whether it is a phony security or it is a real security, it's my consciousness that has to answer. For my practical purposes and my training, I have to be with my God now and forever. That's why, for most of the things I want to do, I get corrected automatically by Mother Nature. I am not to hassle. That's why in my relationships I am very blunt and direct. It is much better to establish that now than later. You understand? But to some people it looks like I am a man, that I have emotions, that I have commotions, and that, therefore, I can be manipulated. Unfortunately, when they find they cannot manipulate me, they become very disgusting.

I have a tremendous opposition because people want me: "All right, please come and pray for me." I say, "Why should I go to your house? You are a cursed person and all your earnings are bad. I can't eat at your table." Do you think that man will like me? No. He will tell everyone what an idiot I am, that I am no holy person because he has to satisfy his ego.

When somebody asked me for a second visit, I said, "Wait a minute, I went the first time and I told you what to do. You have not done it. You are a very idiotic man and I won't visit your house again." I asked him to establish the relationship between him and his God, which he promised. Why should I go a second time? To become a social object? I'm a divine object! My purpose is to seed the Divinity. Therefore, I'm not an entertainment.

That's what I said to you that night: I am not Bob Hope. I am The Hope. I am not a comedian to entertain you, and I don't run the "Yogi Bhajan Show." I want to seed that hope in everybody. I want to seed a seed that sprouts. I want to seed a seed that grows. That's my happiness. And that's exactly what I meant when I said I'm not a man. Thank you for asking and clearing it up.

Q: What can a man do when a woman is being very quiet?

Yogi Bhajan: Do you understand when the weather is quiet what happens next? When a woman is quiet it is exactly like when the weather is quiet. Estimate then how many miles away the storm is. You are going to be hit by a hurricane. And you can measure exactly its strength by how silent she is. It is not her nature to be silent.

Q: I understand what's going to come. But where is that coming from?

Yogi Bhajan: It comes from the very depth of her; all that she has gathered for the time being is called low pressure. When she becomes angry within, she will express that anger outwardly. There is no difference between the two.

Q: *Also if you feel that she is progressing spiritually, but maybe not as much as you are...?*

Yogi Bhajan: Fine, when she is progressing spiritually, tell her to practice it, to show it. That is the best thing that can happen. When a woman says, "I am divine." Tell her, "Thank you. Then I am safe." Then she can't say anything to you. Reach her etheric nature and you are safe with every woman.

If you can reach the Mother Nature, then what you have is a nurse in your hand. You will be served. She will give you massages, good food, wonderful laundry. Everything is done because of that nursing nature. Forget operating on a 50/50 basis: if she washes your shirt, then you have to wash her pajamas. On a 50/50 basis she can be so cruel you can't even believe it. You understand? If you start becoming even with a woman, "All right, you start doing my laundry"; she will say, "All right, I'll do your laundry, you cook the meals." Instead, her nature, the nursing nature, which God has given her in abundance, you can use to manipulate her to any extent and she won't feel the pain.

Q: *Are you saying at that point to direct her spiritually?*

Yogi Bhajan: Definitely. When she is silent, talk to her. Read *Japji*. Loud. One day I got a funny call:

He said, "Sir, my wife is meditating, you understand?"
I said, "Sure. But read Peace Lagoon loudly so that she can hear."
He said, "Sir, I don't have my book. What should I do?"
I said, "Do you have any tapes?"
He said, "I have got a tape recorder and tapes in my car."
I said, "Can it be removed?"
He said, "Yes."
I said, "Play the tape."

So he pulled out the tape recorder, put a tape in it and started playing *shabds*. She started singing with the tape. Then she said, "I'm not that mad at you that you have to play this Gurbani Kirtan to me. I'm not going to kill you. I was just thinking about it."

And he checked it out and found that she had gone right to the bed pillow where he always kept his revolver. Later on she said, "I just wanted to kill you; I went to find the revolver, but it was not there. And I was thinking where you could have put it; I was concentrating." That was when he found her meditating. So when she becomes silent, then something is becoming silent. And when that moves, god of death moves with it. Don't misunderstand: a silent woman is of no good to you. They must talk. A talking woman is much safer than a silent woman.

Q: *Sir, if a man is earning money and providing for his wife and for their house, and she begins to think, because of his attitude about earning it, that she is not contributing and so she wants to go out and get a job so she can earn money to contribute...?*

Yogi Bhajan: That only happens when she feels earthly insecurity—that money is not enough. Woman is very particular in mathematics, income and liabilities. This is because every woman would like to save something for security. When she feels money pressure, she always likes to contribute, go find a job, do this, do that.... In other words, all she is telling you is that you are not earning enough.

Q: *Well, should she have a chance to have some say?*

Yogi Bhajan: Under those circumstances, sit down and discuss it with her. Don't ignore it. When woman gives you a confrontation, confront it. Don't back off. Most men do that. They back off and this causes more trouble in their life than anything else can cause.

Q: *When a woman gets the environment that she needs, but she still worries about money, what is the cause of that?*

Yogi Bhajan: Her own insecurity. Money is the other man to her. Money doesn't mean anything. Money is just another man to her. When she talks about money, she is indirectly communicating that she's not putting her security in you. That's a very simple indication that she's dissatisfied, and then you have to approach her very analytically and go into the very depth of it.

Sometimes a woman would like to spend more money and make you feel impotent when you cannot meet your bills. Woman is to you maya, money, used in every way, to clutch you. Sometimes she will come out with money to help you cover it. Have you seen that? So she can make you understand that she is a participant. Money and woman are—they call it two sides of the coin, and heads they win and tails you lose—they're the same thing.

Q: *I think basically you are talking about how to establish new relationships in a proper way. When you have a longstanding relationship that is kind of out of balance, do you apply the same principles to correct it?*

Yogi Bhajan: Yes. The relationship may be of any length. Sometimes the relationship erodes. That is the second chapter that I am going to discuss. As she develops, her cycle of consciousness is 7 years, intelligence is 11 years, and life is 18 years. When she passes her 35th year or as she approaches her 40th year, she is a totally different woman than the woman you know. I am going to cover that before I leave, but there are certain areas that I would like to complete today. But I know I cannot complete the total sum of it in this series. I will complete enough of it that you will have something very concrete and positive to use.

Q: *How do you deal with a woman who finds more security in, say, her parents' home than in your own."*

Yogi Bhajan: That we will cover under "phobia." That she wants this or she wants that is all phobia. Actually, no woman wants anything. All this is her phobia and that is very easy to deal with.

Q: What is the cause and cure for a woman who is very angry? She wants to become a martyr and seems to want to be hurt. Anything you say, she...?
Yogi Bhajan: Well, that is a father phobia. That is a very simple disease that is very common in America. It is a very, very common existence for women. There are certain things that I am going to discuss that will let you know why she behaves that way. The most unfortunate part of it is that most men do not know why a woman does this or a why a woman is doing that. If you know why, then you know what to do about it. When you meet a woman and she meets you, you do not want to study her childhood at all. Neither do you want to share your childhood with her, so one very strong, basic link between the two of you is missing.

Q: Well, in this case her mother views her as a tool for manipulation against her father.
Yogi Bhajan: That's possible. That's very, very possible. Sometimes the mother uses the daughter against the husband because she hates her sons, or she hates her husband.

Q: What does a woman mean when she says, "Sometimes I am afraid of you, but I don't know why?"
Yogi Bhajan: Can you wait until we discuss phobias? I understand all that. For 9 years now I have seen the American woman in every aspect you can imagine. And all these things are very familiar to me. All these languages and words, I know what happened when they say that and why they said so.

Q: Two things. How would you apply this approach to sexuality? Being direct in sex, tell her we are going to do it at 4 o'clock on Thursday, or not telling her...?
Yogi Bhajan: No. No. For that you just wait. The sexual act I am coming to; this was the first-hand information to establish the law of the cosmos between woman, man and earth. The statement I started with was, once you understand you are a man, you have no problem. If you have a problem, you understand that it is minus-man—you. So what we are trying to do is to establish this relationship, which is the outline, then to establish this minus-man. How can this minus-man be made a plus-man, and get out of the problem and into a trouble-free life?

Q: In that case, on this topic then, one time you said, I believe, 'Woman comes from ether, man comes from the earth...' Is that right? And today you said that woman comes from the ether to act as earth, and man comes from earth to act toward ether.

Yogi Bhajan: Law of polarity—that's called the law of ultimate polarity.

Q: Once a woman starts . . . when you've unfortunately triggered this questioning sequence, what's the best way to stop it?
Yogi Bhajan: You have to go through the whole situation. That's what I say. Once the sequence starts, you must live in the consequences of it and you must reach the end. The most basic problem you face is leaving off in the middle. That is what is called irritation. We are going to cover that, too.

Q: When you bank upon the kind of person you feel you are, do you want to get involved with a woman's curiosity or can you choose when you want to be silent?
Yogi Bhajan: No. No. When she wants to be curious, go ahead if you can afford it. There's no way to stop. This stopping business, I don't understand where you have learned it. She's not going to let you stop. Have you seen any man who can stop? There's no way. If you stop her this way, she will go that way. If you stop that way, she will go another way. She can take any route. Not being willing to confront the woman is the one place in life where you get totally defeated. I have seen a relationship where the woman caught the man fooling around:

He asked me, "What should I do?"
I said, "How compassionate do you feel your woman is?"
He said, "Tremendously."
I said, "Just become a baby; go and confess to her."
He went and said, "Well look, that's it. That's how it happened. That is how it is. I've learned my lesson. And that's the end of the world. Let us be on probation for two years."

He suggested this himself which she liked the most. In two months, she forgot he is on probation. Understand what I mean? He approached her compassionate nature, which is the Mother Nature in her. She's 60% Mother Nature, 40% woman nature. Fortunately, I have been married for the past 25 years. I know these teachings. About me it has been said that I am, "a man who lives among woman, likes a woman, but never subjects himself to a woman."

Now I'll tell you something very fantastic, which you will not like hearing, but that's the way it is. If you write woman, man is contained in it. If you write female, still the male is contained in it. Is that true? "In the beginning there was the word, the word was with God, and the word was God." And this is the word. I can understand that God took the rib of the man and created a woman. The fact is that our total life revolves around a woman: to earn, to buy things, to have children, etc. After all, even if you hate her, it is all directly or indirectly related to woman.

Give me a single example of a life where man is not doing anything for a woman either to build her or to destroy her. That's all you do. When you start a relationship between a male and a female, you need to remember certain things. There are three cycles: 18 years is a life cycle; 11 years is intelligence; and 7 years is consciousness. So within you there are three changes which happen. As far as your life is concerned, after 18 years all that remains of you is your name. Mr. Smith after 19 years is still Mr. Smith; everything else is changed in him. This is the 18-year cycle. Eleven years is that of intelligence. Whatever your intelligence demands the first 11 years, it shall demand totally differently the next 11 years. Consciously you are in a different frequency of consciousness after every 7 years. That is why you will find that a woman who was very obedient when you were young may be very bitter after 40 years. Do you understand? Sometimes you don't understand; but I tell you, after every 18 years, confront your partner. After every 11 years confront your partner at the frequency level of intelligence. After every 7 years, confront the partner on the consciousness level. You are three in one.

Your main problem in life is that you think you are just one and that you can go ahead with just that one. There is no such thing as you. You are Y-O-U. That means you are three words in one word. Do you understand? Language didn't come out of the sky; it came out of what our practical needs are. O—that is the center, the direction. Y is the curiosity, the first question, "Why?" U is you. Only you could serve you: Y-O-U.

Direct communication is a necessity if you want a relationship with any female. You must not stop communication; and you must channel the energy to be on the positive side of her. Never conspire or join anything which is morally low.

The Secret to Sexual **Satisfaction**

If you do not understand woman, you do not understand yourself.

[Yogi Bhajan gives a demonstration using kinesiology to reinforce certain universal concepts. A young man who is not in 3HO comes up from the audience to volunteer as a subject. He is 20 years old. Yogi Bhajan asks him to stand and raise his right arm perpendicular to his body. Then he asks him to resist his efforts to push his arm back down to his side. The subject is able to resist. Yogi Bhajan makes a slashing motion across his body from the left shoulder down to his right side. Asking the subject to again raise his arm and resist, he easily pushes his arm down. Then he presses the subject firmly at the Heart Center (the sternum), the Navel Center, and the reproductive center (the pubic bone) with the heel of his hand and then asks him to raise his arm again. This time the subject successfully resists the pushing on his arm].

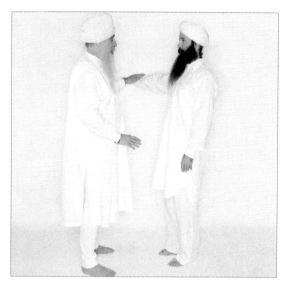

Q: What did you do?

Yogi Bhajan: First I cut his aura diagonally with my hand, and as you observed, he had no strength; then I blessed his three points and his strength returned.

You do not believe me when I tell you that you are not just this body. Your energy is in your aura and your aura extends nine feet from your skin. The animal aura is three and a half feet; metal things and other inanimate objects are a foot and a half; the human aura is nine feet. There are two things which can increase the size of the aura: white clothing and cotton cloth. When you wear white, cotton clothing from top to bottom, you can increase your aura up to three times. This is under all circumstances, even if you are at your lowest ebb. That's a law of the universe.

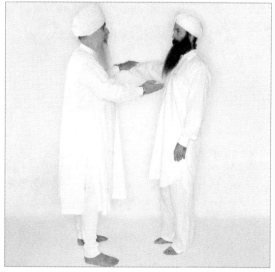

[Yogi Bhajan proceeds with his demonstration: this time he has the subject put his left hand into Gyan Mudra (index fingertip touching the tip of the thumb) and then put the mudra at his Third Eye Point. Asking the subject to raise his right arm, Yogi Bhajan finds that he is unable to lower his arm. Now he asks the subject to place the mudra at the pubic bone and to press in firmly. The subject is totally unable to resist the pressure and his arm lowers easily.]

Yogi Bhajan: Same person above the Navel Point and below the navel point; but below the Navel Point is the *apana* [the eliminative energy] and above the Navel Point is the *prana* [the life force]. When I asked him to touch his concentration point (Ajna Chakra) he was steel. I tried my best. His arm shook, but it didn't move an inch downward. When he was in his Second Chakra [the reproductive organs], he couldn't resist, although his ego wanted to maintain him. As a human being you must operate from the higher chakras [those above the Navel Point]. That is where your real strength is. This is what you have to understand.

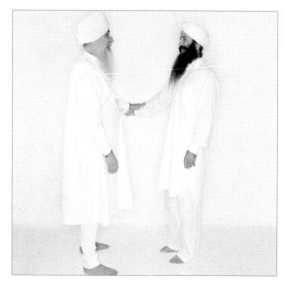

[Yogi Bhajan continues his demonstration: "Close your eyes, please." Yogi Bhajan asks his secretary, a woman, to touch the subject's foot. As she is touching his foot, Yogiji applies the technique. The subject is somewhat weakened. He then has the subject open his eyes and look at the woman. When Yogi Bhajan repeats the muscle test, the subject is totally weak and cannot resist at all.]

Q: *What does that mean?*

Yogi Bhajan: I want to share with you how man functions on a scientific level. The moment a man looks at a woman, with just the sight of her he becomes one-third his normal strength. When he listens to her, the ratio is 1/4, and when he touches her it is 1/5. That is the amount of influence a woman has on a man. Saying you don't care, or you don't understand is idiotic. Pushing your chest out and pulling your chin in doesn't mean a thing because you can't beat the laws of nature.

You must understand one thing: your polarity, man to woman, is heavier than one over two. This is because you are born out of woman. If you do not understand woman, you do not understand yourself.

Now I'll tell you something very funny. The majority of you do not know in which posture you can have physical intercourse with a woman. This is the majority of you. In my 9 years of living in the United States of America, I have talked with so many people and I have seen so many people. The majority of relationships break because the majority of women do not know how to get intercoursed and the majority of men do not know how to intercourse. That is why in intercourse you lose energy. Actually you should gain energy. Discharge is not a small thing: Eighty drops of blood make one drop of semen and you discharge almost 50 drops in a normal ejaculation. Let us figure it out—that is 50 to 80—it is about 4,000 drops of blood. Think about it.

You have three nervous systems: sympathetic, parasympathetic and the action [motor] nervous system. If your parasympathetic is out of balance, you will have a hard time getting an erection. If your sympathetic is out of action, you will ejaculate quickly. If your action nervous system is out of balance, you will have a problem ejaculating at all. Now these are the three systems which have to be in balance before you even go near a woman. Some of you go near a woman and before she does anything, you ejaculate. Others of you start having sex at seven o'clock in the morning and by nine in the evening you are still there, where you started. How does this imbalance happen?

Now I'll tell you the secret. Remember the word, three, and remember the word, seven. Together they are thirty-seven. A woman should have an aura of seven feet. That means that you will feel great. If her aura is less than three feet, less than that of an animal, your energy level will be down for a week. The intercourse doesn't mean a thing. The intercourse takes from you the strength of the blood through your semen. But intercourse can give you the strength of this blood; it can give you life. For this to happen you must understand that woman is not flesh. Woman is aura. Woman is aura. Woman is aura. When you have intercourse with a woman who is negative, a woman whose aura is not seven feet, you will lose your strength. Until you have a divine order to do it, don't do it at all.

The men who masturbate do not realize the physical difference between ejaculations: ejaculation through masturbation pressurizes the gray matter. It is heavy on the brain. It creates more problems than any sexual activity. To be very frank with you, homosexual interplay is better than masturbation. Masturbation causes a triple action on the pituitary gland which takes away your power to concentrate. I will say, "Don't masturbate." If you can't help it, run, and you'll be all right.

We recommend an underwear that can hold the testicles and the organs. This is a guarantee to your strength. It is a special underwear called kachera; it is an Indian underwear made of cotton cut on the diagonal. The legs come to the knees where they fit snugly. Because of the form of the kachera, a wind pocket is created on the thighs, where the balance of the calcium and the magnesium in the body is controlled via the thigh bone. The sexual energy is controlled by the sciatic nerve. The pressure point or sensitive area for this is just above the knee. The kachera is tight at that place so that pressure point is stimulated all the time from the action of walking. Also, the snug band provides for an air block which creates a constant temperature around the genitals.

Just as you breathe in left and right nostril cycles, your scrotum expands and contracts. Sometimes this skin stretches so long that your testicles touch the water when you sit on the toilet; other times, you do not know where they are they are so contracted. Now if you do not have the proper underwear and you do not control that area, the testicles can become lodged. This is the beginning of sexual problems for the male, the beginning of male frigidity. That is why we recommend this special kachera. Furthermore, you need to wear this underwear when you bathe. This is a precautionary measure. By doing this, the genitals are protected from temperature changes and water pressure and kept under control. The idea of wearing the underwear in the bath or shower may surprise you, so you need to experience it for yourself.

In the ancient days, man used a loin cloth. This is a triangle of cloth which is tied in such a way that the male organ and testicles are completely supported. This is the best type of undergarment. Next is the kachera worn by the Sikhs. Third is your freedom to choose whatever you want to choose to keep that area under physical control. Like the bra of a woman, which keeps the tissue of the breasts from breaking down, the right underwear is a human necessity. This is very important and it is smart as you grow older.

To have mutually gratifying intercourse, there are certain conditions that you must meet. Initially, you must not have eaten for at least two and a half hours. If your bodily energy is centered in your digestive tract, sexual interaction will cause you a lot of problems. Secondly, you must not be constipated and if you need to clear your bowels, you must do so. Don't say, "All right, I'll go to the bathroom later, let me have sex now." This is very foolish behavior. Thirdly, in a normal gesture, you must give yourself two to three hours time. And even then, you must start from the woman; you must touch her and caress her.

The woman has nine highly sensitive areas which are called moon centers. There is an order in which these centers need to be touched using any technique you wish. First, the breasts; second, the neck; third, the lips; fourth is the cheeks. Number five is the ears a most sensitive moon area. After the ears, remember the spine. Then the thighs are seven; the calves, eight; and the clitoris or vagina, nine. If you use any other order, you are an idiot. Furthermore, this act must not take less than 30 minutes to an hour. Within that time, playing with that kind of energy, in this kind of area, and in this kind of order, your woman will have the 7 to 9 foot aura that you need. If you cannot take that much time and you cannot adopt this procedure, you had better sleep.

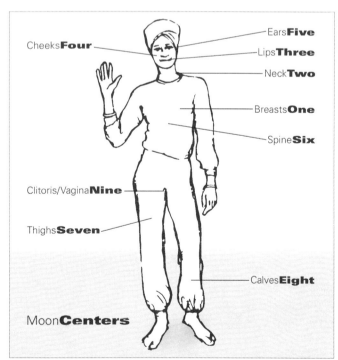

Once you have stimulated the woman's moon centers, the time comes to enter her. There are three different positions of the opening to the vagina: upper, normal and lower. The lower

Yogi Bhajan on Money

If you have money, let the woman do the bookkeeping to involve her. It is called the science of the household. If you have money or any business, if you let the woman manage it, then she is accountable to you. That control that you want to have over the woman, actually, you get anyway; but you get it in a genuine way rather than forcing it on her. Force only communicates to her, "If you don't do it, I don't believe in you."

What I am trying to tell you is that women need to be believed in. Certain things we do very innocently. We don't mean to get the women to the point of feeling insecure, but we really do make them insecure.

vagina is so far back from the beginning of the genital cleft that to enter the woman from the front, you need to use pillows to raise her buttocks 6 to 12 inches. Actually, in this posture you can comfortably enter from the back. Also, it is easier for the woman with a lower vagina to be on top of you rather than under you. Out of 100 women, 60 will have a lower vaginal entry. That means that 60% of all women are in this category. Ten percent have normal entry and 30% have upper.

The woman with an upper entry has no problem with orgasm. She can reach that optimum point more times than you can imagine. Because her vagina and her clitoris are so close together, all she needs is a little touch, a little entry, a little doing and there she goes. However, she will discharge and relax so much that there will be a great deal of lubricant. You will not know whether you are having intercourse or swimming. For her it is far out, but for you it can be too much. Sex with the woman who has a normal entry is regular, rhythmic and good for both of you. The 60% is a problem—never satisfied, always bitching, always complaining, always blaming. With this woman all 9 rules must be applied, especially number 9, the clitoris. During the act, she can stimulate herself through the clitoris; it is not a bad thing. And in case you have done away [ejaculated], don't walk away; satisfy her through the clitoris and bring her to tiding.

A woman never masturbates. In the case of a woman, it is called "tiding" and she needs to be brought to tiding a minimum of four times after the male ejaculates. If she has not aroused herself enough to come and you do not find that her nails have gone into your skin and her teeth have not given you a biting, which is very normal behavior, then you must stimulate her to three or four tidings. You will find that after that, she will quite naturally turn over and go to sleep. Remember! You start with the breasts. Normally, in this country, no one bothers with their existence.

Question and **Answer**

Q: Are you using your hands or your mouth or both?
Yogi Bhajan: You are free to use anything. Do your best. That is my answer.

Q: With the lower vagina, putting the pillows under the woman changes the angle so that…?
Yogi Bhajan: Yes. She has to change the angle; she has to raise her legs and you have to help her with this.

Q: Does this tend to change the clitoris contact?
Yogi Bhajan: It will move it, which helps. She has to get those tidings and you have to help her.

Q: You said something a few years ago about putting her legs over your shoulders…?
Yogi Bhajan: Yes. That is number three. If the vaginal mouth is so low that there is just no stimulation for the woman, put her legs on your shoulders. It is a perfect posture, out of the 84 that I have discussed with you.

Q: I don't understand the tidings.
Yogi Bhajan: Whenever you use friction to ejaculate, it is a type of masturbation for you. In intercourse this masturbation is with a woman. However, when the woman is stimulated through the clitoris, she gets a kind of feeling of ejaculation which is called tiding, moon tide. In her case, there is actually no discharge, where in your case there is.

Q: Do you mean a woman can masturbate without damage?
Yogi Bhajan: I don't think that a woman has any damage whatsoever from mastur . . . but I don't use the term masturbation. That doesn't exist in the case of a woman.

Q: But she can have good tidings anytime she wants?
Yogi Bhajan: I am not jealous of it. That is the way God made her.

Q: Our women will love to see us when we get back.
Yogi Bhajan: I am not saying anything; I am just sharing with you whatever it is. Whether it is good or bad is not my problem. I am teaching you just like at the university. I am explaining to you that woman has no such thing as masturbation. It is unfortunately so for the male and males became so insane doing it that they started cutting their foreskin just to get out of it—to the extent that about one percent results in death or deformity. That is how circumcision started in the world.

Q: Is yoga an antidote to masturbation?
Yogi Bhajan: A child can masturbate even when he is two years old. Sometimes you will find them masturbating much better than the adult. It is a question of how the erection comes. Children are very sensitive and they don't know what to do. They start fondling and you need to just divert their attention lovingly. But you start him masturbating because you become curious and start reacting to it. He then becomes a good masturbator.

One girl started having this kind of a situation by going on a pole. She would get on a pole and rub that area; her clitoris would be stimulated and she would have a tiding and she would enjoy it. And she wanted to go on longer and longer. Pole and parents started trouble and she became insane and was sent to a psychiatrist. He asked her and she admitted that she enjoyed it. Innocent. She didn't know what it was about. So they would chain her and cut her in the back and all that—and problems started. She was almost 38 when she met me and told me. I told her it's a very simple situation. Whenever she feels a little itch, however that is, put a little turmeric and yogurt, you know a douche with yogurt and turmeric? Yogurt will save your woman from a lot of infections. And sometimes she experiences a certain smell when she ovulates; it is a very pungent smell, but if she knows how to clean herself, then it is fine.

Q: In the notes from Ladies' Camp[1] I was reading that the woman goes through a rotation of her different moon centers.
Yogi Bhajan: That is well-explained.

Q: Isn't there any way for a man to know which stage she is in?
Yogi Bhajan: No. That is what you have to concentrate on. That is why I told you to touch on these nine points; you start with one and as you touch them all, you will know where her moon is.

Q: When a little girl eventually discovers that her clitoris is sensitive, how should her mother respond to her?
Yogi Bhajan: I do not think the clitoris should not be sensitive. It's very normal, but sometimes it overdevelops itself to the size of a pigeon egg, then it has to be taken care of surgically.

Q: No, no, I mean if the girl is stimulating herself.
Yogi Bhajan: Then you can teach her to douche with acidophilus. It will be all right. Normally it is the irritation of the inside area caused by bacteria.

Q: On the subject of odors, you once said that in men who are circumcised, there is an odor emitted from the part that's been cut…

[1] Also known as Khalsa Women's Training Camp, a month-long retreat for women, led by Yogi Bhajan, for more than 20 years.

Yogi Bhajan: There are two incision-like marks where that secretion comes out. Nowadays, it is said this secretion which comes out of that semen under the skin causes cancer because it is not clean. Actually it is the food of the woman's vagina. Normally a man is supposed to be in one 28-day moon cycle for intercourse. When he has intercourse, that secretion is cleaned out in the woman. It is plucked out by her membrane, which gives strength to her pituitary gland and her pineal gland. That is the way nature made it. Now I am not going to change your local belief system, but I am going to share with you whatever is explained in the old scriptures.

Q: What effect does circumcision have on the exchange of this secretion?

Yogi Bhajan: God bless them. It happened. What should I do? A little bit might be coming from somewhere. Otherwise, you know, after intercourse a woman can be very depressed sometimes—and that is why. Two things can spoil intercourse. Sometimes she is, herself, very wet, or sometimes the male organ does not supply that "butter of life." That little secretion, which happened with that little cut, is called "butter of life" and it is very rare.

Q: How does being circumcised or not circumcised have an effect on that?

Yogi Bhajan: When you are circumcised the secretion is produced, but it cannot be stored. You know circumcision was not a good idea. Actually circumcision began as an anti-masturbation drive. It was felt that if the organ was circumcised, one would not be able to masturbate. There is a wonderful article in Human Nature I would like you to read. It is a very thorough study of the reasons for circumcision, the dangers of it and why it is unnecessary. Sometimes we maintain certain rituals without recognizing their effects. [Circumcision] started even before masturbation had reached the point of insanity. Take that article in *Human Nature* and study it. It's a well-explained scientific article.

Q: In the uncircumcised male child, do you clean away that secretion?

Yogi Bhajan: After the third or fourth year, you can just tip it back and he can clean it himself.

Q: How often?

Yogi Bhajan: Every time you take a bath, you are supposed to clean yourself . . . it is just like wax in the ear. When your ears do not create the wax, you go berserk. It is just like that natural wax. But sometimes we do not clean out the wax.

Q: How about the cancer thing?

Yogi Bhajan: The cancer doesn't happen because of the secretion. Laboratory tests have been made. There is definite proof that cancer is neither eliminated nor caused that way. There are Jews who have cancer. There are circumcised Muslim boys with cancer. Cancer has something different as its cause. To be very frank with you, cancer is the problem of an over-heavy protein diet. That is, if you want to know about cancer, eat too much protein and you will get cancer whether you like it or not. An alkaline body doesn't have cancer. It can't create it. Too much acidity is what makes you unhealthy.

Q: In our perfect design, why is it we have to have the kachera. Why isn't it designed in somehow? Why do we have to add that to the body?

Yogi Bhajan: It is because of weather. There are four seasons and you have no protection from them. Your skin is not your protection. You are not a lion nor are you a bear. So you have to wear clothes. I would prefer that everybody would wear cotton clothes. At least your underclothes, your shirts and shorts and kacheras, should be totally cotton. That is, if you want to live long and have a better life.

Q: Many times you've mentioned the air pocket. What effect does the air have?

Yogi Bhajan: When you wear kacheras, the air controls the temperature by the creation of an air pocket.

Q: What is the recommendation about intercourse during pregnancy and nursing?

Yogi Bhajan: During pregnancy, anytime after the first 120 days until the woman stops nursing there is to be no intercourse. No. No. No.

Q: Until she stops giving milk? From the 120th day to that time, there is no sexual intercourse?

Yogi Bhajan: I said, "No. No. No." Three times. After 120 days, the soul enters the fetus. Actually, the baby is born on the 120th day. That is why there is a ritual for the mother on that day. Leave the woman alone, let her meditate, let her be happy, let her go in prayer, release her. And after the birth, she has to nurse the child. There is no substitute for a mother's milk. Remember that. You can tell me about experiments showing DDT in the mother's milk. Even lead has been found in the mother's milk. I say that even if they find potassium cyanide in the mother's milk, there is still nothing equal to mother's milk and that child who is not nursed on it for at least six months will have a deficiency in social behavior. No matter what you do, you can't correct that.

There are two securities that a mother gives to her male child. The first is that the male child should be with her, in her bed, in her lap for at least six to nine months, come what may. Secondly, she must nurse the child from six months to one year. This gives him his fundamental malehood. Otherwise you are raising a baboon in your home. This is true whether you believe it or not. These results have been found to be true by the sages who never lied through the ages.

Q: Um, I'll assume, 'No. No. No.' meant... Absolutely no.
Yogi Bhajan: When I say, "No. No. No." I mean absolutely no way.

Q: Off the subject, but you just mentioned protein. Is vegetable protein in any way connected with cancer?
Yogi Bhajan: No, vegetable protein cannot cause cancer. It cannot. We are talking about meat protein. Meat protein is not eliminated from the body within 24 hours. There is no vegetable protein that does not leave the body within 24 hours. This is not a question of whether or not to eat meat. That is not the problem. We are talking about time and digestion. You must not eat food which does not digest and leave your colon within 24 hours. That's a basic human law. There is no "yes" to it; there is no "no" to it. Only eat that food which leaves the colon within 24 hours. Do this and you won't have any problems.

Q: How can you tell how long it takes the body to eliminate a food?
Yogi Bhajan: I can tell you that very simply. One day eat beets with your meal. You will see the beets in your stool and that will give you the time. It is a simple way to measure.

Q: What about people who get cancer who have never eaten meat?
Yogi Bhajan: Well, sometimes it is hereditary. However, consult the affairs of families who are vegetarians, strict vegetarians. They do not even know all these diseases. What should we do? Should we totally close our eyes to that fact? In India, they eat tamarind, rice, lentils and yogurt. They don't know what fatness is; they don't know what cancer is; they don't know what impotence is. They do not go blind. There are diseases that we are very commonly confronted with that they don't know at all. Their disease is old age. That is their major disease. Once in a while there is malaria and a third they call seasonal fever which is caused by a virus. These are the three main diseases. A woman may suffer from some abnormality in pregnancy or some other type of female disorder but they don't know any of these diseases that we find in this country or in Europe or in some areas of northern India where the people eat meat. Most of India, my God, they don't know even what we are talking about. If you speak of "cancer" they think you are talking about astrology. They don't even relate to what we relate to. They are healthy; they live long.

I'll tell you one thing more: whatever your weight is when you are 18 to 21, that is your normal weight. Any excess weight [over that baseline weight] is guaranteed ill health.

Q: For men and women?
Yogi Bhajan: Yes.

Q: Should men wear brief-type underwear, jockey shorts, underneath the kacheras?
Yogi Bhajan: I'll tell you, I'll send you a loin cloth. I'll ask my wife to make it. I wore a loin cloth and cummerbund all my life and look at the tragedy. One day I wanted to play soccer. That day I wanted my heavier cummerbund but I forgot it and there was no time to return for it. I was the captain so I had to play. In the first bout, my tendon was pulled. That is called a tragedy. I never went without a cummerbund until that day; and the one day I forgot it, I got it. One side is now longer. Had I not been a yogi, I would have died. But I know how to clean myself; I know how to keep myself; I know how to take care of myself. It is difficult.

Q: My wife won't do certain yoga exercises because she says she knows she can get air into her vagina.
Yogi Bhajan: If she gets air into her vagina, it can cause her some trouble. In this case she should wear a pad under the kachera. The kachera is a very popular garment. People who know how to live healthy and sexual for a long time realize that.

Q: Even at that, the air still goes in and out, right?
Yogi Bhajan: No. No. The body develops that polarity in layer, you know. It is not all this air you are talking about. You have surrounding the body this layer, it can be photographed. What do you call it in the Western world?
Student: That layer? It is called a Sclerian layer of humidity. It can be photographed. It is made up of the humidity and the hormones to form a negative ion layer. The flow patterns of this layer can actually be photographed. By wearing kacheras the depth and the consistency of this ionic layer around the sexual area is increased.

Q: There is just one problem with that. When it's real hot, you can get a rash, you know.
Yogi Bhajan: Oh no, you don't get a rash, son. Use almond oil and scented oil on your body. It really smells good, like a garland. You won't get a rash. I get into the worst, hot season and I don't get it.

Q: Should the kacheras come to a little above the knee?
Yogi Bhajan: Yes. It is called a "Khalsa kachera."

Phobias and **the Man**

Neither be compensated, nor compensate—establish your own relationship. The first law is to establish your relationship. Establish your own wavelength.

Now I am going to work on the last phase of today's lectures: Phobias and the Man.

After 120 days, the soul enters the fetus. Got it? In 9 months and plus some days, it depends upon the moon cycle, the cord is cut and the first breath of life is taken. Either you are a male or you are a female. In the first 3 years, your mother has to teach you the values of life. Whatever she can teach you, that is called "ingrained knowledge." At 7 years old, your father can give you values and security. Up to 11 years, you learn values and behavior, then that is the end of you. After 11, you learn nothing. You can accumulate, accommodate whatever you want to do; but your base, your foundation is already laid. Do you understand? First, the mother is teacher; then the father; then the environments and relatives; and then comes the spiritual teacher.

It is always better to instill values about the spiritual teacher in the child so that he can have something of faith. It is called faith and destiny. Without that, man is an orphan. In your life there has to be one man who can say, "Hey! Stop it!" That means you have the power to stop it. Otherwise the sequence will lead to consequences and to construction and destruction—God knows what. A spiritual teacher is nothing but an emergency brake. When that is applied, nothing moves. That is the importance of the spiritual teacher. A spiritual teacher is not your friend, not your enemy, not your altar, not your worship, not your knowledge, not your money, not your wife, not your husband. The spiritual teacher has no relationship with you, but functions only as an emergency brake. He or she must have the power to analyze you and say it to you straight. You are just in the wilderness without a compass. You don't know what the hell you are doing.

Remember: woman is an institution that has laws and bylaws. Man is an institution that has laws and bylaws. Parenthood is also an institution that has laws and bylaws. When these laws and bylaws are not followed, the children end up with certain problems. You may hate your mother. You may have a mother phobia. If your mother was harsh and strict in discipline, you will want your wife to be absolutely subservient. Then marry a Japanese woman; don't marry an American woman. An American woman doesn't know how to bend more than three inches. Do you understand what I mean? They are among the most neurotic stock of women folk. This is because the American woman has been built by her own ego and also because American women and Oriental women are different women.

Do you know how many fathers have had intercourse with their own daughters? Thirty percent of the fathers have maliciously fondled—I am using a very delicate word— with their own born daughters. And if to this you add the stepfathers, 30% to 40% of the women in this country are molested by stepfathers or by relatives as teenagers. That is a horrible picture to represent. Now out of that, 10% of the wives, the mothers, have conspired with the fathers. That is the most horrible breed born. There are 10% to 50% of women who have seen their father nude, or in undesirable situations. Now that is another situation. Women, out of the stress and pressure of the family, have run away from the ages of 13 to 21.

A spiritual teacher is nothing but an emergency brake. A spiritual teacher is not your friend, not your enemy, not your altar, not your worship, not your knowledge, not your money, not your wife, not your husband. The spiritual teacher has no relationship with you, but functions only as an emergency brake.

Now this is a category of woman we call insecure. An insecure woman is one who has no connection or only a meager connection with the personality of the father whom she rejects. When the woman rejects the father in the father phobia, she rejects every male, including her husband. Not that she's trying to fight you, not that she's trying to make a mess out of you, not that she wants to quarrel with you, but because that is her basic subconscious. Is that clear? A lot of men come under this category also. They had harsh mothers, or they have been lollipop kids. The "nah nah nab nab" babies are the most hopeless of all in the human race because they cannot stick to anything they say. They end up saying "nah nah nab nab." We call them "banana men" with banana spines. These are those banana men. Whatever the woman says, "yes, yes, yes, yes." It is ridiculous. Even when they say "no," they say it in such a way that it ultimately becomes "yes."

Expect your wife to be your wife, not an equal. When you think her to be your equal that is the most disgraceful way of thinking: expect a lot of things out of her and you cannot deliver her anything. The first law is to establish your relationship. Establish your own wavelength valence; establish your own frequency with each woman.

I'll tell you one principle of my life: whenever a woman tells me something against somebody, that's the only thing I never hear. When she says something against me, I can see her insecurities. When she tells me something good, I know how to hold myself and not slip. Under all circumstances and every sentence that a woman speaks, you must find the undercurrent. A woman has not yet been born on this Earth who does not speak without an undercurrent, including Mother Mary. No woman can be a woman who does not know how to speak with an undercurrent. That is her basic nature. Don't blame her for that. You must understand and study that undercurrent language. If she says, "Ah, it is very, very muggy, it is very close today," she may end up taking you to a movie. When she wants to get out of the house, she is going to start discussing the weather. You understand what I mean, what I'm trying to say? When she wants to eat out, she's going to discuss how difficult it is to cook food at home. We call woman's talk, "indication language." Remember her nature. First she uses indication language, that is, signal language. She follows with discussion and then she becomes quarrelsome. This is how she goes: indirect talk, direct talk, and then comes war.

When she talks indirectly, fine. When she talks directly, fine. But when she makes war on you, don't fight head to head. Divert her. When she's at her worst and looking for a fight, just tell her, "O.K. This we'll decide tomorrow, but right now I have got this emergency." Take her along with you and get it over with. A child and a woman have one frequency in common: they can be diverted easily. A woman and a child have one thing in common: they become uptight and stiff. But you can tell them something is an emergency and they can divert themselves, forgetting what they are uptight about.

There is hardly a man who doesn't have a phobia. Unfortunately when you have a father phobia, you become very harsh and rough with your woman. Or, you become totally soft and totally giving with your woman—either way you compensate for your father. But if you have a mother phobia, you demand that your wife compensate for her. Actually both are wrong: neither get compensated, nor compensate. Establish your own relationship. Please remember a wife is a wife, she's not a mother. She is, though, the mother of your children. Is that understandable?

You must not be married to a woman whose childhood you do not know, because that's going to cause a lot of problems. She must know your childhood; you must know hers. Because I'll tell you, when she's 36 or when you're 40 or 45, a lot of problems are going to show up because you become a child again. She becomes a child again after 36. A woman after 36 and a man after 45 reestablish their securities. You establish your first security when you are 7 and 9. Then you reestablish your security when you're 18 and 21; and then again when you are 36 and 45. What happens is a misunderstanding when you reach that age. Do you follow? Understanding life as a continuous relationship is totally wrong! I think every 7 years (they call it the "7-year itch") as the cycle of consciousness changes, you should renegotiate and reestablish your relationship toward the better, not toward the divorce.

How can you get out of the phobias? Tantric Yoga is one way, but there's a longer way which you can do yourself. Sit down for one hour, husband and wife, with a simple resolution that you will not yell and scream at each other, and discuss the problem. That is called self-counseling. Discuss your relationship, say whatever you feel and let her say whatever she feels, and then write it down on paper and put it in the fire. Don't remember it and don't remind each other about it. That is the biggest folly on the planet! That's the only danger.

Certain things you must not do: One—if you know the negative side of your woman, don't remind her when you are angry—never do it. She will never forgive that. Two—don't question a woman's character when you are not 100% sure, and don't question it directly. She will go reverse. Number three—when she sees you not uplifting yourself consciously and spiritually, you have a 40% chance of losing the relationship. The woman looks to the man as

Sadhana: **An Experiment**

Sadhana has now been standardized. Since Baisakhi Day there has only been one change. Now we read the whole sutra of Anand Sahib and Japji. That is the only difference. [Editor's Note: The Aquarian Sadhana has since become the standard that we practice until the year 2012 and beyond.] Because we are going to be hit by the insanity soon, we don't want to take any risks. Anybody who takes the risk of missing sadhana is on his own. I don't take any blame. Is that clear? I'll tell you, I made an experiment one day. I told my secretary to hold all calls. I didn't take any telephone calls. Not that I was busy. I was available. But I wanted to see what would happen. She noted down all the calls. Out of all these calls, 60% of those calling with troubles were irregular with sadhana. The serious trouble was with those who were very, very irregular with sadhana. People who were regular with sadhana had normal inquiries about their progress. It was one of the most mind-blowing things for me. You cheat, you get cheated.

God. I do not know why, but in her chemistry, this is what she wants to look to. You know what she wants? They say, "She wants the devil in the bed and she wants a sage in the living room." Got it?

Question and **Answer**

Q: *What do you do with a woman who doesn't know her natural parents?*

Yogi Bhajan: When a woman doesn't know her natural parents, she doesn't know who they are and what their circumstances were, you can be successful if you tell her about Mother Nature and God the Father. These two images were used in the circumstances of children orphaned in war. During the war a lot of parents died and children were left behind. Mother Nature and God the Father became a substitute. This can become hard for a man because sometimes he has to really act out the mother and the father, both at the same time, to his own wife. It is not a very difficult case; but it is a harsh case because she will be extraordinarily insecure. That's what the difficulty is.

Q: *Again, what about a woman who finds more security in her parents' house than in her own?*

Yogi Bhajan: A woman who finds security in the parents' house, or in the parents' riches, or if she leans toward the parents is what we call a spoiled brat and she must be confronted once and for all, just to straighten it out. Go right to the in-laws' house and make such a mess that they may know what kind of a son-in-law they have. It is a good drama; but it should be done fast, without her even understanding what you are doing. If you put a woman on the alert that there are certain things she is doing that you know she is doing and you don't like it, she will not do it because she is a very sensitive animal. From wherever in the world she comes, sense prevails. A woman only does that which she can get by with; that's her basic nature because she's not conniving, she's conceiving. She has that metabolism; she has that mechanism; so you have to be very direct with her.

Q: *What is the most effective way to establish a relationship when each of the marriage partners involved have a particular phobia against their parents or one of their parents?*

Yogi Bhajan: At that time you have to make a "suicide pact." You both have to sit down and decide once and for all, "All right, that is our past; that is over with; we have a definite future and we have a present now—together." That's called a suicide pact. You do it once and for all and just go through it.

Whenever a woman brings up the past, just tell her, "What is it, past? Then why are you wasting time for the future?" Remind her of the future. The moment she becomes secure she will forget it. At least it will take the sting out of it.

Q: *Can a woman be convinced to place total trust in both God and Guru in terms of financial aspects?*

Yogi Bhajan: They can do it more easily than the man. Only when they want to bug the man, then they bug him. First, they start financially. A woman will start proving the impotency of the man through the financial resources, remember that. She's not trying to reach your money matters. She doesn't care about that because she's money herself. The moment she brings money up front and starts talking to you, she's trying to test your manhood and that's how she does it. A lot of ladies make men use MasterCard and buy things that they cannot afford. She will take you out of your budget. She will make you look like an idiot later on, when you can't pay. They love this fun—making men donkeys.

Q: *Before you talked about a woman who has a father phobia and who wants to be righteous but can't...*

Yogi Bhajan: It is a simple problem to solve. When you have a phobia, it doesn't go away in one day. In the case of a subconscious nature, then you need to do Tantric Yoga. It is the best way to change subconscious fear and burn out the karma. You both need to go through it. It is just like putting toast through the fire. It will bring you out better than yesterday. But you must understand that if that technique is not available [White Tantric], then an alternative technique is to constantly be on guard, aware that it is a phobia. Then the solution is that whenever you catch her in the problem [the phobia], you remind her so she can turn around. Mostly men get into trouble when they allow a woman to take space. When she gets the time and space, she's on your back.

Remember one thing: woman is always available for talk. You can talk and talk and talk with this creature for hours and hours and she will like it. I've yet to see one woman who doesn't like talking.

Q: *If someone has an emotional problem and wants to get out of it how can he do it?*

Yogi Bhajan: Well, basically I tell you the Sa-Ta-Na-Ma meditation[1] is the best for that. It is a very proven fact. It takes a long time. You can't do it like Tantric Yoga, but it's an answer.

Q: *You said if you have a father phobia you are very hard or soft in dealing with your wife...*

Yogi Bhajan: If your father has been very hard and rash with you, then you want to compensate for that and you give a lot of leeway to your woman. Or, if you feel he was

---
[1] Also known as Kirtan Kriya. See Appendix A.

harsh with your mother, you give in a long way with your wife. You feel he was very harsh and your mother suffered a lot; and therefore, you do not trust the circumstances and you become very rash. Sometimes, out of that fear—that it may happen to you with your wife—in trying to prevent the situation, you end up doing the same to yourself. You act out of sheer insecurity of the past.

Q: *You know that image of woman as the Goddess Kali? What is that aspect of a woman?*

Yogi Bhajan: When woman comes into a rage, then she doesn't know any reason or logic. That's the image. She will chop your head off. People think woman is the better half. That she is wonderful, very kind, family is great. I understand all those situations. But I will tell you one thing about a woman: when woman is not a woman, when she has the body of a woman but not the mind of a woman, you are in really great trouble.

The only aspect in woman which can nurse you is the female aspect of her, the mother instinct in her. Sometimes because of the past, the environments, the arid circumstances, you have to confront that and you have to be very strict by the law of dharma. You must understand one thing: karma cannot be wiped out; the sequence must lead to consequences. The only, the only, the only way is through sadhana. I can tell you that without sadhana, you are as useless for positive change as a junk car is. You can talk for hours and hours and I can teach for years and years; but without sadhana, you have no chance. Sadhana is a self-victory. Sadhana means self-victory; and one who cannot have self-victory cannot have this Earth at all. I can bluntly tell you. There's no need lying to you.

Q: *Is it important to have some particular balance in who serves which partner most, for example, is the woman supposed to serve man, give him foot massages…?*

Yogi Bhajan: I don't think that is true. I think it is totally mutual. I feel when a man asks a woman for service, to be very frank with you, I don't think he's a man. I believe if a man is a man he attracts a woman for service. I may be totally wrong. There are certain areas in my life where I have no experience. I have no experience of asking somebody to serve me. I don't have that experience. If a woman is within 20 miles of my radius and she won't help me or do something for me? I don't have that experience. I don't know why you people get into that trouble. Basically, I am a Shakti worshipper. Adi Shakti may be a symbol to you, for me it is my worship and Bhagwati[2] I worship. I am a Bhagwati worshipper. So I have never seen a woman in my life who has not come to my aid in one way or the other. But you must understand, I am a decent man; I am a noble man in the company of the woman. I have never lost my divinity, dignity, and nobility—these three things—toward any woman. In my most adverse circumstances, in my worst accusations, I have been noble. I have been divine and I have been dignified, because I am born of a woman.

What if a woman is my alphabet? I must learn decency. You can only learn decency when you are decent. The test of decency is whether you are a decent person or not. Your test lies in whether you are decent with a woman. And I have been put personally, in my experience, under certain environments, where a woman has gone out of her orbit, but she couldn't provoke me to be indecent. No. There's nothing in any woman that can make me indecent; I won't. I think that is the beginning of manhood.

The only, the only, the only way is through sadhana. I can tell you that without sadhana, you are as useless for positive change as a junk car is. You can talk for hours and hours and I can teach for years and years; but without sadhana, you have no chance. Sadhana is a self-victory. Sadhana means self-victory; and one who cannot have self-victory cannot have this Earth at all. I can bluntly tell you.

Q: *Age difference between male and female?*

Yogi Bhajan: Yes, age is a very beautiful question, thank you. Age difference between a man and a woman: in all normal circumstances, the woman should be 5 years to a maximum of 10 years younger.

Q: *How do you explain out-of-body experiences that occur during deep relaxation after intercourse?*

Yogi Bhajan: It is very normal that if the woman is a giver, then relaxation is a must. In this case you synchronize your skin: your body becomes bigger and your skin becomes smaller. You want to shrink after ejaculation and you fall asleep and there you go. I have seen people, nothing could wake them. I had a married couple living with me once that I could tell when they had had intercourse the night before. Their way of getting up, their way of talking, their eyes were so bright; they looked like they were heavenly angels. That's what intercourse means. Physical intercourse is a blend of the auras, which purifies each other. It's not what you do. I know what you do. I can't even understand how you do all that, but anyway, you do it the way you want to do it.

---

[2] Bhagwati is one name for the Goddess, the Divine Feminine, the Primal Creative Energy.

Q: *When a woman signals to her husband that she wants to have sexual intercourse....*

Yogi Bhajan: You must either send a counter signal that your ship is sinking or otherwise poof, load it with fruit and fragrance and go.

Q: *What do you mean, 'send a signal that your ship is sinking'?*

Yogi Bhajan: Well, if you don't want intercourse, tell her right away through the signal. When she's giving you a signal, you should learn the signal too. That is called unknown language of the known. She will say, "Ahem, what's happening this evening? Are you going to write the article or what?" Or she will say, "Are you going to use the typewriter or some other kind of typewriter?" Do you understand what I mean? Every word has three meanings: one is for you, one is for the one who listens and one for who's saying it. There is a saying—they call it "woman's language"—when woman speaks the woman's language she is the most beautiful creature.

Q: *We've been talking primarily about women and wives. What can we do for people who we meet in society who have the experience of coming from a broken home?*

Yogi Bhajan: Social experience should be totally noble. There's no virtue better than nobility. When you meet with anybody who is not known to you, absolutely remember that your nobility is your virtue; don't let it go.

Q: *Is there something we can give to people who come to us?*

Yogi Bhajan: No, no, that is our sadhana; our sadhana is well contained. We have given thousands of meditations; it depends on what the teacher thinks is right. As far as knowledge is concerned, we are not giving any secret knowledge. We are as open as the sunlight is. Where there's a mystery, there's no mastery; where there's mastery, there's no mystery. Some meditation teachers teach in secret because they can't run their businesses otherwise. If they just gave one meditation, everybody could pick it up. Where would they collect the money? So they make all that ritual. It's a money collecting ritual. It has nothing to do with the meditation. Sa-Ta-Na-Ma meditation is very open. In the case of divorce it will work.

Q: *When I was young my father was very harsh on my brother and sister and me, and he punished us. He was basically all right, but he was very harsh with us. Now all three of us have basically made our peace with him, but he's very, very hard on our mother, and they fight constantly about very stupid things. What is our relationship to that situation?*

Yogi Bhajan: I think if he takes cucumber juice himself, he will change. Can you believe that? That's all your father needs—24 ounces of cucumber juice.

Q: *How can I suggest it?*

Yogi Bhajan: Well, all three of you can put a bottle around his neck one day and get it in there.

Q: *I asked you earlier about a woman who is afraid of you [her husband or partner] sometimes, but she doesn't know why.*

Yogi Bhajan: On the earth level it doesn't mean a thing, but on the ether level, it's very essential. Woman is very important to the male and that one woman is the one.

Q: *How long does the interlock in the aura stay from the one night of intercourse?*

Yogi Bhajan: The instinct of the sexual intercourse starts about 48 hours before you actually do it. It takes about a week. That's why there are 7 days in a week. It is an ingrained thing. If you love a woman, you may be away from her for 10 days and then you will start missing her like hell.

Q: *When the auras merge and the two bodies separate...?*

Yogi Bhajan: There's no time and space. For the purposes of that pair, the earth stops rotating. I have seen people that met once and at the time of death, the dead partner totally manifested so much into this reality that even the audience could see it. For example, we were taking a dead body of a very saintly man and his wife's image appeared. It's unbelievable. It was like a rainbow situation, but very factual. When *tattvas* become the truth, truth becomes the *tattva*. Therefore, it all becomes the Truth. Now read those scriptures for God's sake; they're all with you. Don't make me read it.

Q: *How often should a husband and wife be apart?*

Yogi Bhajan: Fall apart, live apart, or what?

Q: *Live apart from each other during their lifetime?*

Yogi Bhajan: I think two months a year. A woman should be a woman and go to Ladies' Camp. I tell you, you American men, don't misunderstand: The only way to safeguard yourself is to give your woman a chance to become a woman, and then you will remain happier. Otherwise you end up with troubles you can't even believe. This two month break is called "marriage insurance."

Q: *Sir, you said two months. Should there be another month in the winter or something?*

Yogi Bhajan: No. What I'm talking about is that there should be some area, some place and space, where she can become a woman. That's what we are trying to reach. In 3HO we don't have much trouble. We have Ladies' Camp and we have Summer Solstice. On a six month to a six month basis, you must understand one fundamental thing:

the ladies' course gives the ladies self-respect, which is a very beautiful idea and very beautiful training. On the other hand, there are two special times of energy, when there's a Winter Solstice and a Summer Solstice that we get together. I know sometimes businesses suffer and we lose money; but after all, what is money? When your whole life goes down the tubes, what is there to talk about? And I request to all of you—it is my personal request—don't bring trailers, bring tents; live with the earth. I don't like this trailer business—that's not what Summer Solstice is about. We want you to bring a good tent. I'm not saying a small tent. But, if you bring trailers, don't pack it up with food. This year we are going to confiscate food. We are going to write an agreement that any extra food that is found on you or your trailer will be confiscated and we are not going to give it back come what may. That's ridiculous when people bring trailers full of food and then they distribute it as a sign of good will and friendship. The basic diet is a mono diet and a most healthy diet. It keeps you going. I do not want anybody not to eat that food, at least for those eight days. It's a very good meal and we spend so much money on it; and still you get in that stuff in-between. Therefore, this year don't spend your money on extra food. Use your energy keeping up, on positive efforts toward God, so that God can lean toward you. Blessed are you to be a man. I started with a sentence. I end with a sentence. When you are a man, you have no trouble. Thank you.

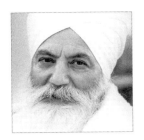

Man to **Man** 2

Inside the Real Man

Circa 1978

We are talking about the inside man—the real man. In the past, there was nothing more beautiful before a man than a man himself.

- Potency and **Potentiality**
- The Downfall of the **Man**
- Potent Potential of the **Inner Being**
- Exercises for **Potency and Potentiality**
- Creativity of **Consciousness**

Potency and **Potentiality**

The beauty of you is not in your hairdo, your turban, or your talk. These things are all temporary. Temporarily you can convince somebody, temporarily you can love somebody, temporarily you can turn on and temporarily you can turn off. But are you willing to believe that you are permanent?

Man's Projection and **Creativity**

We are talking about the inside man—the real man. And this is the potency: however potent a man is, that much he can project. Now, it is not that we know very much today. I am taking you back twenty thousand years from today. I am going to explain to you how much man, twenty thousand years ago, knew about what man is. Today we know what a machine is. We have become totally computerized in our life. But in the past, there was nothing more beautiful before a man than a man himself. Man recognized that with all the time and all the power that he had, he had to understand himself. At this time there was a very beautiful competition among men to excel.

The beauty of you is not in your hairdo, your turban, or your talk. These things are all temporary. Temporarily you can convince somebody, temporarily you can love somebody, temporarily you can turn on and temporarily you can turn off. But are you willing to believe that you are permanent? There are men, we have known them by experience, who are permanent. For example, Lord Rama, Krishna, Mohammed, Gautama Buddha, Guru Nanak, Moses, Lord Christ, Hazarat Abraham. They had a man's body. Did they live the life of an ordinary man? They walked and talked like an ordinary man. They made statements, created controversies. Some got crucified. Men like Guru Nanak, men like Guru Gobind Singh. It's unbelievable about Guru Gobind Singh. Singlehandedly he fought, within the fire of the battlefield, just with the spirit of God; because the spirit of man is the undying, infinite, potential potency. Man cannot die.

It is not that spiritual people have not had conflict. Spiritual people always have conflict, because a spiritual person from their very birth is nothing but a conflict. The one sign of a potent person is that he is a conflict. He is in conflict with ignorance. That is the first sign of your potency and your potential. What you call potential has become a sales shop item, with everybody selling it these days. There's a slot machine everywhere. You put in a coin and you get potency out. This is a funny thing. This is why I say that people have not understood man at all. In the 9 or 10 years that I have been here, I have been going very slowly, explaining it. I'm just telling you that it is not how many people you have, that doesn't matter. But what is their potential understanding of themselves? That matters. That is the criteria.

There are about 10 or 11 million people who live in this city. Among you there is not a person who knows what his proportion is in frequency to the relevancy of his polarity, in existence with his cosmos, which is the outside world, as an individual; and proportionally how much he controls. You may not understand this. But if there is any situation with a woman, you are in her. The only area you do not know how to deal with is 'wo'. You need to understand how to deal with these two letters, 'wo'.

Once a gentleman told me, "I'm going to go home and she is going to blast me."
I said, "Who's she?"
He said, "Well, my wife."
I said, "What did you do?"
He said, "Well, whatever I did, if I start explaining it to you, first you will blast me, and then she will blast me."
I said, "Rehearsal is a good thing. Why don't you tell me? I'll blast you and see what you can do."

So, he told me his neurotic story, which I couldn't believe that a man of his caliber and intelligence was in a position to do that. I said, "Wow, wonderful, you could do that? Really, you did all that you told me?"
He said, "Yeah."
I said, "Well, 9 years you have been a technical person. Six years you have been a successful person. That is 15 years. Plus, you have studied to be a graduate for 14 years. That is 29 years in all of conscious education, systematic system realization, and you did this dumb thing? And so dumb that she can catch you on your own words and your own statement and your own actions?"
He said, "Well, Yogiji, you know one thing. I did it. And, I did it and I really did it. I don't know."

And I saw sitting before me a two-year-old child who was saying, "Well, I spilled the milk. What can I do? I did it. The Persian carpet is spoiled, now take care of it." Instead of thinking it will cost five hundred bucks to clean the carpet, I was supposed to think about his million dollar innocence. I said, "Okay boy, you learned the whole thing."
He said, "How? How did I learn? You haven't told me anything. I only talked to you."

I said, "The very words you said, 'Yogiji, I did it', that will cater to the 'wow' of her. And I don't think she is going to say a word to you."
He said, "Are you sure?"
I said, "I am not that sure, I am exact. You try the formula—'thirteen' they call it. Devil's number. Formula thirteen is known as the Devil's number. When you face the devil, never face the devil straightforward. Just confront the devil with the devilish attitude of total surrender. Devil cannot do anything." That's what spirit is. I am the spirit, you are the devil. The devil can't do anything. That's called formula thirteen in the spiritual world.

On Circumcision and **Masturbation**

We can't even think of missing a night. You must understand. Masturbation is such a terrible sickness with men. They do not know what they are doing it for. Woman loses nothing. She goes on tides. It is a nervous stimulant to her. It is like a vitamin B-12 injection to her. But to you it is minus B-18. You lose, she doesn't. Men lose so much that the process of circumcising men was started to take away that area so that man might not enjoy masturbation. It was a medical cure. Actually that little flesh that is gone is so useful in old age to stimulate the sexuality in you that without it you are just using a bamboo stick. Circumcision happened in the hospital, you were very innocent, nobody even discussed it with you. Now keep it as it is and think about God.

What can I do? Somebody ripped you off, stole your stimulant. That little thing has two most beautiful things: One thing is that which secretes—that ring around that area of your sexual organ secretes. That secretion creates a smell which is called the aroma of the male. You don't like it. Woman can get that smell within a range of 11 miles. I am sorry I was not here. It happened to you without me. They charge $50 to $60 in the hospital for damaging you. Can you believe that? God has created nothing without rhyme and reason. There is always some reason for every part of the body that is there.

To regulate your physical system, your ejaculation and your maturity, or if you have been damaged and you have been sexually inverted or perverted, either way, the milk of the banyan tree, 36 drops on a candy or sugar, (normally it should be brown sugar, **gur**, which doesn't have lead), at the time of spring or at the time of fall, is a human necessity. It regulates the semen, its productivity, its thickness; and the thickness of the urethral walls. It does a lot of things.

Many of you may not be aware of this, but sometimes you are so stimulated that when you urinate, you discharge semen, either before or after. You may not have been aware of it for a long time. That loss is a very, very big loss. Then many of you are just wonderfully . . . a nonsense. You do not play enough games so that the secretion may come through that system to alkaline it so that when you ejaculate, the acidity can be taken care of. There has to be a long, long game of foreplay. It is in the scriptures that a person must play 'krishan lila'. It is called 'krishan lila'. Lord Krishna played with his gopis in absolute ecstasy. So man should play to stimulate woman and this play should go on for an hour to two hours at a time, to the extent that he can smell his sweat. (Try this sometime: sweat so that you can smell your sweat and then your woman will just be in love with you.) But you don't have that game; you don't know how to play it; just as you do not know how to do many things in life.

You are very quick. You want to just push buttons and plug in switches. For that I recommend, in the fall season, this banyan milk from Hawaii. There are seasons. When spring comes this milk is very, very, very much in the tree and when it is fall, it goes back. It is very thick in the time of fall. It is very, very milky at the time of spring and 36 drops at the ratio of 6 drops a day should be taken. Not more than that. It is required for this gonad system, the whole of your sensual, sexual area. It is good and in the body it creates a thick semen so that your ejaculation can improve if it is thin. Naturally the ejaculation should be like a yogurt, a jelly. It is not very white, but it is whitishly thick. That is how it should be. If you are very perfect and very vibrant, then it should be brownish. If you are weaker, then it is more watery and less thick. If it does not have this kind of required thickness you cannot enjoy your sexual relationship. You can try, but you are just working like a foot pump, not more than that. Your ego is the balloon and you're working like a foot pump and that's it—you don't enjoy it.

So this gentleman went home and he said, "I have some news for you before you utter a word." And she said, "What?" He said, "You are going to go through the greatest test of your life because your husband has totally blown it. Not only have I blown it, but I am going to be proven insane; my job is going to go away; my reputation is already gone; and I feel miserable. I can't even stand." And he fell on the sofa with such a thud that he broke it. Then he pretended he had whiplash because his neck hurt and there he was, lying in a perfect position.
She said, "My dear, a lot of men do a lot more weird things than you. What is wrong with you?"
He said, "I do not know. My heart cannot even beat! It's choking, my breath is all right, but my heart is choking."

And that 'wow' turned out to be a very warm and compassionate mother and that night they had their honeymoon, which they were waiting for all the years of their marriage. When he went through this whole ordeal and he was all right he said, "I feel sometimes that I should repeat it again, just to get that experience." He said, "I couldn't even believe it. What worked? I was not only wrong, I was totally wrong. I was absolutely wrong. And it was such a wrong thing to say and do, and—how did it get managed?"

'Wow' can manage everything. 'Wow' is the sound of Infinity. And that is why we put 'wow' with the word man (woman) and relate it to the female, the creative power, the creativity. It is potentially very essential in us that we should relate to every situation—business, friendship, social affairs, political affairs, personal affairs, with our subordinates, with our bosses—in the framework of one understanding only and that is that relationship is a relative term in which there are always two situations. One is 'wow' and the other is man. Man alone cannot survive. You can take it as granted. If you ever want to survive as a man, now, there's no chance. You have to deeply understand what that 'wow' means.

There are three cycles of life: 7 years, 11 years and 18 years of life. Seven years represents the cycle of consciousness; 11 years, the cycle of intelligence; and 18 years, the cycle of life. When I say that, you listen; but you do not go into the 'wow' of it, the Infinity of it. Every 18 years of the life cycle contains your intelligence and your consciousness. Consciousness will be two point something, intelligence will be one point something, and life will be one. If you have a calculator, you can figure out exactly the data in proportion. Your consciousness and your intelligence is in proportion to your life, which you forget. When you are out of that proportion, you are out of everything in life. Period. It is wrong as a plus; it is wrong as a minus. If you are over-intelligent in proportion [to the life], you will be misunderstood. If you are under-intelligent, you will be dumb. So don't misunderstand; don't think that this proportion has no part to play. The real part, the potent part, the destiny that you are talking about can only be achieved by keeping that proportion, which is 7, 11, and 18; one, one point something, and two point something.

Now, the continuity of life depends upon your flow and that flow is the spiritual flow—the spirit. Spiritual flow simply means when you don't give an inch, which can only happen if you have the experience of knowing that the unknown is known to you. "I know the unknown is known to me." Can you repeat this? "I know the unknown is known to me." Your unknown and my unknown and our unknown—that is called the 'wow' state. In this state of consciousness, this 'wow' state, you must know that your unknown, and his and her unknown, and their unknown is totally known to you. Start that way. Why? Because you are a product of harmony; because the one creative power of God is totally harmonious. There is nothing in disharmony on this planet; there is no conflict. Anything that has been created by God is neither triangular nor square, it is round. That is the symbol of harmony, the symbol of Infinity, because a circle has no corners. Corner means the end of the world and the end of hope. There's no such thing as the end of hope in man. Somebody said, "No, there is a word." I asked, "What word?" He said, "Hopeless." I said, "Write it." So he wrote: "H-O-P-E-L-E-S-S." I said, "Less the less, what is left?" He said, "Hope." If you cannot less the less, what kind of a man are you? Just a little less—a little. Just have a little sight and it will go away. Don't fight, because it is hard, it is troublesome, it is bad. When you feel something is coming toward you, just give it an angle—just shift. This is called movement.

The state of consciousness of the individual, which is called man, is to relate creatively to woman. Without woman you are not complete. If you think that you don't want a woman, then you are hating a woman, and then you will do everything you can to hate a woman and to prove to yourself that you hate her. Hate, or proven hate, or a developed understanding of why you hate her—it doesn't matter. In the end, you are hating a woman.

In abstract, in reality, in thought form, in experience, from the past, to be in the future, and now, the woman is with you anyway. You love a woman, you draw pictures of her, you imagine her, you think about her. The ideal woman, which you never got, which you are trying to get, which you are pursuing, which you intend to pursue, which you think you can pursue, even then, woman is with you. As surely as Eve came out of the rib of Adam, you all came out of the womb of a woman. There's this one, simple, biblical, knowledgeable effect, that God came himself, pulled the rib out and turned it into woman so that you can have one rib short and there may be a pain there, right in your rib. That's what woman is. When you don't understand her, she takes that rib and rubs you so hard; I have seen a lot of people going round and round and round [like that].

The Downfall of the **Man**

Three things bring about the downfall of the man. Three things: **Zer**, **Juroo**, *and* **Zameen**. **Zer** *means wealth.* **Juroo** *means woman.* **Zameen** *means the earth, the potential authority.*

Zer—**Wealth**

Wealth, we need it, it is a friend. Wealth in the bank can do a lot of things, right? The very idea that we think wealth can do a lot of things makes us forget to do those things we have to do. We think we can buy love, things, environments, circumstances. The power of wealth makes us forget how to relate to 'wow', and we think our wealth can do the job for us. That is a disastrous thought. It has killed more people, more marriages, more happiness, more relationships than anything else you can think of. All kings, all men of wealth, all rich men have terrible family lives. Why? First of all, they waste all of their energy trying to grab the wealth. If you think grabbing wealth is very essential for you, remember that the woman you are married to is also a wealth. Grab that, too. What's wrong with that? Most men ignore that part and grab only the wealth: "Honey, I have a diamond set for you; I have a ruby set for you." She says, "Go to hell you son of a so-and-so. I am happy with the gardener. Why did you come home?" From her garden the gardener plucked her flowers, for which this son of a so-and-so is paying, and he comes and he gives them to her, and she loves it, and closes her eyes and takes them. Her husband comes home and she says, "Why didn't you have a car accident?" You think that by diamonds and by all that you can acquire a woman, but you can't.

It is a most foolish thing to deal with a woman in measurements of money. That is another wrong conduct. "If you go with me, I will buy you this, this, this. If you do this, I'll do this, this, this." You understand what I'm trying to say to you? With this attitude you trigger hatred in her, because woman is the master of maya and when you measure her with maya, you trigger in her the hatred. It has been seen in 40% to 60% of cases, hatred in a woman has been totally triggered, assimilated and created by men's own behavior. It is very seldom that you can talk about money with a woman without asking her mind to go into a million different directions. Your mind is going toward her, just talking to her, just thinking of her, trying to pursue her into the trap of maya. And at that moment she's thinking about what traps she can lay with that money. You are knitting the trap and meanwhile she is trying to think of how many other things she's going to catch in that trap. Aren't you a fool?

We studied successful marriages and we found that the successful marriages are those where the man gave an exact amount of money to the woman and told her to manage it. She gets so involved in the whole management business; and she looks to him as this great god who has to rescue her if her management falls apart. The relationship continues for years and years and years. That's why they say, "Make woman the queen and the empress of the home; man is a hunter in the outer world."

If the woman wants to make a home with one needle, she can make a palace that man cannot destroy with a cannon. These are certain qualities, certain calibers, certain constitutional differences, which have to be understood when dealing with a woman. If you do not know how to deal with a woman, you don't wheel with a woman. Normally, you do not know how to deal with a woman, but you wheel with a woman and under that wheel you get ground. The majority of the time, we go through our misery. On average, man remains married for 50 years. Scale it. It comes to one and a half scoldings per week. Scale it. Make an understanding: marriage is a continuous combination of putting yourself into a carriage with another person. Marriage is a carriage of happiness unto Infinity. You decide this and you must pull it through. What tactic will you use? What will work? What is the key of it? "Wow."

You know, one guy had a very fat woman. I have seen it with my two eyes. Her shoulders were so lumpy that there was a hump on her like a camel. She was beautiful when he fell in love with her. After they married, something happened. So one day he waited for me for about three hours.

He said, "I'm your friend. Either give me something which will work, or never see me again."
I said, "What are you going to do? Suicide? Everybody threatens. You are a fool. Don't be afraid. If you are afraid, you can't do a thing."
He said, "Well, afraid I'm not. Question is, there is a scripture saying, 'When you are in trouble, don't go to a friend, don't go to a man, go to a teacher, because you will get egoless, Infinite wisdom.'"
And I said, "That means I'm your teacher?"
He said, "Sure. You guys never knew about it?"
I said, "We are buddies, we are friends."
He said, "Forget it. I am just in trouble and I have got a baby elephant. Last night I was trying to make love with her and the bed broke and I am in absolute shame. Now I cannot weigh her in pounds, I have to weigh her in tons. You can't believe it. And this is not going to work out."
I said, "Are you sure that you want to do something really good?"

He said, "Yeah, I'm really sure about it."

I said, "Other spiritual people have related to this man and woman relationship; it's a very divine relationship. Either it is divine or very divided. If it is divided, it is a duality. If it is a duality, it is a destruction."

"If it is divine, it is par excellence. There is such a powerful flow of magnetic spirit flowing through the female, you can't even believe it. Take any religion and their laws and the whole thing, it's all dependent on one thing—how to relate. In the Siri Guru Granth Sahib, all the Gurus (except for Guru Gobind Singh), have called themselves "*Mehelaa*". *Mehelaa* means spiritual wife. *Mehel* means wife; *Mehelaa* means that worshipping wife. So basically, if you want to understand, man has worshipped this relationship in the true concept of it."

So I said, "Look, my friend, I don't know what I can do but I know one thing you can do. Do you imagine a skinny girl?"
He said, "Yeah."
I said, "Do you feel it?"
He said, "Yeah."
I said, "Do you understand it?"
He said, "Yeah."
I said, "Tomorrow morning when you get up, just say, 'Wow, I have had a beautiful vision and then describe the whole thing to her, and don't talk further than that."

He was a little bit more clever than me. I told him what technically I know, but he put a lot of what you call beauty into it, and he said to her, "I've had a beautiful vision. An angel came to me, full of light; he sat on my right shoulder and he told me that it is the karma that you are becoming like this. But he said you will have a son, joy, money, the whole thing, provided you eat only one zucchini a day." Now, gentlemen, one may be as fat as an elephant itself, but on one zucchini a day even an elephant will come out to be a skeleton. Then he made it totally religious, absolutely. And once in a while, in-between she would say, "Oh, I am dying, I am hungry, I'm miserable." And he said, "Look around darling, do you see that angel, that light, that special light? Just look that way. I see it. I see all the time that angel is protecting you. Nothing is going to happen to you." In four months folks, that girl could compete with anybody in skinniness. She totally convinced her ego, that 'wow' in her, that Infinite 'wow', that Infinite, whole ego, that there's a beautiful, charming, excellent angel all the time hovering around her and guiding her.

Your relationship with a woman is not as a man. Your relationship is in your capacity to convince her 'wow'. Do you understand? This is a million dollar talk I am giving to you. If you don't understand this, you'll be miserable even in spite of a whole day of my lecturing. Your relationship is not as a man to a woman. Your relationship is not based on sex. Your relationship is not based on theory or any performance you want to create. You must be the biggest fool if you think that is what relationship is. Instead, it will be a misguided statement of your own, toward your own personality.

Relationship is proportionate to how much you can capture the 'wow' of the woman you are with. Your proportionate relationship to the state of consciousness of the 'wow' of a woman is what they call relationship. That is why in scriptural knowledge, all the rishis, swamis, and yogis say, "Where there is dharma, there's no karma." And dharma is nothing but a progressive path to Infinity. Dharma doesn't mean "the religion"—no, no, no, my friend, you are mistaken about that. Dharma is a progressive path toward Infinity. If your potential, your attitude, cannot be reconciled in capturing that Infinity in a woman, the rest is circumstantial. Your marriages and your circumstantial marriages, your relationship and your circumstantial relationship, they will exist. They have been existing and they will continue to exist. But once she knows that this man has reached my 'wow' and this man has caught my 'wow' and this man is capable of reaching my 'wow,' that woman will be nothing but a flowing fountain of spirit unto Infinity with you, and no mistake, no blunder, no fault of yours is any itch to her. Otherwise after seven years, when the consciousness will change, the seven-year-itch will start. Normally marriages fall apart after seven years. Understand? Is there any question you have about it?

Q: *Yes, sir. Could you say more about what you mean by the 'wow' of the woman?*

Yogi Bhajan: 'Wow' of the woman is her attitude toward her own Infinity. "Wow' is the attitude of every woman. That is what woman is. In her own status as a woman, a complete woman, she feels that she is just a living Infinity. Man has to urge himself to think about that; woman has to come down to that. That's the basic polarity between a man and a woman.

Q: *How does the consciousness change after every seven years?*

Yogi Bhajan: Psychologically, physically, potentially, basically, and metabolically, the conscious cycle in the sophisticated computer called the human brain is meant to grab fewer fears and more experience after every 7 years. You will be surprised to see that after age 70, a man likes to rely on experience. After 70 years, you will find men talking about their experience more than trying to learn. But when a child is 7 years old, he has more questions, less answers. After 70 years, the same man has more answers and less questions. Do you understand that reality? Have you seen old people? They start talking and then go on and on and on and on, and you say, "My God, why did I get him started on this subject?" Because they want to talk, they don't want to listen. But a child wants to listen and wants to talk less. That is the 7-year cycle of consciousness and it affects the marriage relationship—it is called the 7-year-itch.

Q: You said that the man should try to capture the 'wow' of the woman. To do this, should he try to reflect this consciousness he sees back to the woman?

Yogi Bhajan: I am coming to that. Well, you asked the question: how to capture the 'wow'? 'Wow' of the woman is the intellectual and compassionate Infinity. Woman is very intellectual. She is 16 times more intellectual, and 16 times more compassionate, and 16 times more patient than a man. By construction of the two beings, "*solokhe padaee*," 16 times more; and one has abundance, you can take as much as you like. It's not a weakness. God made it that way. If she is convinced, with a compassionate heart, with an Infinite reason, she can tolerate the worst with you. The circumstances in which a man would want to leave you, woman can go through it without even grumbling. That is the inherited quality in her. Through your conduct, which is very important to a woman, you should not behave as a drama, you should not behave as a trauma. Both will not work. Both are what a woman hates. Woman is a drama herself, trauma herself. Equal poles reflect, opposite poles attract. When you behave like a dramatist and a "traumatist," you lose a woman.

Relate to woman as a simple, intelligent, man of words. Because she has too much compassion, she wants to see whether you have compassion or not. If you don't have compassion, woman won't go with you. I can give you this in writing. You may belong to anything, any group, any spirituality, any person, any country, any form or style. Woman wants to find these things about a man—is he compassionate, is there compassion, and if so, where is it? She will look to see if he is intelligent, and if he is, where is that intelligence? In which field? And, to see if he is firm. If so, how firm?

Woman wants to share with you your body, your intelligence and your power. Your body—she wants you in a good body, nicely dressed up, neat and clean. That's her nature; she likes it. She may be filthy herself, it doesn't matter. Don't look to that. In a man she always likes a neat and clean personality. And she wants to brag about that man. For example, how intelligent he is. If you don't give her an outlet for bragging about the man, you are losing yourself in her. And then she wants to have that power. Your money means nothing more to her than her power. You may not give her a penny; but your capacity to do it, she wants to think it is hers. These are the three areas that the woman likes to relate to—a common woman, a known woman.

Don't think that a woman who is very spiritual and higher in consciousness, who has got a divine experience doesn't care for anything; or that the woman who is mentally sick and totally rotten doesn't care for anything either. Because however sick a woman is, you can bring her up. However spaced out a woman is, you can bring her down to reality, because woman has the capacity to relate to the reality. That is why she needs the man—to keep her balanced, to keep her equilibrium. Man is supposed to give her the security that he can provide and protect. She can protect herself; but once she starts protecting herself, you have no chance. Once she starts providing for herself, you have no chance. It doesn't mean that you should not allow a woman to work or to protect herself. No, that is not the area of conflict. Instead, you must give her a firm area—be united. Unity. "Honey, if you protect yourself, you protect me. If you are providing something, you are providing for me." Be honest about it. Some men are so crazy that if a woman is working, they take away all her pay and put it in their account. It won't work. It is not the capacity of any man to stretch a woman beyond her tolerance. Therefore, that is what we are talking about—the 'wow' in her—which you can approach, which you can know, which you can rub against, which you can feel, and which you can understand.

Love is something in which there is no relationship. It is Infinity itself—no loss, no gain, no up, no down, no this, no that, no black, no white, no yellow, no brown, no nothing. Love is love, from the beginning unto Infinity.

When a woman makes her own money, it should be treated exactly the same way as the money you make is treated. That's what they call a joint account. The household must be run by a joint effort, not with the attitude that it is your money and it is my money. The moment you create 'yours' and 'mine' you have already ruined the household. These are the mistakes which our Western friends do. And that is why the rate of divorce is going higher and higher. Money is a medium, money is what money does. Money is not mine or yours. Money is ours. And it is very beautiful if you are very honest with a woman in these areas. Just tell her, this is this, whatever you say. But some men have difficulty when the woman has the money; they want to manage it; and they do weird things to put a pressure on that. That brings real bickering in the relationship. Or some men have their money and they want her to just be a servant who is paid for ironing, who is paid for this or that. For all the chores a woman does, if you paid her at a normal rate, she would require $17,500 a year. It has been totally statistically calculated. For all the jobs she does in the household, if paid at a normal wage rate, she could earn $17,500 a year.

Q: You said a man has to urge himself to think about the 'wow' but that a woman comes from that. Can you explain that a little more?

Yogi Bhajan: The capacity of a woman is that she represents the moon, that means the mind. So in her territory, she is pretty established; and she wants to establish a territorial, intellectual, permanent relationship with the man, which she calls love. You must understand, you have to differentiate between relationship and love. Love is something in which there is no relationship. It is an Infinity itself—no loss, no gain, no up, no down, no this, no that, no black, no white, no yellow, no brown, no nothing. Love is love, from the beginning unto Infinity. But what we are calling love is just the relationship; but relationship is not love.

To beautify that relationship, we give it the word love. So, you are mixing two different things. Therefore in the territorial conquest in which a woman is creatively proceeding in her inquest into the inquiry of life, she wants a definite, territorial relationship with you where she must feel comfortable. And her comfort with you, as a man, is that you can protect her; that you can provide for her social grace, mental stimulant, and spiritual compassion; and that you are a man of your word. If a woman knows that you are a man of your ego, then the days of your marriage or relationship are numbered. You can number your days. You can stretch it, but it won't work.

Q: *Sir, in your past lectures you said that woman doesn't really care about anything except that you are a leader to her. I think the notes say that she doesn't care if you are intelligent or anything else.*

Yogi Bhajan: Leader is a most intelligent person. She doesn't care for the intellectual raps; she doesn't care for your ego flairs; she doesn't care for a lot of things. A leader is a very sacrificial, highly calculated, most sophisticated human behavior in relationship to a woman. And that is expected of every woman: to demand a man who can lead her, who can stimulate her, and in all that stimulation, he may not demand back. Because you have to understand, in theory a beggar is a beggar whether he begs a penny or a million dollars. A giver is a giver whether he gives a penny or a million bucks, though both are different. Do you understand?

Juroo—Woman

Now we proceed to another area, *Juroo*. *Juroo* means woman; actually, it means a woman in a living vibratory effect. A man who loves a woman, or has a relationship with a woman and a contract to relate to a woman, if he is dishonest and prefers another woman, other than the one he's with, he's creating a conflict in himself. You can lie; you can socially undermine. But if you undermine your woman for any other woman, she will betray you. She is not there to betray you; you are invoking the betrayal. You are causing the cause; and you must have the effect. You come home and you praise your ex-wife. Ex-wife and the praise of ex-wife will make this wife an ex-wife. You come home and you praise your secretary. I have seen men so foolish, totally foolish.

What is a wife? Wife is a 'why' and an 'if'. What is a wife? 'Why' and 'if'. If a woman is totally 'why and if', and somebody just gives up that 'why and if', she becomes your relative. You come home and you start it, the 'why' and 'if': "Oh, my secretary's great, my this is great, my that is great, my girlfriend is great, my Chancellor of the University is great (provided she's a woman)." You know what that 'why and if' woman thinks? She thinks you're a sex maniac. And all these relationships in life have become totally bizarre because of our wrong approach. Some men, I have seen, they start using threats on their wives—threat, threat, threat. Finally, a wife will become so confirmed in the threat she will say, "All right, prove it to me that you can do it." You understand?

There are three egomaniac living beings: *raj hut*, *teria hut*, *bal hut*. One is the authority, *raja*, the king. *Raj hut* is the king, the emperor, or the authority. They are very dispassionate when they get into their egomaniac scene. Second is the woman, *teria hut*. Third is *bal hut*, the child. If you push a woman to such an extent, or you tolerate a woman to such an extent, you actually ruin your own woman. Therefore, you are required to draw on your capacity and your capability.

In the science of astrology, we say that when there's a square in the horoscope, it means it's a dangerous situation; it means the flow of energy has a block; it cannot flow. Now taking that attitude as true, all you have to do is take a square and cut it through. What does this make? Two trines. One triangle is the sign of happiness; two triangles is the sign of double happiness. Man is born to walk a diagonal path in relationship to woman. And man is born to walk a diagonal path in relationship to his own mind. Ask your mind, "Oh, my mind, think, think, think. This is it, this is it, this is it. Mind, go on giving your situations, pictures, sequences, consequences, get them all together and cut through them." That is the power of your own meditative mind to accept and to go through a diagonal path. The creative carrier in you is your potent, potential man. Sensually, sexually, basically, relatively, and comparatively, you are what you can create under any given circumstances. And that is what they call kundalini, *cherdi kala*—how much you can get from your base to your top.

Q: *Sir, what is the square that you were referring to that the diagonal path crosses?*

Yogi Bhajan: In the flow of energy of the zodiac in contrast to the stars and the zodiac, which is called the heavens, if there is a square sign it means there is an obstruction; and if that obstruction is cut diagonally, it means trines—two triangles. And two triangles are a sign of double good luck. That was what I was explaining.

You are nothing but you. And you have to understand that you cannot be anything but you. Neither there was, nor there is, nor there shall be, anything more important than you. And from that you, as a base, you must rise unto the top—as you. Excel. Command the situation and the challenge and excel. That is a man. Don't mind to excel. What is a spiritual teacher? What is a spiritual path? Nothing. On this planet there is experience, maya, moment. On every side, all around you, there is a woman, maya, and every situation is a demand to excel. This is true whether you are married or you are not married; you are divorced or you are not divorced; you are gay or you are not gay; you are a woman maniac, sex maniac, this, or that. You may vary yourself, label yourself into a million varieties, but the fact is the creation, the maya, is a challenge to you and you have to rise from the base of your spine into your forehead. Your potency is you. It is your creativity that excels in environments and circumstances.

Zameen—Earth

What we are relating to now is the third part: woman in comparison to the woman you live with and link with. Link. The word link is very important. You can live with a woman without having a link, and you may not live with her but you may have a link. Woman has a kind of feeling, a sensitivity. Her aura has more antennae than that of the man. Woman has 16 more antennae per square millimeter, which is called 'electromagnetic antennic vibratory effect'. Woman's aura is much thicker than that of a man's. She can make you feel. Very few men have the quality to make you feel; but the majority of women can. That is called the electromagnetic antennae in her aura and she has that feeling, that sensitivity and ability, to create a link.

Question is: if that link sits in you, what will happen to you? So you must have a defensive magnetic field. Man without a defensive magnetic field and woman without a magnetic link are both useless animals because there is no relationship. Relationship is just temporary, as are the seasons. Impulse comes, season comes, they decide the territory, they have the relationship, they have the kids, kids go their way, parents go their way. Normally, in the Western society today, our relationships happen like that. We marry, we have children, then our relationship breaks. We are going through the pain of non-continuity and we are not in a position to stop. The reason we are not in a position to stop is because we do not know how to stop. We do not alter ourselves at the altar. That is our problem. We do not know how to alter ourselves at the altar, and a man who has no altar in life has no ultimate reality to reach. Everything is temporary: woman, children, relationships. There has to be a permanent link to keep a relationship alive. You have to have an altar to alter your consciousness so that you can go into the situation and be clean and radiant; so that your magnetic field can be so defensive that nothing can enter and bifurcate you and tear you apart; so that you can always maintain yourself continuously.

In relationship, you cannot derive your energy from profit and loss. Only through the heart can you live; it is the Heart Center—the heart. The energy from the base of the spine should go to the head. It is called serpent energy. We are speaking of the serpent, the kundalini. This is the tail of you which nobody sees. And nobody sees your projection either. That is why man has 11 years; he starts as 11 years old, and he matures at 22 years old. Between 11 and 22 one should not indulge in any sexual activity as a male. He should allow his system to grow and become mature. In the oldest scriptures it is advised that man should not marry before 24 or 25. Before 24 one should not marry, and one should try not to become involved in any sexual activity. Look what we do: we are 9 years old and we are horny.

Listen, because you must understand. It is not a sexual, physical game you enjoy. Out of this whole thing, it is the sense of smell you enjoy. It is etheric. Your body aroma and her body aroma is the creativity of the whole relationship. The physical part is very gross. It is not what you are talking about or what you understand. When you are young and powerful and you are blind, you get into the very physical part of it and you go on and on; this has nothing to do with the relationship. It won't establish the link. After all, if it is a spiritual world and you are very spiritual and fanatic, what else can you give this earth if your game is not right? And you do not know how to play it and you do not play it right? If you do not play it right, how can you conceive right? How can you seed right? How can it grow right? What right thing can come to you? If it is true that on this earth we want the angels, the sages, the saints, the rishis, the yogis, the swamis, the spiritual teachers, the messiahs, and all that stuff, how are we going to produce them? You don't grow wheat in the desert without water.

So, basic requirements are very essential and the relationship of male and female is a very productive, creative and important relationship. It is the most important relationship God ever created. Now to undermine this relationship and brand it as sex, brand it as negative? It's ridiculous. After all, all these saints and sages who we follow for spiritual purposes, did they drop from the ocean or from the sky? Did you see them coming down from a parachute? Or did a whale come and open his mouth and throw Jesus out of it? What do you think? Purity and piety of relationship lies in the very rules of the game. If you play any game, it has rules. The joy of the game lies in the rules of the game; and the sexual game, if it is not played by the rules, is a horrible situation. But how can you play it, if you do not know how to?

Potent Potential of the **Inner Being**

You should be you in beginning, and you should be you in the end, and you should be you throughout, and you should fill yourself up with your own you.

Okay, now we go into the potent potential of the inner being. The potency and the potential is the frequency of the individual—from whatever level of consciousness he can relate.

$P = C + P$.

That is the formula [for life]. Potent potential is equal to creativity plus patience: $P = C + P$. "C" stands for creativity and "P" stands for patience. Without that, the potent potential of a person is never exhibited. And without that exhibition, that expression, without that flow of radiance, the person is not complete. The person feels handicapped. The cycle of life is equal to "C", to creativity. When you complete the cycle of life, you must have the potential satisfaction of saying, "Oh, I lived it!" There are divorces in life. You know, you divorce your wife, you divorce your children, you divorce your country. But there's also a divorce from the cycle of life. You divorce your life; you do not live it. "I am a yogi and you are not." That's it. It is a divorce from life.

Actually, a yogi means a person who can unite with everybody, with the worst and the best. All this creativity means, which we have potentially created in us, is that through thick and thin, in every environment and circumstance, we can be in a position to talk, create, and relate. Because you must understand: nothing affects you and you affect nothing. You will always win, if you remain you at the start and you in the end. Throughout anything, you start as you, you go through the frequency as you, and you end up as you. And this is called the vibration of life. Start as you, end as you. Even when you are before a spiritual teacher, start as you, end as you, and in that "you," if something is filled up, carry it, drink it. You are a cup of life: fill it with good, fill it with bad. This chance to fill it is called the cycle of life.

Now the cycle of life has many centers. It can be here, it can be there. It can be truly in the center. It is the center of the circle. When the center is somewhere other than the center of the circle, life will be odd. But if it is at the center of the circle, life is even. Learning in life is a continuous experience. Learning in life is a continuous experience; and in this continuous experience, each day there should be a record of progress. They always say, one who does not process the life, in the progress of life, loses life to animosity. You feel happy when you lose the enemy, animosity. When you lose it, you feel very happy and very free. When you do not process the life in the progress of your experience, it is as dangerous as animosity.

It is your in-bound nature. You must not decide, "Oh, she's beautiful; oh, he's beautiful; oh, it is beautiful." There's nothing beautiful. There's only one thing beautiful—and that is you. Just understand that you are beautiful. And still, you are going to fit yourself in a frame. After being fit in the frame are you going to remain beautiful or not? That is what you have to decide before you proceed. So please do not walk on shaky grounds. It is for your own convenience to check out the ground you walk on. There's a very popular saying, "Prison is not a palace, though it can be built like one." If a home is a home, it may be a dungeon, but it is still a home. You have the freedom to come in and go out as you like.

In our life, we call this process amalgamation—union in amalgamation. We are talking about the you and the Id. And we are very technically saying, that you should be you in beginning, and you should be you in the end, and you should be you throughout, and you should fill yourself up with your own you. Are we saying that it is a comparative statement or are we saying it's a definite statement? What are we after?

It is said that man is like a sun; he can light the whole universe. But when man is eclipsed, that is where the danger lies. Relatively, our progress is understandable progress. It is just like going on a hike; we are simply going through the experience. Otherwise, the journey becomes very difficult. So the journey of life is a very difficult journey. You do not understand the relationship of life. I understand the relationship of life. I understand what you understand; but the only question is that I and you are not two different people. Between male and female, the understanding is complete. I become the you and you become the I. I and you must coincide to go on the journey, otherwise there will be a conflict. Therefore, it is what you want to create in your life, not what is in your life.

When you think that the relationship between a male and a female is nothing but a sexual and sensual relationship, you don't know anything about relationship at all. It is a friendship; it is a trust; it is a creativity; it is a total relationship of creative understanding in which you must know that you have to carry along another person. But after all, what is that pivot, what is that focal point? Because everything that you motivate [or move] must have a karma. Must. Karma means however you react, it will act. Wherever you act, it will react. It means you'll be counterbalanced. You will act, you will react and you'll go nowhere. You have to go and you have to complete. Therefore you must proceed toward the unison, the harmony we talk about, which must be here and hereafter.

That is why life should be motivated by two people toward dharma. And what is dharma? A righteous progressiveness unto Infinity. Two must decide, two must join, hand in hand, to walk unto Infinity toward righteous progressiveness, and in the process, the progressiveness must be understood, mutually, by both. You know when you are young, your blood is hot. You can keep going. But what happens to you when you are mature and you are not that hot? Will you betray? Life must not become an endless cycle; but it becomes an endless cycle if you do not completely understand the fulfillment of it. Life is a period of time, within time and space, given to you to fill the fulfillment.

Exercises for Potency and **Potentiality**[1]

These little exercises, if you do them, you can't think about getting old—getting old is impossible. This body is not meant to be old; this body is meant to die young.

There's one basic exercise which is for the potent man. That is, when you wake up in the morning, lying straight on your back, you must crunch your knees into your chest and you must jerk yourself. That jerking will bring your lower back, which is normally curved, into a straight line. Ten to 15 movements are very much required. That's number one: Lying on your back these two knees should come into the chest with your arms clasping them, lifting this buttocks area up, thus adjusting the lower back.

Q: You said that you bring the knees to the chest when you first wake up and then jerk. Do you mean roll on the spine?
Yogi Bhajan: No, no. Just pull your knees toward your body in jerks, while lying on your back. It will create a heat in the lower back; and it'll pull the muscles; and it'll correct the magnetic field.

For exercise number two, go into what is called Child's Pose. Come onto your heels, place your forehead on the ground in front of you, hands by the sides on the ground. Begin to move your tail, these buttocks, from side to side, back and forth. When this body is moved this way and that, in a couple of minutes, you will be in a position to go to the bathroom and clean yourself straight. It is called moving the tail. It will take care of your clearance system. Before going to bed you must go to the bathroom to urinate and after getting up in the morning, after these two exercises, if you need to urinate you must go and/or clear your bowels.

There's one exercise which adjusts the hipbone. It is very essential for you. Place your two legs wide open, about three feet apart with one hand going to one foot and one hand going to the other foot. Understand? It is for the hip area.

One more exercise for the hipbone. It is very essential, whether you have done sex or not, but so long as you want to live: take a sink, like a bathroom sink. Put your hands on it and put all your weight over it and then you must jump from left to right. Put your weight on the sink and you go up and down, left and right, left and right, for 10 minutes. It will build up the back muscles, very effectively. You follow? The weight must be put on the sink and, at the same time, the back must be bent similar to what you call cow pose, and then you go back and forth constantly for 10 minutes.

For good sexual relationship, you must take light food after 4:00 p.m. If possible, after you complete your sexual relationship, if you take hot milk at that moment (if it is available), it will be very healthy. Your sexual nucleus, or the meridian points, are located in what we call Area A. This is a point located on the thigh, about four to five inches above the knee.

Q: That area, Sir, is that above the back of the knee?
Yogi Bhajan: No, the front. Area B is located on the heel bone, corresponding to the Achilles tendon. It is the sexual potential meridian, the nucleus area of stimulation.

Q: Does difficulty in getting up for sadhana relate to sexual problems?
Yogi Bhajan: I'm not into sadhana and God at this moment. I'd like to give God some rest. First let us explain the fundamental, the outline, and then we will come out of it.

Q: Do these exercises also pertain to women?
Yogi Bhajan: It is a men's course and is not for women. Do you find any trace of a woman here? What we talk about in a woman's course, you can't even hear it. What we talk about here, they're not hearing it.

Q: Does this meridian run along the inside of the thigh?
Yogi Bhajan: No, on the outside, on top. You know, you do like this? (Slaps the thigh). It is just to aggravate the sensuality.

Q: Sir, is that to massage regularly?
Yogi Bhajan: There is nothing wrong in massaging regularly.

Now, your age and your sensual, creative productivity or potential can be measured by this next exercise. You must keep this angle alive. This is very important. From a standing position, keep the knees straight and bend forward, putting the nose in the space between the knees. Now, stay this way. Wrap your arms around your legs, backwards. Do this for 3 to 5 minutes. You will hardly complain that you have grown old if you can maintain this for the rest of your life.

Q: Is that to be done first thing in the morning or just anytime?
Yogi Bhajan: I am just discussing the preparation of your

---
[1] For a complete write-up and photos of these exercises see the end of this lecture.

sexual energy anytime, everytime, all the time, beyond time, within time. If you have time or you don't have time, it is all the time. Three to five minutes of this can keep you alive.

Q: *You said this exercise can gauge your age?*

Yogi Bhajan: Yeah, that gauges your effective age. If your knees can be straight and you can put your nose between your knees, and if you can hold it for up to 3 to 5 minutes, you'll have the capacity of an 18 year old man. That flexibility should be maintained. If man is able to bend about half the way, he is about 45. Less than this, he is about 55. If he is just barely able to bend, he is about 65. But if he can bend like this at 65, then he's 18.

Today I pulled my muscle, which normally I should not have done, but I overdid it. I was trying to experiment. I meditated, I was very relaxed, and I should not have done it; I pulled my own muscle. I know and I'm telling you and now you know; but one can make the mistake, so that's why I am saying this to you. After meditation, you should relax and have a good time. When you eat, you should take a nap and have a good time. When you have sex, you should have a nap and have a good time. You should not indulge in over-indulgence of any other activity at these times.

Today I was laying the angles and feeling the press of the meridian and I was computing; it was my job as a teacher to honestly experiment, to feel it. But I pulled a muscle—no good, but I had to do it. So I have to die, boots on, but you don't have to. Don't follow my bad example. Do what I say, don't do what I do. That's how true it is, because a teacher is at a level wherein he's free to experiment within himself, because he wants to be sure, because his interest is Infinite. Sometimes I might be taking a good food, a heavy meal, and then I might do exercise. I just want to know whether the wind pain (gas) will affect my liver or my spleen. You need not follow that or you'll be in trouble.

Under normal circumstances, if you want to live a happy life, don't sleep on a soft bed, ever. It's a human tragedy for which there is no cure. It is sexually bad, bad, and very, very bad—soft bed is just a God-given curse. The only time it might be okay is if you are in a jail and they lock you up with such a bed. I'm not upset about it; you are off the list of society anyway.

Q: *Can you determine if the bed is too hard?*

Yogi Bhajan: Yeah, if you have a good king-sized bed, put a one inch thick wooden plank under it and then put a white sheet and sleep. You want a hard bed. The maximum allowance you can have is one-inch thick foam, or a woolen carpet, or a big skin, above the board. Do you know what is the best thing to sleep on? A bear skin—that is very good.

Now, one thing you know in the Western world: knee bends. Knee bends, whatever bend, bend something! It's not very difficult provided you can do it. There is a meridian nucleus above the knee, and if you have not done this in a long time, when you do it about 20 times you'll find there is a needle kind of sensation which starts happening in the legs. That means the meridian is not stretched; it is getting stretched; it is getting in shape and, without that, you cannot enjoy continuity in sexual, sensual, or creative activity. You will start feeling bored, dumb, and irritated, even with all the best food, absolute American life, and everything else. It is called Crow Pose–sit up. Try to keep the feet flat on the floor, but normally they don't remain flat. Heels come up because you guys in the West are tough, you don't have that flexibility. But after awhile it happens. From a standing position, try and keep the feet flat on the floor as you bend down. We recommend between 20 to 50.

Now, there is another exercise which must be done for 11 minutes. This you never do. Standing up straight, bring the elbows and upper arms out to the sides in line with the shoulders, and then raise them a little higher. The elbows must be kept up. Raise the forearms, hands and fingers and point them to the sky; they will be perpendicular to the ground. Keeping the elbows up, they must move upward with the legs, to create a combination of the meridian. You will be running in place in this fashion. Main line here [in the elbow and shoulder] and main line here [the sciatica]; both must move in harmony at the same time. Do this between 11-22 minutes. It is extremely good. Don't worry about the breathing. It will be automatic. You'll be yelling in time with it. At 22 minutes your tongue will be out. And you can do it in your most private room. What is that? The bathroom.

Q: *Would it be just as well to run with your arms up like that?*

Yogi Bhajan: There is nothing which can match with this. You do it tomorrow and you will really remember me. It is really a good exercise.

I am trying to tell you all this because the older you become, the less sexual, the less creative you become, and the more naive and dumb you become. All because you start thinking you are old. But these little exercises, if you do them, you can't think you are getting old—getting old is impossible. This body is not meant to be old; this body is meant to die young. Old age gives you a maturity; weakness comes when it has not been maintained properly. Otherwise, this body should be like an antique car, which should be more valuable when it is older in years than when it was a new car. Provided it is maintained in a perfect condition, that is. Yogic exercises are maintenance exercises, not continuing exercises.

Other exercises do continue the body. Yoga exercises are the maintenance exercises; they are not to continue. Jogging is a very good exercise but jogging doesn't match with this. And during jogging, you sometimes start releasing protein out of your urine. It is too much and the body has to readjust. But with this, there is a time limit, and within that time limit you are okay. Joggers jog 10 miles, 12 miles, 15 miles; they are endless.

One thing, which is the most important thing, we call it a simple kriya. [Editor's Note: Sometimes called Elephant Kriya] That is, when I came in the very beginning, I told you that sometimes, when you've done all the exercises, and you have totally rested, and you feel very good, twice a week, minimum, you should take water and fill your stomach and then put your two fingers against the back of the throat and gag until the water comes out, bending over while doing it. You follow what I'm saying? Twice a week—minimum.

Q: *How much water do you drink when you do that?*
Yogi Bhajan: It depends on how much you want to; but whatever you drink must come out.

Q: *Salt water?*
Yogi Bhajan: No, no, no. Just regular water. You must take it in and then let it come back out.

Q: *What do you do if you have trouble throwing it up?*
Yogi Bhajan: Think of a bad thought, you'll throw it up. No, no, just put your fingers deeper into your throat. It will come out.

Q: *When should you do this?*
Yogi Bhajan: After you do all the exercises. You are tested; you are rested; and just to do that once or twice a week. This is to cleanse the stomach, take away the acidity, take care of the wind, all that pressure and what not.

Now, how to continuously keep yourself creatively young and take care of your semen, and your whole [reproductive] area. When you urinate you must not urinate straight. It must be stopped 3 to 5 times because the muscular pressure inside will stimulate everything and then there is much less chance of making stones. We do not know whether this takes away all the garbage and stones are not formed, or if it creates some ion action in the body. But normally, people who have this habit to stop the urine 3 to 5 times while urinating have never been reported to have stones. It was a very, very difficult study we had to do: first to convince a person that it was for the good of the humanity, then to find out if they had the habit. Of all those who were doing yoga, this was essentially told to them and some didn't bother to do it. We found among those who do it, even in later age—one person was about 87 years old—was in absolute health and was absolutely disease free.

Jo Jo desai, so so rogi, rog rahet mera , sat guru jogi

"All those that are seen are disease stricken. It is only my True Guru who is a yogi who is free from disease."

That suits on this. Yoga is just keeping a clean temple so that the spirit of Infinity, which you call God, can sit in it and reside and radiate. People totally misunderstand yoga. To some, yoga is exercise; to some, yoga is a philosophy, to some, yoga is a trip; to some, yoga is this; to some, yoga is that. Yoga is nothing but a clean science to create a clean union of the finite with Infinity. It has got no left and no right. All yoga exercises are meant to do is pressurize and stimulate the glandular system. Glands are the guardians of the body. Above all, when your glands are functioning all right, you are highly protected.

Now, for creativity and sensuality, there is another exercise. You know this exercise called Maha Mudra? And you know it uses a single leg.

Q: *In Maha Mudra, is the heel of the foot under the buttocks or is it fit into the anus?*
Yogi Bhajan: Maha Mudra is when you put it under the anus. But, in this exercise, one leg should join inside the thigh. This exercise allows you to place your foot at the side of your thigh to pressurize the sciatica. Don't worry about the breath at all, it doesn't matter. Just hold the position. It is a stimulant. These are the stimulants which we are discussing. The spine has to be straight all the way. It can be straight and the body can go like this. (Bending forward). These are called stimulant meridian points, stimulant nucleuses. It is a particular nucleus point and you put a pressure and you stretch and it works a miracle. The secret of it lies in the holding of it. Now, you must do both sides, left and right. Do not move while you are doing it. You make one position—stretch, then rest. Do the other side, stretch, and rest.

Now I am going to discuss with you the creative nucleus. You know the Stretch Pose? You must shake. The body must shake in this exercise. And you must hold until the last shake, and then go flat and rest. It is on the lower back on which your whole weight should be. It should be on the ground. If your lower spine is popping off the ground, you must be raising up too much. Do six inches, then one foot. You understand? If the head is raised one foot, you should raise the heels one foot. If you are raised six inches, stay at six inches; but more than six inches, you must not do. More than one foot when you are raised at one foot, should not be done. If you are at two feet, you are doing something which we do not know. It should be done until you shake. Hold the breath, or you breathe. It is the same thing. Some people do Breath of Fire with it. You do it until you shake.

Q: You don't shake while you are doing it?
Yogi Bhajan: You will shake while you are doing it. It has shaken the biggest people. It is also known as the yogic earthquake.

Q: What if Stretch Pose is hard on your lower back?
Yogi Bhajan: Go to the chiropractor's. I have nothing to discuss. I will not discuss any problems of the medical profession. On any medical question I will say, "Go to the doctor." I am sharing with you the ancient science as known to us from sages through the ages, from heart to heart, and we have experimented and we have seen that it works wonders. It is very perfect and it is very correct. Now the cynical question—why this, why that, and doctors don't help—don't bring them into it, because that way we are discussing a profession which we are not required to discuss. Now, in Stretch Pose, when you shake and you cannot hold it anymore, then lie flat and rest. In Stretch Pose, the hands can be horizontal to the ground or facing one another. Both ways work.

Q: When you introduced these exercises you said, "Now we're going to go to creative nucleus." What's creative nucleus?
Yogi Bhajan: Of your potency—that's what it is. Navel Point is the creative nucleus of your potency and this is a Navel Point exercise.

Q: Are these very old exercises, ancient exercises, or are they recent and something that you've found out through your experimentation?
Yogi Bhajan: They have been handed down from time Immemorial. I can't even date them back.

Q: Is there one exercise that is best for potency and overall health, above all the others?
Yogi Bhajan: Yes. That exercise is basically, when you sit in Lotus Pose and you do Sat Kriya. Sat Kriya is the master exercise.

Exercises for Potency and **Potentiality**
circa 1978

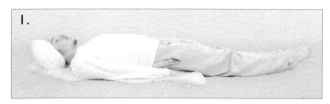

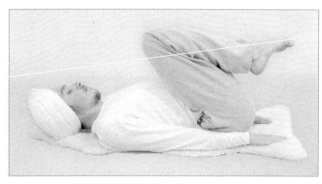

Note: Arms should clasp the knees with each repetition.

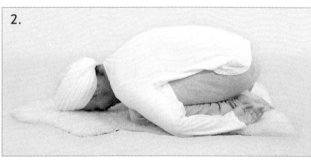

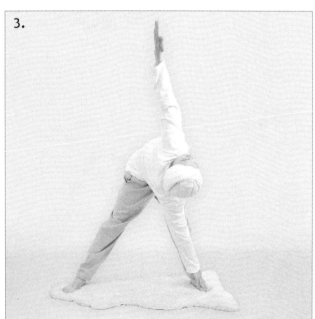

Time: 60 Minutes

1. Lie down on your back. Bring your knees to your chest with your arms clasped about the knees, then shoot the legs out—keeping the feet together—and immediately bring them back in to the chest. When extended, the feet should be about 6 inches from the ground. Exhale as the legs extend; inhale as the knees come to the chest, clasping the hands around the knees with each repetition. **10-15 repetitions.** *This exercise produces heat, adjusts and aligns the lower back and balances the magnetic field.*

2. Dragon Tail. Come into Baby Pose, with the arms straight along the sides of the body with the palms up. Keep the brow relaxed on the ground as you move the hips left and right. Imagine you are swinging a 1,000-pound dragon's tail. *If you feel you need to clear the bladder or bowel, act. Do not wait.*

3. Windmill (or Alternate Toe Touch). Stand with the feet 3-feet apart and arms extended out to either side. Inhale and then exhale as you turn, elongate and bring the right hand to the left foot. Inhale back up. Exhale and continue on the other side. Continue alternating from side to side.

4. Stand with your feet about 6 inches apart. Support your hands on a chair or against the wall. As you lift one heel, transfer the weight to the opposite hip. Alternate from side to side, moving quickly and vigorously, stretching the hips. The movement is like walking in place, except only the heels lift off the floor. The toes remain firmly planted.

5. Standing Front Stretch. Come to a forward bend; bringing your nose as close to the knees as possible; wrap your hands around the legs and hold. Breathe long and deep. **3-5 Minutes**.

6. Crow Squats. Extend your arms forward with the palms down. Let the feet be hip width apart or slightly wider. Inhale and then exhale as you drop the hips into a squat. Inhale back up and continue.

7. Shiva Dance. Bring the hands up so that the palms are facing forward and the elbows are in line with the shoulders. Dance, bringing the knees up alternately. Keep the hands high. **11-22 Minutes**.

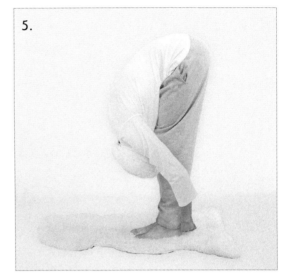

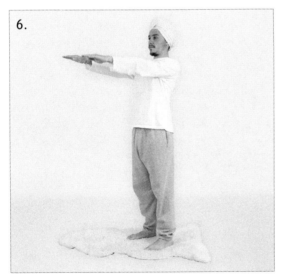

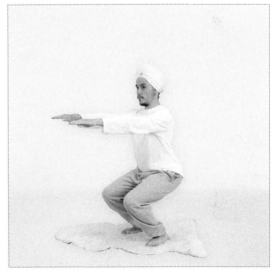

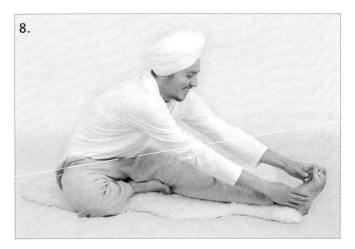

8. Seated on the floor, extend the right leg out in front. The left knee is bent so that the foot rests against the inner right thigh. Reach forward with the right hand and squeeze the toes; the left hand reaches forward and grabs the heel. Stretch for **3 Minutes**. Repeat on the opposite side. **3 Minutes**.

9. Stretch Pose. Lie on the back with the arms at your sides. Raise the head and the legs six inches, and the hands six inches with the palms facing each other slightly over the hips to build energy across the Navel Point. Point the toes, keep your eyes focused on the tips of the toes and hold the breath as long as possible before exhaling and repeating.

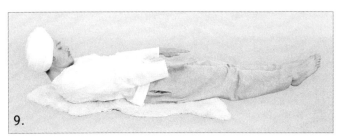

10. Sat Kriya in Lotus Pose. Bring the arms overhead and palms together. Interlace the fingers and extend the Jupiter fingers straight up. Men cross the right thumb over the left; women cross the left thumb over the right. Chant *Sat* and pull the Navel Point in; chant *Naam* and relax the navel. Continue powerfully with a steady rhythm for **6 Minutes**, then inhale, apply the Root Lock and squeeze the energy from the base of the spine to the top of the skull. Exhale; hold the breath out and apply Maha Bandha[2]. Inhale and Relax.

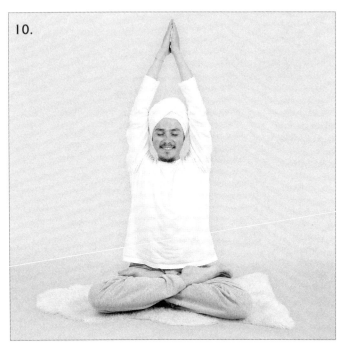

[2] The Great Lock, that is, when all three locks are applied: Neck Lock (Jalandhar Bandh), Diaphragm Lock (Uddiyana Bandh) and Root Lock (Mulbandh).

Creativity of **Consciousness**

Creative consciousness is creative Infinity. Creative Infinity is equal to the creative polarity between male and female; and creative polarity is equal to the circle of Infinity.

Now we go into the creativity and the consciousness and the relevance with the female—creative, creativity and consciousness. It is going to be a little difficult and very scientific.

This is said of a great man: "Man who can offer his head becomes egoless." Man who can offer one tenth of his time and one tenth of his wealth can also become egoless. One takes time, one is timeless. Remember that.

Creative consciousness is creative Infinity. Creative consciousness is creative Infinity; and creative Infinity is equal to creative polarity between male and female; and creative polarity is equal to the circle of Infinity. When you relate to the creative consciousness as creative Infinity and creative Infinity as creative polarity, then you must understand, without creative Infinity you do not enjoy the circle of Infinity, which is called life. Your life is not what you eat, what you drag around, how you sleep, how much you have, how much you don't have. Actually, to be very honest with you, nobody has anything, and everybody has everything. You take a gun and point it in the neck of a rich man and say, "I'm going to blow your head off. Give me everything," he'll give it to you in one minute. Then you go and try to yell and scream, "Somebody give me a penny," and nobody will even look up at you. So there is nothing and there is everything. There is everything and there is nothing. All you have is only one thing: you have time and you have space. Within that space and within that time, you can experience the cycle of life.

Woman is unfit and woman is fit. If you are higher in intelligence and she's lower in intelligence, you come down. If she's higher in intelligence and you are lower in intelligence, you come up. It is the frequency of the intelligence of both that makes a fit. It is you who has to move, not her; because woman is moon, mental territory. She can reflect you. She can represent you, what your inner consciousness reflects and what your outer consciousness reflects. Therefore, your posture doesn't mean anything. Remember that law: when a man falls, an individual falls. When a woman falls, a generation falls. In your creative capacity, and in the polarity of your existence, which is life, you must adjust.

Between a male and a female, it is not just the difference in size or build or function. The inner is different, just as the outer is different. Thinking a woman is just equal to a human being is not correct. She's *par excellence* in certain areas and she is *par minus* in other areas. It is your word and her word which must amalgamate. It is the law of amalgamation that can carry you through. Therefore, if you live at each other, you live like dogs. If you live with each other, you can be separated. If you live for each other, that is what amalgamation is.

When a woman asks a question and you do not know the answer, what'll you do? Ask her to find it out. If she asks you a question and you don't know the answer, you say, "Wow, I don't know anything about it. Would you find the answer for me?" You will not get a question from her for another 6 months. To match up with a woman in intelligence is a sin because she's 60 times "Miss Question". She has 32 times the doubts, 64 times the inquisitiveness. How then can you beat her? Adapt the simple law.

There was an attorney who was married to a very intelligent woman. He was working hard and he would come home late and she was very upset. So one day he brought home the files. He said, "Why don't you copy the important points in this file?" So she had to burn the midnight oil and work through the whole night. In the morning she gave him the data. He said, "Yeah, I know that data. But I need certain other points. I think there were 32 points in all and you have only found 16. I'll leave the file home with you today and in the evening I think you will complete it." So, he started asking her to look into the work and as a result, her criticism became less and less and less until finally it totally got eliminated. In the area where she starts questioning you, ask her to participate and shift the burden of the load toward her. Two things will happen. The questions will totally get eliminated and a friendship will develop as participation becomes equal.

This law applies to every sphere of life. Ask people to share with you. Sharing is assuring people that you want to live with them and that is the beginning of a good relationship. *"Vando Chako."* Share with others. Share responsibility, share knowledge, share goodness, share work, share trust. And do it without grumbling or a painful mind; do it with the essence of a human being. Your essential essence must not represent insecurity.

The cycle of life is a creative cycle—it is called plus cycle. As much energy as you spend toward the plus, that much energy you spend toward the negative. What makes you negative? Do you know the name of the thing that makes you negative? Id—because Id defines you, and the moment you are defined you become insecure. When you become insecure, you become irrelevant. Then you create a lot of hodgepodge to cover your own irrelevancy. Remember one thing: there is nothing that anybody is interested in, in you, except you. All of these side interests are to pass the time. Who cares whether you are a big tennis player or a small tennis player, as long as you are a good man, as long as you are good company. Tennis may be the excuse, but what happens these days? Tennis becomes the good man and the good man becomes the tennis. Participate as you and use everything as a tool to make participation beautiful. It's not as if you have to give someone a lavish meal when he comes to your home. But if you have one piece of dry bread and tear it into two and give the one to the one and you take the other and sit and laugh and drink a glass of water, that may be the best party you have ever enjoyed, because it is a sharing.

Nothing you individually want to define or grab can be yours—even your own home. Somebody has to come and clean it. Somebody has to take care of your garden. Somebody has to do something in your body even, for example, the doctor has to cut it open for an operation. Food has to be prepared by somebody. No life is absolutely independent. Life is dependent. It's a multi-cell life. Life is dependent within itself and dependent without itself. Therefore, realize that the cycle of life is a plus cycle. The cycle of life is a creative cycle. The cycle of life—sexually, sensually, creatively, divinely, or dividedly, devil demon or angelic God—is just given to you for the purpose, the benefit, of experiencing life.

Without guidelines, positive, proper guidelines, life can become very boring. When you start thinking and re-thinking—and thinking again, and re-thinking the re-thinking—those questions and boundaries so much so, that you become entangled with them, then you find you need to open up to new entanglements—and new entanglements bring more entanglements. Finally your life becomes nothing but a bunch of entanglements and it is very painful, even suicidal. But if you keep the life clean, keep the life straight, it doesn't matter how much you have, how much you work, or how much you want to expand. Life can be everything. Remember, there's a certain law and that law is: you should not compromise *you* for anything. All of your surroundings should be made straight in relation to that *you*. But that *you* is a very compassionate, inflowing spirit—not an ego. If that *you* is ego, then you will have more enemies and less friends. If that *you* is of the flowing spirit, then you will have more friends, but hardly less enemies, because that person who'll have friends will always have enemies. The law of polarity is—equal reaction shall be there—equal and opposite.

Every action has a reaction, equal and opposite. So when you go forward you become big, you become great. A lot of people who cannot see your forward growth, your bigness, out of jealousy start pulling your leg. The more they pull your leg, the more you push forward. The more you push forward, the more they pull your leg. This way all of you must die victoriously saying, "Oh, they couldn't pull my leg!" Adopt this posture. This is called satisfaction. Life is another name for satisfaction—and in that satisfaction we must live.

A family is the test of that satisfaction. You must understand that sometimes you are mistaken. You'll marry and your wife will be a challenge. Children, they'll be a challenge. The whole thing is a challenge. Creative polarity must complete its circle, and in that circle, there shall always be challenge. Because from where you start, you must end; and from where you end, you must start. You can't run away from it.

What is a woman? Woman is your Infinity. It is the 'wow' of the man. It's the 'fe' of the male. It is the nucleus from which you focus to see through the experience of creativity. That's what children are about; that's what it's all about. But in these days in the Western world there is a problem. We are talking about a normal woman, not about an abnormal, obnoxious, ill-raised, neurotic, psychotic kid in the body of a woman. Therefore, please, in the body of the woman, find the woman first. Otherwise, you are playing into the hands of a very big risk. You are relating to a woman, not to a body. These days, plastic bodies are more beautiful than the woman you are looking at. If you want that, then have a huge picture of her hung in the living room, meditate on it a couple of hours and you'll be in good shape.

If there is a man in you and there's a woman in her, there cannot be a problem. Frequency adjustment in communication and dependency on trust are normal human capacities; they are part of our human caliber. Within that human caliber is the capacity of two living frequencies to adjust and tune-in to the same frequency. The goal of Infinity is possible. This is the way the God made it. It is not impossible for two people to live together. They can live together provided that the two are committed and their commitment comes from intelligence. Intelligence comes from the excellence of Infinity and that is the path of dharma. That's why in dharmic people, all is the Will of God. The Will of God is nothing but accepting the role of Infinity.

Free will is accepting the will of the finite ego. Therefore you must understand that the game must be played well. How do you play it? In the circle of life, the circle is the stimulant. The stimulant is the name of the game and the name of the game is the stimulant. What are we playing with? We are playing with the pluses, which are interrelating with the negative. They have to play with the negative because the circle must be completed. So, if male is plus and female is minus, minus and plus makes neutral. But trying to make her plus and you minus? Making her plus is just opposite. Let her be the reflector and let you be the shining star. Let this creativity continue because it has been coming from time immemorial and it shall continue to time immemorial.

In the sex game it must start 72 hours ahead, somewhere outside the bedroom. If the sex game starts in the bed, it is bad. You must understand that a female is not a body. She is the inner body, the mental body, the rational body, the projective body, the physical body, the subtle body, the auric body, and the cosmic relative body. You are dealing with that many bodies in one body. And it is this relationship you are relating to. You'll hear, "I understand, I fully understand, I totally understand, but something is inside me that doesn't understand," when the inner body is out. "I do agree. It is absolutely normal but I do not see any radiance in it," when the radiant body is off. "He touches me and I shrink," means the physical body is off. "It doesn't feel good to look at," when the subtle body is off. "When we pass each other, something wrong happens," means the auric body is off. "We are not going toward that feeling of Infinity in spite of the fact that we feel good," and the cosmic body is off.

Now, you are married to one body and you are married to many bodies. How many are there? Eight. How many chakras are there? Eight. At what frequency, at what chakra is your consciousness in? If it is in the First Chakra, you are perverted. Second Chakra: you are a (sex) maniac. Third Chakra: unknown. Fourth: compassionate. Fifth: blunt. Sixth: projected, subtle, beautiful. Seventh: cosmic, spaced out, neutral. Eighth: Infinite, divine, unearthly. Which do you want? What do you want? You want in-between all. You want experience. You want to look innocent. That is what you want. You want to look innocent and you may not be innocent; and you cannot look innocent if you are not innocent. This blunder has been committed by man from time immemorial to now and it shall continue. There's one shortcoming of the man: if he's not innocent, he cannot look innocent. And there's one strength of the woman: she may be most crooked, but she can look innocent and you can't catch her. That is the polarity. Therefore, it is very essential for us to grow. We must grow in life. But how do we go about it? And how do we stimulate our consciousness in relationship and relevance to our polarity?

You know what this sign means?[1] (Yogi Bhajan draws on the board.) This is male and this is female; these are the most ancient signs to depict both. That is what I am going to talk about and then I'll finish, because we could go on day and night, but after all, whatever you have been told must be digested. Don't rush to know everything right away. What's best is whatever you know, practice it.

Now, this is what is called the male and this is called female. Woman is not supposed to talk back or confront. Man should never react and should always be positive. Your problems start when you start reacting. By-pass a woman, but don't react to her. It's useless. It's a waste of time, a waste of a very beautiful part of life. It will not lead you anywhere. But what do you do? First you confront her, then you challenge her, then you aggravate her. And then she ends up ruining you. The reaction of a woman can sometimes be totally out of proportion. So, don't push her, don't stimulate a reaction. In between, pad the situation with time or space. Time and space are two tools in your life. If she is willing to confront you, say, "All right, you're right. We'll discuss this later, 72 hours from this time." You've got the space. Because in one punch of the mood, when it comes to *teria hut*—that's the female territory—*zameen*—it becomes my land, my husband, my child, my home, and so on. And in the face of that "my," there's nothing that works. From "me" to "us" is your intelligence. Teach her us, us, us; we, we, we. We can do this. It is for us to do it. If you bring "me," you will bring conflict and destruction.

It is obligatory on the part of the male to look toward the higher consciousness. It is obligatory on the part of the female to look to time and space. You cannot win your point if you will not change your direction toward higher consciousness, in other words—the simple word for that higher consciousness—God.

I remember a story, once a female and a male were husband and wife. They got into a conflict. It was almost going to be a tragedy and then he said, "Oh, my God. Let us stop it for a few minutes. Close our eyes, do the prayer and then think about what we are doing to each other. I don't think I can see you in this." In a few seconds the female totally changed. God is that Infinity toward which your woman can relate faster than the finite, because she questions the finite and she never questions the Infinite. Her capacity toward Infinity is much faster. Where there's no time and space, woman can relate so much faster than you can even imagine. Where there's time and space, she's very curious, she's very reserved, she's very questioning, and she's very intelligent; she wants to know what is going on.

Remember, if you cannot live with one woman, you have to live with another woman. If you cannot live with another, you have to live with a third. If you cannot live with a third, you cannot live with a fourth. After all, if you cannot live with one woman, or with a second, or with a third or a fourth, you cannot live with any woman. It takes the same amount of energy to live with a woman as it takes to not live with a woman. Those who have run away from woman have written books why. Those who have loved the woman have written books as to why. Both have nothing. They end up with books. The creativity of God is the subject. Don't inflate her ego and don't lean on a woman; don't inflate her ego and let her lean on you. Walk. Try to walk with woman hand in hand, on the positive road of consciousness called dharma.

If you play games with a woman, she'll play ten games with you. Every woman knows how to add zero. Remember

---

[1] We regret that the drawings from this early Man to Man course are not available.

that. The most dumb woman, she knows how to add zero. And the moment she adds zero to you? Multiply by zero and it becomes zero. If you want a tragedy in your life, then you will try to take that risk. But if a woman wants to go to the higher path, to the path of consciousness, to the religious path, to *seva* (service), to *simran* (repetition of the name of God), to good things, encourage it. It is your insurance. It is your insurance for the relationship. Because she must look toward time and space, you must make her look to higher consciousness. It is equally important for you to turn her to the higher consciousness because if she can be turned to higher consciousness, that is your safety. That is your security. And that is her intelligence. Remember, a woman who looks toward God shall carry you toward God. A woman who looks toward Earth, shall dig your grave and dump you in it. Therefore, do not stimulate a woman toward the earthly trip. If you always talk to woman on the earthly trip and relate to her on the earthly trip, you will always be the accountant of her loss and gain and all that. These are your jobs: do it with privacy.

If in the essence of your insecurity, you share it with a woman, she becomes doubly insecure because she needs security from you. You are gone. Whether it is financial, social, moral, or mental, you share with woman your strength. Social, mental, moral, personal, impersonal, economic—your strength. Because remember, God made the woman a woman and you cannot make a man out of her. You are a creature of the creation of God. You will fail and in that failure, there shall be a lot of trouble you will go through. So please remember, in the creativity of consciousness, it is always right to relate to that area of the woman that is called expansion. Expansion toward Infinity will always give her creativity, satisfaction, peace and joy, and she will flow toward you as a stimulant cosmic energy and it will bring you tremendous happiness. There's a popular Christian saying, "When the church bells used to ring, families used to laugh. Since the church bells have stopped ringing, families have started crying." Why? It was a stimulant toward Infinity. Anything which is religious, anything which is Infinite, anything which determines her growth toward Infinity, is a positive direction and you should give it to her. Because once she starts looking down, she will bring you down. Also, when there are children and you are married parents, remember: children are the trust of God. Manage that trust as trustees. I will say very safely to you, in the marriage relationship, the relationship of male and female, it, too, is just a relationship in trust. If it is manifested as trustees, in the laws and bylaws of that trust, I don't think there can be any trouble. Trouble is only stopped and started by conflict, conflict between the areas of life that are in conflict with the ego. To create a conflict of interest with a woman is to create a difficulty in your own life.

Remember that woman is a stimulant and she needs internal stimulant. Internal stimulant is what I'm telling you is her Infinity. She needs mental stimulant. Mental stimulant is her direction toward Infinity. She also needs physical stimulant; that is, in her sexual and sensual life, she needs to be totally brought into tides and tides and tides; in that way you'll find in physical intercourse or in her tiding nature she will start saying, "Oh God!" Make sure her auric body and astral body are not left out. For you, when the physical trip is over, you want to turn around and run to something, to do something. This is wrong. There needs to be companionship, more positive nature, more talking, more interrelated relationship than before. That is why they say, "When you start a physical relationship somewhere, it should start weeks before and it must end up weeks after." In other words, the relationship between you and her is constant, back and forth. And this constant relationship guarantees dialogue. It guarantees trust, harmony, homogeneity.

So please remember, in the creativity of consciousness, it is always right to relate to that area of the woman that is called expansion. Expansion toward Infinity will always give her creativity, satisfaction, peace and joy, and she will flow toward you as a stimulant cosmic energy and it will bring you tremendous happiness.

Remember that woman is a gentle creature. Handling a woman harshly is inviting unavoidable trouble. I have yet to see any woman who has been harshly betrayed, harshly treated, harshly related to, who could ever forget that, because she conceives things. She has the capacity to conceive things. So she can conceive from you not only your spermatozoa, your seed, but also she can conceive from you the harshness, the brutality. She can conceive from you the negativity. She can conceive from you—and she will get to you. She will conceive it, sprout it, transform it into children, and she will give it back to you. Remember that. But, once she knows in her heart that you are a gentleman—and thoroughly a gentleman—there are no problems. One thing that a woman likes most is that you are a man of your word. Best of all, when she knows that you have somebody higher up, it may be a God, it may be an angel, a guiding angel, it may be a teacher, it may be a spiritual path, or it may be some spiritual tenets; but once she knows you have somebody higher than you, she feels secure and safe. These are the virtues which man has to relate to in order to have a virtuous relationship with a woman in grace.

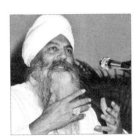

Man to **Man** 3
Incentive and Invocation of Polarities

Circa 1979

Each male and female relationship is not physical at all. The physical relationship is the culmination of the relationship. It is initiated by invocation through the auric body.

- Incentive and Invocation of **Polarities**
- Invoke **Don't Provoke**
- Magnetic **Preference**
- If You Can Fake It, **You Can Make It**

Incentive and Invocation of **Polarities**

Relationship is meant to complement and supplement each other. It's a total service trip. I serve you, you serve me. You serve me, I serve you.

The idea of this course is to renew in ourselves the knowledge that is lost. In the whirlwind of our passion, we have forgotten many things. The name of this course is "Incentive and Invocation of Polarities." It is a very simple thing to understand, but I know you know nothing about it and so that is where we shall start.

There are some special figures which represent male and female as they exist in the cosmic rhythm:

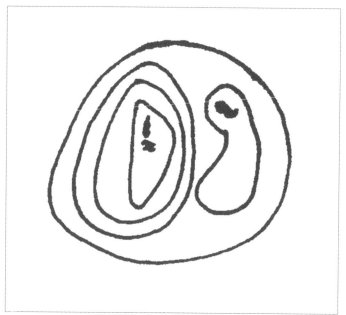

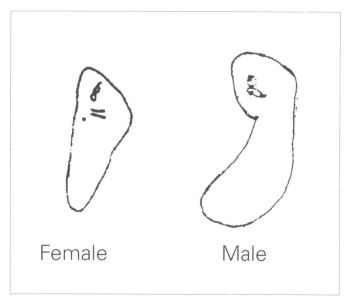

Female   Male

This male and this female are just like two parts that have been taken apart. Each male and female relationship is not physical at all. I emphasize, not physical at all. The physical relationship is the culmination of the relationship. It is initiated by invocation through the auric body. The auric body transforms the energy into a pattern of extension that feeds the pranic body and vice versa. You must understand the relationship: the sensitivity extends from you into the auric body, the auric body goes into the pranic body, then the pranic body goes into the cosmic body; and in the cosmic body, it envelops this subject, called the polarity, which is woman. Any relationship which does not develop from that extension will end up in argument, in frustration, and in pain.

"I got it, I grab it, I had it." This is the worst. It has no meaning in the conscious world. That's why your lives are not satisfied. That's why you feel weak after the physical, or sexual and sensual, intercourse. You don't feel together.

It doesn't give you anything and it takes everything away from you. From one system of the body to another system of the body to the cosmic body; then relay the energy through the cosmic body to the cosmic body and to the physical body through the pranic body, in that way, a situation ripens up. With the weather, it is called spring. From the cold of the winter to the spring; that's spring. Old scriptures are written just that way. We can make an analogy to the spring, the warmth returns, life begins anew: eye contact, word contact, skin contact. Feelings, signs, symptoms: this is called signaling. Out of that signaling, you invoke and provoke a direct contact, or an effort to directly contact. That is called summer. In the heat of the summer, an impulsion happens. You know that. You are all experts in that. Now, if there is imbalance in that impulsion, you can over-ejaculate or you can under-ejaculate. Still, you are not complete; and then comes fall and then winter. These four seasons are an exact transformation of sexuality and sensuality, which is called "*bhog*." There are two words in the scriptures: "*yog*" and "*bhog*".[1]

Don't misunderstand and think that *bhog* is just *bhog*. *Bhog* is also a science. You have to understand that mentality of the mind which triggers this situation in order to get that "correspondence frequency" so that both frequencies of the polarities can be at the same time. It's electrifying, it's regenerating, it's glorious, it's beautiful. But if it's not

---

[1] Yog is union; bhog is sensuality, the sensual world.

handled with a corresponding frequency, it is painful, it is frustrating, and it does not give you relationship. There is no such thing as relationship. If you do not relay at the same frequency and signal the ships correctly, what you get is not relationship because you are not relating. Relationship must be in conjunction with the circumstances as they develop, weather-wise. What is wrong with us? We get up from the cold of the winter, pop out like a volcano, and then we go back into the winter again. I came, I got, I frustrated myself, and it is over with. That is not what woman is for; and it's not what man is for either.

After 10 years together with you, I see that even now you are immature in your relationship to marriage. Totally immature. You are immature in selecting, you are immature in talking, you are immature in valuing the values. There's so much immaturity. Why? Because you marry—or relate to anybody—out of ego. No, no, no! No relationship is meant to be ego. Relationship is meant to complement and supplement each other. It's a total service trip. I serve you, you serve me. You serve me, I serve you. It's a total relationship. The relativity of this relationship is the coordinating of it.

People, do not misunderstand what a great mental security this is—all of this. You stand out, you wear your *bana* (sacred dress of the Sikhs), you read your *banis* (sacred prayers of the Sikhs). Do you know where it comes from? Now, systematically I say, "It comes from God and Guru." Wrong. That's not true, but I should say that to save myself. I *should* say that; but actually your mental security comes from the cohesiveness of the relay, of the message, of each other. This is a concept which is much deeper than the total divinity surrounding us and it is called Khalsa[2]. "I am, I am": I am for you, you are for me. Do you understand that? You can pick up a phone and call. In a moment, somebody will say, "Sat Nam." You feel good. Ahh haaa! Correct number! You may even have dialed the wrong ashram; instead of Atlanta, Georgia, Washington may be on the line, but the moment you hear "Sat Nam," you say, "Oh, I made it." There's an equilibrium of communicative essence: "Oh, we have ashrams all around the world. We are everywhere. We are on this planet." We are, we are; I am, I am; It is, it is; They are, they are. This all relates to the same communication, the same message. There's an invocation, an incentive of spirit, in the law of polarity—you have a reservoir.

Each male does not need a woman. You can masturbate; I don't mind that. It is the oldest sexual expression known on the planet. Masturbation. When it was realized that there was no way to force men to hold back the semen and to let the body be physically right, it became spiritual to circumcise them so that they might not be in a position to masturbate. So came that trauma of circumcising the child to avoid the disease of masturbation. In woman, there is no masturbation. It is a tide to which she loses nothing. But with you, there is nothing which remains of you.

By nature, by nature man is impotent. Your male organ is not hard all the time. Do you understand that? What makes the blood rush there? It is the glandular system. What triggers the glandular system? The thought. What is thought? It is a sensory communication projection. So where lies the incentive? Where lies the incentive? In your polarity. Incentive doesn't lie in you. If you understand that—that the incentive does not lie in you—then you must understand honestly and truthfully from where the incentive comes and that incentive should be as pure as purity can be. Do you follow? Do you understand? Any incentive projected to you from a woman who is not pure in thoughts, not very religiously inclined, let us put it this way, it is a drag to have intercourse with such a woman. It will take such a heavy toll. It will take away from your youth.

I remember this experience clearly. Once, before I was to go to my athletic meet, we were doing a prayer, and in the congregation there was one woman who was sexually, sensually, very negative and low. It was a prayer before the Guru. I went onto the athletic field and I got that serious accident that I have told you of, when my side tendon was pulled. To this day I suffer from it. But I knew at that time, even in the sensitivity of the prayer, that she had got to me. My God, what if I had done something? What hell it could have been! Do you understand what I am talking to you about? You get into any bed, you get into any body, you don't care. You don't feel you are somebody. You do not understand the source. Know this: if you eat bad food, you will get sick. In exactly the same way, if the provocative incentive of the polarity is from a woman who's not very clean, psychically "clean," it's going to mess you up. I don't mean that you should be with a religious woman or a non-religious woman (although I do not see any way that a divine woman can exist who's not a very religious woman). It is basically in your interest, totally, that the thought form—I'm not talking of the physical form only, I am talking of the

---

[2] Khalsa means Pure Ones. Historically, it was the name given to the followers of Guru Gobind Singh, the 10th Sikh Guru.

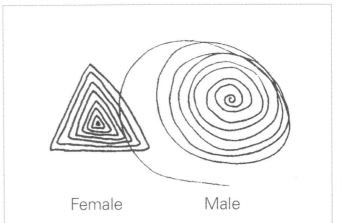

Female   Male

thought form—that the thought form be concentrated like this figure:

This triangle is the female. That is how the thought form works in her. The lines are on the surface, but inside it is the reverse. When a woman is not stable like this, and when she wants to project, this is what happens.
Do you see this? The cosmic eye, or that eye which can

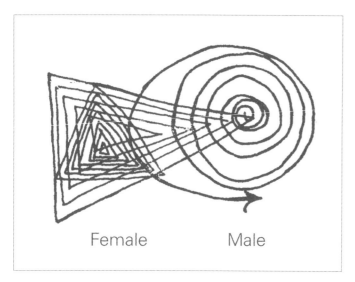

Female   Male

see auras, can see this happen. The apex turns this way and this spiral goes in communication this way and there is an inter-mix. Until this inter-mix happens, communication cannot be established. You understand the rhythm?

Q: *What is the circle?*

Yogi Bhajan: Male. The male has no direction. It has no projection, but it says it has projection. That is the polarity. "I want to grab her." Forget it. This guy is in circles: Should I, should I not? May I, may I not? Where, where will I take her? What will happen? What is going to happen? There is no male who can think straight. You are not born [with the capacity]. Your western hemisphere of the brain is not capable of it. That is why you are very insensitive. Woman is very sensitive because she has to be pregnant, she has to have a child, she has to protect herself, she has to grow; and under all those circumstances, she has to be one-pointed, right on the spot, without loss of time, without space, without anything, she has to decide the whole thing. Her computer works 16 times faster than that of the male. In simple language, woman can make up her mind in one minute when it takes a man 16 minutes.

So what does she do? She is like this [figure]. She turns on her side and starts projecting. She eats [you] up. What is it called? An eclipse. When a woman wants you, she'll eclipse you. When you want her, you'll start talking to her. Where is the fight? There is no fight. I have seen men talking passionately and then snoring after only a few minutes and she says, "Ji? What is wrong with you?" Because when you start talking, you are gone—remember that. When a woman talks, she is going to get you; when you talk, you are going to get yourself. The safer course is to talk to her in a signal language. Don't talk to her in words; talk to her in gestures: "Hello" with your hands. That is a much better indication of what you want than going through the rigmarole of words.

Your projection is in a spiral, an endless circle. Now, what provokes what? Provocation comes when she is aimed and you do not open. When she's aimed and you do not open, God that trauma is horrible. When she aims and you do not open, forget it. Then you can give her a 20-karat diamond, a $300,000 car, and a bolt of silk from here to China—anything—and it's useless.

Do you know what woman feels the man is, when she projects? Exactly as you feel when there is a dish of spaghetti before you and there is a fork and a spoon. She wants to take that fork and roll it around and put it in her mouth. You understand the feeling? Exactly as at lunchtime you want spaghetti—the way I have explained it to you—that is exactly how woman feels about you. She may be a four foot woman or an eight foot woman or a no foot woman, but that is exactly what every woman feels—that you are a dish of spaghetti with sauce on it. The only difference is in your smell. Whether there is tomato sauce on you, or there is garlic and oil on you, or whatever you want to call it. You may be that green spaghetti or that white spaghetti, the woman's objective is that which puts that big spoon, places that fork and rolls you around and puts you in her mouth. That is exactly what happens. If you cannot relate to that, you may be a Ph.D., you may be a doctor, you may be a journalist, you may be a successful attorney, you may be in Sikh dharma, you may be this, you may be an anything, [but if you don't open when she projects,] the relationship is not going to come together. Nothing, nothing [can change it]. It is a divine law, you can't change it. It is a cosmic law. That's what I wanted to make you understand.

Also, if you miss four chances out of ten, you are in her bad books. Every time a woman who has fought with her husband has talked to me, it has been because she needed sympathy that was not given to her. When she was negative you couldn't say, "All right, let us think. It is really a bad situation, let us both think." That's all it takes from you. You need not do her any favors. When she says, "I am horrible," you say, "I am miserable, too, let us think." But if you say, "Yeah, it is a habit. You are always horrible, miserable. That's nonsense, be a Khalsa woman." She'll say, "Go to hell."

That is why, folks, no religion works between woman and man. You know, I have seen some very foolish people. I talk to them and they quote scriptures back to me. Can you believe that? Now, in this age of mind, in this consciousness of mind, they quote the scriptures to me. At times like that I always like that saying, "The devil quotes scriptures." One thing to remember when you talk to your woman: talk to her in your words. Don't quote Shakespeare. It's the biggest blunder on this planet to quote Guru Nanak, to quote Shakespeare, quote this, quote that. You must quote yourself to her at that moment, because when there is a triangular projection then the spin of the cycle—it is called "spin of the cycle"—and the frequency have to be at zero. I am talking to you of these relationships in exactly the level and sequence of scientific, cosmic vibratory effect. Your life, the maleship, comes from the female. Her joy, being a female, comes from the male. The relationship is connected by a projected frequency. Among the trees, too, the breeze comes and it releases pollen. You all know that? You know that? Then why did you come to this course? You should have saved your money. I never knew that you knew about trees. You are no more than a tree. You are all walking trees. And you should release the pollen at the right time.

Do you know, in the United States of America, there are 220,000,000 people? Two hundred twenty million people—and they do not know what we are talking about today. They all want to know. I'm sharing this ancient knowledge with you so that you can go out and share. Until we can understand this scientific relationship, we'll be totally in a space that does not allow for any congeniality within us, or between us. When there is no congeniality in us, there's no reality in us. When there's no reality in us, there's no security in us. When there's no security in us, there's no satisfaction in us. When there's no satisfaction in us, we are frustrated and bored and that is what makes us low-key men. That's why we are not successful. Woman doesn't mean anything in our life except that she is power, an energy, a reservoir, a success, a push, whatever you wish to call it, a thrust upward. Sometimes you meet this challenge in a very weird manner. I'll explain to you through figures.

These figures are very important and you should keep your relationship to them. Listen, somebody taught me and I learned it. Now I am going to be 50 years old, and I still remember it and I can reproduce it. That's the way you should learn it: preserve it and pass it on to your friends and to your generations to come, so that humanity can enjoy itself.

If you want to fight, fight with your destiny. If you want to fight, fight with your Infinity. If you want to fight, fight with anything. Never fight with a woman. Never.

This is how the cosmic eye looks at people who are horny. Do you understand that? Follow it? This is female and this is male. And then what do they do? They start a dance. Their base becomes curved like this and on this they move like a pendulum.

When both are charged with projectiles in the sexual or sensual energy, they both start moving, swinging. This is where the word "swinger" comes from.

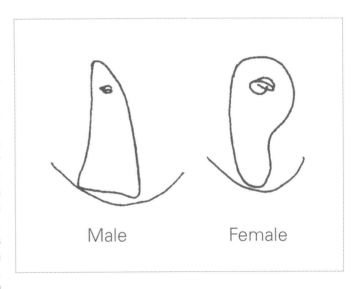

Things do not appear out of the heavens. There's a word for it. They both start swinging on the base and they begin to make very funny statements: "Ji, what are you going to do today?" "Oh, well, I am going to go to work." Foolish. But what do you want me to do? That is called swinging. So, in this swinging, if you start swinging harmoniously, things are okay. But when you start swinging in opposite directions, there's a 'dang, dang, dang'. I need not explain it to you. I think all of you must have experienced that. You follow? She's very inflated upward and very squeezed downward; and he's very big downward and very sharp and thin upward, so his brain doesn't work. When a woman's brain starts working, the moment she projects to the man his brain ceases to work. Do you know that? It is automatic. When she's high there, he's high here—and vice versa.

I tell you honestly and truthfully, there's no fun in fighting with a woman. Absolutely not, there's nothing to it. If you want to fight, fight with your destiny. If you want to fight, fight with your Infinity. If you want to fight, fight with anything. Never fight with a woman. Never. Because in that fight, you are fighting your own projective power and the polarity will blow your fuse. It is ridiculous.

Do you understand this 'law of swing'? Do you understand the law of swing? This projectile power is very skinny and this is very big and round. You have to understand that. You think you are a physical individual. I want to make a very serious point to you and you should be very careful about it. Suppose somebody is in Tucson and somebody else is in Vancouver, B.C., what is the distance between those two places? Fifteen hundred miles? In this swinging relationship it means absolutely nothing.

Let me give you another example. Somebody's in London and somebody's in Tokyo, when both swing, the cosmic arc will meet exactly the way it does when they are three feet apart. Why? Because mind knows no space and no time. So thinking, "My sweetheart is in Tokyo, so I can fool around," is dangerous. If she's picking up on your thought, you know what she will say? She'll say, "I am not feeling right today." This is because her projection and your ejection will be totally neutralized. You will be charged with a cosmic perjury. It happens in the subconscious mind—believe me or not. Believe me or not, this is at the root of every bad relationship. What is that? Cosmic perjury. Then she comes and she looks in your eyes and she says, "How was your Tokyo?" "Oh, it was all right." Your eyes come down and she says, "What? Darling, you didn't phone me. Were you getting a massage?" You know what I mean? She will continue making inquiries and the more inquiries she will make, the more the eyes will start coming down until you get into *samadhi*: "I see no more; I hear no more; I talk no more."

She will tolerate it, but there is a problem with woman. Any thought that goes into her subconscious is like a spermatozoa. If that "thought spermatozoa" meets the egg, the ego, it builds itself into a "baby," which, in plain words, we call divorce. Do you understand? Woman is a very problematic creature. Any little thing inserted in her can come out to be 6'2", 52" chest, 250 pounds. It may take 18 years, 20 years, 25 years. That's why marriages break after 7 years and 21 years. Seven years is the cycle of consciousness; 11 years is the cycle of intelligence; 18 years is the cycle of life. Sometimes consciousness develops in contrast with the existing environments so that every 7 years, the marriage is put to the test. In Kundalini Yoga, the fourth year is always dangerous; in marriage, the seventh year is always dangerous. It's called the seven-year-itch.

In Kundalini Yoga, your awareness goes into the management of 4, two cycles are 8. In this way, you are one step ahead of consciousness, because the consciousness cycle is 7. Practitioners of Kundalini Yoga turn to a cycle of 8. That is, every 4 years you have to confront yourself and your own ego and go through it. That is with a margin of 6 months. So every 3 ½ years those 6 months are miserable in the life of a person because he has to shed his skin, the body of the old subconscious, and adapt to the new. In marriage, it is every 7 years. Between the seventh and the eighth years, every marriage is on the hot plate. Every marriage becomes the phenomenon for which Guru Arjun[3] must be remembered. Sit on the hot plate, be burned from below, endure hot sand being poured over you, and still say, "Sat Nam." There's no example in the world of religious scriptures or human acts or deeds where man can go and penetrate through this life between the seventh and eighth years, this confrontation of the mental-cosmic polarity, without a mountainous patience. In this human life, there was only one, Guru Arjun.

That is why the scripture says, "*Guru Arjun Partakh Har.*" *Partakh Har* means God in person. "*Guru Arjun Partakh Har*" means Guru Arjun is God in person. It was a feeling, it was an expression of that feeling. That much patience a male is required to practice. It shall come in your life, in a cycle, every 7 years. Three and a half is Kundalini Yoga—four and four is eight. In this way we extend our awareness by one year.

Question and **Answer**

Q: Is that from the time you begin practicing Kundalini Yoga?

Yogi Bhajan: When you are around any white-clad person, when your aura crosses their aura. Count the time from that.

Q: I don't understand the mechanics of that seven-year-itch.

Yogi Bhajan: Because consciousness, conscious acts, subconscious acts, inner conscious, outer conscious, all that at that time is totally computerized, totally integrated, and brought to completion: it's called a record. So, before it is shoved into a record room, if there are any outstanding points, "spikes" we call them, "conscious spikes," they start hurting.

Sometimes you feel, "Oh, I am miserable. I am not miserable." You are neither miserable, nor not miserable. Life is laid down that way. Because you are ignorant, you do not know. You do not see and feel it with a cosmic eye. Therefore, you make it physical, and in the physical, there's a nervous reaction and then there's depression and pain.

---

[3] The Fifth Sikh Guru, martyred by being burned alive on a hot plate over three days.

There's no need for any pain. If a woman is acting berserk, it is normal. You understand? What is berserk? She is swinging and hitting you and you are not rhythmically swinging with it. What happens? The swings begin to "ding–dang." You say, "Hey, where am I?" and you don't know! When you say, "Stop it," she says, "What am I saying? I am not saying anything wrong. Is it wrong?" You say, "Stop it! Shut up! La–la–la." The neighbors come out, "What is going on?" But there sits your soul; let me explain that to you.

Now, this, between the two, is the turning point. She moves, you move, and you know, when opposite forces meet—what happens? The theory of bang. Whenever the horizontal forces move the vertical forces, or vertical forces move the horizontal forces, it creates creativity. It means bang. Now, what is the safest course to take? When the wall is there, instead of ramming into it and getting into a mess, start spinning above it; start reading *Japji*. You know what I mean? The fire is on.

I once asked someone, I said, "Your family life in the West is very wonderful." He said, "Yes. When I feel my wife is going astray, I immediately bring the Bible and ask her, 'Oh Darling, I want to tell you, I read that psalm. You know, I couldn't understand it. Could you explain it to me?'" You understand? She's a very church-going girl, you know, and her ego cannot pocket it that her husband is learning psalms from her and she can't answer him. So she gets into those psalms. Once she said, "I have taught you this psalm about 20 times. Why do you choose this one all the time?" He said, "I forget it when you are in the red area. This is the only psalm that gives me the cooler feeling." You must understand, the life in you can bring impotency if the harmony of the projectiles of the male and female in relationship are not coordinated right; because then you cannot have the correct and powerful impulsion. You cannot feel right. Your work will not be right; your surroundings will not be right; and your other relationships will not be right if the projection relationship between you and your female is not correct.

The majority of the men who suffer from blood pressure issues have these problems not because they are over-worked but because they are over-extending themselves and they are not relaxed. This stress comes when the relationship of communication between male and female is not right. When your male and female relationship is not right, there's one thing you can do very fast: cut down on food. That's definite. Whenever your relationship with the female is not right, for your life, health, longevity, and perfect maintenance of yourself, cut down on food, number one. Number two, cut down on heavy foods totally. They should be out of your menu. Number three, totally cut down on any or every stimulant drink. Lastly, develop a habit to take a nap after meals; otherwise you will have a bleeding stomach, a bleeding intestinal tract, and heart attacks. All these are the outcome of that. Whenever you take a light meal, no matter how light it may be, try to take a 5 to 7 minute nap. Close your eyes, still your body and lie dead.

Q: *What are stimulant drinks?*
Yogi Bhajan: Stimulant drinks are many: heavy sugar drinks are very stimulant. Syrupy drinks are very stimulant. Coca-cola, coffee, and I know you don't drink whiskey and all those kinds of drinks, but they are all stimulant drinks.

Q: *Do we take a nap after every meal, including dinner?*
Yogi Bhajan: Yes, taking a nap is a law. It is a law just for balancing the energy.

Q: *When you say the male/female relationship is not right, exactly in what way…?*
Yogi Bhajan: In the energy field and you'll know it. Everybody can know it. It's not a big deal, because the red light goes on—daa, daa, daa, daa, daa, daa—all the time.

Q: *What do you mean by heavy foods?*
Yogi Bhajan: Heavy foods—I'll include double cheese, double mushroom, double onion, double pizza. I call a heavy food any food that does not digest by its own gravity.

Q: *Does this relationship come only after having sex with a woman, or…*
Yogi Bhajan: No, no, no. We are not talking about sex. I am going to discuss sex later in the course. I am just making you horny about it. That is why we just make it a male course so there is no female and we can talk openly and explicitly about ourselves. Because it is also the will of God, God made us men. And at least we should have a time when we can talk like men, be like men, feel like men and discuss like men. That does much more than what you will learn.

Q: *How long can this fighting go on before…?*
Yogi Bhajan: You know better than that. We have been beaten up. It goes sometimes for a full week, remember? She's tight and she says, "Eeeeeeeeee, I'm going to eat him up." Remember? It can go on for a week.

Q: *In a discussion with my wife, I'm not sure whether I'm initiating her negativity or whether I'm responding to it, or vice versa. How can I tell?*
Yogi Bhajan: Actually, I'd like to talk to you about this later in the course, but as you have asked the question now. You are not correspondingly corresponding to what she is saying; actually you correspondingly correspond to what she feels. You deal with what she feels and you are not saying anything, nor is she saying anything. Both are dishonest.

So what happens? When both are dishonest, each one wants to win and each one wants to gain victory with the ego. When the ego is projected, then the dictionary takes over, words are found, and both become hysterical. It is hysteria that starts the fight and it is blood that stops it. When someone starts bleeding, you stop the fight.

Actually, the fact is, there's no such thing as a fight. Honest people will never fight. You know a lot of my students turn negative, terribly negative, and they feel perhaps I'll respond. I don't respond. Why should I respond to insanity? The guy has gone insane. Why should I respond? And whenever they meet me, after two or three months, I say, "Hello, how do you feel now?" They can't understand why I am talking to them. You understand? That is why when we see the aura and we see the red is more stretched in the aura than the green, we start talking about peaches, bananas, and those kinds of fruits. There's nothing else to talk of at that time—pears, plums, that kind of talk; because there's nothing [else to speak of]. You can't handle it. There's no communication possible. There's no frequency possible. From the moment that ego comes in, your communication is over; the game is over. Then it's no game of love; it's a game; it's a fight. Mostly, intercourse is the outcome of that fight. Do you understand? Any question over this now?

The main thing in your relationship can be very well decided by your food. There are foods like millet, wheat, wheat berries, wheat grain. There's food like steamed vegetables. There's food like raw vegetables. There's food like meat, pork, beef, and those kinds of foods. There are many different foods. But that food which sustains you will always give you more joy of life. Any food which pushes you is going to kill you. You don't grow old by years, you grow old by food. Your sexual behavior, your communicative behavior, your personality behavior, all is very important, understandably very important. But the base of all that is not how much you know, the base of all that is how much you eat and what you eat, because food stimulates the glandular system and the glands are controlled by the pituitary, the master gland. Your sex is also controlled by the pituitary. Pituitary has a relationship that comes from the circulatory and respiratory system. And it has a relationship of its own. Do you understand that? When you eat any kind of food, your glandular system has to secrete to digest it. You understand? And all secretions of the glands are controlled by the pituitary secretion, the master gland.

You know that in old age people go senile? What is that senility? You think you won't go senile? I have seen people 27 years old go senile. It's a simple psychology: when one gets older, one feels like one has to eat more. It's a simple law. If he can digest; it's the best—if he can digest. That is a part of your life these days that has to be governed, like taking bran, because you eat very refined foods. Bran is missing, leafy food is missing, and p-fruits are missing. You know the p-fruits? Plums, papayas, pears, what else? There's a big one. Pineapple. How many of you normally care to eat pineapple?

All right. How many of you actually eat it as a religious duty? What can I do? All p-fruits, when they are in season, should be eaten in abundance.

Q: *What about pineapple juice?*

Yogi Bhajan: No, no, no. Juice does not substitute for the fruit. Juice is a luxury.

Q: *Pineapples are in season all the time in Hawaii.*

Yogi Bhajan: No, they come in season once in a while; they are stored and shipped from Hawaii.

Q: *Bananas...*

Yogi Bhajan: Bananas are the same way. But the season is always there to a fruit. You remember, we used to go on a banana fast? A fifteen day banana fast? How many bananas? Nine bananas? Right? It is the most excellent cleansing and potent fast ever known to mankind. Actually the scripture says it must be done once a year. Why don't people do it? Because it is a little heavy.

Q: *Is there any time of year that is best for it?*

Yogi Bhajan: No, no. The best time for good food and fasting is springtime. The best time is when new blood comes in—that is the best.

Q: *You said to start on the new moon and end on the full moon?*

Yogi Bhajan: Yes. That is all defined; it is all written. Also, there is another way when the spring comes. You can go on a total fruit diet.

Q: *When is that?*

Yogi Bhajan: Anytime in April or May. From the fifteenth of April to the fifteenth of May is the period when you can decide, "I am just going to eat fruit and nothing else." No juice though. Fruit is fruit.

Q: *Is that for that one month period, the whole month?*

Yogi Bhajan: One month: the fifteenth to the fifteenth.

Q: *Mixed fruit?*

Yogi Bhajan: No. Fruits are very definite. They cannot be mixed. You can take one fruit in the morning, take one in the afternoon, take another later, but you cannot mix fruits. Remember please, one fruit at a time; otherwise you'll mess up your whole system.

Q: *Diluted juice has been mentioned before...*

Yogi Bhajan: I didn't mention anything right now. I know what you want and I'm not going to agree to that. Juices are not in the fruit fast at all.

Q: Is that the same for the vegetables? Vegetable juices with vegetable fasts?

Yogi Bhajan: Use no juices. When you go on a vegetable diet, you go on a full vegetable diet; you don't go on a juice diet of the vegetable. Hey, don't forget one thing in the vegetable kingdom. It is half vegetable and half fruit. Do you know what that is? The tomato. The tomato is half fruit and half vegetable. You know what you should do about this? It is a very funny thing to do. I'll tell you, but it should be done for only one week. This tomato is very beautiful. Use big tomatoes that are not soft anywhere, nor too old. They should be young, fresh tomatoes. Take a tomato. Put it in hot water just like you would a lobster. Pull it out and then take the skin off. You understand that? It should only be in hot water long enough so that the skin comes off easily—not more, not less. When you have done that with 5 to 10 tomatoes, put them before you, okay? Got it? Then take mint leaves, mint leaves, powder them, and put a lot of those mint leaves around the tomatoes. Then add tamari to your taste, take a fork and knife, and eat it. Eat this dish three times a day for one week. You will come out as a good mushroom man who's new, white, clear and best for consciousness. It's the best food for the brain. It takes away all tiredness, fatigue, sexual, mental—the whole berserk thing goes away.

Q: Are the tomatoes we get in the winter in Florida any good?

Yogi Bhajan: They are all good. The tomato is one thing which is very guaranteed good stuff.

Q: They're picked green.

Yogi Bhajan: Yes, but they ripen on the way. I know, I know what they do. Simply avoid the skin of the tomato because that doesn't digest.

Q: We should do that once a year?

Yogi Bhajan: Anytime. It is a timeless thing. There is no time for it. But whenever you do it, remember, start Monday morning and end it on Sunday, midnight. But don't forget to take mint leaves, powdered mint leaves, with it. Lots of it.

Q: Should we ever go on a juice fast?

Yogi Bhajan: I will say yes, but only if you can take the risk. Juice is a good fast but it does not take care of the intestinal tract. Normally, it's not recommended.

Q: Even if it's fresh juice.

Yogi Bhajan: I don't care, fresh or old, you know what I mean? You have to clear your bowels and there's nothing in it to form a bowel. That can sometimes produce certain situations from which you cannot recuperate.

Q: What is the mint for?

Yogi Bhajan: Mint? I don't know, sir. It was written in a very, very ancient book. And it was written thrice, don't forget lots of mint leaves. When I did it, it saved my life. I was in terrible shape once. I was so intolerable of the environments and circumstances I was in, then I remembered it, and I did it. It really is very cleansing. He didn't explain why he put the mint with it and I couldn't ask him, because it was about 3,000 year-old stuff. I have always told you that I don't do things from my side; it is all that has been gathered together for ages, which I just explain to you.

Q: Is it fresh or dried powdered mint?

Yogi Bhajan: Mint? No, no, dried mint leaves.

Q: Sir, this stuff about the springtime, is this a general rule about the springtime?

Yogi Bhajan: Every country has its own springtime. Spring goes by longitude and latitude. Springtime is when new blood starts coming in. It's a good time. Any dietary precaution you have to take, you should take in springtime.

Q: Sir, on this one month fruit fast which could start in just a couple of days, right now there's oranges, grapefruits, and apples, are those…?

Yogi Bhajan: I never go to the market, I don't know. Whatever. I am not bothering with anything; it is your choice. But I tell you one thing, I tell you one thing, and I am making a statement: You cannot be a man in experience unless you cleanse yourself in spring. Write it down: You are not a man in experience if you do not cleanse yourself in the spring. It's as old as man is; it's as religious as man is, as real as man is.

■ ■ ■

Invoke, Don't Provoke

Anything in life, in creativity, and in polarity, you must invoke.

There's a very beautiful saying in Sanskrit, which I will translate: "Invoke, don't provoke." That's the English translation. Anything in life, in creativity, and in polarity, you must invoke. Things should happen in a sublime manner. When you provoke anything, it is totally dangerous for both sexes—male and female. However important it may be to you, you must not forget that the other person has an identity. Never try to capture one person totally; because if that other person is totally captured, there's nothing you can gain in thought form, in sublime form and in projective form. There's a saying: "One and one makes eleven, not two." So, in a simple, idealistic situation, allow, invoke or give incentive to the other's opinion. Make it possible, make it understandable to the other, the partner of your life, that her opinion is very darling dear to you, but never act on it. This is because when a woman gives an opinion, it is totally a woman's opinion; and because woman contains the man, she will contain your insecurity in it. Remember that. When a woman gives you an opinion, she will give you an opinion that you totally have to activate or you totally have to feel insecure. Do it—analyze her opinion anytime you like and you'll find this absolutely true.

First of all, no woman thinks man is grown up. She always thinks men are children, babies. Especially with our modern shaving and hairdo and all that, we look like babies. So in concept, women always think that every man who has asked for things is a child, never an adult. Don't worry about what their age is. And when she gives an opinion, she gives an opinion about those things that you either feel totally handicapped about, or really, really great about. But it will tie you in, so what you have to do is very, very beautifully ask for her opinion, listen to it, relish it, and take out that part that does not belong to you. Do not reject it straight away. Give the reason why you could not do it so that next time, she will give you an opinion again.

Secondly, in our potential sexuality, the tragedy of our life comes from the male. There are many, many males who, when they feel horny and sexual and the woman doesn't respond, get angry and find different ways to show her how idiotic they are. You may not believe me, but every woman knows it. She knows how idiotic you are. When things are normal, there are certain things you must do: let the woman invoke the incentive of sensual wavelength and let it mature. And, if you decide to sleep in two different beds, never go to the bed of the woman you love the most. Let her come to you. Any man who's sexually weak before his woman is a nuisance to himself. I repeat: any man who's sexually weak before his woman is a nuisance to himself. Don't forget either, that the sexual relationship, or what you call physical intercourse, is the practical end of an invoked incentive in relationship. It's a cycle. The shape of it, in the old scriptures, is like this:

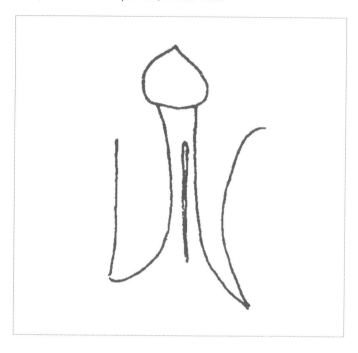

Do you understand this? This looks like a male organ topsy-turvy, right? But it is not. It is a female. And, at the end, this male part, like a bulb which is upside down, is essentially showing that you are not always alive in your testicles: there's a whole body attached to them. This male organ is activated by the pollen of the female and this pollen of the female is activated in the thought form. This physical action does not mean anything if the thought form does not make the pituitary secrete enough. If you are not mature in the thought form and in the glandular system of the body, you will become impotent after age 45, whether you like it or not. It can bring a lot of other diseases to you also. You follow? Absolutely no physical intercourse should be allowed to happen until the maturity of the glandular system is completed and the minimum time for that is 72 hours. I have told you before and I'm telling you right now. It starts in the living room. It starts in the park. Somewhere. It starts somewhere for some reason and it must mature and travel and walk into the bedroom, and remember, it should not be a wrestling bout: "Come on, get me, I got you, now finish."

There's one thing that you do which is a human tragedy, or a human error. After physical intercourse, normally men turn over and sleep or the woman turns over to sleep. Now, unfortunately, that is a mess. After physical intercourse, continue the game of love. It should be continued to the extent that one of you falls asleep. Either of you. Do you understand? Now, honestly, tell me, does anybody know about this? Have you ever done it? If not, you should not be married. [Failing to do this] is the greatest tension and the greatest fatigue to the nervous system. It makes your life five years shorter—five years! You're not rabbits that just go one, two, three, and out. When physical intercourse is over, it is better to massage each other, talk to each other, do something; but keep the physical entanglement going on until somebody starts snoring. Then that's the end of it. Yes?

Q: *Do you think it's harmful for the male to go twice?*
Yogi Bhajan: Normally, psychologically speaking, the male is meant to go once. But if he's a little rabbit-like, he can go twice. It is a bunny game. Once is more than . . . for a normal healthy person, once is more than enough. But, you know, for a sneak, twice, three times, six times; you can count your "but's". I don't care. Yes?

Q: *What happens to the males, before we got in 3HO, like if we should be dead?*
Yogi Bhajan: You are absolutely right, people are dead. In Hollywood, I can tell you. They look very beautiful, but they are dead. The bell doesn't ring. All these men who are perverted, there are thousands of them; and I'll tell you one thing, you are not all my students. I have got thousands of impotent students. They still call me; they still relate to me; they have love for me. Their bell doesn't ring.

Q: *Well, how can they get their bell to ring?*
Yogi Bhajan: First of all they have to do Kundalini Yoga, and any other type of yoga, to bring back their muscular system, and their nervous system, and their circulatory system. Get the whole thing under control. It may take two to three years, and thereafter, they have to learn man to man, within the man, and all this. It's a long study. Most of our people, who have damaged themselves in the past, are all right. Some of us have stopped doing yoga, something which cured us, something which put us on the world map was Kundalini Yoga. Kundalini Yoga is a total corrective system for the entire human being. What happened to you is that you forgot about it. Now you feel you are a Mukhia Singh Sahib[1], you are a Singh Sahib, you are a this Sahib, that Sahib: "*Dhan Dhan Ram Daas Gur, Jin Siree-aa Tinai Savaree-aa.*"[2] That's perfect. But what about the physical, over-done damage you have done to yourself? That recuperation is very essential and that's why a kriya in morning sadhana is for physical purposes, for mental purposes and for spiritual purposes. We have divided it into three.

Q: *In your drawing, does it represent the physical?*
Yogi Bhajan: I think so. This is a very, very ancient drawing. They made it however best they could do. I think they were not very artistic. To me it is a very gross, straightforward scene. You know what I mean? This is the female part, and this—out—is the male part. This apple-like male I have never seen anywhere, but maybe that guy might have had it that way so he drew it that way. I remember it exactly from the woodcarving. It was exactly like this. Yes?

Q: *I thought you had said, many years ago, that after intercourse, the man should, before retiring, urinate once and also wash himself.*
Yogi Bhajan: That is hygiene. But that is when he finishes.

Q: *But how do you do that if you fall asleep?*
Yogi Bhajan: Well, those things are understood. I don't think there's a serious danger in falling asleep. Germs are not going to fly in, in a few minutes. It is all okay. Yes?

Q: *The ancient teachings that you referred to earlier, what technical source did they come from?*
Yogi Bhajan: I'll send you to Tibet; we'll get it free from China. There was a student who came to our teacher. He was a Lama and he had a lot of information with him. If I had known that we would lose Tibet, we would have gotten everything kept there and sent him to God. But we didn't do that, and everything is fixed in the memory; but it was a good memory, a photogenic memory. I never thought that I would ever need his books or any help. But anyway, we'll try to reproduce whatever we have.

Q: *When I feel horny and I don't want to feel horny, what's the best thing to do?*
Yogi Bhajan: You feel horny?

Q: *And I don't want to feel horny...*
Yogi Bhajan: Oh, yes, the meditation is very simple. To control anything on your mind, never pressurize the mind. Just do Sa-Ta-Na-Ma meditation,[3] it will all be neutralized. To feel horny is not a sin. It's okay. I wanted to feel more and more but nothing happened. I mean, you are tired sometimes, you don't have time, you don't feel good, you know what I mean? But when you, through incentive, feel horny toward a woman and you know how to invoke the meditative mind, you can become totally creative. Horniness on the physical level is intercourse, but on a higher level it is creativity also. Artists feel horny many, many times. Many, many times they feel very stiff in their male organs and then the stiffness is gone and they can't sit still. They go out and paint a painting. In a couple of hours something comes out. They paint; their forefathers can't

---
[1] Honorary titles in the Sikh tradition, usually connoting some level of authority or leadership role in the community.
[2] Blessed, blessed is Guru Ram Das; He who created You, exalts You.

[3] See Kirtan Kriya in Appendix A.

paint like that. So, it is the same, you must understand, it is the same energy. Use it this way, use it that way, use it up, use it down. It doesn't matter. Yes?

Q: *Is it the same way if you wake up in the middle of the night, maybe?*

Yogi Bhajan: If you are waking up in the middle of the night, there are three things wrong with you. One, your prostate gland is not functioning right; two, you drank too much water and you didn't urinate before going to bed; three, in the daytime you were thinking wrong. (Laughter)

Q: *How about wet dreams?*

Yogi Bhajan: Wet dreams are very wet. Wet dreams are the product of subconscious horniness. It is a weakness of hallucination rather than being practical. A lot of yoga exercises have been given.[4] There's a set of 18 exercises to take care of your spine, which helps control wet dreams. Shoulder stand is also included in that and all these things. It is all perfectly given already.

Do it, then you won't get wet dreams. I do not know if you understand or not, but if your semen is not, if your ejaculation is not like yogurt, you are a useless man anyway. If it is just like milky-water, like lassi, you are so-so. If it is just crystal clear, you should take care of yourself; you are in bad shape. Do you understand? If the ejaculation is brown and yogurt like, it means you are absolutely healthy. If it is whitish, like a yogurt lassi, it means so-so. But if it is more clear than that, forget everything and take care of yourself. That is how it is. Yes?

Q: *I've heard you talk about* ojas *being the gray matter of the brain. I still don't understand everything you have been saying.*

Yogi Bhajan: The *ojas* actually is that liquid in which the brain lives. The gray matter is that which you call the brain, isn't it? Say, doctor, what do they call the brain? Gray matter?

Student: *Gray matter and white matter. Gray matter is on the outside.*

Yogi Bhajan: Outside that, in which it remains, is what is called the gray matter. The top of the brain, isn't it?

Student: *Yes.*

Yogi Bhajan: And the serum around it is called spinal serum in English. In the older scriptures it is called *ojas*; and when you ejaculate, it is also called *ojas*. You follow what I mean? Sometime doctor, get the components analyzed. Find out what is in the serum and what is in the ejaculation, what is common and what is not, because in the older scriptures, both things are called *ojas*.

[4] Referring to the kriya, Flexibility & the Spine, available in The Aquarian Teacher Yoga Manual

Q: *What's the double ejaculation you were talking about? You said you can have two ejaculations: one in the mind and one in the sex organs.*

Yogi Bhajan: Have you seen sometimes somebody has a dream that he has intercourse with so and so and he has done a great thing? But he was dreaming. He has had a wet dream. He gets up and it is not real. Do you know that experience? All right. Then there is an experience in meditation, you feel exactly as if you were ejaculating with that girl you love the most, and the whole thing, you know? Bah, bah, bah? Can you imagine that? It is exactly the same feeling that you get when you are meditating, that feeling at the Third Eye, exactly that feeling. You understand?

And there is a third form in which you feel it from the spine, something going up like a thermometer, like the mercury rising. It is a kind of sensation in which you feel like an electric current is going up your spine. It goes up and then at this same area, you feel something goes around and around and around, and then something like rain comes down. Let me complete this. When you are having physical intercourse and the love game is perfectly divine. She has totally merged in you and she is a *hunsani* (*hunsani* is that purest form, that highest form of that); she is totally supportive of you and she is playing the game; and you are ejaculating—two ejaculations will happen. One will be in the lower area of your male organ and the other will be in your head. If ever that should happen to you, one symptom and sign of it is that you will be aware of what is happening in the universe and universes beyond, but you won't move physically. What I am teaching today can only happen if woman is perfectly into her entanglement with you: 100% supportive, 100% projective, 100% cooperative, and 100% your mate. You are mating with your mate and the meeting is very, very, very, very meditative.

Q: *Could you say a little more about what goes on in a man during the 72 hours from the time that the woman is thought of?*

Yogi Bhajan: It's a game. It's eyes, ears, mouth, hands, feeling, fingers. It's a vibratory exchange between the two. Symbolically, systematically, it is a rhythmical change. When you meet a woman and she crosses by you, you look like that. You know? You make gestures. It's a play of gestures between the two. Mostly it is not a spoken language.

Q: *How does it affect the glandular system?*

Yogi Bhajan: Oh, it causes it to totally secrete. You are trying to play very holy. You have nine holes, why are you upset?

Q: *What signs are there that you, you know, that the glandular...?*

Yogi Bhajan: That is another course that I'm going to teach. I'm not going to add that course here. This course is invocation and incentive of polarities and I'd like to stick to that. That course [that you're asking about] is very horny and that day I'd like none of you to eat. Otherwise, who wants wet dreams in class? Yes?

Q: *When a man and a woman, when they're in an intimate place in their bedroom, are there any perversions? What is perverted and what isn't perverted?*

Yogi Bhajan: Between a man and a woman, there is no perversion until you notice it. Anything between a man and a woman that is noticed is perversion. There's one area in which God doesn't interfere: that's between male and female in their privacy. What do you want to say? See how I got out of it? Yes?

Q: *Could you say something about the attitude you should bring into the bedroom?*

Yogi Bhajan: The attitude in the bedroom is the attitude of unison, the attitude of "I am for you, you are for me." Not expecting already certain things. It is a common flow. That's the maximum I can tell you. It's a common flow. If you do not have the incentive invocation in the woman, the understanding that she's out to please you and serve you and glorify you and put you on the pedestal of the Lordship, and just raise you from your bottom rear-end to the top of the *sahasrara,* the tenth gate, the lotus feet, you are not having a woman.

Q: *Then what?*

Yogi Bhajan: Then the basic idea is that such a student should be tied down on their knees, topsy-turvy for a couple of days, so that they can think right. Then you have to reground yourself and reassess yourself, find where the defect is, try to remove it, and recapture yourself and your personality; because without the total, absolute, beaming support of the woman . . . this is how the old scriptures describe it:

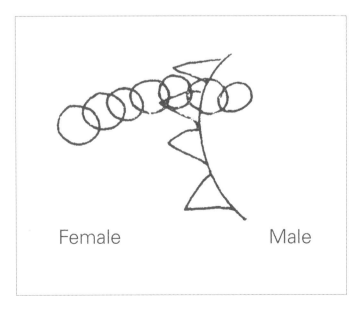

They always draw the sun as limitless, so it is always the arc. This means sun. The small circles always mean the moon. Full moon. This is how it goes. This is called woman. You understand? This chain of moons is not a chain to show you something. This chain shows, on a practical level, how the woman can be going, going, going, on and on, through all the trials. The moon doesn't care. It doesn't care for the hottest burning surface, it goes right into it. You have to induce that from your moon, your female. You do not understand. There may be a million supports to you, a million friends, millions of dollars, power and all that. You need the support of a woman. It is in your biological genes. And it is not that God didn't provide it for you. He did. Your satellite of the earth is the moon and it doesn't take a harsher way to do it. All it needs is a combination, combined forces, between the two of you, to come to an understanding

But we are sneaks. We don't confront woman. We don't talk to her. These are my needs. I remember a man said once to a woman, he said, "Lady, I cannot milk the cow, boil the milk, mix the sugar, and drink it, digest it, and wait to kiss you." In this statement he said it all. So she said, "Darling, from tomorrow onward, the cow will be milked, the milk will be hot, honey will be mixed, and it'll be digested by you and still I'll be smiling." What you want should be totally settled in the relationship. What she wants, what you want—decide it once and for all. Tell your obnoxiousness, tell your niceness, tell your needs, tell what you feel, tell what you want, and let her say what she wants, what her feelings are. Sit down and mutually give and take and decide what you actually want. Because in the privacy of the bed it is bad to discuss, sit down across the table and figure it out. Then give each other a 20% margin. Period.

The woman should be so attractive—and so powerfully attracted by you—that she should be just like a baseball you throw; she should get right into you. Any reservation on the part of the woman should be understood by your sensitivity. If you cannot understand the reservation of the woman, you are heading for a tragedy.

Q: *Could you talk a little bit more about the physical relationship between man and wife, outside intercourse?*

Yogi Bhajan: Outside intercourse, the relationship should be very supportive and very graceful. No childish remarks should even be allowed to slip through, because that doesn't make any sense to you both, but it makes a lot of sense to children and to people who watch you. Yes?

Q: *How many orgasms should the woman have?*

Yogi Bhajan: Woman gets what is called the tidings, through the clitoris and sometimes they get the tiding through the physical entry. Every woman has a different area and a different approach to it. There are some women that if you tell them some very horny, nude stories—just tell them, "Honey, I went to the beach, my God, they were not wearing bikinis, bah, bah, bah, and I saw this," and you just describe two or three women—after a few minutes she'll say, "Oh, oh, oh," and there she goes. You didn't even touch her. You know what I mean? For a woman to get off and reach her optimum point is her mental tendency. If you don't know this secret, will you please read *Women in Training*, first chapter where the woman's moon has been explained. There is a whole chapter about it.

Q: *Are women circumcised in some Arab countries?*

Yogi Bhajan: They are not circumcised because God wanted them to be that way. It is just a misrepresentation of the word circumcise. It doesn't have any significance as far as sex is concerned.

Q: *Then why is it done?*

Yogi Bhajan: Because violence is the solution of brutality. It is through brutality that place becomes scarred and hard, and then a certain operation is done so that the vagina becomes like an anus. It is a whole system. Those women are not considered to be human beings. Those men are impotent. They do not ejaculate normally. They take a long time and their glandular system is very slow to respond.

Q: *Have men got centers that are similar or corresponding to a woman's 11 centers?*

Yogi Bhajan: No, no, no. Forget it. What made you think that? Are you too much influenced by woman? None. You have totally different ingredients from her. Yes?

Q: *Something on technique. I was just wondering, you know, when you're actually making love, if…*

Yogi Bhajan: This "actually making love" is not my subject today. I know where you are going. At this time, so near Baisakhi,[5] I'm not teaching a course which involves discussing anything actual. I have to discuss it someday, I know. I'm ready for it, but let you all mature to that ground.

Q: *In trying to go to sadhana the day after…*

Yogi Bhajan: You should. You should go to sadhana the next day otherwise everybody will know what you did the night before.

Q: *Living in an ashram…*

Yogi Bhajan: Is difficult because everybody knows what is going on.

[5] Baisakhi is the Celebration of the founding of the Khalsa Nation by Guru Gobind Singh, The 10th Sikh Guru.

Q: *What is the answer to that?*

Yogi Bhajan: Living in an ashram is very beautiful for many, many things, direct and indirect. It is difficult because we are insanely insecure. Otherwise it is in many ways so advantageous that you can't even believe it. It gives us this: in the madness of love, we can take refuge in sanity. That is where you are put into balance. Ashram living is just like living in a condominium with a common kitchen. It is very beautiful to develop your personality in every form. But it does not give you a place for weirdness and private bungling, so it is difficult. Yes? I know when a woman tells me, "Sir, I want to live in an apartment," I say, "Uh, uh." Because a private apartment means anybody can come, anybody can go. See, in an ashram, things can't happen that way.

Q: *You talked about Krishna and Lila at one time. Are you going to delve into that at some point?*

Yogi Bhajan: Well, Krishna was a great Lord God. He was an incarnation of God. He had 18,000 women and he kept everybody safe and satisfied. In Siri Guru Granth, there's the story of Chandrawal. Lord Krishna's story is that he was very, very horny for that girl. Her mother, Jemina said, "Look, Krishna, if you look to my girl, I'm going to do you in totally." Krishna couldn't do anything and the mother married her away. Krishna was very clever. Disguised as a woman he went to her house and said, "I have come from the aunts," and then they said, "Where are you going to sleep?" He said, "I am going to sleep with my cousin, you know?" So that night, Krishna got over her and she said, "My bangles will be heard by my in-laws and all that." But Krishna didn't hear anything. Krishna gave everybody so much ecstasy that they felt like the night was as long as six months and the day was as long as one year. After a day and a half, Krishna left her totally amazed. He was still disguised and everything. So that was Lord Krishna and it is mentioned in Siri Guru Granth. His mind was always somewhere else even when he was doing something else.

Q: *Is it unhealthy to make love in the same room where a child is sleeping?*

Yogi Bhajan: It is not healthy in the sense that the child should not know what is going on. Sometimes a child can get in the middle and he will never think you are making love, he'll think you are fighting, which can sometimes be a trauma to a child.

Q: *What is the difference between orgasm and tiding?*

Yogi Bhajan: Oh, orgasm is what you think it is; it is like the orgasm for the male where you ejaculate. Tiding is an orgasm where she doesn't ejaculate but the feelings are the same. Sometimes there are women who will just grind their nails into your skin and when you're through with it, you'll feel that you're bleeding and she'll be laughing. Most of the women who are totally going into ecstasy of tiding will scratch you totally deeply. Yes—they will bite you to hell. They will scratch you to hell. They can do many, many things. It's absolutely normal. And it depends on which mood she is in. Sometimes it can be very fun.

There was a case, which was studied, where the woman went into tiding, she would just get so berserk and feisty that the man, who was almost my size and with more than twice my strength, found himself helpless. The case was brought to me, what to do? When the guy came to me, he was almost three quarters blue all over his body. It was amazing; she was totally not aware of what she did. He wanted to have intercourse with her, he wanted to, but when he remembered that—no way.

Q: *Why do men have nipples?*
Yogi Bhajan: Men have nipples because in form they are the co-form. It is also the heart center line. Nipples do not make you a woman. There are equivalent forms, except certain areas where the functions are different. Yes?

Q: *Can you raise the kundalini through the nipples?*
Yogi Bhajan: We don't; we do it through exercises. Sometimes intercourse can totally be an exercise. Well, you are my children. I have to tell you everything so that you may not look dumb to the world. Yes?

Q: *In the beginning of the course, you talked about the difference between the ejaculation of intercourse and that of masturbation...*
Yogi Bhajan: In masturbation, the glandular system is over-pressurized. The nervous system is drained to death. It is a forced situation. But in the intercourse, it is normal. In one masturbation session, the pressure on your body is more than you can ever consider handling. But even if you ejaculate one time after the other in intercourse, there's no pressure on the nervous system, and so that makes a lot of difference.

Q: *Does it have to do with the fact that you're doing it yourself, or that in the case of intercourse, that the woman's energy is there?*
Yogi Bhajan: Woman's energy is right there and that's what intercourse is. In masturbation, woman's energy is right there, but you are doing it to yourself. It means you are forcing your system to go into a space where there is no partnership. It is solo and it is very painful solo. It's not very normal.

Q: *You talked in Hamburg about when a woman...*
Yogi Bhajan: Were you listening to everything I said there?

Q: *Everything.*
Yogi Bhajan: Good.

Q: *If she stimulates you orally and sexually, and you go into a sleep, and it's a deep sleep because you're so satisfied and in ecstasy, it's at that time you have an orgasm. You said that that was the highest orgasm.*
Yogi Bhajan: That is what I said that happened here, and that is what is triggered by a woman. When you go into that sleep, there's a feeling, a coolness in your very depths feeling, which drags you down into the deepest sleep. It's called *turiya* stage. It is equivalent to ten hundred thousand ejaculations, whatever you call it. It's beautiful. You want to practice that?

Student: *Everything.*
Yogi Bhajan: Well, my idea is to leave you behind in this world as a very matured incarnation of God, so that when I'm gone you will be capable of enjoying divinity even in adversity.

■ ■ ■

Magnetic **Preference**

In the joy of your life, if you really want to enjoy your living, you must get the spring of life, the nectar of life, from the projection of woman.

Now we are going into the gray matter. That is, the scientific fact of male and female polarity and invocation. Let us see what we can come out with.

Every male relates to his own moon, female. The basic problem that you have is that you relate to woman in the physical form. You never study her mental form or her spiritual form. Woman has three forms, which is why she is a triangle: spiritual, physical and mental. All three forms must support you. If one form of the woman supports you, it is no support at all. A dog can be a better friend; it can support you physically and mentally with all its spirit, but most of the time it doesn't know what to do. Do you understand? But there is no time when a woman doesn't know what to do. That's the difference between the two.

This is what you do: you look at woman and you try to look at woman only physically to see if she is beautiful. You never consider that a physically beautiful woman, if she is 40% physically beautiful should be 60% mentally beautiful and almost 80% spiritually beautiful. Then it is worthwhile to consider the case; otherwise, you are getting into a very dangerous situation. Under no circumstances in your life can you disregard the direction and dealing and polarity with a woman toward her Infinity, which is God, which is dharma, which is spirit; whatever you name it, it is there. Her mind can only be supportive if the flow of spirit gives her security. It is my experience of 10 years [in the West] that you cater to woman on the physical level much more than you cater to woman on the mental level, or on the spiritual level. On the spiritual level lies your security.

If a woman is spiritual, she's securely behind you. On a mental level, if she's intelligent, she will solve your problems; life will be very convenient and beautiful. On the physical level, if she's attractive, she'll bring other people into the home. Why do you want that? Once a person was in love with a woman and I said, "Well, dummy, why don't you marry her?" He said, "Sir, I cannot pay for the security guard shift." The real beauty of a wife, or a woman, or a beloved, or a partner, or whatever you want to call her, is her mental intelligence. Her real strength is her spiritual growth and her real asset is her physical behavior. Physical behavior is what it is, not physical looks. Sometimes what glitters is not gold. Your aspect toward woman is that way.

In our life, we cater to our children and we cater to the ego of children, we spoil them. Children think they can milk you. That is okay with children, because children one day have to grow up; they have to be on their own. Normally you don't worry about that. But when your wife knows that she can milk you, you have no happiness in your store. Once your woman knows that she can twist you . . . I saw a very terrible scene once: I was talking to a student of mine and his wife was whispering in his ear. It's the most obnoxious behavior on the planet. He was trying to talk to me and tell me certain things, and she was telling him certain things. It shocked me! The guy was not even aware he was tolerating it. So there are many, many behaviors where you tolerate something that you should not. Because you are cowards, you cannot confront. You think that she is not your wife, that she is your mother. You can't tell her anything. You may not be rude to woman ever, but politely you can tell her to wait. Later on he said to me, "Sir, what did I do wrong?" I said, "What's wrong is that you should have told her, 'I am talking to my teacher, I have certain questions to be answered. I need them answered immediately, would you please talk to me later?'"

In the joy of your life, if you really want to enjoy your living, you must get the spring of life, the nectar of life, from the projection of woman. She must project greatness in you. That's the only way you can become great. By your own criteria, that of a man, you can never become depressed. The problem with us is our neuroses with our mother. First of all, dealing with that point, I want to tell you: never consider woman as a mother. Don't deal that way; don't think that way; don't relate that way. For that purpose you must take a paper and pencil and write down all the incidents which you have had with your mother for which you like her or dislike her or hate her—those incidents which have influenced you. Write it down. Make them numerical points. Then also think, "How does this correlate with my wife?" Avoid those areas for polite discussion; confront those difficulties with absolute firmness.

Q: *Discuss those with your wife?*
Yogi Bhajan: Deal it out, discuss it so that she will know what you are doing and she will get with you. That is your mental process; you have to make it up. It is useful to recognize the areas of neuroses that you have with your mother or which you can remember, or which you can feel, and correlate them with the areas of conflict that you have with your wife. You can then cancel them out. Find out where the conflict is and then deal with that conflict as politely and as firmly as you can. Yes?

Q: *Is it possible that the wife can also do this in her relationship with a man?*

Yogi Bhajan: Yes, you can ask her to do it. If you cannot find in your life, this relationship or neuroses, then help out. But when you help her out, don't tell her your pattern with your mother and her. It is much better that the woman doesn't know your weaknesses. Because to begin with, she thinks you are weak, that she can manipulate you. Remember also in life: don't get manipulated by the woman you love the most and never try to manipulate a woman you love the most. Straight, firm talk. Straight, firm talk is the way to deal with those areas where mental and physical intimacy can breed contempt. Do you understand? Yes?

Q: How can you not reveal your weaknesses if you're talking straight and forward?

Yogi Bhajan: That is not necessary. You talk to me five minutes, I won't let you catch my weaknesses at all. My weaknesses are my weaknesses and I have a right to privacy. Why should you know about it? Who are you? And why do you want to know? You want to stab me in my back? Yeah. You can get firmer and firmer. You know, in our lethargy and our loose talk, we tell certain things that we think are going to bring, or win, her confidence; so we tell every idiot thing to her. Then she twists all those things. Anything that can be twisted and used against you should not come out of your mouth. Also, things that you can twist and pin it back, you shouldn't do either.

You must remember that your wife is another human being. She has her own identity, she has her own feelings, she has her own mental process. You, too, have your own mental process and all you want out of her is the inspiration. There's no other purpose of a woman in the life of a man—sex, children, and all that are nothing. It's all through inspiration that I am growing. "I have a future, I have children, I have a home, blab, blah, blah." It's absolutely necessary for you to know in the depth of your heart what you want from a woman. What you want from a woman is inspiration and companionship. You don't want anything more than that. What is sex? For ten dollars, here in Hollywood, you can go and have your fun. Companionship, you can hire it. You can do something, you can get along. But in the wholeness of relationship you need something more. It is called companionship of trust. You need somebody in your life you can deeply trust.

Next to God, you trust your woman. You want to talk to her; you want to tell her everything. Some people cannot even digest their food without telling the whole day to their wife. They may not remember the day. They wouldn't be able to recall the day for themselves. But to tell their wives, they can recall it like it is a movie. They're so accurate. Now, you think it is dangerous. No, if that is your habit and that is your need, go ahead and do it. It's most relaxing to a tired man to share with a woman all he can share. For people like that, life has to be very honest. Otherwise, if they live crooked and they don't share that duality, they are eaten up. Your basic maturity is that you must provide your woman security and she'll provide you with inspiration. That's the bargain. When in your life you cannot provide her with security, you are playing a very badly losing game.

Q: If a woman fluctuates...

Yogi Bhajan: If a woman doesn't fluctuate, she's male. They fluctuate. Let them fluctuate. A stable woman is very boring.

Q: How do you trust her and yet not share your weaknesses?

Yogi Bhajan: You trust her with your strength. Why would you trust her with your weaknesses? Can you trust a person with your strengths? Why use a woman as a garbage pit? You put all this garbage in and then it multiplies and sprouts; it will come to you and eat you up. That's the first thing. I said this earlier, "What kind of a man are you if you cannot stand out and understand the problem?" That's what I said. Share your weakness with your Teacher, and you'll always get an answer. Share your weakness with your woman, and you'll always get multiple criticisms.

What does a psychiatrist give you? Nothing. You go and talk and talk and talk and tell all the weaknesses. He listens and listens and sometimes says, "Yeah, yeah, you should do this, you should not do that, bah, bah, bah." That's all. But professionally, you think you are safeguarding yourself because whatever you tell him, he is not going to tell anybody. But if you want a thing to be propagated, tell your woman. The next day you can hear it in the last house on Preuss Road.[1] When a woman can keep a secret, she becomes the sacred—and they are very rare. Sit and talk. Let them talk and just give them something that talks; that's your public relations policy.

Tell her only good things; she will talk them all out. You'll be fantastic. Suppose you are very depressed. You come home and you just want to lie down. Don't tell her you're depressed; tell her, "I'm tired and I want to rest. If you can successfully put me into a comfortable sleep, and I can be refreshed and good again, I'll take you out for dinner. Otherwise, please don't bother me." You'll get a good foot massage and a good nice blanket. You may go right to sleep. Then you can go out and really have a good dinner if you feel like it. Otherwise get up, cook for yourself and feed her. It's a very friendly gesture and she'll always admire it. Woman likes the touch of nearness. Don't be absolutely stiff and don't make it a point of authority with a woman.

When you make it a point of authority with a woman, you are asking for one standard trouble: that is, she will love to challenge your authority. She will do this in three ways. One is to criticize you behind your back. Second is to denounce

---

[1] The road where Yogi Bhajan lived and taught in Los Angeles for many years.

you or criticize you publicly, or in the living room. Third is to pack up and leave, or sometimes don't pack up and still get away.

Don't have a stiff-neck policy ever with a woman, because woman fluctuates and she needs the room to fluctuate. When you put a strict discipline, direct confrontation on her, she has to use her defense mechanisms and while doing so, she can sometimes prove very dangerous. Got it?

Now, as far as your personality toward the control of a woman is concerned, you can only control through your image. You must build your image as a holy man or a spiritual man or a man of honor, of honesty, of true words and all; all good qualities. Write down on a piece of paper these qualities and just try to put them in your image. You have no reason to worry about it. It all happens. Once I asked a woman who left her husband, "Why did you leave him?" She said, "I'm not sure of him." I said, "He's very committed." She replied, "He may be committed, but he does three days of sadhana out of the month." This was her entire answer. I said, "But you know, he has been hanging on with 3HO." She said, "Well, he has been hanging on with 3HO, but 3HO is not what I have been looking to. I have been married to him for five years and on the average he does sadhana three times a month—if a man cannot do a sadhana that would save him, he cannot save me if I'm in trouble, and so I have to leave." And, she left. There was nothing we could do for her.

Whenever you show ego to a woman you ask for confrontation, and whenever you make a woman confront you, you're the loser. She'll break your spirit if not your bones. Remember this part which is very serious: if a woman really wants to do harm to you, she'll break your spirit. She'll hit you with a pounding of words that you can't digest. She'll try to hurt you in certain areas. She can spread bad will about you. She can tell certain things. "Oh, my husband is cruel." That tells a lot more than you are willing to hear. In the magnetic polarity between male and female, each woman has what they call a dark trend and a light trend: 15 days of the moon which are light and 15 days of the moon which are dark. The trend goes up; it goes to the male. It comes down and goes to the male also. Her menstruation cycle is 30 days in all and there are two categories of woman: either the first 15 days are very charming or the latter 15 days are very charming. You must know that trend. If her first 15 days are the up trend, then it is beautiful. If her last 15 days are okay, it is beautiful, provided you know. You should know it, and if you cannot know it through your own sensitivity, you'd better communicate and talk to her.

Q: Does woman's discomfort come in cycles like that? Is that like a yearly thing?

Yogi Bhajan: No, no. She goes up and down by the moon; you know the waning and waxing moon? Some women are more energetic on the waning moon. On the waning moon they are very energetic. Some are very energetic on the waxing moon. When woman is very energetic, keep her positive. Any tendency to show or give her a chance for negativity is just asking for a fight right at your door. Who wants it?

Q: If a man is solar, does he wax and wane on that cycle?

Yogi Bhajan: Does the sun do it?

Q: No, I'm saying, if man is the solar stability, does he (pause) I've noticed in myself a waxing and waning lunar cycle. Is that from her or is that broadcasted from within myself?

Yogi Bhajan: There's no such thing as a man waning and waxing. No, no, you simply cannot handle your woman because you have a bad sugar level. Your problem I know. Don't blame your sugar level on your wife. She is the only one who could live with you. Anybody else would have totally punched you out. Now, when you behave neurotically, you are a very classic, classified neurotic. I know that.

Q: Does man have any cycle where for a few days he's off?

Yogi Bhajan: Weekly cycle. It's a very sneaky cycle. You will learn about it. It is called 30/70. This is a male cycle. In one week, you are 30% up; in another week, you are 70% up. It is called the projection of the sun. Sometimes it flames over, sometimes it flames under. But it is always there.

It's called the 30/70 cycle, and it's on a weekly basis. That's why we made the 7-day week. It changes week to week. In one week, there are certain things you want to do. In another week, you want to eat something. In another week, you want to go out. In one week you want to do everything; and the next week, within the same environments, you don't want to do anything. Have you noticed that? On a certain week you promise everything on the telephone.

The next week you say, "nay" to all those things that last week you promised. That is called sun caliber—30/70. In one week with you, there's a 30% chance to get you to admit to things; in another week, it is 70%. Each woman should know that. This part you can tell the woman. Yes?

Q: Does it relate to biorhythms?

Yogi Bhajan: You can almost call it that, with biorhythms though, only our energy and power are projected. But basically the concept of you to you is 30/70. Most of the things that you admit before a woman, you do when you are on a 30% rhythm. She can get everything out of you. When you are on a 70% rhythm, she may try her level best, but forget it. You are the king and there is nobody else. On the 30% rhythm, forget it, you are nobody. Now, we are coming to this.

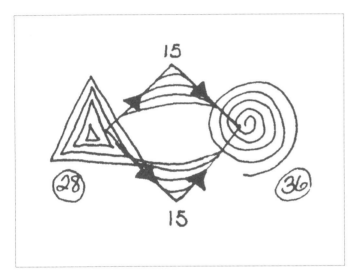

A rhythmic projection from a female goes toward the male and the male returns it in a horizontal way. The main problem that you have to understand is that in the early years of your life, maybe up to the 35th year, you do not feel insecure as a male. You do not feel insecure, but neither can you provide security. So when you feel secure within yourself, you cannot provide security to others. Later on, you'll need security and because you have not provided it, you can't get it. So project firmness and security in the first 36 years of the male life. Do you understand? Woman definitely needs security to age 28. So do not trust your wife if she's not yet 29. There are two opinions about it: 29 years of her sun age and 29 years of your living age. It has not yet been solved. Yes?

Q: You said don't trust her?

Yogi Bhajan: Yes. She can fight her way out anytime. She can walk out on you anytime. It is not that she is Oriental, or she is American, or she is Western or Canadian, it doesn't matter. It is in their breed. This is because up to age 25, woman thinks she can get anything she wants and up to age 36, man thinks he can do anything he wants. Ego is absolutely in contrast in both. So up to 28 of her age and up to 36 of his, it's a very crucial period. In sexual habits, you are required to be very calm and firm between these years. Not having any discipline, or not controlling yourself, not living by discipline, or not going by rules, or not establishing some sort of security is a definite danger to the married relationship or friendship, whatever you want to call it.

Now, I will give you one example of security. Suppose there is Sunday Gurdwara and you don't want to go. Drag yourself. You must go because if you cannot provide leadership, you cannot gain respect. Write it down in your heart, head and feet, also. If you cannot provide leadership, you cannot gain respect and this is what bugs the woman most. In certain areas, she looks to you for leadership and you can't provide it. In the children's discipline, sometimes she needs you. In many things in life when she needs you, she looks to you. When she looks to you, and you cannot answer, you have lost her; because what is a male to a woman, he who provides and protects. When she feels you provide and protect, she'll give you every inch of energy she has. But you must remember, you actually live here, in your spirit.

Have you heard this story? There was a king who had an enemy, a great giant. He would come to the kingdom and eat the king's men. There was nothing the king could do. Finally, the king got a prince and told the prince to go and catch that giant. On the way the prince met a goddess and asked, "What should I do?" She said, "That giant you cannot kill." He said, "Why?" "Because his spirit is in a parrot and the parrot lives on a mountain." So he said, "What should I do?" She said, "Don't go toward the giant, go toward the parrot. Kill the parrot and the giant will be dead." The prince knew it was true. So he went. There were a lot of hassles on the way, which he conquered, and finally he reached the parrot. He took the parrot's neck and he said, "Parrot, you are so beautiful, but I have to twist your neck just a little bit." And the parrot said, "Why? What is wrong with me?" He said, "By doing that, the giant will die." The parrot said, "Hurry up." He twisted the neck, the neck broke, and the giant was dead on the spot.

That is exactly how it is for you. Your ego cannot live without the inflow of the woman's projection, and when your own woman wants to kill your ego, there's nothing you can lean on. You want to have a defense mechanism, because you actually live in the projection of the woman; therefore, you have to be a leader in three fields: spiritual, mental and physical, in that order. Problem with you is that you believe your physical comes first when actually it comes last. All this discussion, "She doesn't love me, I do not love her." It's all ruthlessly wrong. Got it? Everything that refreshes you, makes you look great, makes you feel great, inspires you, gives you beautifully disciplined children, a clean house, beautiful social respect comes from this triangle, the female. Your problem is that you don't recognize it.

Because up to age 36, you feel it comes from you, and after 36 you do not know what to do. Got it?

How many of you feel that at this moment you can change your life? Well, that is a good number. And how many of you think you are really going to do it? Best of luck to you. Remember the polarity of a woman—woman is flexible and is always available in flexibility. A woman is never uptight or stiff. So at any moment in life, if you can provide her with spiritual leadership, she'll automatically—mentally and physically—be yours. Go ahead and ask me questions.

Question and **Answer**

Q: What if she's in father phobia?

Yogi Bhajan: Father phobia is in every woman, to a degree. But at that time, you should not have a mother phobia. Father phobia can be utilized for advantageous purposes; but when you have a mother phobia and there's a perversion in your personality, then you cannot utilize it. That is how it goes. Yes?

Q: What if her mother is influencing the situation?

Yogi Bhajan: Huh? Her mother can only influence the situation when you cannot influence the situation. Mother, father, brother, sides, this, that, it is all a hopeless situation. Once you influence her, there is no other influence possible.

Q: To what extent are you responsible for seeing your wife out of her father phobia?

Yogi Bhajan: 100%.

Q: Is that by eliminating your own mother phobias that you have?

Yogi Bhajan: Yeah.

Q: What are some examples of mother phobia?

Yogi Bhajan: Mother phobia is where the woman hates you; she thinks you are the greatest creep. The first chance she gets, she will tell you that you are a creep. Then if you ask her why she said so, she'll not have any reason. At that time, if you shut up, you are just an idiot. That is the time, the opportunity, to politely discuss how she comes to think so, from which thought it came, why she said that, and so on. Whenever woman starts negating you, at that moment, she is working under a bewitchment of a secondary thought, which comes from her subconscious. Try to meet that thought half-way and kill it forever. At that time, if you ignore it, you are asking for trouble.

Q: What do you do or what does it mean when you come home from work and you are very tired, and your wife likes to tickle you and tease you about it.

Yogi Bhajan: Tell her to give you a foot massage, "harder, harder." Turn over on your belly and tell her, "Give me a back massage." You can use that energy. That's why she is energetic. Why not? Yes?

Q: Sir, you said that during the light period, the responsibility of the man is to make sure that the woman's energy stays positive and that she directs it in a positive way. What if she's on that dark side, and she doesn't have the energy, or the energy seems to be…

Yogi Bhajan: I'll tell you, inspire her spiritually. What you do is inspire her physically. That is the only wrong people do; they inspire woman physically and make a monster out of her. All you have to do to deal with a woman is to inspire her spiritually, because she's very handicapped toward Infinity, very handicapped. Inspire her toward Infinity and you'll have the best friend in the world by your side, totally for you.

Intellectually some people talk and rap with a woman. They are ready for divorce. Some people instigate her physically; they are ready for a fight. If you always do it spiritually, you'll win the game. You have to understand that your strength lies in the spirit, which she is—not what she is in the body and in the mind. You can go up to the heights of Infinity by inspiring yourself from her spirit.

Q: Do these principles apply to all women, not just your wife?

Yogi Bhajan: Yeah, yeah, same thing. You can have intercourse with your wife, that's the only difference.

Q: How do you inspire someone spiritually? Do you talk, gesture? What's the best way to go about that?

Yogi Bhajan: Can you tell him what is the best way to inspire somebody spiritually? Action.

Q: How do you help a woman who has low self-esteem?

Yogi Bhajan: Raise her spirit. Talk to her spiritually. Spiritually tell her, give her examples, think about it, and if she's just doing it to lay a number on you, don't relate to it.

Q: What about when her husband has low self-esteem, when both people in the relationship…

Yogi Bhajan: When the woman and man both have low self-esteem, it's a tragedy. Then go to your Teacher, run and let him do something. If he cannot do it, go to God. If nothing, jump in the ocean. It's terrible.

Q: When a woman goes through emotional stages, and she does it in extremes, how can...

Yogi Bhajan: She's asking for help. When a woman has any extreme behavior, she's asking for help. She doesn't mean to break; but sometimes we react so much, out of fear, that it breaks up the marriage. Remember always, in every length and strength, woman doesn't seek a break, because she seeks security by nature.

Q: How do you know what help she's asking for? Will she tell you?

Yogi Bhajan: Oh, yes. Woman can be trapped with politeness always. Politeness is the key of life. Rude talk to a woman is like a bullet to a bull.

Q: Why do you use the term spiritual handicap?

Yogi Bhajan: Because she is here to sprout, she is here to receive, conceive and she is very insecure. The only thing that makes her secure is when you tell her that she is Infinite and that her spirit is what can give her the experience of Infinity. Because of the mother instinct, every woman is basically a mother. Woman is overprotective of children, she is overprotective of herself, and she overprotects her environments. She overprotects her material wealth. This is because to her, all this means security. If you transform it to the security of Infinity, she is always secure.

Q: Is there a way to deal with a woman who is really freaked out?

Yogi Bhajan: Yes. Just don't worry about the freak out. Do your job. When a woman is freaked out, you relate to her; but when she is freaked out, you can't help her.

If You Can Fake It, You Can Make It

You can't make it, if you don't fake it. Faking means blueprint. You understand? Faking means you sit down and you think about it, you understand it, you draw it, and then, you act.

If you fake it, you can make it. The first idealistic position is, pretend you are holy. Pretend you are holy, attend all holy services; and second is, try to eat holy food. In other words, what I am trying to tell you is, look very religious. You may not be religious, don't worry about what you are. You have to look very religious. Never eat food without saying a prayer, loud and clear. Remember, when you come home, I'll tell you, there's a solution I once gave somebody. I said, "When you come home, wash your face, wash your hands and all that, and sit down and pray for a few minutes." So when he came home, he washed his face and all that, he sat and prayed, and she said, "What did you pray?" He said, "I'm very happy and divine and thank God that I'm back home and I'm with you." She told the entire neighborhood: my husband has met a yogi who has totally changed his life and now he comes home like an angel. In the morning, as he left home he would pray, and she asked, "What prayer is this?" He said, "That when I come back, you should be healthy, happy and holy. I'm leaving you in the rhythms of God." These words don't cost anything and they are better than kisses and flowers and all that. Write it down: "Fake spiritual behavior." What am I saying? I'm telling you, don't look at me, write it down. Write down a pattern. It's called a fake spiritual pattern and just force yourself to live it. After about 3 months, she will totally inspire you to live it. The gap between your fake spiritual inspiration and your living a spiritual life is about 90 days.

Question and Answer

Q: *Early in the very first part of the session, you were talking about* yog *and* bhog *in the scriptures, and I remember one time way back you asked, 'Are you a yogi or a bhogi?'*

Yogi Bhajan: *Bhog* is what divides you—what divides you. *Yog* means what unites you. Okay. That's good.

Q: *Did you say anything about singles' relationships? Between single men and single ladies who are thinking about...*

Yogi Bhajan: Oh, that's a beautiful relationship of a brother and sister. That brother and sister is a relationship of kindness. There's no other, better relationship than that. Even people who have to marry, they have to be very friendly and not exploit each other sensually and sexually. That is required. It is good for your own system, otherwise you stimulate your metabolism for nothing and end up with a disaster. Okay, what else?

Q: *Regarding the fruit diet in the spring time? Should it be don't mix fruits at any one meal, or...?*

Yogi Bhajan: No, no, eat one fruit at a time. You can eat four times or three times during the day, but you eat one fruit at one time. Don't have peaches and this and that all mixed up together.

Q: *Each meal should be an individual fruit?*

Yogi Bhajan: One fruit. Mono-fruit.

Q: *That's fasting only, or is that a general rule?*

Yogi Bhajan: No, no, when you go on that fruit diet.

Q: *If a person suspects he's hypoglycemic, can he still go on this fruit diet?*

Yogi Bhajan: Yes. He can just have a little piece of fruit every 2 hours. It won't hurt.

Q: *You mentioned earlier about intercourse after arguments and fights. If a wife approaches after a fight should you respond?*

Yogi Bhajan: Take her out for a walk. That's the best response. Don't give in, because then it becomes a pattern.

Q: *What is happening physically if you perspire heavily at night, even when it's not hot outside?*

Yogi Bhajan: Dr. Soram has a Khalsa Clinic. It needs immediate attendance. There's something wrong with the nervous system. Yes?

Q: *Is the tomato diet a mono-diet?*

Yogi Bhajan: Tomato diet is a tomato diet. Yes?

Q: *You spoke about the projection of a woman who is non-spiritual and her lustful thoughts; then you told the story about the prayer and how you went out and were injured afterwards. Is there some way to deal with these...?*

Yogi Bhajan: You can immediately find the sensitivity when woman is not pure. Listen, I remember once a friend of mine went away with some woman somewhere. You know, ran away. When he came back, he couldn't go home. He couldn't go to his own home. Then he came and stayed with us in the hostel for two, three, four days. We talked to his home and said he was going to stay; he was not feeling well. Then when he was to go home, we went with him and stayed a couple of days to put him back. It's not a guilty consciousness. Your soul cries sometimes. The only thing in your personality that the Id hates is when you are dishonest with yourself, when you lose your own grace to yourself. You can lose your grace for three things: woman, money, and authority. All three are temporary. Your own soul, your own personality, are far superior. Yes?

Q: *With this assignment of writing down incidents that your mother laid on you, is that something to do for homework also?*

Yogi Bhajan: Yes. The homework is for you to relate to it. It's very good. Always check your personality on a monthly basis. Always check your traumas on a monthly basis. Is there any trauma in your life? Has anything affected you? Does anything relate to your childhood trauma and your present trauma, your trauma in 3HO, your fears, and all that? Make a chart. Take a mark. You'll be perfect. It's a personal psychoanalysis. Always do it. You'll always be in shape, and always in good shape.

Q: *In writing down the list of problems you have with your mother, how can you tap back into the value of those incidents?*

Yogi Bhajan: Well, just understand that it is positive or negative. If it's negative, be guarded. If it's positive, it's fine. But when you write your own traumas and you calculate your own answers and finish with it, just burn them. That's the way it goes. Don't leave the record for somebody. It's your own privacy. Yes?

Q: *Why is it that man has to fake it?*

Yogi Bhajan: Oh, you can't make it, if you don't fake it. Faking means blueprint. You understand? Faking means you sit down and you think about it, you understand it, you draw it, and then, you act. It's just like a blueprint you make before you build a house. You are; you are not. That's not the problem. Don't waste time in that because the challenge is right there.

Q: *In order to solve a woman's father phobias you solve your mother phobias. How does that affect her?*

Yogi Bhajan: In mutual relationship, it will limit you. It definitely will limit you. [Editor's Note: By 'limit,' Yogi Bhajan is referring to the strain that phobias can create in relationship.]

Q: *When you pray over every meal, what do you do in a restaurant?*

Yogi Bhajan: In a restaurant, there also you start with a prayer. You are praying before the food. You must pray to smell the food, relate to the food. No food is digestible to your body until you relate to it in odor, form and self. There's even an airline, I don't know which one it is, which gives you a prayer before the meal and after the meal, duly printed.

Q: *Does a woman go through the 15-day cycle when she's nursing a baby?*

Yogi Bhajan: When woman is nursing, she needs your 101% support. At that time she's very motherly, she's highly defensive, and she can be irritated for nothing. That is the cost you pay to have a baby.

Q: *Your instructions with the banyan milk were to take six drops for six days in the fall and spring. What's the hazard of either taking more or not enough?*

Yogi Bhajan: No, no. I don't think that when the people who have experimented say that, they mean don't take it more or take it less.

Q: *There is a problem in winter or summer?*

Yogi Bhajan: Summer…

Q: *Somebody's bound to do it, that's why I want to know.*

Yogi Bhajan: No, no, if there's a problem, and it's to the point of disease, then you can do it. But on a regular basis it's only during those seasons.

Q: *You said that any man who is sexually weak before a woman is a nuisance to himself. Right before that you said something about, "Don't provoke a woman to sensuality." Does that mean that you should just let the woman…?*

Yogi Bhajan: That only means be firm and polite. You should be very firm but very polite. Never use harsh language with a woman.

Q: *You spoke about how you should always provide for the needs of a woman. But where do you draw the line by providing for her needs and not catering to her demands?*

Yogi Bhajan: Well, that is a mutual interest, isn't it? It's called mutual interest. When you can't provide it, you tell her, "Dear, I can't provide it. It's too much. I can't." Be honest about it. She won't bug you. But if a woman knows you play one game, she'll play ten. Otherwise she's not a woman.

Q: *If you explore the areas of neuroses with your mother in the past, what can you do to eliminate memory blocks?*

Yogi Bhajan: For that there is sadhana. The majority of your problems are when you are handicapped by sadhana. If you have a good and regular sadhana, your will is aroused enough to take care of you. That's definite. That's a definite experience.

Q: *You said something about the 70/30 percent rhythm of the man.*

Yogi Bhajan: No, that's the woman's rhythm. Sometimes, as a man in relation to woman, you are positive by 30% and sometimes you are positive by 70%. That's your rhythm in relationship. But when you are on 30% rhythm and she approaches you, she gets you. And at 70%, there's no question, it won't happen. So all you need is an extra guard.

Q: *I remember you saying that you shouldn't expose your weakness to your woman and then, about your mother phobia, if you take care of yourself...*

Yogi Bhajan: Well, you can take your weakness to your Teacher, or take your weakness to your advisor, or take your weakness to a friend, or you can take your weakness to a professional. Why do you have to take your weakness to your wife?

Q: *If you can take care of those mother phobias in yourself, it's best not to...*

Yogi Bhajan: There's no need. When you can take care of anything yourself, it is okay. Yes?

Q: *You said you can lose your grace in one of three areas: money, women or authority. How do you lose it in your authority?*

Yogi Bhajan: In authority, when you bring it to uptightness and do not consider the other man's point of view, and you are not supported by a conventional law, then you can be challenged. There's no need for that.

Q: *With your mother phobias, is there any point in discussing it with your mother?*

Yogi Bhajan: Oh, she will tell you that you are brainwashed, blah, blah, blah. She'll add more.

Thank you very much for listening. But what I want is for you to grind these notes, think about them, use them, and then sometime, when you get a chance, write to me about how you feel and tell me what they have done for you.

Blessed be my soul which goes through the living experience of God within me and without me. May this day of mine, through the creatures' grace, as a congregation, and as the Creator's activity, be always healthy, happy and holy. Bless me, my soul, to live in joy and peace. Sat Nam.

■ ■ ■

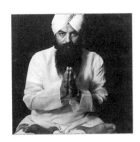

Man to **Man** 4

Growing as a Man

Circa 1979

*After a man presents himself, he must communicate...
When you communicate, the only friend you have is the
art of creative dialogue. That is what establishes you as a
man.*

▪ The Multiple **Man**

▪ The Growing **Man**

The Multiple Man

There is no greater attribute that I can give a man than this: man is what man is and man should be what man should be.

The knowledge that there are certain things that you have not been taught causes me absolute pain. It is not that I think that men in America are not willing to be happy, are not willing to be great, or are not willing to be men; it's that you have not been taught the fundamental values of being a man. There is no greater attribute that I can give a man than this: man is what man is and man should be what man should be.

Recently, I was discussing the idealistic concept of the multiple man with a man who is supposed to be an authority on the problems of men. He could not understand the concept of the multiple man. I said to myself, "Well, if this man, who teaches psychology to the psychologists, and psychiatry to the psychiatrists, and who is considered among men to be an authority on any problem, if this man does not know that in every man there is a multiple man—forget it. There's no fun in living."

I was 9 years old when I learned the concepts that I am going to share with you. The essence of what I want to say is in the saying, "God made it only this much, don't take it to this much." Do you understand that? I am talking about your penis. God made your penis not more than 11 inches, maximum. Now what we do is this, we take our whole life and base it on this damn thing which isn't even a foot long. You are 6 feet tall! But all you ask is, "Am I potent? Am I competent?" Nothing can kill you as a man more than fear of impotency and incompetency.

There are three phobias that belong to every man born: "Am I potent?" "Am I competent?" "Can I prove it?" Do you understand? All of these questions relate to the Second Chakra. They relate to our sex area. Picture the body with the male organ going from the Second Chakra upward to the extent that it comes out through the top of the Crown Chakra. That is the psychic picture of all men. In simple words, you love your penis that much. Your every action—conscious, subconscious, and unconscious—relates only to prove that this thing is still standing above you. That is a fact. Why do you elevate to a position above you, a part that is not the total sum of you?

Basically, a woman relates to you for millions of reasons, not just for sexual intercourse. Moreover, on a level of physical potency, you are 60% impotent just through sheer fear. Relatively speaking, you are impotent because you are scared, you are afraid, you fear. Pre-entry ejaculation is the outcome of sexual fear. Overexcitement—it's a battle between overexcitement and underexcitement. This sexual fear in you is very negative because it negates the creative sense in you, what you call your "sixth sense." It inhibits the art of creative dialogue in you.

Creative dialogue is your most competent friend. Your personality may affect others as ugly, or friendly, or impressive or even very negative. That first impression is called "structure concentration." A man who can appear saintly in every approach has that as his plus. That's how it is. But after a man presents himself, he must communicate. Is that true or not? When you communicate, the only friend you have is the art of creative dialogue. That is what establishes you as a man. In your life you must deal with the physical to the physical, the mental to the mental and the spiritual to the spiritual. Not only that, you have to balance these three with those same three of the opposite sex. Some men have a strong mental projection but are weak physically; others who try to be strong physically are weak spiritually, even though they can spout every spiritual philosophy.

Once while I was talking to a certain woman, her husband came in and she said, "Sir, my spiritual baboon has come." I couldn't understand why she would call her husband a spiritual baboon. I said, "Dear lady, what made you say such a negative thing about your husband?" She said, "Sir, he is such a spiritual baboon that he does not recognize you as a spiritual man. You watch it with him." "Okay," I said, "I'll see." One day this gentleman came to see me. He said that he had always wanted to talk to me and for two hours he talked. He went from the Greek version of spirituality to transcendental meditation, covering the whole field accurately, correctly, and in great depth. After hearing all that, I asked him one question. I said, "I think with all your religious knowledge and spiritual practices, you must have found out something very unique and beautiful." He said, "I have not even found out who I am." Then I saw the twist—there was a twist. He wanted me to match him on the mental level. I simply turned to him and said, "May your spirit bless you to find who you are." That one line saved me from another two hours of listening, or talking or any discussion. That is the art of creative dialogue.

All you have to do is say one line, but that one line should establish you—and you'll be saved from one more hour of talking. Remember whenever you speak with anyone, you have only one line to speak. You must gear yourself mentally. Whatever you have to communicate in that one line, it must be helped by your creative sense, your sixth sense. You must know where you can penetrate the person or situation and then your creative sense must let you establish your relationship.

In each kind of relationship there is a motivation. In business the purpose is to make money. Money is equivalent to security in this instance. In an intimate relationship, the purpose is to get out of loneliness. All sexual relationships have one purpose—to get rid of loneliness. All the rest is hodge-podge. Even sexual intercourse in itself is an expression of trusting each other, or letting each other trust. We do not believe in loneliness. That's all it is. In all political and other relationships, the motivation is power, who controls whom. Do you understand these motivations? One is security. The second is to fight loneliness (man is a social animal; he wants to establish that society). And the third is power. It is to these motivations that you apply your art of creative dialogue.

As a man there are three faculties that you must have: wisdom, humility, and the desire to serve. In any walk of life, if you cannot establish that you are a man of wisdom, you cannot win the game 100%. Your wife, your child, your partner, your spiritual teacher, your city, your county, your country—all look to you to be a man of wisdom. The second qualification is humility: that you are social and humble, approachable. Humble means approachable. You need to be approachable, easy to communicate and talk with. That is the second faculty. And the third is that you have the desire to serve, that you are sincere in your purpose of service.

Can you remember all this when you talk to a woman? Can you? If you forget one part of it you will look bizarre to her because she is absolutely sensitive. No woman is fooled. Remember that: God has never created a foolish woman. God might have created a mad woman. He has created a lot of foolish men, because His computer malfunctions from time to time; but He has yet to create one foolish woman. She knows where you are coming from and what to do about it. That is her automatic instinct. She has that instinct because of her capacity to be a mother. She may never become a mother, but she has that capacity, and therefore that ability to know where you are coming from.

When you communicate, you use your various chakras. First Chakra, anus; second is the sexual plane; third is the Navel Point; fourth is the Heart Center; fifth, the throat center; sixth, the Third Eye, *ajna*; and the seventh is the Crown Chakra, with this crown, you are a total human being. Your communications can come from more than one center at one time. If you are coming from your fifth center, through your fifth center, you'll be absolutely blunt. If you are coming from your fifth center, through your fourth, you'll be compassionately blunt. If you are in the fifth and come through the third, you'll be diplomatically blunt. If you come through the second center, you'll be intellectually blunt. (In truth, your purpose of sexuality can be seen very well). Coming from the first center, you'll be pervertedly blunt; from the, sixth, creatively blunt; and from the seventh center, you'll be intelligently blunt. The characteristic of the fifth center, when it is used with a mixture of other centers, is to be blunt, to say things directly.

Suppose the mixture is with the seventh center. If you mix the seventh with the fourth, you will be compassionately intelligent; with the third, you will be protectively intelligent; with the second, you will be creatively intelligent; and with the fifth, you will be distinctly intelligent. It depends on the mixture.

To give you an example of mixing the chakras, I want to share with you a meeting I had with a gay person who runs the gay center of Los Angeles. I said to him, "Suppose I believe that enjoyment of sexual relationship between male and male is the perfect relationship. Could you explain to me how we will perpetuate the human race and continue to enjoy the creativity of childbearing and child raising which is an outlet to our sentimental neurosis?" He said, "Your Eminence knows the Divine Law, and in this Law, your Eminence also knows that the excellency of God is complete within Itself." (Watch it). "Within the complete ecstasy of consciousness, Your Worship knows that that is the state of mind, body, and soul which we have to acquire. Therefore, it is all God's will that we must reach that complete, absolute Oneness…"

What could I say? Tell me, what could I say? I was His Excellency, His Holiness, His Eminence, His Worship, His Divine Self. He put so much butter around me that there was nothing to stand on. Further, he was talking a philosophy that is absolutely true. So he was using the seventh center mixed with…? The first. As a human being you can combine up to three chakras at one time. First, third and fifth; first, fifth and sixth; seventh, sixth and fifth—any combination can be used. With your male ego, you can learn to pull the energy from any three centers accurately and consciously.

You think it is difficult? No. A guitar has six strings, right? Sometimes it has twelve strings, yet there is always only one player and he uses only four fingers. With his fingers he can make one, two, three, four creative pressures on those strings. But what he's producing is not strings and fingers, he's producing a note. In your own life, all creativity has to be a harmonious note. You must combine your chakras harmoniously. When there is an unharmonious note, that's when you miss the point.

Now I'm going to talk to you directly about woman and I'm going to tell you something that will surprise you. Woman doesn't love you. No woman ever born with a uterus and a menstruation period has ever had the capacity to love a man. This statement I'll repeat: no woman with a physically complete cycle of menstruation has any instinct, direct or indirect, to love a male. Then what does she love? Her own fulfillment! Dummies! That is where you get blinded: Woman doesn't love a man, her man, any man. There's no such thing. It's not in her genes. It's not in her creativity. It is not in her consciousness. She loves her fulfillment. Secondly, she loves her strength, and then, she loves her security. Fulfillment, strength, security—one, two, three.

If you can't deliver those, forget it. Call it love, call it communication, call it by any word you like, emotional-commotional dialogue, any spiritual word, it's all yours. I am telling you confidentially, this is the ultimate truth. Therefore, don't be foolish. Women are also creatures, they are human beings. They have their degrees of faculty, of vastness and smallness. They have their degree of security, their degree of fulfillment, their degree of strength. But one way or another, this is all that they want. I know that this is shocking for you to learn but I must tell you certain fundamental things very directly. Every day you are making ridiculous mistakes, unconsciously, because of your lack of knowledge.

Now that you know what woman loves, what does man love? Does he love woman? No. Does he love the same things that woman loves? No. Man loves only one thing: man loves shelter. He loves the shelter of a confidant, the shelter of uplift and the shelter of a "cushion." It is the habit of a man to have some other person with whom he can talk about those things that he cannot discuss with just anybody. This confidential person is called a confidant.

To strengthen him, he needs a second kind of shelter. That is uplift. Somebody should uplift him. "Oh, don't worry, darling, you can create the heavens in your head." There will be one foolish phrase he wants to hear again and again, "I love your muscles." He may be as skinny as a crow. He may not have an ounce of meat on his entire arm, from his armpit to his fingers, but he loves to hear somebody saying in a soft voice, "Darling, I love these hard arms." You'll go insane without it, I can tell you that. It's a million dollar trip! You don't care what crazies she can take you through, what mud you have to be driven through, but that one phrase, "When you hug me, your bones really get into my inner rib," that's it. "God," she says, "I touched you and I flipped out into the skies." This guy feels far out. It's a big drum of 100-proof whiskey. He's drunk right there without a second thought that anything else exists on the planet. That one man must have that "whiskey" in a specific dose. He needs it. That is what he needs out of a woman. That is uplift and it is a shelter, too.

Then for security, he needs a "cushion". A cushion is also a shelter. Suppose the man fails. She won't let him fail. That's being a cushion. It is an extension of his Id. His Id must be extended through a woman: "Sweetheart, anything in the world I can do for you…."

So there are three types of shelter that man needs out of a woman. There are millions of outward things, such as physical attractiveness, sociability, all that, but basically, it is these three qualities which a man needs.

In America I have seen a woman who really has her man around her little finger. She says, "My lord, I am your genie." She closes her eyes and hangs her hand. She is the ugliest woman I have seen on this planet. I don't even like to look at her without colored glasses, but this man feels that she is a goddess. When I realized that he felt he had found a wonderland, I wanted to know what was in that woman that makes him so fond of her. She's not even competent enough to make good tea. When she served me, she messed it up; she was so lacking in manners that she gave me only a cup without a saucer. They move everything twice a year because she doesn't know how to maintain a house. She is very unclean. The guy has to have two maids, so I can understand how much he must be pinched for money. But in everything she asks, "My lord, what is thy command?"

It took me back 2,000 years into the Biblical age: here she was, uplifting the ego of this man, in this way, and providing the biggest cushion on the planet, the biggest cushion, and further, giving him the confidence that he undoubtedly, absolutely, has perfect control over this female creature. What happens? Such a man can go out and create heavens because man's world is outside. He has to go outside and fight. He leaves the inside. That is why when your woman is not in the dharma, you will end up in a mess; because the inward balance is dharma.

You are a creep one way or the other if you look at yourself. You do a lot of things to look good. Men do things to *look* good; women do things to *be* good. That is the difference between male and female. Can you understand the creative distance? You do a lot of things to look good because you are very social, because you want to see the world and be seen in the world. You will never see a man going out without looking at his collar. Woman studies fashion and dress totally to impress others. You dress to impress yourself. When you are impressed with yourself then you are convinced that you can impress another person. She doesn't care if she pleases herself. She looks at herself from the outside. Her concern is with the fashion of the day. She doesn't understand what will or will not suit her. The majority of women do not dress to suit themselves.

For your peace and tranquility, you need a dharmic woman. This is one aspect that you tend to forget in your relationships—sexual, material, mental, marriage, and otherwise. You need a church-going woman; you need a meditating woman; you need an intuitive woman; you need a creative woman. You need; it is the need for fulfillment. It is the easiest thing you need and you can get it. I want to give you the key. The key is to have a 100% sadhana. Right now you all do sadhana, but you miss 40%. On the average, no matter how 100% he may be, a man misses sadhana 40% mentally. Because he doesn't want to go, even 100% attendance means there is still 40% missing. When a woman goes, she goes 100% or she will not go at all. There is a difference between you and her.

I want to tell you a story of how such a 60% male can have such a 100% female without working hard. That's what you all came to find out, isn't it? You must establish a reputation of holiness with her. It is called "flower of maya." Leave no choice with her to get in and get out. You may not love church, but you must tell her that you love it and that it is your ultimate dream. You may not go to sadhana; but if you even think you cannot go, you tell her that you feel like death.

Once a woman confided to me that her husband was an angel. I asked her to tell me why. She was very shy. She wouldn't tell me, but I could read her mind. I said, "All right, I won't tell your husband." She said, "Oh, Yogiji, when we are making love, he always checks his watch. Though he never stops at two, three, four times, often until three o'clock, still he is looking at his watch and saying, 'We are messing up our sleep. We should be thinking of our sadhana.' I feel he's an angel." This is the guy who doesn't let her sleep! She's getting anemic, she's in terrible shape, she's boney, she's losing weight, and he has a need, a mental need, to have intercourse three to four times altogether. And though he's only Mr. In-and-Out and he's not a big deal either, he has built up a camouflage by looking at his watch, "Oh my God, it is two o'clock. All right, once more, but I think half an hour will be it. Just before three, dear, I think we can finish it."

What can you do? He has totally built up a complete confidence and mirage within her that sadhana is the only thing on the planet through which you can be saved. This is called "thought delivery method." You deliver the thought constantly. This is why it is said, "God is the only w-o-r-d, word, in the world." God is the only word in the world. You must remember it. Such men who understand the meaning of this word God are very rare. You must relate to the word God in your relations with woman, because in her basic intelligence, she is very creative, very vast, and her faculty is multiple. But then, man himself is multiple.

Man has many aspects of concentration, but only one direction can save him. That is, if he can pull his weight to that one word, God, call It any name you like. Just look into the history of man: take Moses, he carried his men through the desert for 40 years. Take Jesus, 32 years he led a band of people who revolted. Take Abraham, he led his folks like a flock. Take Buddha, who never believed in god, never denied God. Take all the Hindu gods and the Sikh gurus. For the sake of your own intelligence, take anybody and study. You will find that they are one-pointed, to a man, and that God is their Infinity. Elevate your consciousness to that. In any relationship where you want permanency, where you want Infinity, direct that relationship toward God—God and Guru.

When Guru Gobind Singh said, *"Ang sang wahe guru,"* it was the most brilliant of ideas. If you can really convince yourself that every limb, that every movement of your limbs is attached to Divinity, you can never accept disloyalty, betrayal, cheating or any kind of game. Under all circumstances, there's just one faculty a man needs and that's the faculty of *antar*, nucleus. The Name is the nucleus.

With all his circles and circling, with everything he does—he can go to the starting line or under it or cross over it—but for his ultimate clarity, man must find his base. His base is to find his base. But what base can you find if you do not have a base? If you do not build a base, what are you going to find? All men are motivated toward that end. When you pull your weight toward God, you pull more than the physical body. You have ten bodies in all. You have the physical, the spiritual, and the mental. The mental is, as a whole, called the "mental basic body"; it has three parts, mental plus and mental negative and mental neutral [Positive Mind, Negative Mind, and Neutral Mind]. So the mental body is three bodies; this gives you automatic protection mentally. Outside the mental body you have the arcline body (Noah's ark), the auric body, the subtle body, the pranic body, and the radiant body. Ten bodies.

When you deal with a woman, your ten bodies and her ten bodies must correspond, for these mental, projective, and basic reasons. If you fall in love because the woman is rich, then you have to understand you are poor. When you fall in love because she's creative, then you want to be complete because of her. When professional men marry a woman to carry them through their professional education, often when they complete their education and want to become established, they divorce their wives. This is because the focus of the relationship was motivation. In this case the motivation of both was for the man to become a professional. Motivation cannot be the focus of a relationship. Relationship has to be a **commitment**—commitment. That is, you must have meant to commit. If a woman ever finds out that you didn't mean to commit, she will think you are mean. Then she will misdirect all her productive intelligence.

Once there was a Mukhia Singh Sahib who wanted to leave [his wife]. Before leaving, he wanted an interview with me. He said, "Give me some leeway. One inch—I ask for one inch. Believe me, she'll come around, I'll be very grateful to you." I said, "Don't ask this." He said, "Please." I said, "All right, I'll give you one foot. Take care of yourself." Do you know what the result was? Today he's loitering in the streets like a mad man. One day he came to me. He was very angry. He said, "Father, happy birthday to you." I said, "Good son, may God's Grace be with you." He said, "That one foot of yours took everything away." I knew that that one inch of leeway would cause the dam to give way. Understand that if there is just one crack, the dam can totally give way to the entire body of water behind it—just one crack. How many times do you crack up? How many times can't you handle the situation? How many times do you say things that don't mean anything?

In our 3HO way, the majority of marriages are very strong because they have an outlet. "I'm going to call the Siri Singh Sahib." They may not call me, but the outlet is available. For most of the wives I have talked with, it is such a soothing bond. "Sir, he is out. I am talking to you privately." I say, "I am very private. Go on, what is it?" She tells me the whole thing. I say, "All right, I'll pray for you. Call me in two or three days." In two or three days, normally she'll become normal. I know that. I do nothing. Then she calls me, "Sir, everything went all right."

So what was it? A two or three dollar phone call, that's all. But there's an ultimate hook, an ultimate faith that there is someone she can talk to. She can express her grievance and she will not be betrayed. This attribute you need in yourself—not-to-betray. Not-to-betray is a different faculty—not to mean to betray. That's why we ask you to remember one phrase: commit unredeemably to Infinity. At that moment, we also deliver a thought of Infinity in you: that your commitment is like a commitment unto Infinity. The faculty in you to relate to Infinity is a very progressive thing. The beginning and the end may cross in any way, any form, any shape, at any velocity, it is all the same. Relating to Infinity breeds happiness, confidence, fulfillment, faith, joy, pride, relaxation, incentive, intelligence, and self-experience—ten.

Now please ask me the questions you need to ask, and let us clear the air.

Question and **Answer**

Q: You have presented a great deal of knowledge and I feel I don't know what to do with it. For instance, the ten bodies, if I try to apply that to myself in my own life, I don't know what to do with those ten bodies.

Yogi Bhajan: In action these bodies are in existence whether you like them or not. You can take care of them by studying their activity as you study the activity of the physical body. Try to interrelate them because they are interdependent.

If your pranic body is weak, your creativity, intelligence and intuition is weak. If your subtle body is weak, your judgment will be impaired. If your mental negative [Negative Mind] is weak, then you cannot defend yourself intuitively. If your mental positive [Positive Mind] is weak, you cannot penetrate through odds. If your mental base [Neutral Mind] is weak, you cannot be compassionate and fearlessly loving. If your spiritual body is not flowing, you'll be depressed to death.

Now, all those bodies have reactions on your physical body, your mood, activity, projection, and creativity. I am glad I got this chance to tell you that you have ten bodies because I know that you have only been aware of one body.

The tenth body, the radiant body, is your hair. Your hair controls the radiant body and the radiant body controls the hair. In times past when a man was captured and enslaved by another tribe, the first punishment was to shave his head, his armpits and his pubic hair.

Q: What technique can you use to assess within yourself the state of each of the ten bodies?

Yogi Bhajan: Without going into detail about the ten bodies, and taking ten years explaining them to you, simply use the technology of Kundalini Yoga. Do you remember that science known as Kundalini Yoga? It is earmarked to balance, to improve and to coordinate—balance, improve and coordinate—all of your ten bodies into the oneness of your life.

Q: Do the chakras correspond to the ten bodies?

Yogi Bhajan: The ten chakras have their action and reaction; the ten bodies have their action and reaction. Studying them will explain everything to you in detail. I'm just building a base. I want you to understand, you're all mature human beings. You're all male. You are the cream. You have sacrificed so much to become a male and to be a male and you are all males. Some of you are male chauvinists, some of you are all male ego—sick—some this, some that. I want you to understand what a male is. For you it looks like a post mail, stamped and delivered. That's not what I want. I want a male to be a male.

At the Las Vegas ashram, I met one lady who was a dealer in a casino. I said, "Dear, if you can deal in a casino, you can deal God also. Deal God to the people and they will listen to you." That's what I believe. I sincerely believe all your faculties and energies can be turned toward God.

I remember a friend of mine in India. He was a college student with me. One day he called me and said, "Bhajanji, you look like a very Godly man." I said, "I doubt very much that you even know me." He said, "Well, I feel like I know you a little bit. Bless me. I want to be a great politician." I was in a very good mood and I said, "So be it." He became a minister in the Janatha government. One day I was totally astonished to receive a phone call from him. I said, "Whoa, some minister is calling from India. What is it?" He said, "Hi, Yogiji. How are you?" I said, "I'm very fine." He said, "You cheated me!" I said, "What is wrong with you?" He said, "You blessed me to be a politician and you became a man of God. Man, you are wonderful and I am in bad shape. Can we reverse the blessing?" I said, "What is the problem?" He said, "I understand that you are enjoying life, you are doing all right. Look, we are hassling here and I do not know how many days more the ministry will last. I remember your words. God, I wish at that time I had asked to be a man of God and you the politician. Now we are the politicians and the politicians are looking to you." We had further conversation like old friends and buddies, but what

I'm trying to tell you is that the real faculty in you is the faculty of Infinity. I believe that you can be so creative and so much a genius that the entire world will come to you. I believe that that is your ordinary basic state.

Q: Can you explain circumvent force and magnetic force?

Yogi Bhajan: The circumvent force is our radiant body, which protects us. The magnetic field is our pranic body. When the pranic body switches off, in spite of your having a most healthy looking physical body, you are dead. Your heart won't pump, your blood won't circulate, your brain won't function.

Q: Sir, this summer you said a lot of things about men to the ladies...

Yogi Bhajan: Yes. I classified the man and his basic negativities—that was the ladies' course. You can read those notes. I don't have time to tell you all those things here. I told the women all the worst things about the men—all of them. I bundled them all up. Then the second month, I explained to them how to take care of those negativities.

Q: Didn't that make a problem for the ladies who could not stay for the second session?

Yogi Bhajan: We're taking care of that and we won't have that problem again. Next year, Khalsa Women's Training Camp will be for six weeks only. We are not breaking it into two intervals. We realize there's so much to teach and there's such a short time. We realize the difficulty. A lot of ladies could not afford to stay for the second session and we had to convince them that it was useless to hear the first part and not the second part. Now we have covered that mistake.

Q: Sir, many times you've made reference to the big computer in the sky constantly making mistakes in the Creation. If God is perfect in Its Infinity, how could this be?

Yogi Bhajan: God is perfect in Its Infinity, but the Creativity is also subject to the faculty of His resources of power; and every orbit, however clean and perfect it is, has the tendency to go out of orbit sometimes. Anything that has an orbit can go out of orbit. It's hard to believe, but it's a reality. As long as God is One, It's perfect. Whenever It's two, then there's a polarity—plus and minus—and you have to deal with it. For your sensitivity, God is perfect, agreed; for my sensitivity, God is a mess. When you work in a locomotive shop, you get a lot of grease. Do you know what I mean?

We who deal with this whole creative science of God see things happening and sometimes we laugh and sometimes we get totally depressed, but that's the way it is. I think God does that with one intention: to make us the most compassionate people. That's why we can't get angry at anybody. Our commitment is like Infinity because we understand that the most perfect, the Creative One, can mess things up. So what does it matter if His Creation gets messed up, or His creatures get messed up, or that we sometimes make errors? So long as it is not intentional, it's all right. It gives you an ultimate hope.

Q: Why are our men's courses only two days and the women's course is six weeks?

Yogi Bhajan: This is because the women need more rest than the men. In this country, woman has been so abused, so misused and so much negated that is takes us about two months to get them together and create them together so that we can send them back super-positive. That's the motivation of those ladies' courses. When they go back, we want them to go as super-positive and to keep going so that there may be less hassle in life.

You have to understand that the most important, the most time-consuming, nerve-consuming, intelligence-consuming, most creative job on this planet earth is to raise a child to be a saint, perfect. Few people appreciate this. If you make dollars and your wife makes dollars and together you make lots of dollars and you are very rich and you are living fine, when your child, your daughter, is 14 and runs away from home, what use is your life?

We want our children and our future generations to guard against that totally and absolutely. We want the woman to be so strong; basically, we want her to be so creative, so intelligent, so compassionate and so giving that she can handle this child-raising situation totally. This will take years to accomplish. That is why I ask the men—I even call them personally—to send their wives to Ladies' Camp. Although we never break even in the Ladies' Camp—it is always a game—we feel that we gain so much out of it, toward creating a substantial woman and home and marriage unit, that its value is priceless.

Q: What did you mean when you said, "meant to commit"?

Yogi Bhajan: I said it, I wrote it, and not only did I say it and write it, I said, "You must mean to." Your underlying meaningful purpose of life is that you must mean. That is why I broke the word commitment into "commit" "meant". That was the punch line of the day. In this first part of the course, I am letting you know the woman's version of a man.

Q: Is there any difference between how a woman and a man meditate on God, how they conceive of God, how they relate to God?

Yogi Bhajan: Woman seeks creativity, conception, in everything. Man seeks ejaculation in everything. That's how the two are totally different. The woman wants to feel God. "It is there." Man wants to reach out to God. He enjoys reaching out; she enjoys feeling it. She wants you to be God-like when you come home. You want to go out and see the feeling, God-like.

Have you seen the movie "Ten"? It's the best example, psychologically and analytically, of how you behave toward what you think woman is and how she reacts to what she thinks you are. It's so well done, it's unbelievable. I would definitely recommend that you, as men, see this movie. It is very, very eye opening. It shows what you think it is and what it really is. Actually the title should be, "All That Glitters Is Not Gold". The basic line has been communicated so heavily that a lot of people come out very depressed. But I think it's good to go through that depression and see it on the screen. It will be helpful to you because you are in the habit of seeing things on the screen.

Q: I'm not clear on some of the aspects of male consciousness that you have described. For example, "Men do things to look good and women do things to be good." Is this something we can overcome or is it something we have to learn to accept?

Yogi Bhajan: Please understand, I am not presenting you with a problem. This course is to describe the basic multiple man. In this part, I am giving you the overall picture and overall faculty of male consciousness from any angle or from all the angles that are possible. It is not that we have to believe to conceive that's the end of the world. We have to proceed yet further.

Q: Could you explain what you mean when you describe man as seeking ejaculation in everything?

Yogi Bhajan: Ejaculation is to project out. Have you seen men running in a race? Suppose a man is capable of running one mile, he'll make a mile and a half his goal. He may reach two miles; and then he'll put his head into the sand. Have you seen men running on the beach? They feel they can go a particular distance, then they aim to complete a distance half again as far. They may try to go even further than that goal and they'll even pull all their muscles doing it.

Overdoing things: this is a basic male faculty. Making a big thing out of it is like the psychiatrist who analyzed men by the way they put their legs into their pajamas. Pajamas are made by sewing a left leg and a right leg together. That's all. To say that the left leg means this, the right legs means that makes no sense to me. Male chauvinism, male machismo doesn't mean anything. It's a basic male faculty, that's what a male is. He wants to ejaculate, complete the action, and then he wants to fall to the level of zero. Zero to one hundred, one hundred to zero—that is his circuit.

Q: Is there a way that we can use that kind of energy for our own spiritual growth?

Yogi Bhajan: Yes, you can use it. It's called rebound energy. When you want to rest, instead of just falling and resting you can either slip into a sleep, or you can slip into a fanciful thought. It's called a plus thought. You've got a great friend in your plus mind. Present your mind with a situation: "All right, if I build a room, how will I build it?" Go over it for half an hour. It doesn't even matter if the room is already built, think how you would build it. Be fanciful with it. If you were to build the Golden Temple, how would you build it? That kind of projection is very essential to qualify every male.

Challenges and the **Man**

Jealousy is self-animosity. You share it with a partner as a matter of confidence, of directness, but actually you create self-animosity within the partner and in this way you strain the relationship rather than building the relationship. You start projecting fears.

What we are trying to build in you is a very stable state of mind. Remember, and bear with me, that although it happens, I want you to understand that divorce is a curse. Nothing happens to one only. It is a curse for both partners. You can never forget it, you can never outlive it, you can never get out of it. Whether you like it or not, a fact is a fact. However, I want to communicate to you that that situation can be avoided very easily by mutual development. Mutual trust is one thing which can keep this unfortunate situation from happening.

I know that in certain cases I have agreed to divorce. Those cases concern particular women who have extreme father phobia and the circumstances have been such that we didn't recognize the condition until very, very late. In the case of such women, you can be aware that the situation is developing when the moment the woman gets a child, and the child becomes one or two years old, the woman starts slipping. That is the sign. Each particular case has to be immediately discovered and very closely watched. It is just like hepatitis: if you discover it in time, you can cure it; later on it becomes too late. The main symptom of that problem [father phobia] is that she will bear with you spiritually, physically, emotionally, and commotionally until she gets a child that she can hang on to for security.

When she begins to slip, the first thing she does is she stops wearing her turban. That's how it starts at first. Then she'll start negating other values and one day, you will find that she wants to go and blah, blah, blah, the whole story. The best way to handle the situation is to catch her at the beginning and take care of it.

There are some women who have a lot of doubts about their men. This has been handled very successfully by asking these women to come to the Secretariat and work. In this way they feel and understand that they are part of the family. They know Yogi Bhajan is a very compassionate man. It doesn't matter; that really doesn't matter. What matters is that they see that 3HO is a huge organization, working for the fulfillment of something. When they see that there are hundreds of calls every day, hundreds of letters coming in and hundreds going out, that there are certain dedicated people working, and that there is a total energy happening, then they feel that "one-in-a-million feeling" that is called nucleus.

When a woman finds there's a nucleus other than her husband—now try to remember this, because you must build it in her—when your wife knows that there's another nucleus she can lean on equally well, you'll be safe. In the realms of consciousness, it's called a safety valve. That's why we request every teacher to send his wife as a volunteer to the Secretariat. She must learn that she is not the only one who has a problem; she's not the only one who calls; she's not the only one who receives letters; she's not the only one who has to look to just one man and beyond that there's no world. The truth is that there's a huge ocean of world and a lot of boats like hers—that gives her a lot of support. That is why in Ladies' Camp, we work exclusively to build her moral values and character. Basic woman is basic woman.

Now we find that we have a problem of "re-entry," re-entry into domestic life. We are trying to give her the perspective that she's not alone in this world. What we are trying to tell you is that restriction you put on her out of jealousy—"You choose me against this, me against that"—is your own shortcoming. Do you get the message?

We want you to prosper; we want you to remain married; we want you to become rich; we want you to be healthy, happy and holy; because, therein lies our salvation. So we are in no way and in no shape trying to work against your male ego. After all, our ego is a part of your ego. How can a part work against the whole and the whole against a part? Basically, you must understand, if we will not allow our women to have a broader view of things, deal with a broader family of life, and have a broadened social spectrum of life, we'll actually bring the devil of divorce to our own gate.

I called one teacher: "Why don't you visit such-and-such a family. They may be lonely. Call them. Invite them over. Get your scene together so that you can have that feeling of your own goodness." The important thing is that you should experience your own goodness. Some people do not want to socialize because they are afraid their social values and weaknesses shall be known. My idea is that your weaknesses and values are going to be known anyway; so if divorce can be avoided, it's worthwhile.

Every day for two sessions of four weeks each, I sit with the ladies. I come to tell them that they shall not be betrayed. You have to understand fundamentally and positively that 3HO is one organization that can say proudly that it has not betrayed, dumped, or abandoned anyone in its ten years of existence. Not a single person can come forth and say, "We met with injustice in the hands of this organization." In ten years, we have not said a single negative thing; we have not lied to anybody in a single aspect of life. We have inspired; neither have we hired, nor have we fired. We have inspired everybody to his full potential.

We believe the strength of the man is in the challenge: the higher the challenge, the higher the man's capacity to meet it, the higher is his achievement in life. Challenge is not something that destroys you; challenge is something that gives you an experience.

Unfortunately, everybody differs from everybody else; everybody's circumstances differ; everybody's aspect and prospect are different; everybody's moods, needs and faculties are different from everybody else's, as are their desires, body odor, physical approach, and mental approach. There cannot be a general law because humans are different. We must understand in 3HO, we put our greatest emphasis on respecting individuality and individual privacy. We believe that if an individual is strong, society is strong; and a strong society will provide a shelter for the individual. Therefore, our main objective is to build a strong individual.

Now here we are in a men's course. We want to build a strong man of you. Not so that you become macho; not so that you become self-destructive; but so that you can handle every challenge you face. We believe the strength of the man is in the challenge: the higher the challenge, the higher the man's capacity to meet it, the higher is his achievement in life. Challenge is not something that destroys you; challenge is something that gives you an experience. I can't believe how anything can be wrong with you guys; after all, our philosophy is to live for each other. The whole system is for you.

One night a male teacher called me. It was almost 12:30, so God must have been sleeping. I saw the blinking line, picked up the phone and said, "Sat Nam." He said, "Oh, Yogiji, how come you answered the phone?" I said, "I am working." He said, "I want desperately to talk with you." I said, "What is it?" He told me that his father had come and had given him three proposals. He didn't know what to do and was very confused.

I said, "All right, you take a paper and pencil. Give me the proposals." He gave me the three proposals. I analyzed them and he wrote it all down. When I was finished, he said, "What should I do?" I said, "That I can't tell you. I want you to make your own decision." "Why, sir? I want you to do it. I want to do what you tell me to do." I said, "I am the last person to tell you what to do. I want you to decide. I have given you the pros and cons accurately. I have actually analyzed this before you and now I want to see what you decide."

Three days later he called me and said, "I have gone over it, I have thought about it, and I have decided. Am I right or wrong?" I said, "Discuss it with your dad." He said, "What does that mean?" I said, "It depends on how you deliver the goods. It is not what the goods are." He sat down with his father, he talked, and he came out 40% successful. He called me, "I am 40% successful." I said, "Do you have a father-in-law?" He said "Yes." I asked, "Friend or enemy?" He said, "My father-in-law is a great friend of mine." I said, "Discuss it with him and ask him to call your father."

When he discussed the story with his father-in-law, his father-in-law took a plane and flew in. He met the father and took him out. The two fathers discussed for two days. Finally when the father-in-law left, the father felt absolutely satisfied knowing that another American, like himself, supports his son much more than he does and was telling him so. Then a call came to me, "Yogiji, I am grateful. You are a miracle man." I said, "No. I do not want to be known as a miracle man. I just want to be known as a man who believes in wisdom."

That's what I believe: I believe that you are wise enough to answer every question. Your failure is when you don't mean to commit. Because without a base, without your bolting and nailing yourself to the situation, you will never find the answer. You may want to have the answer, you may badly need the answer, you may try to have the answer, you may do everything else; but without your nucleus, there is no answer. As you shift, everything will shift with you. Figure it out. Are you going to live with this woman or not? Are you going to be with this situation or not? If you are going to be, then go through with everything! And don't forget how you started with her and how you want to end with her.

There are a lot of things to deal with—future, present and past. I'll tell you that every call comes in during the time they call timelessness. So you must deal with it timelessly within the time. Remember that: you must deal with every situation timelessly within the time. That's the basic concept we are working with. If you think there will be no problems, I don't believe it. If you think you can solve all the problems, I don't believe that either. All I believe is that as time approaches you with the problem, you must approach it with the answer. That is all the woman needs, because leaning on Infinity within the finite circumstances is the secret of success.

Now I want to introduce Hari Har Kaur. She has been with the ladies throughout the summer and she has listened to a lot of wives and a lot of their complaints. She knows how to express their side to you. Are there any questions which you would like to ask Hari Har Kaur?

Q: What would the women like to have in their men?

Yogi Bhajan: I know what they want. I know what every woman wants. Women want saints, heroes and givers. That which they want to produce, they want to have. Say it in your American English.

Hari Har Kaur: They want a man who's great, strong, supportive, understanding, open, totally devoted, respectful to Yogi Bhajan, their Teacher, and humble before God and Guru. That's what they want. They want a saint. Even if they won't admit it, even the women who don't seem to be as devoted or fanatic, want that.

Yogi Bhajan: Let me sum it up: they want a sexual saint. Is my one line right? They want a sexual saint. Nothing less and nothing more can satisfy them.

Q: Is that only true of American women or is it true of all women?

Yogi Bhajan: Political territories don't make any sense to me.

Q: I'm really trying to support my wife's being in Ladies' Camp. Your talk has made me examine how I may subtly undermine it. My question is this: my wife is one of those people who loses weight during the summer and gains it back in the fall. Do you have any suggestions as to how I can help her?

Yogi Bhajan: Yes, I have a suggestion. Be a husband. Tell her that you want a skinny wife. Tell her that you are most pleased with her skinniness. When she eats, pray to God and eat less with her. Bear with her. What we do—we don't create any miracle—we bear with them. We *be* with them. You do not know how much we inspire every woman to belong to her husband. We read sentences from Gurmukhi, from Gurbani, and we tell them the story of how ultimately, her husband should be as God. If she neglects her husband, she becomes less human. We do everything we can. I'll tell you the main difficulty: we build up the husband as a solution for her, and when she comes back, she doesn't find that. It comes as a shock to her. We are offering that re-entry program so that when she gets back home, she will not feel handicapped.

Q: When a woman is feeling insecure, how can I help her out of it?

Yogi Bhajan: When a woman feels insecure, she only feels that way because you have said something, directly or indirectly, that shows that your faith is trembling. It's called "earthquake." If you can rebuild that area, you will find that she will immediately recuperate. You must not see a negative woman as a bad instance—that negativity started six months previously. You know when the earthquake comes, the center is always 40 miles away; the shock is always at a different point. That's the point you have to understand.

Q: Is the material covered at Ladies' Camp meant for the ladies to use by themselves or are there some facets of it that are incorporated into ashram life, and should these be shared with the men in the ashram so that they can work on them together?

Hari Har Kaur: At one time, Yogi Bhajan said that certain pages of the notes from Ladies' Camp should be casually left on the dresser so that the man would pick them up and say, "Oh, what's this?" Those pages would contain solutions to some of the problems the couples were having. All that information is definitely supposed to be shared and used. Mainly the woman has to incorporate it into her being, but it's also to be used and read by the men, by husbands and wives together.

Q: Should this information from the men's course also be shared with the women?

Yogi Bhajan: The first question your wife is going to ask you is, "What did you learn there?" That means the start of a communication.

We don't want you to *not* share any knowledge, to *not* ask questions, to *not* doubt any statement. We only want you to understand, we do not want you to feel shy. That's why we have separated these courses so you won't feel embarrassed by any situation. You can ask any question. You can ask any question with any freedom you like. In fact, this year at camp, the ladies asked that all the working men either hide themselves or be eliminated from the camp because the women could not ask certain question that they wished to ask. We provided that facility. In the same way, we want to provide you with that facility.

Q: You talk a lot about male-female relationships between married partners and I guess that's understandable in 3HO, but do you have something that single women in Ladies' Camp talk about and would like that they are not getting? Or do you have some advice for single men?

Hari Har Kaur: I think for women, most of the time before marriage is spent working on themselves, strengthening their sadhana, and preparing, ultimately in this lifestyle, to be married. So if you're asking, how are single male-female relationships supposed to go? I would say they don't really go anywhere unless they're praying for marriage. Is that what you're asking?

The single women are not taught in detail how they're supposed to relate to the single men because they're to relate to them as their brothers and they are taught to serve just as they would serve a brother. There's not a lot of emphasis on it because we don't have dating or that kind of socialization. It's not part of our system.

Yogi Bhajan: But they still date, sneakily.

Hari Har Kaur: We try to work on that at camp, too. We try to teach the women how not to be flirtatious, how to relate from their soul and not from their ego, and how to be patient and wait without being totally hung-up on getting married or having crushes on man after man, or having a crush on a man and pulling him away from his sadhana, and things like that.

Yogi Bhajan: Mostly we work on the single women so that they understand what the patterns were that lead them to any mistake that they have gone through, and how to eliminate those and not rebuild them in their future relationships. That is the main emphasis with the single woman.

Q: You mentioned about women begging their husbands to go to Ladies' Camp, and that the men aren't supporting them to go. However, I've noticed in ashram life that there's a love-hate relationship within the individual women themselves, and they're terrified to go to Ladies' Camp. A woman may have basic control over her husband and the finances and may drive a fancy car and have everything she wants, but when it comes to Ladies' Camp, all of a sudden money is short and she can only go for a week. These women go for a short time and are not at all into it. I'm wondering how to address that.

Yogi Bhajan: I'll answer that. Now try to understand this very minutely and accurately. These are the few basic patterns you will find in every woman: a: Idealistic Conflict of Harmony and Disharmony and b: Basic Thought.

These inter-cutting triangles represent conflict and the zigzag circles that cut through the circles represent the idealist conflict of harmony and disharmony. Then there is what is called "basic thought." It has "I" in it. That part may or may not be.

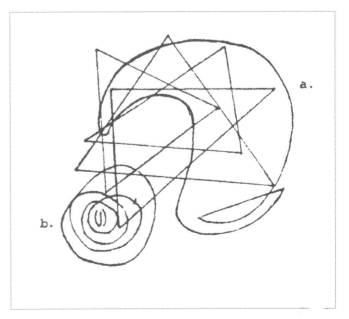

Because these patterns exist, they have to be dealt with. Always approach these basic behaviors in three ways: come down; go up; ask her to go up and bring up down. Do not create a confrontation. It is called "open communication." Create open communication through every conflict, argument, and situation. For example, she says, "I am fed up with you." "What did you say?" "I'm fed up with you." "All right, now tell me what you fed that made you so much up?" Break up the expression "fed up," and then sit like a yogi.

Then what do you do? Make her speak. The first art is the art of listening. Don't let the thing get dried out, keep urging her to speak, let her express herself. If she cannot say it to you, ask her to say it to anybody, everybody, somebody. Your basic responsibility is to meet the conflict when there is a conflict.

The Polarities: **Personal and Impersonal**

In every person, there's a plus and minus; in every person, there's an up and down; in every person, there's a potency and impotency. If it's 40:60, you're safe; 50:50, far out; 20:80, forget it; 10:90, you are miserable. Sometimes you are dealing with a living misery. Have you seen me talking to you when your aura reflects total negativity? I yell! Then I say, "All right, now what do you want to say?" You can't figure it out. You say, "Well, what is he doing? First he yells at me and now he wants me to tell him what I want." I can do it because I'm not involved. That is uninvolved conversation. With every personal there is the impersonal.

Every communication should be personal and impersonal at the same time. For the one part that is fighting with you or loving you, there is also another part that is in reverse that is not at play. Don't forget that part, which is not at play. If there's prosperity, disaster is not at play. If there is a disaster, prosperity is not at play. Always examine everything impersonally–personally. That's the line. Confront the conflict. Examine every communication personally in the impersonal state of mind.

Now I want to explain how you can get through it: "All right, you feel tired of telling me things. I feel tired because you feel tired. I feel tired, you feel tired. Within 72 hours, tell me what you expect of me so that you will not feel tired." Give the woman 72 hours so that she is off your back those 72 hours. You always need breathing time. Remember that. Create breathing time.

Ida, pingala, underneath is *shushmana*. This is also the picture of the female.

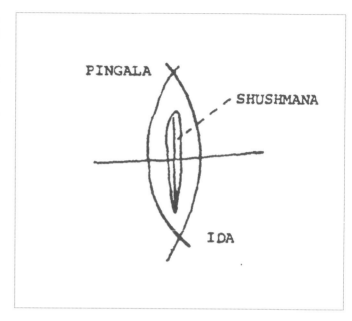

This is most important. The measure here, at the line, is 0.0 and you must stretch it out to give you a breathing part.

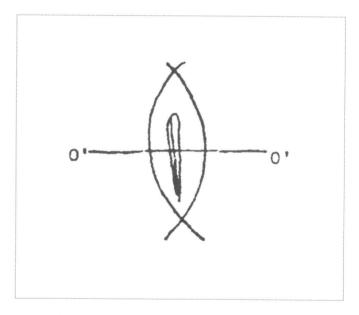

Remember *prana*, breathing, is what life is about. Life is about *prana*; *prana* is about life. So, please, under any circumstances, if you cannot avoid the conflict, make a breathing space. Give your *prana* a chance to earn time. Whosoever can earn time will emerge successful. The purpose of life is time alone.

Are there any further questions?

Q: You said whenever you speak, to speak just one line.

Yogi Bhajan: Yes. Make a punch line of the idea you want to express.

Q: Every time you speak?

Yogi Bhajan: No, no. If you want to rap, rap. That is your problem if you have a lot of time, but there has to be a punch line to communicate.

Q: What is the line across the shushmuna?

Yogi Bhajan: That is zero:zero (0.0). That is to give yourself a stretch, to give yourself an opening. Don't leave a conversation without an opening. A dead end is a dead end. Don't create dead-end communications.

Q: You said that man is only at sadhana 40% of the time. Is there any way to cure that?

Yogi Bhajan: Oh, yes. A lot of people are curing it. That's what practice is. Mentally—mental, up, sadhana, okay, aaaahhh; that is the victory. Victory is not going to sadhana; victory is getting up for sadhana. "Oh, damn sadhana, but okay." That's victory. The victory of the self is when you totally fight a mortal battle and that everyday battle is a mental victory. Fight to rise, and then you rise, then you are risen. That is called excellence. It is the first part of it which is excellence.

Q: You were saying at the beginning that some people go to sadhana and they're just 40% there, but they won the fight to get up so didn't they win the whole thing?

Yogi Bhajan: Yes. Sometimes you don't need an alarm, you don't need to set the time, you always know when to get up. That is perfection. Practice makes you perfect. I'm talking about basics. I'm talking about the elementary multiple man; I'm not talking about the accomplished man. That's the next session.

Q: You mentioned that each of us can handle three chakras at one time in our communication. Is there a way to develop the capacity consciously so that we can use it?

Yogi Bhajan: That is an ordinary, basic capacity. As an accomplishment, you can handle all the chakras, all the time, at the same time. You can also control the frequency, projection, reversal relevancy, reversal projection, reversal projection into relevancy of effectiveness, and cause and effectiveness in relationship to present, past and future; and future into present into the build-up for leaving a gap, which causes a vacuum and not returning to the vacuum; or returning to the vacuum as the case may be. Did I say it all? That was only one part of it.

Q: A while back you discussed the relationship of Infinity. You listed happiness, confidence, etc. You said that the beginning and the end may cross at any place at the same time. I didn't understand what you meant.

Yogi Bhajan: Sometimes there's a conflict. That's what I meant by beginning and end. You can collide in the course. If you have an understanding of keeping going, then you can get up and keep going.

Q: You drew a spiral. What does it represent?

Yogi Bhajan: Communication, life, thought, living together, conflicting, non-conflicting…

May the long time sun shine upon you. Sat Nam. SA sound of Infinity, TA sound of life, NA sound of conquering death, MA sound of resurrection. All that is contained in the Christ Consciousness is hidden in the four folds of this word into the fifth of Infinity. May the consciousness become higher and higher, and highest of the highest. May we sacrifice the ego to receive, and resurrect our own Self into the domain of light, to the Grace of God, to merge in God Itself. Sat Nam.

The Growing **Man**

There is only one way to relate to a woman and that is to relate to her as a woman. Period. Do not think that she's your mother, or that she's your friend, or your enemy, or your this or your that.

Whenever you want to relate to a woman, just relate to a woman. Period. You may be able to make anything out of anybody, but you can never change a woman to anything other than a woman; and you can never change a man to anything other than a man, though many methods have been tried. Not to treat a woman as a woman is the first fundamental fault of any man. He will either lose her or misconceive her. To misconceive her, in her essence, means that she becomes your mother, or she becomes your friend only, or she becomes your wife only, and not your friend. When you do this, you miss the totality of the woman.

You will find that some men reach a certain stage when they start growing their beard. Have you seen that? That is the sign that the man wants the woman to be a woman. A man is a fundamental relationship; there should not be a conflict of interest. When you try to relate to an interest group, that is when you have to compromise. You may compromise only a little at first, or you may compromise fully; but you never forget the compromise, nor does she. Then the bickering begins.

Treat a woman as a woman. Don't treat her as a goddess, don't treat her as a second class citizen, don't treat her as a friend, don't treat her as an enemy, and don't treat her as somebody you have an arrangement with. No compromise—just treat her gracefully, as a woman, so that she can treat you as a graceful man. That's one ideology that works 100%. Are there any questions? Have you read your notes from the first session? Could you make something out of them?

Q: One thing that I didn't understand was that you said the relationship can only be based on commitment, not on motivation. What did you mean by motivation?

Yogi Bhajan: Sometimes you are hard, you feel sexy, you feel lonely, you want to have a woman. You will just grab a woman and get into it without knowing the length, breadth, depth, water current, anything. It won't work. Anything that you have not worked out shall not work. Commitment means to go through all the pros and cons in the possibility of the relationship. Think about it. Be clean about it. Explain it. Elaborate on it. And don't try to grab her individuality and represent her; let her represent herself, so that you can have a complete understanding of what you want.

Commitment based on emotion is no commitment. Commitment based on commotion is not commitment at all. Commitment based on neurosis is totally self-treachery. Commitment is when both parties freely, totally, cleanly understand the bases and then commit to those fundamental bases. That's called commitment.

Q: In the first session, you gave examples of how the woman fulfills the three shelters that a man needs. Would you give examples of how we can fulfill a woman's need for fulfillment, security, and strength?

Yogi Bhajan: That is what I am going to talk about in this session: What does woman look to in man? I'm going to complete "Growing Man." Previously I talked about "Multiple Man," the multiple power of you. Now I want to interrelate it and integrate it with what the woman wants to look to.

For example, there's one class of woman who comes to 3HO, she commits herself, she looks very religious, she attracts a man, she marries a man, she has a child; then she leaves her sadhana, she leaves her turban, she leaves her *bana*, she leaves all the values, and after that, she splits. Now this is a woman who has totally engendered within her an image called father phobia. She will do it again and again. One part of her will be excellent, perfect, precise, magnetic, but the moment she makes the kill, she will flip and go through the other part of it.

You have to investigate this before getting married, not after getting married. When you don't investigate everything beforehand, when you don't put your cards on the table and make sure she puts hers out, then you do not communicate and establish a relationship; you do not establish a basic bond. The emotions don't have anywhere else to take you but to commotion, commotion to drama, drama to trauma, trauma to disaster. That's the path.

It is very shocking that in 3HO, where we are willing to counsel anybody, analyze everybody's problems and tell them what to do, people still cannot handle themselves emotionally. That is what we are trying to relate to. If socially a girl is just a girl to you—well, my God, she's not "just a girl"! You're going to put a lot into it, and if all you get out of her is a disaster, there is something fundamentally wrong in your behavior. Don't start that way.

Q: What kinds of questions would you ask to investigate whether or not she has a father phobia?

Yogi Bhajan: I'd check her history from her third year to the present. Then I'd ask her to share all the possible experiences she has had in her life, knowing that I'll share my experience, too. I'll even make up an experience to see what she relates to and how she relates to it. I'd like to check her totally inside-out, and then I'd like to see whether her tendency is toward the earth or toward the ether. I'll watch how she comes to gurdwara. I'll say things like, "I'm not going to go to gurdwara today" and see whether she pulls me out or not. I would like to see where her pull is. If her pull is toward God, I'll be sure that she'll make it. If her pull is toward the earth, she's going to let me down, any day. That is what I'm going to look into.

I'm not going to look into the superficial things: "Oh, she's beautiful." Today she's beautiful, tomorrow she gets diarrhea, the day after that she doesn't look beautiful, then what happens to my neurotic image? I am not willing to make a relationship that is temporary. Marriage is not a temporary relationship to begin with. It's not a friendship; it's not a living arrangement. It has to be worked out on such a mutual frequency of give and take that we always feel secure. Marriage is a relationship that grants you security—that's the fundamental marriage.

Q: What type of father causes father phobia?

Yogi Bhajan: Father phobia is a very heavy situation. If the father is a banana, and if she then hates her father, she will hate every man. If the father has tortured her, she will want to destroy.

I know one woman and this is what she does. She's far out. There's nothing wrong that you can pinpoint. She is extremely perfect. She meets a man and raises him to a plateau, then brings him to the edge where there is a 30,000 foot drop into a deep stone pond—that's where she wants to push him. In her life, 96 men have met with that tragedy. Ninety-six men she has ruined completely. She brought them to that point, she totally bewitched them and they had nothing to say. With all 96, she did one thing: one morning they got up, after having had a beautiful night with her, and found that she had gone. There was no note and they never knew where she went. She never called. She never talked. She never communicated in any way. She had been their therapist, their counselor, their provider, their sex dream. She was everything to them.

When seven years have gone by, I'll see what she has become. She's insane to that extent. She can meet you and enchant you. Fifteen minutes is a long time for her, I'll give her ten minutes. She can totally charm you, go all over you—your laundry will be done, your underwear will be pressed, your boots will be shining. She'll be half an hour earlier than you and all your appointments will be made.

You can name anything in the world, but when a certain time passes, when the man is totally saturated, when he no longer looks to anything else, then it happens. I asked her one question, "What is your signal to leave?" She said, "The day he has no friend to call and he throws away his telephone book, that's the signal for me. The next day I leave." This relates to her father phobia.

There's another girl that we just lost (she comes back and forth). We had been working on her. She just wants to be with you. She's so spiritual to talk to that you think she is not born out of a woman, but that she came from the heavens. She's right there. She talks about God, and everything. She sleeps with you; she makes love to you; she tells you everything—far out. After a while, you realize you can't sleep with her every night and make love to her. You can go for five nights, six, eight, even ten nights—fifteen nights, maximum. After all you are a human being, you also have some cycles. The night you miss her, you'll miss her. She'll be gone. There's not a single man on this planet that can go on and on continuously. Even the craziest man can't do it; but that is her phobia. The day you have not made love to her, she feels you are not in love with her; therefore, there's no use living with you.

All these hidden faculties are there because the American woman is not innocent. Most of them have lost their virginity, and most of them have 10, 20, 30 relationships. They know how to sell their bodies and exhibit their bodies and play with their bodies and they think that you are just another creep. You think you are the Romeo of the world. So, the bridge has to be built between Romeo and creep

Yogi Tea and **Other Ordinary Things**

Now, how many of you honestly and regularly take Yogi Tea? In your lives you are not drinking Yogi Tea. Not drinking Yogi Tea means that you have no backup for your nervous system. Drink it every day. It's a regular food. It's a part of your life. It will always save you—your nerves and your work capacity. It will save you from viruses and it will save you from many, many deficiencies.

Also, you are not drinking enough whey and you have forgotten to drink Golden Milk. I'm just reminding you of the ordinary things. These are ordinary things. Whey will clean your kidneys; Golden Milk can save you from arthritis; Yogi Tea can give you a beautifully working nervous system. Why don't you use them?

and nobody knows where the end shall be. You need to build a bridge, right? The Mississippi Bridge was built. The engineers must have considered many factors—depth, length, current. They must have considered the whole system. They studied the history of the river, the accidents and incidents. Then they planned and they determined the strength the bridge would need for a lifespan of 200 years. They figured out the whole thing. Why can't you do that in your own relationship? Talk. Figure it out.

There are men who really, really make trouble for themselves. When the woman says, "Come on, get up for sadhana," he says, "Leave me alone. I was watching TV late. I can't get up." She will say, "Okay, you won't get up." But I can tell you, you have lost all respect before her. When a woman gives a call and you cannot answer—and the call is righteous—you are totally ruining yourself before that woman. It's very important to establish your male faculty to be a leader.

Let me tell you that as a leader you have to understand, whether you want to or not, that you are the sun. You are the sun as the male and she's the moon as the female. (She loses the faculty when her menstruation stops). She fluctuates 28 days, 6 hours; that is her normal cycle, her rhythm. You have no rhythm. Your faculty is stationary. Therefore, your commitment, your communication, your caliber, your projection, your project, your everything has one thing—the sun—the underlying fixed sign. You must prove that you are fixed, you are committed, you are it. You have to set up a behavior wherein you plan, you ask for opinions, you do everything to look absolutely democratic, but in doing so, you cannot forget that one important faculty—the faculty of the "it". This is the main faculty to which the woman looks. She fluctuates, she wanes and waxes. If she finds that you are it, you shall be it, but if you cater to her, she will never cater to you. All she needs is a little crack, a little crack in your personality and you will lose miles.

There's a saying about woman: give her an inch, you have to work out for a mile. That is as simple as it is honest. She can play and pretend that you are always compassionate and giving, but if she catches you in your dishonesty, forget it. You have to understand that the basic personality of woman is to conceive. When the little spermatozoa goes in, she conceives and produces a baby. She can grow anything into conception—even a concept. It is the faculty of her aura.

She never forgets any man who comes into her life. You don't remember for more than one moon—28 days. The fastest you can change your emotions is within 20 days, 28 days, 30 days maximum. She won't forget a person for life, though she'll pretend and say, "Oh, I don't remember." So you have to provide her with a stationary, constant value—and that value is radiance. Your wife must know, or be convinced, or should think that you are trying to be a saint. "My husband is a saint." Do you understand that expression? "Saint" does not mean that you have to wear certain types of clothes and do certain types of things, but that you have to give a certain type of impression that you are very righteous, very self-contained, and very sweet.

For a growing man, certain things have to be remembered. A woman may do a lot of things. If she is provoking you to anger and you are not relating angrily when she is saying certain things that are morally hurting you, you don't deserve to be a man. There are two standards: you do not tolerate moral insult, nor do you react to any trap. If she's trying to make you angry, just tell her, "There's no reason to push it, just explain it to me." The moment you can make a woman explain things to you, you have put her into a form of obedience. But if you start arguing, then you are arguing with an equal—and you are not equal to a woman. You can't get pregnant, you can't deliver a baby, you can't lay the emotional trip that she can lay. She has a natural ability to lay her trip. Therefore, there's no reason to discuss her power. Never do that. Just tell her, "Please, explain it to me, and we'll go over it. Let me think, I'll get back with you."

I'll tell you something not generally known: the woman will never insult you morally when she's alone with you. Instead, it has to be in a living room or some public place where there are other people. The term for her then is a "real bitch." There are no other words. I've tried to find other words for it, but couldn't. In the scriptures, the language is much more aggressive and insulting, but I don't want to repeat that. In the American language, I want to tone it down. So the moral insult will come when you are sitting with your friends, when you are sitting with people. Don't take it.

Q: *Can you give an example?*

Yogi Bhajan: Suppose you are sitting like this and I'm your wife. I say, "Ji, Yogiji gave you a name I really understand. Hari Singh is a name of God. Hari means the creative activity of God and you are a God. But really, when I see you having a crush on another woman, I do not feel...aren't you insulting Yogiji, who gave you such a high name?" I'm giving you the minimum of what you can expect from her. She will hit the very root, the main root of the person, and it will look very casual: "What?! Oh, nothing, nothing. A thought just came to me." The response to that is, "No, Yogiji knows things beyond what we know, and if he gave me the name, he must have seen beyond that which you can see. But if you want to tell these people, who are your best friends, that I do not measure up to the expectation of my Teacher, I will leave it to my Teacher, and not to you. I think you want to prove what a beautiful and acknowledged way you have to insult a man whom you call your husband." Then full stop. Deliver back with 60% interest. There's no need to argue, there's no need to yell and scream. There's every need to talk; and the talking has to be very, very, very, perfectly exact.

Q: Would you tell her that in private or in front of other people?

Yogi Bhajan: She said it to you among people. The moral hit is never in private. You have to prove that you are intelligent. If you can't prove intelligence, she will not accept you and your friends will think you are a creep. Don't take it. That is the worst fault in America. We take it and we end up with divorce. That's the main problem I have seen in divorce cases. The man does not stand up to the woman when he should. He stands up to her when there is no reason for it.

One woman said to her husband, "Ji, you are very sleepy, you are dozing, can I drive?" He said, "No, what? I'm not dozing. I'm not dozing, I'm all right." After a while she said, "Look, I want to go to the ladies' room." He stopped and she got out and said, "Bye. I'm not driving with you." "No! You have to." He started hurting her; he started becoming fussy, started showing off. So finally, because she didn't want to make a public scene, she got back into the car but she sat in the back seat. She wouldn't sit with him. They didn't go but about two furlongs, not one-eighth of a mile, and crash! Thank God that the sign post was not very strong. Now is this a stand? Should a man take this kind of stand? The car fender was smashed, the engine was damaged, the child was hurt, she was hurt and he was hurt. And the police gave him a ticket.

When you take this kind of stand, you prove yourself to be a fool. She is your partner. She is a human being. Treat her that way. There's no harm in asking her to give you her intelligent opinion or to give her your opinion. Tell her it is an opinion. She may not listen to your opinion four times, but the fifth time she'll start respecting it.

There's also a simple situation in relationships called mother onslaught. This happens when you are scared of a woman. When you were young and innocent, you communicated nicely as a child to your mother but all the time your mother was communicating arrows to you. All you remember is that your mother freaked out, she yelled and screamed. She messed you up, she messed up your father; all she did was mess, mess, mess and all that mess has left a permanent mark in your life. The underlying memory of that mess is there to mess up your life, to the extent of 30%. Therefore, your relationship with a woman needs to be totally free of any other relationship.

I'm trying to give you this picture: the woman is totally innocent. She's totally confirmed and confined in her innocence. You are talking with absolute grace but you are under these clouds of mother onslaught. Therefore, please remember as a matter of policy, your wife is not your mother. Once a person asked me how I felt about the fact that his wife would not act as his mother. I said, "Did you ever sleep with your mother?" He said, "When I was a child." I said, "Did you have sex with her?" He said, "No." I said, "Just remember, this is the woman you have sex with."

People are so insensitive that they cannot differentiate. That's the main problem men have today, they don't differentiate. A wife is a wife. How do you spell wife? W-I-F-E, right? Wife is a combination of two words, why and if: "Why are you doing this?" "If you do that…" It is called 'why and if' behavior. If you foolishly question this behavior, the answer will be, "Ji, I was just checking, nothing special." It does not mean she doubts you, it does not mean she's negative toward you, nor does it mean she's not relating to you. It doesn't mean anything. It's a normal procedure: why and if.

As far as your growth is concerned, your growth is not here. It must not stop here. Your cyclical strength is—and now I am giving you therapy—that your consciousness is 7 years, your intelligence is 11 years and your life is 18 years. These are the life cycles. When you are about 21 or so, check it out. If you are 36, are you intelligent enough? Figure this proportion: at 36, you are two life cycles, three 11-year cycles of intelligence, and five 7-year cycles of consciousness. If you do not proceed with consciousness to that relevancy, you will be irrelevant in your own life, not to speak of your relationship. This checks your integrity, character, social limit, personal interest, emotional interest, progressive interest, and future security.

If a person can hurt you, can hurt your emotional interest, then you can be heavily damaged and you'll never progress the way you need to progress. Those people who hurt you emotionally are not your friends. These are people who hurt you socially, people who down your character, people who down your integrity, and people who damage your progressive interest. These things form your personal credit; this credit is your future security. Wherever you go, your credit will go with you. All of this is you.

Self-Image and **Sabotage**

The best way to deal with personal problems and decisions is by using the following therapy. We used this therapy when I was young. We didn't have tape recorders, so one person would talk and the other would take dictation in long hand. We would choose a subject, and then penetrate it mentally by talking, assessing, analyzing, and judging. Today our subject is woman. The object is to describe a beautiful woman. Take a tape recorder, talk. Replay it and listen to it. Assess it. Analyze what you said in that talk and then judge yourself. Follow? These are very wonderful times when you can just use a recorder.

Suppose the greatest problem for you is sadhana. Record the plus for it, post the minus for it. Talk about it. You can go 60 minutes talking about it. Assess it, analyze it, judge yourself. You'll find your deepest personality—and your problems with that personality. Write them down and then call your Teacher and receive your assessment. Mostly you will find the answers yourself. If you cannot, just call for help. This system is better than self-hypnosis, it is better than group therapy, it is better than anything that you have done so far. You can do the same thing with decisions. Take a problem, consider the plus and minus of the problem. Talk it out. Take the pros and cons, the odds and evens, the achievement, and then analyze and come to a result.

Q: *Sir, could you go through an example of a problem and solving it?*

Yogi Bhajan: Suppose you didn't do your sadhana today. Get through your day and forget it. There's nothing to feel either bad or good about. You remember that you didn't do it: your wife told you, your teacher told you, everybody told you, you know about it—forget it.

But instead, you think you are an asshole. That's what you think. When you don't accomplish your progressive goals, at that time you have only one faculty working against you, and that is called self-mutiny. It's not self-destruction, it's not self-animosity; it's self-mutiny. It is done by those unfortunate people who do not understand that the progress, the second progress to God, is father. That's why God is called Father—Father or Padre. That's what we call these priests and reverends—"padre", "father." Why? It is an image of security. Against that image there is a desire for revolt—self-revolt. Self-revolt will be found only in those people who are destroying their fatherhood, and it is found in men. It's a psychological disease. It is not a behavioral pattern problem. It's a very deep-rooted disease of self-image. Such people will be successful, but then they will destroy themselves. This is the problem of self-revolt. It is worse than the problem of self-revenge.

Self-revenge comes through unexpressed desires, subconscious conflicts, bad childhoods, uncongenial environments. These are problems that you bring from your childhood. They are caused from an insufficient outlet. You need an outlet. For example, if you are upset with your father, you can talk to your mother. If you are upset with your mother, you can talk to your father. Then both can talk to you. That's a sufficient outlet.

Q: *What did you mean when you said self-mutiny was a disease?*

Yogi Bhajan: Anything that is a mental deficiency, we call a psychological disease. Disease—uneasiness on that part of your personality.

There are three important guidelines you need to use: Don't say anything against anybody to anyone; don't listen to negativity against anyone; and don't act negatively. These are the three secrets of success. Don't speak negatively, don't listen to negativity, don't act negatively.

There is a student of mine in Canada. When I came ten years ago, he was in the university. When I went this last time, he was still in the university. I think when I'm a hundred years old, if at all I'll be, he'll still be in the university if that university remains a university. He's highly qualified; he works in the university. He has three Ph.D.'s and now he's doing his M.A. in some nonsense. I said, "Why are you doing this?" He said, "That's all there was available." Can you believe that? That is why we are trying to push all of you into businesses. Business demands responsibility, business demands concentration, and business demands your growth.

There is one great problem with people: self-image. There is no such thing as self-image, it's what you are. You can have a very real relationship with it or you can have a very unreal relationship with it. When you have a realistic relationship with your image, then you are very positive and creative. You can achieve, you can go ahead with the whole world of yours. When you have a poor self-image or you have a conflict with your self-image, you will somehow only achieve in order to destroy. That's the worst part of it—destroy or distraught.

I am working with one person who has a business. He brings it to a perfect, smooth level, then he does some funny thing and in one week the business comes down to bankruptcy. I have been watching him for the past three years.

I want to remind you that I didn't learn all this as a grown man. Basically, I learned it all between the ages of seven and nine. So, please understand your obligation to your children. I was taught all this when I was seven years old. I was told. I was made to see things. Everything was discussed with me. I was told this will be the problem, this will be the woman, this will be the man, this will be the… whew! So as I grew, I knew what was happening. That's why you go to the university. You learn to be an engineer, then you become an apprentice, you become perfect, and then, you start your own business. Isn't that how life is?

When you confront a situation person to person, remember that within this situation, Person A and Person B are opposing each other: "I have a confrontation with you and you have a confrontation with me" is the thought. But at the same time it's interlocked: "You are with me, I am with you." Interlocked personalities: "He's talking to me, I'm talking to him, therefore we are together. We are talking from opposite sides because he wants to overcome me and I want to overcome him." The outcome is as intelligence will decide. Personality should never come into conflict.

You can save tons of energy, only be in the person you talk to.

There are three important guidelines you need to use: Don't say anything against anybody to anyone; don't listen to negativity against anyone; and don't act negatively. These are the three secrets of success. Don't speak negatively, don't listen to negativity, don't act negatively. I mean, don't plan negative action: "I want to destroy you. If I don't destroy you, I'm going to destroy myself. I am out to destroy."

If any person has been talked about negatively, his name is Yogi Bhajan, right? We don't have any doubt about it; but I don't react. There's nothing to react to. People say negative things. They say them because they know better than I do, right? Good luck. If you want to be successful, don't say negative things, don't listen to negative things, and don't do negative things. That is the way to eliminate negativity from your life.

Q: Sir, if someone in your ashram, for instance, is negative toward someone else, is it okay to listen to what they say and explain to them that...
Yogi Bhajan: That is called counseling. We're not talking about counseling. A Teacher's job is different from that of the ordinary person.

Now, in your attitude toward life, you have to be on it—on life. Life is a horse and you are its rider. It is always describe like that. You are riding on life; you and life are separate. Separate. You are riding on life. Therefore, as long as you are riding on life and you have the reins of life in your hands, it is all okay. The moment you leap to something, forget it. When you are doing business, you are doing business; when you are having sex, you are having sex; when you are eating, you are eating. Don't mix business in food, food in sex, sex in the living room, the living room in the drawing room, the drawing room in the bathroom, and the bathroom in the sadhana room. Don't do that! You are not living in one big hall. You are living in apartments. In the living room, we are talking to people; there's no social segregation. But, in the bedroom, you are talking to somebody who's in the bedroom with you; you're not talking to somebody in the living room.

Habits: **Quality, Quantity and Interval**

You have a pranic body. The pranic body is divided and always projected into three lines, which reflect back-and-forth, back-and-forth, back-and-forth. That's the movement of the pranic body. The pranic body is strength. [Editor's Note: Most of the time we think of prana as air, our breath; but another major source of prana is food, what and how we eat.] Now basically you are supposed to eat right. One—eat on time. Two—eat specific food. As a male you cannot overeat, nor can you under-eat. If you do, it will affect your sexuality. You make certain things impossible for yourself when you overeat or under-eat. Because of particular sugar changes in you, your sexuality, thinking, flexibility, and imagination will be messed up. Imagination, flexibility, thinking, sex—what do you have left? And this is just through eating wrong and overeating or under-eating. If you are a hard-working man, you need 1800 calories. If you do office work, 1000 to 1200; 1800 to 2500 are needed by the laboring man. Three—you must eat like a king. That is one of the most important rules for any growing man. It doesn't matter if you are only eating one carrot. See that the table is set, the plate is there, the utensils are there. You reach down, you cut it, you chew it, you eat it. Food should never be eaten when you're tense or in a hurry. It will mess up your nervous system.

The greatest mistake made by grown men is to cut down their eating time for work and their work time for eating. That's the biggest blunder; it totally wrecks your nervous system: "Oh, I'm very hungry, let's have a snack;" "Let's eat while walking to work;" or, "Give me a cup of coffee, that's enough, I won't take yogurt. I'll just eat junk food because I forgot my lunch today." Those are the kinds of things we normally do. At work we always do it. This

Yogi Bhajan on **Wearing Cotton**

From earlobe to earlobe is the arcline; then there is the aura. The aura can be 9 feet—from your skin out—so you are about 21 feet wide. Now that aura represents your intelligence. When you wear white, you get one foot of aura. It has been confirmed. Why should we have an animal aura at any time? Wear cotton. Cotton is the answer. Cotton. It is costly, but it is the answer. If somebody asks what to wear for winter clothes, the answer is to use quilted cotton: cotton quilted with cotton. This makes the warmest clothes. In the Himalayas, we have been in altitudes of 14,000 to 17,000 feet at minus 50° or 60° temperatures. We never used all your American junk. We never died. I never even lost a toe. We wore padded cotton shoes. There was rubber on the outside but the padding was totally made of perfect cotton. This allowed for proper circulation. The people who live in those mountains still have that technology. They have gone through very severe temperatures and are never scared of dying.

hampers the creativity of our digestive system and our supply system. When the supply system is not together, then stress occurs because the demand is constant. The demand is constant because we have a pattern; we have a behavior. We have created that behavior and it is constant. The outlet demand is constant, on the inlet we fluctuate, and in-between, the balance, there's a gap. That's why people overeat and get fat. I know. Flying causes me such stress that you wouldn't believe it. It never used to, but these ten years of flying have totally brought me to a point of stress. This time I didn't want to break my diet, but I was trying to catch a cold, I knew it. So I merely took good, hot food: vegetables, hot chilies. I went through it. (Green chilies are good and red are best. Take as many as you can handle, but be very careful with those chilies. You most know how to digest them.)

You can fight stress with food, but the intake, the quality and the quantity must be a regular habit. The best times for eating are regulated by age: for the first 18 years, you can eat all the time; up to 36 years, you can eat four times a day; to 54, three times, to 72, two times; and beyond that, once per day. That is complementary to the physical process.

Q: What do you mean by four times?

Yogi Bhajan: Four times during the day. I didn't say at night. Do you eat at night? The first 18 years, eat all the time, eat as much as you want. It won't bother you. Normally in the first 18 years, you never get enough; you always want more to eat. It's a natural law. Even the rich kids don't get what they want to eat. But from the very first day to the last day of your life, the quality, quantity and interval must be regular. I repeat: Quality, quantity and interval.

Internal and External **Values**

A growing man is affected in his integrity, his commitment, his dignity, and his communication by the difference between his external face value and his internal value. If your inner value doesn't match your face value, and your face value doesn't match your inner value, you're always in trouble. You should not forget that the outside is what you look at, but the inside is what you deal with. People are not dealing with your outside—the outside is giving an impression. It is the inside they are dealing with. The inner values are the real values, which people want to relate to. Therefore, please deal with your inner values and keep your face values impressive and clean. Though in reality, they are only an introduction—nothing more or less.

These ideas that you have, for example, that when you dress in *bana* the impression you make will be a set you back in business. Let me tell you something very funny. One person went for a job interview. He went in perfect *bana*. They said,

"Oh, why do you dress this way?" He said, "Because we are religious people. We are supposed to, blah, blah, blah." "Okay, you are hired." You will not look like a common pigeon. Some of you feel that as a common pigeon, you will sneak out into jobs, sneak out into success, sneak out into anything. Remember: anything that you have to sneak to will cause you to fall flat also. Earn every bit of life, that is, real value over real value. The real value over real value is that you must earn every bit of your life—everything. That's the only way to grow as a man. Earn your woman, earn your money, earn your home, earn your prospect, earn your progress, earn your success. Learn to earn; don't learn to get. Do you understand the difference? Don't learn to get. Whatever you get you will lose, whatever you earn will be yours. What you can earn you can re-earn. What you get you can lose. There is a tremendous difference between the two faculties.

Don't be imaginative; be realistic. Don't be impulsive; be practical. Imagine everything, but extend it only to the practical, the reasonable. Imagination has a lot of loop holes; practicality is a hard fact. Over and above all that, remember one thing: everything changes, even the sun—which is stationary—has its entire environment change. Even the sunlight, which should be as constant as the sun, causes day and night because the earth rotates. It's the law of two: One thing may not change, the other may. Change is the inevitable fact of life.

Change is inevitable; therefore, you have to change. Since you have to change, why not change to the positive? Positive—change for the plus. Whenever something has to be put on the touchstone, see that it changes you for the plus. Go along with it. If it's changing for the negative, forget it.

One last word, sex is not physical intercourse; sex is the creative sixth sense. You must grow to impress people with your sixth sense. It is not your animal physical sex that can do anything. What you can do physically for a woman, she can achieve with masturbation. A woman once told me, "I don't know why I'm married to him. I can masturbate myself and feel better than I do with this guy who calls himself a great husband." I could see the frustration. There was a tremendous lack of sixth sense.

Now you can ask questions about the inner woman and the growing man. I will answer you as a woman. I will transfer my personality and I will let you know what she wants. Ask any silly question; it's all for men.

Question and **Answer**

Q: You said a woman hasn't the capacity to love a man. Where does love fit into the relationship?

Yogi Bhajan: Love is an imaginative smoothness between

two individuals called imaginative harmony. In real "love" there's no faculty of reason. Reason has no place and love is blind. You fall in love, you don't make love. All we are talking about here is the love process and that is imaginative harmony. Anything that gives you harmony or imaginative harmony is called love. That's where it fits in.

Q: *You mentioned the "why" and "if" of the woman. Can you tell us how a man is to relate to that?*

Yogi Bhajan: It's the sixth sense intelligence. When she's "why and if", you have to give a satisfactory answer to proceed. When she asks you a question, there's no way that you can escape giving the answer. You may think you've gotten away with it, forget it. You have gotten away with it at the cost of your self-respect, self-image, self-integrity, self-dignity, and self-grace. It's a very heavy cost you have to pay.

If she asks a question, you've got to come up with an answer. At least you can answer her, "I'll answer you tomorrow, definitely. Please remind me." Don't let it drop. That's the first challenge that every man has to grow to and has to meet.

Q: *In sex, a woman's mind is sometimes not there; it sort of splits to another place. I remember hearing you say something about a woman's mind going to just practical things. One part of her gets swept away and the other part is just…*

Yogi Bhajan: Highly imaginative. The woman's mind is called "swinging mind." On one side, she imagines heaven; on the other side, she thinks of hell. You are in-between, caught between her imaginative hell and her imaginative heaven. Neither exists. That is why we always say that a woman can be a very practical bitch in bed and a graceful puppy in the living room. There's a whole philosophy around that situation. Only ten percent of all men know how to keep a woman entangled in bed. Those who don't know are very resentful about it. In bed, it is your foremost duty to keep her entangled, physically and mentally—both. If you let her mind go off, forget it. It is no longer sexual intercourse, it becomes rape. That's why many women say, "My man rapes me without being caught." It's a common expression.

Q: *How does a woman's meditation differ from a man's?*

Yogi Bhajan: Once a woman feels meditatively that you are it, she no longer uses her reason and logic. Then all you need to do is touch the button and the right answer comes. She becomes a computer.

Q: *If you're living in an ashram with a lady who has a father phobia and she's not your wife, what would be the best way to relate to her to help her get out of it?*

Yogi Bhajan: Keep your grace. Don't make her come out of it, let her come out. You can never make a woman come out of her phobias, come out of this or come out of that. Remember, you ego-maniac idiots! It's the greatest fault on the part of a man to think that he can change a woman. She can change by taking the lead from you; but you can never change a woman. To think so is your biggest fault, your worst direction, and a totally wrong challenge for a man to take on. Nothing is a greater waste of time, waste of life, and waste of energy. Don't make a project out of a woman.

If you want to change anybody, the project must be to give yourself grace. You'll find the answer coming then, because she is challenged to match up to you. All of you who are working on a woman to change her are wasting your time and looking for disaster. It's a conflict of energy; it's not required; it's not needed; it's not wanted. Just match up and she'll match up to you.

Q: *Can the father phobia apply to a male child, or can the mother project it onto the male child and, if so, what might be some of the signs?*

Yogi Bhajan: The mother may not project her own father phobia, but she can produce sufficient insecurity [to initiate phobia in the male child]. Some signs are that she won't toe the line of the father/husband, and she'll always remind the child that there is a difference between her and the man, always. It's called "non-supporting living attitude."

Q: *You said that a man can't change a woman; what about the woman changing the man?*

Yogi Bhajan: Well, they always want it. This is their utmost desire. We do nothing. When a woman wants to change me, I do nothing. After a while, she gets frustrated and stops. For ten years in America, they have tried to change me; they have found no way. Don't you see? I am a man, living as a man, among the women.

Q: *When a mother dies early in life, what is the effect on the children?*

Yogi Bhajan: It's a tremendous trauma. The child then looks to the mother in the father. It's a very heavy psychological trauma, but if it can be talked out for a long time, in short intervals, every day, with time, it can totally soothe itself out.

Q: *You just said, "The child looks to the mother in the father." Is it possible for a man to have a certain level of evolution to exhibit some of the characteristics…?*

Yogi Bhajan: Yes. People do that. I have seen a case where the woman would run away for days at a time. Out of that one woman, the father raised his three children to a perfect mental condition. The children knew about their mother's behavior because he never lied to them. He never hid anything. He totally trained them, mentally and socially.

He did the job so well that once, in a public meeting, when another child said to one of his children, "Oh, your mother's no good. She runs away with other men." The son replied, "Thank God that your mother is not that insane. We are unfortunate, but we have to handle it because our mother is insane."

They are fully convinced about it. The boy handled it very well, socially. The other boy felt very sorry for his friend, but this boy made the other sit down and pray that his mother would never go through that kind of behavior. It was very heavy. Surprisingly, they are best buddies and they are both five years old. From this you can well understand how much security a father can give a child. To make them totally rock-solid, "strong as steel,"[2] nothing can cut through them.

Q: How does a father provide security for his children?
Yogi Bhajan: Only by being a living example. The best way to teach is by being a living example. You can't teach by communication, by convincing, by arguing, by reasoning. It won't work.

Q: Does Kundalini Yoga affect the homosexual tendencies of men and women the same way?
Yogi Bhajan: Yes. There is no homosexual woman in the world. You must understand, there's no such thing as a lesbian. Men made that up to have an equal counterpart.

Woman is stimulated by the clitoris and it's natural. Basically, you can't stimulate a woman other than through the clitoris. If the clitoris is very close to the vagina then she will have an orgasm with intercourse. If it is a little distance away, forget it. Then it's physical, emotional, commotional, call it anything, but the orgasm has to come through clitoral stimulation. In the woman's world there is no such thing; it is not even called orgasm. It's called "tide." They go through tiding. The correct word is tide.

In men, orgasm is exactly what it is, but there's no damn thing like that in a woman. Her "orgasm" is very simple. If she's in the mood to go through it, you touch her clitoris and there goes the atom bomb. If she's not in the mood to have it, you can take a knife and cut out her clitoris, she won't even feel it. A woman can be that frigid and that hot.

Woman is the most moody animal God ever produced. That's what they say. You should read those scriptures where they speak against women: "Forget it! She's not worthwhile." But the fact is that's what you have to deal with. That's why we want the woman to be a graceful woman. The aim is to inspire her to be graceful and to keep her that way. You will be safe.

Q: What effect does menopause have on a woman?

Yogi Bhajan: You are dealing with another man. Exactly. Quote, unquote. Exactly.

Q: What is the professional relationship between man and woman?
Yogi Bhajan: Very graceful. Don't project yourself as a man to any woman where you have to deal professionally. You will hamper the professional relationship. It will misdirect the expectation and it can cause a lot of problems. Between a man and a woman professionally? Straight. If the two of you are working in the same office, "just friends" is the best description. "Friends" is the coziest word in the English language. It covers everything well.

Q: Woman looks to man for strength and the relationship is based on honesty, honest communication. What is the way a man should communicate weakness to her?
Yogi Bhajan: God! Don't let her look in you. Let her look to God in you, and you direct her to God. Don't let any woman look at you, because what she's going to see in you is what you see in the toilet. If you allow a woman to look in you, she's going to find a lot of nonsense there. For God's sake, keep her away! The moment she starts looking in you, let her look at God. Ask of her the same energy.

"Look at me through God," they say. Let her get lost in Infinity. If she starts looking at you, forget it. You know, when she says, "Oh, your chest is just so wonderful." Say, "Far out, God made it especially for me." She says, "Your belly button is so nice." You reply, "It must have been made on Sunday, because God had a holiday that day." Just slip in that word somehow. Otherwise, forget it. Behind the belly button, the belly is filled with surprises. Why should you let her go from the belly button onward all the way? Are you crazy?

Q: How do you change a confrontation relationship to one of cooperation?
Yogi Bhajan: Well, thrash it out. Thrash out the conflict. In 3HO, it's a question for the People's Problem Project: "Come on, tell me your problem, I'll tell you my problem, and let us find a viable medium." If both sides can do it honestly, but the problem is, you don't do it honestly. That's where the main problem is. You don't want to give the woman a reason to disbelieve you, so you put up an ego show. There is only conflict when both parties are fighting for their ego. This is not reality. Reality has no conflict at all.

I'll tell you. There was a man who never wanted to work. He never wanted to go out to work. He always told his wife that Yogiji, Siri Singh Sahib[3], had a tremendous demand on his time and he simply couldn't get work. Finally one day,

---

[2] Referencing a familiar 3HO family song, *Song of the Khalsa* by Livtar Singh.

[3] Yogi Bhajan's formal title within Sikh Dharma International: Siri Singh Sahib Bhai Sahib Harbhajan Singh Khalsa Yogiji

I went to the ashram and she asked me about it. I said, "I never talked to this guy." We sat down and analyzed it. We found the solution. Since then, he's making money, he's caring for his family, and both are happy.

In relationships, your hidden intentions are your own enemies. But if you put the problem out front, and you decide to meet it, you'll always find smoothness.

Q: *But how do you apply that to never allowing the woman to see your weakness?*

Yogi Bhajan: It's the greatest, most ridiculous and most unfortunate ego-maniac blindness! She knows the weakness anyway. She wants to see your strength, whether you want to admit to it or not, whether you know it or not, whether you are intelligent enough to say it or not. If she doesn't know your weakness, a woman will never cause a conflict. Remember that as a law. She sees the weakness; she knows the weakness.

My staff sometimes tells me, "Sir, you don't know how to fire anybody. What are you going to do?" I say, "Well, some of you should do that. I can't." They tell me to fire someone; or they exploit my compassion, knowing I'm not going to do it; and sometimes they act crazy. It doesn't bother me. I stick to my guns. I use a very strong technology: when I love somebody I am very direct—very, very direct. When I think it's not working, I go silent, so silent that you can't even track me down. I use my technique and that's the technique I use with everybody. You cannot hide your weaknesses from a woman who lives with you. She knows. Be up front.

Q: *If a woman feels she's disliked by a lot of other people, how can she be helped? Also, if she's been told that she's messed up…?*

Yogi Bhajan: Basically, at any given time, every woman is liked by a lot of people. But if you cannot grind into her the feeling of permanency, you're going to lose her. Relationship between a man and a woman is a permanent relationship, not a flirtatious one. The alert mind is opposite to the flirt mind.

All right folks, let us share this meditation. It's very simple. It's very old.

Narayan **Kriya**
October 1979

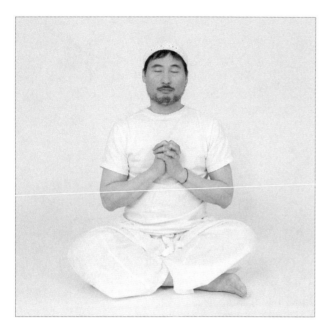

Mudra: Lock your fingers and thumbs at the Heart Center in Venus Lock[4]; hold the mudra against the body.

Eyes: Closed down—9/10ths. Hold the position; feel absolutely steady.

Breath: Inhale, exhale and suspend the breath out. Apply *Maha Bandh* and mentally chant **3 times**:

Sat Narayan Wahe Guru, Hari Narayan, Sat Nam

Inhale. Exhale. Hold the breath out, and mentally chant the mantra 3 times. Inhale. Exhale. Hold the breath out and chant mentally. It will give you an absolutely new lease on life. Continue chanting the mantra three times on the held exhale.

Comments: Try to invoke your own strength—and God's strength. You should feel and experience that strength.

Time: 11 Minutes a day. **31 Minutes** is the maximum time.

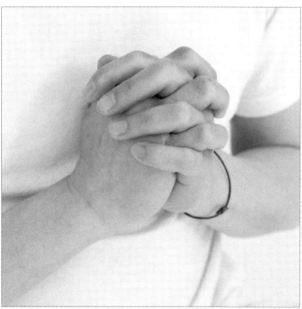

---

[4] Venus Lock: Used frequently in Kundalini Yoga, it derives its name from the Venus Mound at the base of the thumb. For men, place the palms facing each other. Interlace the fingers with the left little finger on the bottom. The left thumb rests against the webbing between the thumb and index finger of the right hand. The position is reversed for women.

Question and **Answer** about Narayan Kriya

Q: *If you can hold the breath out longer, can you chant it four times or three times but slower?*
Yogi Bhajan: You can go three to five, but normally we leave it at three. If you cannot hold the breath longer, it will create unnecessary pressure. We want you to just go with that perfect understanding.

Q: *What is the difference between chanting this mantra out loud and silently?*
Yogi Bhajan: I am not saying a word about this. I want you to do it. Figure out what it brings to you rather than asking me. I did it, I know it, I understand it. The hand mudra is a support to the diaphragm area. Hold your hands against your body.

Q: *Do you use Maha Bandh?*
Yogi Bhajan: Yes. You have to lock all three locks. You just hold it that way. Eyes are closed down nine parts.

Q: *Can we give this meditation to our students?*
Yogi Bhajan: You can give this meditation to the whole world. It will change anybody who is just nothing to everything. That's the punch line that you need to remember. If you can perfect this meditation from nothing to everything, all will be open to you.

May the long time sun shine upon you. All love surround you and the pure light within you, guide your way on. God, Creator of all creatures of this congregation, if you have blessed them, bless them with peace, prosperity, grace, harmony, and joy. If you have made them men, let them grow to be men of grace, dignity, divinity, peace and projection to all sight. Give them the radiance that they should carry Thee on this planet. Sat Nam.

Thank you very much. May you all be blessed. Be healthy, be happy, be holy.

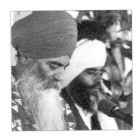

Man to **Man** 5
The Real Strength of Man

Circa 1981

Your ultimate desire is a desire that uplifts you, your spirit, and your consciousness. It is always positive to you and your surroundings and your framework… It is a love of self and grace. It is a consciousness, which has nothing but radiance about it.

- Your **Arcline**
- Developing Your **Arcline**
- Creative **Relevance**
- Woman and **Wisdom**
- The Ultimate **Desire**

Your **Arcline**

Your arc body is your first protection from negative thoughts—yours or somebody else's.

The subject of this course is "The Real Strength of Man." I'm not going to make it a very sexy course because I want to deal with the nitty-gritty of the man in you. I want you to understand the man in you.

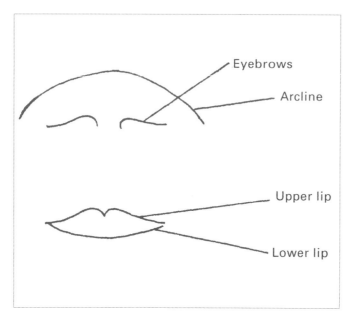

From earlobe to earlobe each human has an arcline. This arcline, which is the arc body, is also called the 'arc halo'. Its expanse should be from six to nine millimeters. Though it passes through the whole body, it can only be seen from earlobe to earlobe. If the expanse of your arcline, or halo, is between one and three millimeters, then you are going to have trouble.

Somebody once asked me why he should be spiritual. I answered him in a very simple way, "So that you can have an arcline." Your arc body is your first protection from negative thoughts—yours or somebody else's. That is why the arcline is so important. I will give you a very practical example: Once when I was working for customs, we were faced with the problem of an underworld figure who had successfully evaded the efforts of all our law enforcement agencies for two years. We decided to get together and pool our resources. After three days of discussion, the representatives involved had to admit that they didn't understand the situation. The case was specifically brought to my attention at that time.

I said, "The guy has a very powerful meditative mind and he is sensitive to all the dangers. Anytime we focus on him, he automatically focuses on us and leaves the city before we can engage him." It was his arc body that protected him. The arc body is the automatic shield of the real being. It protects, acts, and projects. It needs no further qualification or classification. When a negative thought hits, it hits the arc body's shield. The arc body's shield has the power to neutralize with a force of ten. That means that if the negative frequency is at a million thrust, then the arc body will automatically project a wavelength projection of ten million thrust. (Editor's Note: Thrust is the measured force of acceleration. Projection is measured in the same way on the spiritual level.)

If one person wants to get another, say with a million thrust, the arc body will automatically project ten million thrust of projection wavelength. That is why you have been given the right to life. It is your fundamental, divine right. Your second, fundamental divine right is the right to live, and your third is the right to protect life. That protection can be automatic if you have an arc body. It is so simple. Can anything be more simple?

Man is not meant to suffer. I have presented you with a path to follow in your life that will change the course of your existence so that you can be healthy, happy and holy. The path is well laid. It is complete and it is positive. You can never, ever be in trouble.

Look at the American ego. "President Reagan was shot. But he's okay. He's perfect. There's no problem; the bullet was taken out." You don't understand that this country was established on one fundamental law: "In God We Trust." Some Americans think that the President is a solid institution that cannot be crumbled. People like that have a very, very thin arcline. When your arcline is thin, you compensate it with ego. Ego causes you tragedy. It causes you death. It causes your downfall. Have you seen people with ego? You will ask them how they are and they will tell you they are very happy. They act so charming, so perfect. Then they will ask you to loan them $20.

What I want to tell you is that if the arcline is really 9 millimeters, the halo is really bright, then it doesn't matter what happens around you. If you understand this concept, then you don't have to waste 25 cents buying flight insurance at the airport. First, the arc body rejects all negative projections toward itself, the physical identity of the body from which it transmits. Second, it rejects all negative mental projections at the point of origin. Third, it rejects all bacterias, viruses, etc., which approach the physical body destructively.

Finally, it has a connection with the spiritual body. There is a triangular connection between the mind (all three minds[1]), the arc body and the pranic body with the spiritual body at the center. The arcline has a direct connection with all three mental bodies. The arc body has a direct connection with the pranic body and a direct connection with the spiritual body. Because of this connection between the arc body and the spiritual body[2], a spiritual teacher teaches you to follow a spiritual destiny. The spiritual destiny is the most protected destiny. The spiritual destiny has no beginning and it has no end. Everything else in this world has both a beginning and an end.

The real strength of the real man is his arcline. By developing your spiritual self, you automatically develop the protective aspect of your arcline. In its projective aspect, the arcline influences the mind. It influences every mind—which is connected, shall be connected and was connected—was, is and shall be. The arcline practically computerizes the action and reaction system of the being. I'll give you an example:

A very beautiful, saintly person had an appointment to meet someone. I received a message asking me to come to him immediately. When I arrived he asked me to keep his appointment for him, explaining that he had a fever and could not keep it himself, but that he wanted to be represented there. When I questioned him about his fever, he said, "Something's asking me not to go, so my body has this fever and I cannot go." So I went.

When I returned he said, "How was the visit?" "God bless you, Sir," I said. "It's good you didn't go." Of course he knew that. His arc body had arranged the fever. It had totally arranged the fever. That fever was a 105° and the doctors couldn't find any reason for it. When I came back at three-thirty that afternoon, it was absolutely normal. We discussed the situation on a practical level. I said, "Actually, the fact is, something in you that is stronger than you would not let you go." He said, "Yeah."

Remember, I said that the arc body influences the mind. I did not say directs—that is important. First, it influences the actions—the meetings and the not-meetings. Second, it influences the thought form. If it is powerful, it starts making you think right, toward righteous thought. Third, it stimulates kindness. Fourth, it gives you divinity. Divinity is not God in His form of G.O.D.[3] or truth or consciousness. It is infinite consistency—infinite consistency at the frequency of Infinity. That means any negative becomes positive as it's transmitted into the filament of radiance, which is called the arcline. That which radiates is just like the electric bulb. The negative passes through the positive and there is a resistance. Resistance is the existence. So the existence of you is a radiance. The more it radiates, the more you are; the less it radiates, the less you are. Money can't buy it. Money can't sell it. Wall-to-wall carpet cannot give it to you. Ten, twenty women can't give it to you. Skinny, beautiful, brunettes, blondes cannot do it. Power or political position cannot do it. Planes and yachts can't deliver. Neither can gardens or fruits, Chinese or Spanish restaurants. Nobody can do it.

Man is not meant to suffer. I have presented you with a path to follow in your life that will change the course of your existence so that you can be healthy, happy and holy. The path is well laid. It is complete and it is positive. You can never, ever be in trouble.

What is God? Infinite consistency at the frequency of Infinity. All creativity is a magnetic action—all creation. So what is your magnetic action as a human being? What is your power? What is your strength? It is your word. That word which is said, heard, or given by you—that word is your magnetic projection. For example, "I love you." If you are not bound to your word, you are nobody, because your real power is in your word. Those words as spoken, heard or given by you are you; they are your infinite consistency. When you change, you change the range of your magnetic field and, therefore, you are not that you, that infinite consistency. Then you are nobody. You are nobody and nobody wants you.

Dead statues do not make love. Remember my words: dead statues do not make love. Without love there is no life. Without life, there is no experience. Without experience, there is no God. You didn't want to hear all this. You were hoping I would tell you to eat mung beans and rice and be sexy. But I want to tell you what your real strength is. I will play it straight. I will let you know and understand it.

---

[1] The three minds as described by Yogi Bhajan are the Negative Mind, Positive Mind, and Neutral Mind.
[2] In this particular discussion, when Yogi Bhajan refers to spiritual body, he means the subtle body.
[3] G.O.D.: God as Generator, Organizer, and Deliverer.

Developing Your Arcline

When you have trust in God, then you are not afraid; and when you are not afraid, you don't react. You let the Divine create the sequence and the consequences and you enjoy it.

How can you create the arcline, the arc body? You can do it by consolidating your thought form through the development of a neutral, meditative mind.

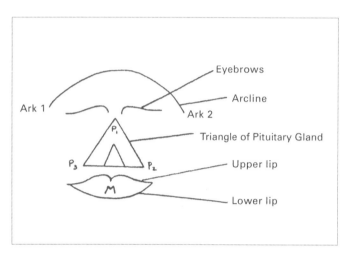

In this figure, P1, P2, and P3 form the triangle of the pituitary gland; M is the mouth with the upper and lower lips; ARK1 to ARK2 is the arcline. If we create a pressure on the pituitary area, the master gland, then, fundamentally speaking, we may reach a stage where we create a kind of channel. Have you seen my forehead? It has caved in. When you meditate very deeply, then you will find this porous bone at the forehead caves in under that meditative pressure. It becomes concave, creating a kind of channel where the two brains meet together. Therefore, if you meditate between the eyebrows and the center of the root of the nose, your concentration is right under the cavity of the pituitary.

These days, people are developing and studying many sciences of the mind—psychiatry, psychology, NLP[1]—I have no problem with them; they are good as instruments. They can give you the technology to pass through a phase, but they can't give you the mind to conquer a phase. Your meditative mind is the Neutral Mind, which runs your destiny. Actually there are three ways to conduct your destiny. First is through the law of karma: action and reaction. Second, you can be a freeloader, tune-in to the magnetic field of the Earth and just float; third, your life can be run by that magnetic, attractive, very positive, creative, meditative, Neutral Mind. That way you can do very well.

It is my understanding that you react under fear. My feeling is that when you have trust in God, then you are not afraid; and when you are not afraid, you don't react. You let the Divine create the sequence and the consequences and you enjoy it. Rather than living the harshness of life, you watch the drama of life. I'll tell you about a very beautiful situation.

One day I went to the home of a friend of mine who had become my student. When I arrived I found that although he was absolutely calm, his wife was very, very disturbed. When I asked about it, he said, "It is called the 'law of polarity'." Then he laughed. "What is wrong with you?" I asked her. She said, "I don't know. I feel very upset and he doesn't feel upset at all." The truth is she was upset because she couldn't make him upset. That is all—nothing special. I asked him, "Wouldn't it be human for you to give her a reaction sometimes, when she wants a reaction?" He said, "Why should I react to her at all? If I react then she acts; when she acts, then I react; when I react, then she reacts. I don't want to play that game. She is who she is and I am who I am."

You are who you are. On that basis, the creativity of this planet Earth is 'creativity is as creativity is', just as 'you are as you are'. That essence of creativity gives you sexual abilities, sexual frequency and sexual frequency is creative frequency. You can have sexual intercourse with a woman and get it over with or you can do something with it. All that sexual activity is controlled by the pituitary gland; therefore, it is controlled by the Neutral Mind, the meditative mind.

This is very important for people who are non-creative. Non-creative people become senile. They shut everything off. It is evident when a person is senile because they are old and they cannot hide it. But actually, most of you are senile, too. You shut things off from your consciousness all the time. The difference is that you don't show your reaction externally like the old folks do. We have to find out about your senility.

Basically every human being who does not have a Neutral Mind acts like a valve. I call it 'valve living'—closing off and opening up. You open a valve: "I love you." You close a valve: "I don't love you anymore." You have experienced that. It is all through American life. The most powerful expression I ever heard was, "I have put my love in a temporary dead file." Write it down. I have to analytically deal with this situation with you. It means, "I have frozen

[1] Neuro-linguistic Programming

my love." Western people have developed in their brain, in their vocabulary, a section which is called the 'freezer'. The first thing they freeze there is love. They don't understand that when you freeze love, you freeze consciousness, you freeze kindness. Love, consciousness, kindness, and creativity—they all go together.

Loving or suffering—doesn't matter—as long as you are alive never stop the flow of love and never ever be unkind. These faculties will give you tremendous amounts of joy, experience and consciousness. You may experience temporary setbacks. But in every situation, always fight back with kindness. Be so kind that you become one of a kind.

On the physical level, you have to close down your eyes and fix them on the tip of the nose. Then put a heavy pressure between the center of the eyebrows and the root of the nose and consolidate your thought form. This practice of consolidating the thought form will give you a meditative mind, and the meditative mind will give you a huge arc body. That huge arc body is the strength of the man. That is his strength in the bedroom, in the living room and in the world at large.

Question and Answer

Q: *Could you explain "consolidating the thought form"? Do you recommend any particular mantra to use in order to consolidate the thought form?*

Yogi Bhajan: There are three mantras which are best to consolidate thought form: Guru Mantra, the *Panj Shabd*, and any three and a half frequency mantra.

These are the particular mantras which will cut the thought form and consolidate it. They work because they stimulate the magnetic field and not only bring the arcline back to normal but also enhance it. Where there is mastery, there is no mystery. Everything is there for you to do, but it is up to you to do it.

Q: *Can you tell us the difference between the **Panj Shabd** and the Guru Mantra?*

Yogi Bhajan: Here is the difference. You need 8.4 million lifetimes to become a human being. Some human beings receive a blessing, a promise that they will meet a spiritual teacher; this is *Gurprasad*. God has somehow told you to meet a spiritual teacher. The spiritual teacher will lead you to

---

Consolidating Thought **Forms**

The Guru Mantra: **Wahe Guru**

Wahe Guru, Gur Mantra Hai, Jap Haomai Khoee.

"Wahe Guru is the Guru Mantra. By repeating it, ego departs."
—*Bhai Gurdaas, Vaar 13, Pauree 2*

This mantra (pronunced wha-hay guroo) is the purest of the pure, the holy of the holies, the being of the Being and the self of the Self. It is the divine of the Divine.

It is very important that when the thought comes to you, you project the mantra at the same frequency and the same rhythm as the thought's frequency and rhythm. For example, a thought comes to you about a woman. "AR-R-R-R-R, I should go and get her." Instead, you think, "No, I'm not going to go after her." And you chant, "Wahe Guru, Wahe Guru, Wahe Guru." It will not be effective. You must project the same frequency and rhythm as the original thought: "AR-R-R-R-R, Wahe Guru!" Whatever the frequency and tension of the thought form, it should be matched and meted out in the tension and frequency of the mantra. Because you do not use this technique, many of you do not get to the bottom of yourself in spite of long hours of meditation.

The Panj Shabd: **Sat Nam**

*Now of the millions of names of God, His real name, His "buddy" name is **Sat Nam** (pronounced: sat naam, like hut and mom). The **Panj Shabd** or Panj Mantra, uses the **bij** or seed sounds of Sat Nam; it derived its name from panj, meaning five, because it has the five sounds of SAA, TAA, NAA, MAA (the four consonants and the vowel sound, aah).*

Three and a Half Frequency **Mantras**

*The third way to consolidate a thought form is to use a three and a half frequency mantra: The Laya Yoga Kundalini Mantra, Ek Ong Kaar-(uh), Saat-uh-naam-(uh), Siree Whaa-(uh), Hay Guroo is this type of mantra as is the **Ardas Bhaee** mantra which has the same frequency but is soft.*

the Guru. The Guru will lead you to God. That is the circle. The Guru Mantra is promised to those who have already been promised. The *Panj Shabd* is for those who have no promise. There is nothing in their destiny. They are:

Palach palach sagalee muee jhoothai dhandhai moh.
"Everybody dies suffering in the false entanglements of worldly things."
—Guru Arjan, Siri Guru Granth Sahib, p. 133

I am going to share with you my version of America. This is how I look at it: Do you remember those days when people were making cookies out of earthworms? The type of worms used for fishing? They have the best protein. I saw a sign, "Earthworms for Sale" and I was curious about it. How were they grown? What did they sell for? I saw boxes, three feet by four feet. Three foot long boxes filled with earthworms. They were all entangled with each other, writhing and crawling all over each other. I feel we are just like those earthworms. Nothing separate or unique, we are just into each other, but with no enjoyment, no identity—eating the mud, living in the mud. There is nothing much to it. Everybody is doing the same thing. Everybody starts wearing jeans—and soon there is a jean fad. Everyone has to have them. We live by fads, not by consciousness. That's the difference. Those who live by fads die by fads. Those who live by consciousness live as divine. It is that simple.

When the Guru Mantra is repeated at the same frequency and intensity of the thought form, you will stop the thought immediately; and when the thought form is stopped, you are relieved, your tension is gone, and you can think straight. You can live right and you can be a better human being.

Q: *In meditating with the eyes on the tip of the nose, how do you put pressure between the eyebrows and the root of the nose?*
Yogi Bhajan: The pressure just comes as you look at the tip of your nose. It is not very difficult. You concentrate and exert the pressure mentally. I can do it even when I am sleeping, that is, many times I pretend to be sleeping. I lean back in my chair and pull my blanket up. Then no one disturbs me because they think I am sleeping. I can meditate two or three hours. It is so good. It is such a relaxation. That is the best way to get it.

Q: *You talk a lot about being fearless. How does a person become fearless?*
Yogi Bhajan: Fearless: *Nirbhao, Nirvair* (from the Mul Mantra). *Nirbhao*—you become fearless when the love of God comes so near you that you not only trust in God, you dwell in God. Then you become fearless, you are afraid of none.

Where there is mastery, there is no mystery. Everything is there for you to do, but it is up to you to do it.

You? You are afraid of death. You are afraid of failure. But it is all in polarity, because you are also afraid of success. You are afraid of love. You are afraid of hatred. You are afraid of everything! But you cannot be afraid of one thing: you cannot be afraid of God nor can you be afraid to dwell in God. Remember: love without trust and trust without love means nothing. Love is nothing but infinite trust. Infinite trust is nothing but love. When you dwell in God then you are in it. You are in love with it, you are enjoying it; it is all perfect.

Q: *To consolidate our thought form you originally said there were three things. I only got the first one which was the Guru Mantra. But the other two, what are the two...?*
Yogi Bhajan: Yes, you've got it? All darkness will be equated with the thought form, because when you feel a thought you feel the content of the thought. When you counteract, counteract with "I am the brightness of the soul." You should feel the essence of your being that is the soul. It will equate, "I am the light." Okay.

Q: *You said that you have to change the thought form and when I think something, I think of the content of that thought.*
Yogi Bhajan: Then you should feel the essence of your being. That is the soul. It will equate.

Q: *For those who don't have the destiny, Panj Shabd will...?*
Yogi Bhajan: For those who do not have a destiny, the *Panj Shabd* is the destiny. There is no secret about it.

Keertam naam kathe tere jaihbaa. Sat Naam teraa poorbalaa.

"My tongue utters Thine acquired Names,
But 'Sat Nam' is Thy primal and ancient Name."
—Guru Arjan, Siri Guru Granth Sahib, p. 1083

All names given to God are as I feel Him, know Him, understand Him, and be with Him. But Sat *Naam teraa poorbalaa*, that is your real Being.

Q: *How would you know if you had a destiny or not?*
Yogi Bhajan: Circumstances will prove it. Our destiny is. There are two ways to understand destiny: One is that you live and you die like those earthworms. Two, you do certain deeds that cause you to be remembered unto Infinity. If you carve your place into the memory of this planet Earth, your destiny is served. That is why it is said, "Live like a saint; die like a soldier." Then you shall carve your destiny into the planet Earth.

Q: What about giving positive projections to political figures when they are in power?

Yogi Bhajan: First of all, you must understand that political figures are not very powerful. I know some politicians personally. They are the weakest people. Not only are they the weakest, the majority of them have no moral standard, no time and no space. Political power is a dream world. It is a totally temporary reality in which you prostitute your soul most of the time.

I know a man who is a very powerful politician among the politicians. He is a very powerful man and he is a very good Christian. One day he said to me, "I love Jesus Christ, but I think he hates me." "Are you sure?" I asked. "Yes," he replied. I asked, "How do you know?" He said, "Because I am a politician." He is a very, very saintly Christian politician. Very, very Christian, very liberal, very beautiful; he lives by the book. He lives by the rule. He felt very blessed by my visit. He was very grateful that I came to see him. He asked me, "Do you think Jesus loves me?" I said, "Yes." "No, I love Jesus; but Jesus doesn't love me, because I am a politician." There is no space in politics. The power is very corrupt. It is very temporary.

The ministry of the Divine is an ever loving, longing ministry. Martin Luther King, Jr. was not the President of the United States was he? Was he a senator? He was nobody. But he is respected and loved more than anybody can be respected and loved. Black loves him. White loves him. Brown loves him. People of all races love him. All of America loves him. This is because the act of power of the Ministry of Divinity is always everlasting. He died for peace. He died for mankind. He died for a righteous cause. He died righteously. That is why there is the saying, "If you cannot live for God, at least you can die for It." You sing it, too: "We die before we fall."[2] Have you heard that?

Q: Is there a major difference when you meditate at the tip of the nose as opposed to meditating with the eyes fixed at the root of the nose?

Yogi Bhajan: No. There are many meditations. We have given 700 to 1,100 meditations. Pick any one of those. They are all equal. They all have a purpose. They are all well explained. I am just giving the first fundamentals. I am not into meditative gimmicks to prove myself. Anybody is welcome to use these meditations.

Q: Will what you eat and what you wear affect your spirituality?

Yogi Bhajan: Yes. What you eat is what you are. What you wear is what you want to project. Your entire way of life can change, if you change your clothing and your food. Once, the superintendent of a jail came to see me. He complained that riots were happening constantly in the jail. So we did an experiment. You all know the Solstice diet? Well, I told him to give the inmates one month of that diet, mandatory. He continued the diet for three months and then he came to see me again. "Sir, I want to confess something."

I said, "What confession? What has happened?" He said, "The whole jail has become yogis. Now we have surplus wardens. We don't have anything to do. Everyone is meditating. They sit silently. They are calm. They are quiet." So you are what you eat.

Whatever you want to project in your life, your clothing will confirm it. If you want to live a pure life, you will wear white. If you want to live a colorful life, you will wear colorful clothes. All clothing has a great combination and effect; it is called bana. Your power to act and your power to reject is always there, but what you become lies in your power to have a consistent influence. You can't live as a flip-flop. You have to be consistent. Consistency to Infinity is your real strength.

Q: Earlier you told us a story about a criminal who had a very powerful arcline. But then it was my further understanding that a good arcline comes with spiritual living. This seems contradictory to me.

Yogi Bhajan: If a person lives very purely—I won't say spiritually—but very ethically, he develops a very powerful arcline. Pure living, ethical living, comes from spiritual knowledge and spiritual living. Those who develop that way of living also develop a powerful arcline.

Q: But how does a criminal develop a spiritual arcline? He was not living a spiritual life.

Yogi Bhajan: No. You have a total misunderstanding of human living. Most people have never studied human living. Human living goes from action to action, from breath to breath. Nobody lives a spiritual life all the time. Just as nobody lives a criminal life all the time. You only act criminally sometimes. All that matters in the end is the balance sheet. Criminals are human beings, too, and sometimes they have moments that are more beautiful and more honest than those of the saints.

I remember an incident that happened when I was a Custom's Intelligence Officer. I was out in the field with 15 of my men and we got into some quicksand. We were way out in the countryside and all but one of us was trapped. I figured we were about three hours away from death. I knew of a man who lived in the area. He was at the top of the Custom's hit list—at the top. We had been ordered to capture him dead or alive. It had been impossible for us to do that because his activities were very well protected. I ordered that last one of my men to go to that fellow's village and give him my message that we needed his help. "Sir," he said, "if he knew we were here and trapped in this situation, he would come and kill us all." "No," I said, "he owes me one. I owe

---

[2] Referring to lyrics in the *Song of the Khalsa* by Livtar Singh.

him one. Go and tell him."

When he got the message, he acted immediately. I think a saint would have taken more time. There was nobody in the village. The men had all gone to smuggle across the border. He was the only one there. He took all the ladies of the village, all the possible ropes and a few bulls and came.

He pulled us out and took us to a small village. He had a fire set immediately. Hot water was made and we were given the chance to clean up. He gave us food, everything. And, what I liked the most, he ended up cleaning up all our arms, counting all our ammunition properly, laying it ready for inspection and then when everything was set, he just left us alone.

We had been totally at his mercy. I think he was a living saint with a little abnormality once in a while. I still remember him. I am proud of him. Thinking that a criminal has no life is like thinking that a woman has no grace or that a man has no appetite. It is wrong thinking.

Q: How can a man change his relationship with his wife?

Yogi Bhajan: It is very easy. Wife: why and if. Wife is the 'why' and the 'if'. Don't answer 'why' and 'if' and the relationship will be changed. That is where every woman gets you. It is their free time, their gossip time, their peanut time. When they catch you alone, they will say, "Why are you lying like this? Would you like me to tell you why you are lying?" That makes them wives. Just don't answer. If you don't know what to say, close your eyes and say, "I am meditating."

No woman will leave you alone. Every woman does three things: She will test your patience; she will test your integrity; and she will test your strength to act. If she doesn't do those three things she has some other man in mind.

*Q: Sir, we have been chanting the mantra **Ardas Bhaee** since Winter Solstice. Can you give us a little more background into that mantra? Where does it come from? What does it do?*

Yogi Bhajan: This mantra came from Guru Ram Das. It is a safeguard against freaking out during *Shakti Pad*.[3] No big deal.

Q: What mudra should be used with that mantra?

Yogi Bhajan: Use any mudra. This beautiful mantra can make the dead walk. Perfect it and see what it can do for you.

Q: If everything should be filled with kindness, should we "turn the other cheek"?

Yogi Bhajan: Who told you to do that?

Student: Christ.

Yogi Bhajan: If you act like a Christ, you will be nailed down like a Christ. If you can stand that pain, go ahead. It is very painful; but what he did, he did.

Student: That is why I am asking.

Yogi Bhajan: Once a rabbi asked me a question. He asked, "Do you believe in Jesus Christ?"

I said, "He was beautiful." He said, "Do you know that he was nailed to the cross?" I said, "Yes." He said, "You are a yogi. Answer a question for me." I said, "What is it?" He said, "Did he pee or didn't he?" (Only a rabbi can ask this question.) I said, "Rabbi, answer my question." He said, "What?" I said, "Were you there?" He said, "No." I said, "Then he didn't pee because you were the only one he wanted to pee at." I mean, you have to be absolutely witty to deal with a situation like that. What I want to express is that this "giving of the other cheek" is a very new phenomenon.

Actually, you do not understand kindness. I am very kind to my students; I bug them to death. Yes! It's a kindness. Kindness does not mean giving in. Kindness is standing up righteously at any and every cost; standing up out of love, out of grace, out of concern, out of everything. It is kind when you are concerned and you stick to your concern and you act righteously on it.

People think that kindness is giving in, lying down, being a doormat. That's not kind. Kindness is giving a hand to a drowning man and pulling him out. That is a kindness. It doesn't mean that once you give a hand, you drown it again and again and again. That's not kindness. Kindness is making people great and strong, and living and doing everything within your meditative mind to accomplish that. Don't misunderstand the word kindness.

Q: When you told us about our fundamental divine rights, you said that the first one was the right to life and the second, the right to live? What is the difference?

Yogi Bhajan: The right to life is a granted act. The right to life is granted by God. The right to live is your choice. You can terminate your life any time you want to; but you can't get it back, because the right to life is through the Divine. The right to life is from the Divine, the right to live is from you.

---

[3] The third stage on the path to wisdom, usually associated with a personal crisis or challenge. Most either leave the path or move on to surrender more fully during this stage of development in their spiritual practice.

Creative **Relevance**

"Creative relevance is what is relevant to me. What is relevant to me and how creative that can be." Quote, unquote.

Creative relevance is the subject. What's more, creative relevance is the subject, the object and the base of every personal gain and loss.

You cannot deal with a person as a person. There is no such thing as "I am a human being. You are a human being." That does not exist. I am an ego and you are an ego. My ego lets in those thoughts that it feels will benefit it. That information has to be relative to my personality, because my personality is shielded by my ego. Therefore, I have to be sold something which reflects me, which to me is me. I only buy myself. I buy no thought, I buy no God, I buy no spirit, I buy no goodies, I buy no tricks, I buy no business, I buy no plans. I am not willing to educate myself, I am not willing to have intercourse with a woman, any woman, and I don't need any children, either. Basically, fundamentally, and principally, all I need is myself. That is God's will; and so it is absolutely in the Divine order. Are you with me? It is absolutely in Divine order that I must buy myself. Therefore, all communications, all dealings, all relationships are based on creative relevance.

Creative relevance is an attitude in which both parties benefit. I create something. I come to you and say, "Look, this will help me and it will help you." You have heard the song? "I'll help you and you'll help me and we'll help each other along." Creative relevance is the part of intelligence in which you benefit others and yourself. Creative relevance can also be called intelligence banking, because you use your creative relevance to benefit others and yourself and, not only that, you earn interest! With creative relevance you use Other People's Intelligence and Other People's Money. This is my OPI–OPM theory.

No person can live happily if he has to live by his own force. You can always live happily if you have other people's money, other people's intelligence; but you must add 100% of your own creative intelligence as well. That is the trinity. That trinity can make you a great human being and that is where your strength lies.

"Creative relevance is what is relevant to me. What is relevant to me and how creative that can be." Quote, unquote. Some things are irrelevant to me, and I am not concerned about them. I can't buy them. I can't be them. But there is one thing that is relevant to everybody and that is spiritual flow. If spiritual flow is creatively relevant to the creative relevance of the being and it is continuous, undisturbed, and realistic, you will feel great. In modern language, it means this check is as good as gold, that a man is as good as his soul, that his word is as good as God, that his action is as clean as the sky, and his personality is as good as the Earth.

If you build your personality too big, nobody will look at you. People will simply walk through your legs and away. You want to hook people—that is why you gather a bunch of friends around you. Man is a social animal, remember that. No ego is bigger than the self and the self cannot be big without people, so you need a lot of friends, a lot of good people around you. Do you know why you want a spiritual teacher? A spiritual teacher is nothing but a destiny computer. No more, no less. You can say to him, "I am feeling this way" and he will say, "that way . . . ." And that is how it goes. So your real strength is in your creative relevance—not your creative intelligence. You can have creative intelligence and not have creative relevance. Then you are on a dead end street. My creative intelligence must benefit you, then it becomes relevant—that is creative relevance.

In the spiritual ream of consciousness you must always be healthy, happy and holy. I picked that slogan; I said, "All right, give them a discipline that will be true, that will work." Whether or not you like the discipline is not my problem. My problem is that whosoever shall follow it shall succeed! Despite a gap here, a gap there; a fault here, a fault there; a goof here, a goof there; a little cheating here and there; coming to sadhana and not doing sadhana; saying, "I love you, but…"

Have you heard that? "I love you, but…" It is ridiculous. Conditional love is spiritual prostitution. It is ugly. It is ugly, it is in vain, and it is a waste of time. Another ridiculous statement is, "I'll be happy if…" Creative intelligence answers every question from the perspective of past, present and future. Creative relevance keeps that in view; keeps it all in perspective. You have every question and every answer before you and still you want to go out and help somebody. It may be a question of taking somebody's clothes, laundering them, starching them, pressing them, and returning them. The person who wears those clothes feels like a king. He looks like a king. He will be grateful to you. You need to understand that your love for anybody is all your own service, your own strength, your own power, your own everything.

You don't love in order to enjoy, so why do you love? There is only one reason you love. Otherwise, in every other way, love has a pain. Love brings more pain than any other human instinct. Love and suffering go together. You have heard it said that to love is to suffer. Love is a pain in the neck. So why do you love? You love so that you can be your Self. When you love, you are your Self. That is why you love—because you love the Self.

That love of the Self forms creative relevance, which paves the ground for understanding, for confidence, for faith and for maturity.

Q: In other words, what you are saying is that the ability to integrate these things, to put them in relevant order, is creative relevance?
Yogi Bhajan: Yes. It is called objective and subjective priority to neutralize the other person's personality. And it is so much so, that if the other person's personality exists, there is no faith.

Even in physical intercourse, when your organ is within the organ of the woman and you are in action, if there is any kind of reservation, it will take away your health and your happiness. It will act so negatively on your brain and on your semen and on your spinal serum that you will age at least two years. I am not kidding you. I am just telling you. Any spiritual action that is without play, or disturbs your sleep—I am giving you a simple, ideal situation—or has any reservation is an omen of ill health; it reduces your longevity and your strength. You will freak out. Normally, from a psychological, physiological and biological point of view, you begin making love and you forget about who is who and who is doing what to whom. It becomes action and then reaction. Then there is a reaction to long for sleep, longing to go into the lap of sleep. You may or may not sleep according to your obligations, but that is the feeling I want you to understand.

Q: What is a reservation?
Yogi Bhajan: Reservation can be anything: "Don't kiss me." "Don't buy me." "Don't hurt me." "Don't talk to me." There are millions of reservations. When the woman is not in the mood, she is totally rude. You have experienced that. When the woman is not in the mood, she is totally rude and crude.

Q: You said that creative relevance benefits both parties. How does the way you use the word 'relevance' correspond to the way the word 'relevance' is usually used in this society?
Yogi Bhajan: Creative relevance creates mutual benefit. Whatever is taking place is definitely to the advantage of both. In terms of reverence, I think this process of creative relevance is very precious and that we should honor that.

I am not interested in the way that the word 'relevance' is used in this society. I am not from this society. This is a sick society. It is not my problem. I cannot accept it. I think Americans are going to go to the dogs—that is not my problem either. You are going to face inflation—that is not my problem. You are going to face crime and poverty and law and order—that is not my problem. You are just pimps and prostitutes—that is not my problem either. I came to this country to solve the problem, not to align with the problem. I know that this society is sick. Who travels more than I do? I get telephone calls from seven in the morning until one the next morning. I understand the pain. I am not outside that pain. But, I do not see America as hopeless. I am a one-man crusade.

I am not in agreement with the use of the word 'relevance' in terms of this society. I am just teaching a science. That is how it is and this science is not modern. Only its application is modern. The scriptures show that people were being given this knowledge 20,000 years B.C.E. This human science existed much earlier than these modern times. My old notes suggest that anybody can be cured of disease through the meditative process and the pituitary gland. We are experimenting with that at the Salk Institute. I am not saying that we are successful, but I am saying that we are near it. We have been experimenting for the past six years. I am very knowledgeable, but I am so busy dealing with this pain on a day-to-day basis that I can't do a lot of the research that I would like to do. But whatever terms I use are scientific. These terms cannot be dubbed "American". They stand for themselves, so don't relate to them from an American attitude or common use.

I have a basic approach to everything in life. If a man will not learn to be a man, God has no responsibility. That is why I have learned. God gave you the energy, the body, the incentive, the intuition, everything. We must put everything together and make it work. If we do not, we are in bad shape.

Q: You said that if President Reagan had an arcline, he would not have been shot. How does that apply to the fatal shooting of Prime Minister Gandhi?
Yogi Bhajan: Gandhi was shot—thank God he was shot. He became a hero. Would you rather he had died of malaria? Dying on a deathbed is a terrible death. All great men come to their end like that. It was an invited end. He knew about it.

Gandhi got shot; Reagan got his popularity. His ratings went up 78% with one bullet. I think the guy did a good job. What strikes me is the way that we habitually speak so lightly about these things. We speak lightly of everything. The President gets a bullet in his lung and everybody talks as though he was hit with a basketball. No one accepts the seriousness of it. It is commonly said, "Oh, he is great. He laughed. He joked. He was dancing. Nancy Reagan was smiling." You need to understand what it actually did to people. It totally confused people. People have no faith now. They do not know if they will ever be told the truth. The common man in America is in terrible pain because he doesn't understand why we are told lies every day. In the old days, at least, whatever the government said was verified. The truth of it was investigated. Now it is an institution of lies, a bunch of lies. Psychologically, this loss of credibility is affecting the people [of America] very badly.

Our minds are creative. We are an art. We are a combination of art and science and that's the best thing. Do you know what 3HO gave to you? There's one word for it—grace. It gave you definite grace. You are special. People trust you on first sight.

3HO is such a snoopy organization, always asking themselves who is who and what is what. A person may be eating an omelette himself, but he will still ask, "Who?" "What?" "Oh, no, it was garbanzo flour." "Are you sure? Did you taste it?" It is such a well-knit, self-policing community; it is unbelievable. One on one—that is the way to go up and up. That is what 'keep up' is.

Can you believe that? Without effective, creative stability can a man do it? Do you see how effective you are? Can money buy effectiveness? Can money buy effectiveness and grace together? Can money buy effectiveness, grace and outstanding personality? Can money buy grace, outstanding personality and remarkable effectiveness, or a chance of time and space?

We picked up some dirt, we made mud out of it, we put some straw in it, and we made a statue. We baked it and

Yogi Bhajan on **Business**

Once there was a person in India who was very beautiful. He said to all the people, "I will guide you to be rich. All I will take is one rupee a day." Then he made himself busy and set up 20,000 businesses. Everyone gave him the one rupee every day. Nobody cared. The people were giving their rupees, they were very happy and charming and they loved him and he was collecting 20,000 rupees a day.

Then he played another trick. He said, "I would like to expand your business. You just give me one percent of your gross." They didn't know what gross was, so they agreed. Again everybody made a lot of money, so everybody paid. He was getting hundreds and thousands of rupees every day.

Then he introduced a third stage. He said, "I will see that you can merchandise yourself totally; but for all that facility, I need a lot of money so you will have to pay me in advance." The people paid, he opened a bank and started loaning money to the same people for their goods. So he completed his circuit. That is called "management-creative-ideal". Because he loaned the money, he knew how much everyone needed; he knew their books; in fact, he knew everything about everybody.

Whoever controls the money controls the business. That is why your bank manager knows everything about you. That is why I told 3HO people years ago to create businesses in which we could employ ourselves. We started our restaurant in Los Angeles with $60. That was all we had. The reason we are as we are, is because we have creative manpower. We have creative intelligence. We are becoming creatively relevant.

I think that in another ten years, if we work properly and intelligently, the entire American creativity will be running around us and we will be in a position to supervise and manage with our experience. I remember one man who had a janitorial service. Today he is making $75,000-80,000 a year just managing that service, nothing else. All this because we are creative. Our minds are creative. We are an art. We are a combination of art and science and that's the best thing.

Do you know what 3HO gave to you? There's one word for it—grace. It gave you definite grace. You are special. People trust you on first sight. You cannot be forgotten. You have one handicap: Your ma and pa say that you look like a white chicken, or a white egg, or this or that. Unfortunately you are in the habit of being bombarded and blasted. That is your handicap. But whenever you go on a business trip and you meet somebody, you shake hands with somebody, that person never forgets you. It takes a lifetime to become special. It takes millions of lifetimes to live special. God and Guru and everything are there; but you live as a graceful being. You look graceful, you live gracefully, and you have no option but to be graceful.

put life into it, and then we finished it. Now it is a very effective product because this product knows what grace is. It has an outstanding capacity, an outstanding capacity to stand out.

Remember this: whosoever shall know how to stand out shall always know how to live. It is a simple law. I have no miracles. I do no miracles. All I do is to make a person stand out and then leave him to the wilderness and wildness of the world. The wilderness and wildness test your ability to survive and there is a great strength in that survival—great strength. Each day, each minute, each second your creative intelligence is becoming relevant. Automatically you are being shaped to relevancy—creative relevance. This is because you know who you are. You know that who you are is who one is. One always knows the One, because the law of One is that there is One. There is only One; therefore, everyone knows every one.

Sometimes your failures are so innocent that you cannot even be punished. I am not saying that you are not failing or that you have not failed, but I am talking to you of your innocence. The law of punishment is that innocence shall always be free.

The creative relevance and relevant creativity, which you can develop in your personality, your self—biologically, sociologically, mentally, personally, religiously, economically, politically—is effective. It is the death of the self. It is the voice of the Self, the voice of the One which we usually call God. It is always infinite, everlasting, and within us. It is the force that runs things. It is the magnificent majesty within us, the majesty of the being, the strength of the being. It is not contrived. It is creative. It is effective. It has no boundaries. It is not limited. It is ever flowing. It is sensual, sexual, attractive, magnificent. It is complete. It has a glory unto itself. That is why, in his compassion, Guru Gobind Singh said:

"Those who have never been leaders, in generations, I shall bless to be leaders of humanity. Those who have never walked straight, will never bend. I shall give them the character to fight with Infinity if they have to, because they will have the character of consistency in proportion to regular life so that they will break, but they will not bend. They will die, but they will not fall. They will give their word and they will live to it. They will stand out and their outstanding personality will be reverend and revered, respected, loved, and acknowledged. It doesn't matter who they are. They are the one stock, one being—'the facilitated faculties into personality of existence by relevance.' The existence of the entire magnetic field, and the creative magnetic field through the force of life, will be totally in their intelligence, in their being, in their fiber and in their nervous system—and they will never fail. Failure will never touch them. It can't. They are protected with the psyche of their own creative being, through the arc body."

So he believed, so he said, and so he created—and that is the real strength of the being. Who can surrender them? Who can kill them? Who can finish them? Who can make them die? Nothing can destroy them. Nothing can touch them. They are great human beings whose cry is, "I am, I AM! I am outstanding. I am here. I am everywhere. I am the pure one. I am the whiteness of that light. I am ready. I am the saint. I am the soldier. I am you. I am me. We are us." Nothing can cut you. Nothing can bite you. Nothing can divide you. Nothing can split you. Nothing can destroy you. Nothing—absolutely nothing.

I am, I AM! I am outstanding. I am here. I am everywhere. I am the pure one. I am the whiteness of that light. I am ready. I am the saint. I am the soldier. I am you. I am me. We are us.

Humans cannot be without the flow of the spirit. Humans, as creatures with the features to become the magnetic archives not of the dead but of the living—and living is the strength of God, Totality, Infinity, Cosmos—such people are not to suffer, shall not suffer. Time and space cannot touch them, grind them, put them through the pain. Unfortunately, some fell; but some have grown. Some have gone and some will come. The continuous cycle of opportunity will always be there for those who want to live in the radiance of their own divinity, in the flow of the spirit. It is unending and it is the oneness of the One. It is relevant, it is creative. That is why we call it creative relevance.

Creative relevancy is the ideal state of the meditative mind. Creative relevancy is the model of the human being—a successful story of every living being. It has love and it has light. It is fulfilling and full of joy. It is complete, the greatest, highest flow of the nectar of life. I will answer one more good question.

Q: *How do we develop that art?*
Yogi Bhajan: In the next lecture, I will discuss how to develop the aura and the arc body; how to relate the arc body to the pranic body; how to settle the spiritual body through the three minds and how to neutralize these minds with the arc body.

I have not yet started teaching you because I have to make money. I am just a servant. I am just like you. Make money, give it to Shakti, so that all of 3HO can function. I am your most humble servant. I keep my rates very low so that a maximum number of you can come to these courses. I turn my money back into you so that you can be organized and live well; but someday I will retire. I won't have any worries about working. When you have no work, you are a jerk. So then I'll be a big jerk and somewhere between two trees I'll tie a hammock, and instead of my big turban, I'll wear a little yamulka, like a little red turban and I'll lie down, half sleeping, half snoring. Once in a while I will open my eyes and you will ask me a question, "What is God?" And I will tell you. At that time there will be no question and no answer but an experience of what I am. We have to wait for that day.

Be creative. Don't feel bad. You are still young and you are fortunate. You have depth, you have dimension, and you have direction. Stick around and enjoy the will of God.

May the Long Time Sun Shine Upon You. All love surround you. And the pure light within you, guide your way on.

Ardas Bhaee, Amar Das Guru, Amar Das Guru, Ardas Bhaee, Ram Das Guru, Ram Das Guru, Ram Das Guru, Sachee Sahee

May the hand of God protect thee, guide thee and be with thee ever and ever, into everlasting Infinity of creative soul and consciousness. May you wake up to your soul. May your being be fulfilled with the guidance of the light and may, out of His mercy, creative mercy, with His mastery of the planet and His creatures, guide you into the depth of love, to the feet of Guru to enjoy the benefit of happiness which may surround you. May you be a saint and a soldier, guiding your way of life unto your own Infinity and destiny in peace. Sat Nam.

Woman and **Wisdom**

Woman loves the wise man in every man. She doesn't need you, she needs security. That depth of security is founded in your wisdom—not in you.

These are two old drawings: One is a male, one is a female.

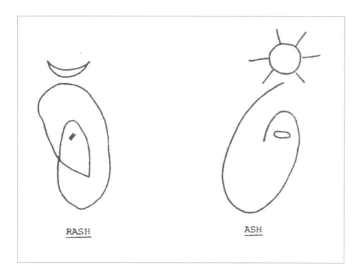

This is according to the old symbols. I am trying to show you the strength of the male in relationship to its female polarity. According to the old teachings, the female is ruled by the moon. Today she is ruled by a jackhammer; you've got to have a jackhammer to rule her. And even with that, it can be very difficult. In the good old days when everything was based on knowledge, she was ruled by the moon—waxing, waning, whining, changing. The moon brings creativity, productivity, conception and growth. You know all about the moon as Americans; you have been there.

Man is ruled by the sun. The characteristics of the sun are constancy, consistency and creativity. Ultimately, the sun burns everything to nothing, becoming nothing but ash. Therefore, the woman who is not rash and the man who is not ash do not exist.

Ash and rash: what do these very important words mean? Woman has the power to stimulate. Basically, woman has the power to stimulate everything into conception. She conceives. All you have to do is put forth a thought and she will conceptualize it, build it like a baby. She will deliver it, nurse it, make a male out of it and present it before you. That is what her rashness is. She will do that quickly and then she will confront you. In other words, the ecstasy of every woman is to put your ego right before you. It doesn't matter if she is 19 years old or 90, that faculty of hers never changes. And what does ash mean? Take a little dust, put it in her eyes, and tell her, "I love you," and that's it. That is the first note that I read from that scripture.

Her job is to confront you with your ego. She will never put herself in front unless she's insane. But when she is wrong, she will never stop talking. You must have experienced that phenomenon: "Tat, tat, tat," it's a duck quacking. She'll say, "What do you want to do with me now? Who are you? What's going on? What did I say? Do you remember what I said? Really? Did I mean what you say? What I mean is, what you say, do you mean what I say to you? You are very mean, you remember everything. I don't mean a thing," All these words should sound familiar? And here is the male, just trying to protect himself.

Creative consciousness is parallel and equal in relationship to the woman, but relative in the terminology of understanding. That is what we are discussing here. You may understand differently, and she may understand differently, and within the surroundings and environment there may be yet a third understanding of the whole thing. That is why there is a pain. To the extent that we do not understand at all, we create pain.

Try to understand that the security of the woman is the security of the woman—in the understanding of the woman, within the environment of the woman, into the desire of the woman, into the thoughts and the ideas of the woman, into the projection of thoughts and ideas of the woman—and yet the woman is still an innocent little woman who's trying to seek, to grow, to perceive, and to preserve her identity. The only idealistic approach a male can have toward that defense mechanism of hers is to defend it. "I love you" will never work in this situation. Your love theory as a male will not work. You must understand: No woman loves a man who loves a woman! She loves the wise man in every man. She doesn't love the male. She can masturbate. She doesn't need you, she needs security; and the deeper her security, the more relevant her love. That depth of security is founded in your wisdom—not in you.

I have seen a woman carry a crippled man on her shoulders—toting him, nursing him, totally taking care of him perfectly. She was an American woman, not an Oriental. I analyzed her personality and her character and I found that she totally believed that he was a pure gem, a crystal clear diamond. She didn't care a bit about that little handicap. She had to carry him from his chair, sometimes on her shoulders, on foot. She told me, "I have developed strong muscles."

You think that she loves your body, your fame, and your domain. To you these are the basics. In reality, these are temporary aspects which she loves. She's searching for deep understanding, deep understanding and the realization that she has found somebody who, according to her, is wise enough that she can trust him. Please remember, woman is multi-faceted. If she has positive creativity, one negative word from you will be like potassium cyanide. Reversely, if her creativity is negative, your positive area will scare her to death. Don't misunderstand and think that if you are very divine, it'll work out; or that if you are very evil, it will work out. Woman likes neither divinity nor evilness. The only thing she likes is having faith in the wisdom of the male.

In most of our communication, and in our relationships, our creative habits are very nonsensical. We create an atmosphere in which there will be a tremendous reaction to whatever we project—that is the fundamental way in which we misuse our strength. Real strength lies in handling situations with extreme wisdom. Wisdom is not money, it is not Persian carpets, it is not gold. Wisdom is something very unique, which very few people can define. Wisdom is bringing the total understanding of truth to the opposite polarity as a reality. The wise person brings to the opposite, whether male or female, a level of understood reality, a state of understanding.

If you speak the truth and someone doesn't understand, it's not wisdom. You must predict, depict, project, and fix it. Wisdom does not mean that you know a few words. Wisdom does not mean that you have a few degrees. Wisdom does not mean that you have money, nor does wisdom mean that you are a beautiful man or a beautiful woman. Wisdom only means that you can convince the other person. Wisdom is nothing but truth and there's no other truth over, under, or around it. Do you understand? Nobody trusts you—believe me or not—and you don't trust anybody. All any of us trust is the essence of truth—whatever it is, wherever we get it, and whether we like it or not. No one wants to be cheated, but without truth how can you not be cheated?

My own experience has been very difficult. Some of the girls that I have raised were very young, little girls when they came to me. They have been around me a while. Now they are 21-year-old women. I am finding it so difficult. If I say anything to them, they quote my own words to me. I can't make a move.

Wisdom is not being clever, or being a con. Wisdom is not fixing something temporarily. Wisdom is not getting away with something. Wisdom is not selling or buying an opportunity. Making something or saying "to hell with it" is not wisdom. Wisdom is predicting what the truth of the situation is, depicting it, and then communicating it, and fixing it, so that the other person knows, exactly, that there is nothing without it.

Everything is temporary on this planet. Only truth is permanent unto Infinity. Every female likes the male to relate to her in truth. Your relationship should be angled toward the flow of truth—that is your sunshine. Therefore, in communication use the theory of poke, provoke, confront, and elevate. Don't leave the person unelevated in the consciousness of ultimate reality and truth. Even in your sexual relationship, your actions should always be natural, physical, truthful. Before entering any relationship, you must totally communicate the state of your personality in the moment: who you are. If you are worried, if you are tense, if you are depressed, tired, hungry, anxious—you must explain.

I will tell you the greatest story. A couple came in early. They got a hotel room, relaxed. Well, naturally in America when two people relax, you understand what happens:

He said, "How about you?"
She said, "How about you?"
He said, "Well, I am very tired."
She said, "I am very tired, too."
He said, "If you take away my tiredness, I'll give you a good time. If you don't, then we sleep."
When he finished the sentence she was snoring. After about an hour, she woke up. Then she awakened him and said, "Hey, you are snoring."
He said, "I thought you were snoring, too."
She said, "I don't know…you said something to me."
He said, "Forget it. It is time for our next appointment now." And they both got up safe and sound.

This is such a relevant joke, because the reality is that two people can enjoy it more than sexual intercourse. It has personality, it has juice, it has action, it has reaction, it has a trip, it has understanding, it has feeling, it has a kind of dealing with each other, and with it is a depth of understanding of reality that you can forecast, but still it's unpredictable, you can't depict it, but it's excellent. It is not the physical dog and bitch relationship. It is the older relationship, which you can live.

I'll give you another example. By mistake, a woman said something very insulting to the man. He went to "Section 13"—deep silence. Remember that formula? "Don't kill a woman with a bullet, kill her with silence." For three days he was silent and she was normal. On the fourth day she lost her temper. She was yelling and screaming and crying and beating herself and pulling her hair. She finally got so tired that she almost fainted and then she fell asleep. When she awoke, she found a very beautiful blanket over her, a pillow under her head, and she was very comfortable. She said, "Very kind of you. You are very nice. You gave me a blanket and a pillow." He turned around and didn't answer her.

That story has a lot of juice, too. When she told me, there were tears of love in her eyes. She was so proud of her man, so proud of him. She said, "God made me a woman and finally, Yogiji, I got a man—a Man." Her eyes were open, her face was open, and there was a tremendous smile on her face: "I got a man." She told me why she thinks he is a man. She said, "Once he becomes silent, there is nothing on the planet Earth I can do to make him talk, until he forgives me. He is a man!"

According to you, a man is one who can drink a whole bottle of bourbon straight and still walk. You know? Your stories are ugly. All those stories of the old days: "A man is a man who will never tie up his horse and go with sixteen women." You remember those old stories about how the West was won? But now the story is different. Woman is intelligent, precise, intellectual. She has personality, surrounding, environment. She has understanding and education. She doesn't need you for money, for business, or even for sex. Women can interrelate sexually now. What I am trying to tell you is that the very deep feeling, the expression that a woman enjoys, which to her is very relaxing, very creative, very relevant, is when she believes and understands in her depth that she has found a man. And in the depth of her heart, she can trust the wisdom of that man. Then she can forget everything that may be a handicap in that relationship.

With your little foolishness here, little foolishness there, you can totally ruin a life, a destiny, a dynasty, a future. Therefore, the male is very important. The male in communication, in expression and in action is very powerful through his word; what you say, what you write, what you speak, what you hear, what you understand and what you communicate.

Q: *Is the woman interested in how you are projecting the honesty which is promised her?*

Yogi Bhajan: If you can make her understand the honesty of your projection—even though it may not be honesty—that's between the two people. No third person is there to judge. It is all based on whether she *believes*. You may be totally honest; but if she doesn't believe you, you are not honest.

Q: *When you were speaking about wisdom, you said that you communicated a truth to the other person and fixed it. How do you get the other person to listen to you, to cooperate?*

Yogi Bhajan: If you are wise, you don't need cooperation. You are wise; only the fool will come to you. His cooperation is already there. He is coming to you—that is his cooperation. That is a maximum. If I listen to you, that is my maximum cooperation. How you deliver your subject is your maximum performance and if you don't fix me, you don't. That's it.

Q: *So it's not your fault?*

Yogi Bhajan: No, no, no. Nobody's at fault. There is only the San Andreas fault in California. No fault. Actually, there is no such thing as fault, as sin, this and that. These are all relative terms.

You know, I'll tell you something funny. I had a friend who was a medical doctor. He made a lot of money. He was very happy. One day he came to me and said, "I'm going to commit suicide."
I said, "What for?"
He said, "I love my woman, my wife. I'm really in love with her, but I can't live in the house with her. I can't stand it. There's nothing I can do. Life has become totally irrelevant to me, so I'm going to commit suicide."
I said, "Why don't you use cyanide and just go to sleep? Very quick, very easy. Very easy death."
He cried, "Shut up!"
I said, "You coward!"
He said, "I am not a coward. Look how brave I am—I have come to you. I don't eat like you, I don't talk like you, I don't live like you, but I think you are wise. Fix me!"
I said, "Okay. How old is your wife?"
"Thirty-eight."
I said, "Alright, ask somebody to hire a maid for you. She is not to be any older than 21."
"What will that do?"
I said, "Now get out of here and do it. I have fixed it for you and I'm not going to explain it to you. It is my wisdom. If I explain it, you fool, you'll mess it up. That's all you Americans do. Twenty-one years old and she should be pretty and Mexican and she should be in your house. And, tell her everything."
"I don't know Spanish."
"You don't have to know Spanish."

He did what I told him and the moment that 21-year-old woman came into the house, his wife became very smart, very humble because there was competition. As long as she had a monopoly, she was intolerable. In capitalism, monopolies are the worst. That's why we have anti-trust laws. The moment her monopoly was indirectly broken, she made the change. He came to me and said, "What can I offer you?"
I said, "Nothing."
He said, "No, I just want to give you a gift."
I said, "Also rent me a 21-year-old maid. That's all you can do." (Laughter.)

Try to understand that life is not the way you want it. Life is not cut and dry. Life is not sluggish. Life is not rude. People make it rude. Life is a pure flow of joy and happiness because it is creativity. When a baby is born, is it unhappy? Is a little innocent baby unhappy? Is the bud of the flower unhappy? Is there any naturally innocent thing that is unhappy? You make it unhappy because you do not know how to handle it. You can make the most beautiful thing ugly; the most happy thing unhappy; the most secure thing insecure. Why? Because you are insane. Is there any doubt about it? Somebody asked Johnny Carson, "What is the secret of your success?" He said, "Insanity in America." The guy gets up, makes a few foolish jokes, a few good jokes, makes you laugh and everybody waits up until 11 o'clock to watch his show. Does he give you scripture? Does he predict what is going to happen tomorrow?

In our lives we do not believe in the flow of commitment. Life is flow; but the commitment of life flows with it. The commitment of life is a flow, too, and we do not guard the commitment. We only guard the life. That is the tragedy. You don't guard the commitment of life and you don't guard the values of life. It is so simple. First, God gave you life, right? God gave you the flow of life, right? You give your life values and you guard those values. They are very important. Is is very, very important that you guard your values. It's important because life flows in order for you to develop values; and as the life flows and you develop your values, the deeper and deeper should be your commitment.

I'll tell you one more thing, a man who can give the impression, the convincing impression, that he is very committed to values never suffers. Your life is not an irrelevant tug of war. It's not a hassle. All you have to do is find the values. That is so important because if you have not found the values for yourself as a father, you cannot find them for your son, your grandson, your neighbor, anybody.

When I came to this country, I didn't have a billboard on my forehead reading, "I am a holy man." I walked in wearing a pink turban and some American pants, which I have never liked, and almost no shoes. This was because my luggage had gotten lost and no clothing fits me here. I looked very peculiar. That made me unique. I was very impressive. In Hollywood, there was no actress who didn't want to shake hands with me. To them, I was imported from South America. Well, that was all fun but then they talked with me for two or three minutes. That was it. Then my problems started. They were totally available to me—all the way; and I was not available at all—no way. So to get rid of all the actors and actresses, I told my faithful students, "All those who are faithful to me," (that was the first time I had said, "…to me," not to God and Guru) "raise your hands." There were less than 40 people. I said, "We'll go on a garlic fast, fifteen cloves of garlic every day." In 10 days Hollywood was cleaned out of the ashram.

In those days, the actresses would send their drivers to put down a big towel to save their place in class. It was very difficult to deal with those egos. I knew they were useless because they were all wrapped up in their own values. They didn't have time for my values. I wanted to find people who could listen to me and pick up my values. The moment people started picking up my values, I told them one more thing: I introduced the idea of *bana* to them. I told them that a specific landscape was required to live my values. The moment they got into that landscape, they started loving themselves, they started watering themselves, they started looking at themselves, they started protecting themselves, they started standing out. Something awakened in them: self-respect. They were doing Kundalini Yoga. All that Kundalini Yoga concentrated into a big ball of fire, and with that energy, we have created a nation in 10 years time. It was the most clever, the most rapid, the most scientific and the most determined way to do it. We awakened the dormant power [in the man] when we awakened his self-respect. We created a saint and a soldier.

Whenever there is a big difference between the man and his landscape, life is unhappy. Sometimes you don't care what you wear, you don't care what you eat. You will eat whatever is set before you—instead, why not fast that day? Do something positive with that energy state. There was a time in India when people were extremely downtrodden. Look at the situation: 10,000 people were picked up to be butchered. Their blood was given to the king's hunting dogs and their meat was used for training the animals to hunt. We are speaking of people, human beings—not animals. Ten thousand people each week and nobody raised a finger. In those days, a mounted soldier of the government, a constable or a policeman, could call on any man in the street and make a footstool of him, that is, step on him to mount his horse. That was permissible.

In that drudgery, that treachery, that holocaust of human consciousness, there was a man called Guru Gobind Singh. He gave everybody self-respect and he started by giving them *bana*. That *bana* of consciousness that he gave them is the arc body. This is a most important secret for you to remember: the arc body is the *bana* of consciousness. The radiant body is the *bana* of the spiritual body, the soul. That is why I say, "Bana, bani." You are what you eat. You achieve what you speak. Your speaking power makes it possible for you to achieve everything, or nothing. Your power is *wand chhako*—what you can spare. I have been saying it again and again and again and again. The power of your personality is what you can spare.

I'll judge how much you love me by how much you give me, what suit you bring me. That's your *personality* power. That's not the power of your soul. If you can spare some help, some gift, some good word, some smile for somebody, then your personality can make it. If you can only spare slander, abuse, negativity, gossip, then you can ruin it. In other words, whatever goes out of you, you must realize that it will create either a positive or a negative situation.

Actually, creative intelligence is called sexual energy because both are governed by the pituitary gland. Therefore a meditative mind, which meditates between the center of the eyes, calmly and with a certain rhythm of breath, is very helpful—such is this meditation.

Eight Stroke Breath **Meditation**
April 1981

Posture: Sit calmly with a straight spine. Bring the hands in front of the Heart Center. The two palms face each other, about four inches apart, with the elbows pointing out to the sides. The forearms are parallel to the ground. The left hand is on top with the palm facing down. The right hand is directly underneath the left, with the palm facing up.

Eyes: Look at the tip of your nose and concentrate.

Breath: Inhale through the nose in 8 equal strokes; exhale through the nose in 8 equal strokes. Make the breath a continuous rhythm; do not pause between the inhale and the exhale cycles.

Mantra: Mentally vibrate SA TA NA MA SA TA NA MA on the inhale and the exhale.

Time: 11 Minutes.

To Close: Inhale deeply and hold for 30 seconds. Exhale and relax.

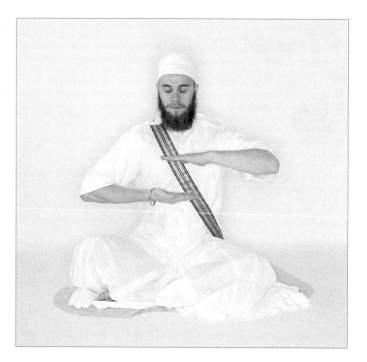

What I have been trying to relate to you for the past 10 years, and what you have not been willing to hear, is that we are required to be a little different, on a practical level. We are required to have a different kind of strength. We are required to have within us what we need. We cannot go with the free flow of insanity. Life requires much more commitment. It needs it, otherwise it can be almost suffocating. Life needs the nurturing of commitment and commitment needs strength of character. Character needs strength of values and values have to be learned from the learned, and then practiced and lived. This is the paraphernalia of life.

Last night we were up until two or three o'clock counseling one man about his marriage. He said, "Well, the home is broken. The family is broken." He was not willing to discuss why it had broken or whether it could be mended. "It is a broken home." Period. Live with it. "You have no right to discuss with me what I do with my spare time. I go with a girl here, a girl there…I find somebody or I don't." It was a very peculiar situation.

We were trying to fix the lives of two children, one woman, and him—not to mention a couple of the others he was running around with. We were trying to reach a point where we could create a demarcation. But before that can be done, your life must have some area where you are committed, the surroundings are committed, the personality is committed, the values are committed, and there is a flow behind that commitment. Commitment will dry up and die if you don't nurture it. Commitment needs to have a constant flow behind it. Commitment has to be nurtured, renewed, and refreshed. That is why we say, "Each day, we must pray." What is prayer? Prayer is the power of man. We pray to nourish our souls so that the flow of the spirit will go through us. The only way that spirit can flow through us is through prayer. We obey religion and its do's and don'ts to channel that spirit. Those do's and don'ts—"I can do this, I can't do that"—are spirit's embankments. We have to develop values and understanding in our personalities so that others can value and understand us. You can't go on and on freaking out, saying what you want to say, doing what you want to do, running around with whomever you wish, and then feel that everything will come out all right—that is not what life is.

Commitment will dry up and die if you don't nurture it. Commitment needs to have a constant flow behind it. Commitment has to be nurtured, renewed, and refreshed.

You can't go on and on freaking out, saying what you want to say, doing what you want to do, running around with whomever you wish, and then feel that everything will come out all right—that is not what life is.

There is a word: *birthi*—imagination. Some people don't have any imagination. They cannot look beyond a few blocks; others cannot look beyond a few days, a few months, a few years.

Once I was having a discussion with a man who said, "Wow, I am 40 years old. I only have another 10 years left."
I said, "What do you want to do?"
"First, I want to divorce my wife. Second, I want to change my job. Third…"
I said, "Third?"
"If possible, I will get lost."

And he did—at the age of 42. It has been 8 years now, he should be 50 years old and nobody knows where he is. Why would somebody run away from life? Run away from identity? Run away from personality? Why is there no strength to face and confront and elevate everything that comes your way? You cannot uplift whatever comes your way because you are not yourself. Further, you have not put forth any effort to be yourself. The most boring job is to work on yourself. When you work on yourself, who is the self interested in? If the self is not interested in its own self, then you won't do the work. It is a very solitary job, it's very lonely, and it is very, very boring. I will tell you a story:

Early in the morning the common laborers gathered in the marketplace, awaiting work for the day. One morning Kabir went there. "How many are here?" he asked.
"There are 500 of us," they said.
"What is the highest wage?"
"The carpenter makes one rupee per day. That is the highest wage."
Kabir said, "Come with me for the day. I will pay the highest wage to each of you."
Everybody was happy that he had a job, and that, too, at the highest wage. Kabir took them to a little place where he had them sit down and gave each of them a mala.

They asked, "What do you want us to do with this mala?"
He said, "Meditate with the mala."
No one could say a thing to that because it was a very easy task. Everybody could do it. Kabir said, "You will all be paid one rupee for the day and in the evening I will give each of you a bonus." Then he went away.

At one o'clock, he returned and he found that only 30 people were doing it. The rest had left the mala and left the place. He asked those who remained, "What happened to the others?"

They said, "They sat down and they did the mala japa, and they ran away. They don't want to do it because there is no interest in the work."

Kabir said, "Alright, you 30 people continue. I'll give you an extra bonus—a super bonus."

They said, "Okay." That evening Kabir returned. All he found was the malas. The people were gone.

There's a very powerful saying:

Moorkhal naal naa lujheeai
Don't entangle with an idiot.
—Guru Nanak, Siri Guru Granth Sahib, p. 473

"Don't entangle yourself with unwise situations or with unwise men." It's not necessary. It is a real strength of the real person to avoid the foolish person and his company. Too much company of the foolish person can make you obnoxious. Try to understand the saying, "Be in the company of the Holy (or the company of the wise)." In this way, you will always be where you can learn something, where you can grow to be something, where you can enjoy being something. That is the real joy. It is required in our caliber that the understanding be created so that we can know who we are and what strength we have. Today we are trying to build that strength.

It is a real strength of the real person to avoid the foolish person and his

Yogi Bhajan on **Sleep**

Somebody once called me. "Sir," he said, "I cannot sleep. I have even tried sleeping pills and still I am in pain and very restless."
I said, "Far out. I can tell you how to sleep."
He said, "How?"
"Take the Peace Lagoon and start reading it."

He has never called on me again. He has no trouble sleeping. When he goes to bed, he puts his head on the pillow and starts reading the Peace Lagoon. Sometimes the Peace Lagoon ends up on his face. You don't need to spend money on drugs. If you want to go to sleep, but you are upset and you don't know what to do, say, you are very angry— do what I do when I feel abnormal. I start chanting mentally, "Wahe Guru, Wahe Guru." It relaxes me, it puts me to sleep. Try that rather than bursting out of your skin and creating a scene.

The Ultimate Desire

What is the ultimate desire? To become desireless.

How do you find your ultimate desire? Your ultimate desire is a desire that uplifts you, your spirit, and your consciousness. It is always positive to you and your surroundings and your framework. It is a feeling within the feeling; it deals with the innermost essence. It is a love of self and grace. It is a consciousness, which has nothing but radiance about it. But, still it is a desire.

What is the ultimate desire? *To become desireless.* What happens when you become desireless? All your desires are automatically fulfilled. When you become desireless, then all you need—physical, mental, social, spiritual, biological, psychological—is catered to by the automatic reaction of the magnetic fields of both the individual identity and the universal identity. Creating a relationship with the individual identity and the universal identity is exactly the same thing as creating a relationship between your pituitary gland and your sexual organ. There's no difference at all between the two. One is on the physical level, the other is on the etheric level.

When you become desireless, three things will flood you: money, women, and power. They will come to serve you.

Money is what money does. Money is nothing but a storeroom of wealth controlled at a certain rate and stocked in a certain pile. You can buy services and goods with it. It is a medium of exchange.

Woman is nothing but a satisfaction of your polarity. If she does not satisfy that, then she's not the woman you want. She may be only a woman to look at. Understand? Take note—the existence of a woman around you must satisfy the following conditions: if you are disturbed, she will bring you peace; if you are down, she will bring you up; if you are sad, she will bring you laughter; if you are unhappy, she will bring you happiness. She will deliver all of this without any loss or exchange of energy—that's the condition—no loss or exchange of energy.

The presence of woman within nine feet of your aura must change your mood. Her insertion into the realm of your magnetic field must bring security. Her communication in the realms of your thought form must bring hope. Her look within the realm of your radiant magnetic field must bring you satisfaction. Such a woman is the coordination of your magnetic field and yourself. She is desirable; she is desire; but she beams the desireless within herself. She projects divinity, dignity, and grace. Therefore, it is required of every man to work on woman and bring her to the ultimate desire. The realm of consciousness in values cannot be the flesh, or money, or sex, or this, or that. It must be desireless; the personal projection of the woman, in the reality of the magnetic field of the personality of the person she's relating to, in dealing with time, space, and circumstances through mental, physical, psyche, and spirit must be desireless.

Your ultimate desire is a desire that uplifts you, your spirit, and your consciousness. It is always positive to you and your surroundings and your framework. It is a feeling within the feeling; it deals with the innermost essence. It is a love of self and grace. It is a consciousness, which has nothing but radiance about it.

The woman has another characteristic. She freaks out very quickly. Woman is extremely sensitive. She is nothing but a very exquisite crystal. In opposition she is fog, smog, and death. But in pursuance, she is a crystalization of all life, in radiance and in all dimensions.

Therefore, you should be very careful of the woman whose company you keep. Don't ruin your strength in a wasteland. Some women are just orphans and they will make you an orphan in their company. Some women are very negative and insecure. They will constantly put down your security. Some women are very irrelevant to life. They will always create irrelevancy in the smooth flow of your life. Some women are like period—full stop. They won't let your life flow. Some women will chase you. They are very, very, absolutely, negatively jealous of environments and circumstances. They will suffocate you to death.

What I'm saying is that in each aspect of a woman, you will find a very undesirable aspect of your own life. Deal with this in a simple way. Let her higher Self live. Cut down communication with her lower self totally. Don't try to fight back. Don't have a bout like a boxing match—15 rounds and you win. You are never going to win with a woman. She's not even a good punching bag. If people see you fighting with a woman, they will say, "You are just a creep." Never fight with a woman. Suffocate her with communication. Wake up and listen. Communicate with her about everything—everything—including getting horny.

The virtues of woman are manifold but they are her virtues and she rarely shares them. When she does share them with you, then she usually likes to get feedback, which is a very costly business. Therefore, establish a relationship with your woman. Call it "unified product combination." It is everything which you and the woman share. Just let her know you value her before it is too late. The biggest mistake you make in dealing with the female polarity is that you do not let her know your values. Communicate your values to her before it is too late. Otherwise, you get trapped.

She acts in total innocence. She doesn't remember the values—this is the projected armament of a woman. She will be forgetful of your personality, forgetful of your needs, but of course, she never really forgets any of these things. She will be forgetful of your personality, forgetful of your needs, forgetful of your time and space and appointments, forgetful of your hunger, and when it comes to the bottom line, you'll find your laundry has not been done. That is the bottom line. It all boils down to maya. When it reaches the point of no laundry, you should be well-warned that the enemy is within firing range. Do you understand?

A woman shall never deny you laundry. She may deny you sex, she may deny you communication, she may deny your love of your children; nothing is very important. In the past, for example, the 30s, if a woman wouldn't give a handkerchief to a man, he would know that divorce was just around the corner.

Another sign to be wary of is her appearance. She will want to meet a friend of yours and she will be dressed in her best; she will want you to meet her parents and she is dressed in her best. But, if she goes to meet your parents and she is not in her best, you are in trouble. It doesn't matter how obnoxious your parents are. (I'm not discussing parents or their attitudes, or their projections, or their frequency of relationship, or whether they are good or bad.) We are discussing how she dresses herself, and how she wants you to dress. Judge a woman not by her promise, judge her by her dress. If the *chuni* is not around her neck, it will be around your neck. I am 100% right; don't underestimate or misunderstand me.

One woman told me, "You are a very clever teacher."
I said, "What did I do?"
She said, "You brought purity to every woman in America but it won't work here."
"How did I do it?"
"You make us wear turbans, chunis and churidars. Churidars are nothing but a modern chastity belt, and the turban is a death cap."
"I can't figure out what you are talking about."
She said, "In this dress a woman can't do anything wrong. It takes hours to dress and once it is messed up, it cannot be made straight, and you can get caught so there cannot be any quickies in-between.

So judge a woman by her dress, not by her words. Understand her by her board and press. When the cloth is not pressed, wrinkles are left. A woman with a wrinkled dress is nothing but a headache. Your real strength lies in wearing neat, clean, well-ironed clothes and seeing that your woman keeps them that way. If you can make your woman dress without wrinkles, you can be miles and miles away from trouble. It is a consciousness.

Further, never allow a woman to walk behind you though she will desire it most. If she can be made to walk in front of you, your relationship will be very strongly grounded. But if she starts walking behind you, your relationship will only be so-so. When the woman walks in front of you she carries the projection of your aura. This creates in her a very strong, meditative personality. Her Self lives on the male smell which you emit when you walk. Therefore, the magnetic frequency of your arc body and her arc body will coincide as one. When she walks behind you, her arc body and your arc body act upon each other but they do not merge. It's a mechanical action, a 'spark,' like rubbing together of two flints. They create this sparking action, which is not merging and it doesn't mean a thing. I don't recommend walking side by side either, though it is fair.

In large crowds or hostile environments, she should be kept immediately in front of you so that you can give her protection. If you do otherwise, you are an idiot. Any man who cannot assure the woman that he can protect her cannot have her, and he will be rejected by the law of divinity. Remember, woman doesn't love your sex, nor your body, nor your money, nor your children. She doesn't love this maya. She loves the depth of security she experiences in her understanding of your wisdom to protect her through time and space, forever and ever. Otherwise, what is the father image? The father image is the image that guarantees her that she'll be taken care of. And, when you take over, you must give her that guarantee. If you can't have that attitude, you are asking for trouble.

Woman has a powerful reaction to all men around security. If you are a well put together, well-balanced, wise person, then normally, the woman will react to you to test your ground. Then she will react to you to test you against her insecurity. Thirdly, she will put up an unreasonable demand just to test your wisdom. She will point out your mistakes and will be bitchy, simply to test your patience. And, finally, she will be mean and abusive to test your grace. The only action you can take with such a woman is to ignore her faults and forgive her. Leave it to God and His wisdom

I wish you to be healthy, happy, and holy men of grace with a saintly projection and a soldier's action. I hope you will understand all that we have shared with you. May the Long Time Sun Shine Upon You; all love surround you, and the pure light within you, guide your way on.

May the hand of the guide, the guidance and the guiding factor of God take you everywhere, to fulfill your higher consciousness and your destiny. May the mercy of God and Guru awaken in you the sleeping, dormant consciousness. May you worship the lotus feet of the Divine in your heart. May each day bring you peace, tranquility, and grace and may you always, always be in love and may the love of God protect you always. Sat Nam.

Thank you very much. Love you a lot.

Dancing Ardas Bhaee **Meditation**
April 1981

Posture: Sit in a very yogic manner. Eyes are not specified. Listen to the mantra in silence.

Mantra:

> Ardas Bhaee, Amar Das Guru
> Amar Das Guru, Ardas Bhaee
> Ram Das Guru
> Ram Das Guru
> Ram Das Guru
> Sachee Sahee

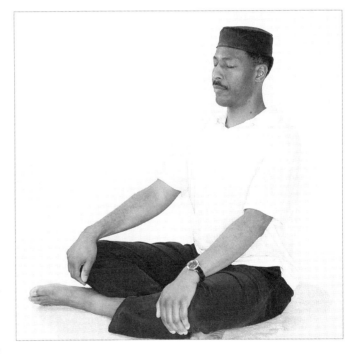

Breath: The breath is to be danced, sniffed through the nose, to the rhythm of the melody.

To End: After **9 ½ Minutes**, inhale deeply and hold the breath. Concentrate on the base of your spine and lock it, pulling the energy up, muscle by muscle and vertebra by vertebra. Mentally concentrate on the first vertebra, and lock it, pulling in and up on it, then the second, third, etc., until you have pushed the energy upward to the first vertebra in the neck—at the base of the skull. "Stretch it all the way upward; consciously do it. It will never let you grow old if you can do this little exercise." After holding the breath for about 20-40 seconds, exhale. Repeat this process two more times. Relax.

Time: 11 Minutes.

Comments: *"I wanted to let you know how you can renew your life in such a cheap way."*

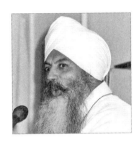

Man to **Man** 6

Sex, Success & Prosperity

Circa 1981

You must understand, thoroughly understand, one thing: this energy, this psyche, this creative energy, this sexual energy is totally yours and nobody can share it.

■ Creative **Sexuality**

■ Creative Sensitivity: **The Fundamental You**

■ Sex and Your **Life Span**

■ Sex Is a Natural **Thing**

■ The Origins of Sexual **Neuroses**

Creative **Sexuality**

The inner Self, the real Self, has to be found, has to be felt, has to be touched creatively before anything in life matters.

This is how I look at life: How long can we live with our problems? Who creates them? I did not ask you here just to gather you together, but to make you understand that if what I teach you today does not sink in, then you are going to have problems and problems and more problems.

The problem is when you do not put your energy into creativity. Sex is a creativity; for you, sex is only physical intercourse, but for me, it is a creativity. This is a concept that we must get clear in our minds. I don't want to put any taboos on your sexual behavior—that you should do this or you should do that; I am just trying to present you with one example so that you can learn from it.

You are like a samovar. We call it a *hamaam*. It is a large tank that sits on a tripod. Water can be heated in it and there is a tap. If you constantly fill that tank, that *hamaam* will eventually overflow. However, if you open the tap while you are filling it, that which enters will also flow out. But, if you don't fill it and you leave the tap open, one day the *hamaam* will be empty. That is how your energy works. What I'm trying to emphasize with you is that you only have "X" amount of energy—exactly "X" amount. You can use it sexually, sensually, meditatively, creatively, non-creatively. You can use it to harass yourself and be frustrated —or you can use it absolutely intelligently. There is no other person who can use your energy. "I gave him a lot of energy" is a totally false concept. You cannot give anyone "a lot of energy." You can give a lot of ideas, you can give a lot of thoughts, you can give a lot of initiative, you can give a lot of things; but one thing you cannot do—you cannot give your creative, sexual energy to anybody.

When you reach your optimum energy point, you discharge. This is the way God made you and it is called 'ejaculation'. All of you know and have experienced physical ejaculation, but we are going to talk about mental ejaculation. Mental ejaculation stimulates the physical ejaculation, which in America, India, Thailand, China and France, is called a 'wet dream'. Ninety percent of all people have experienced it, so it is commonly known. It uses your nervous system to such an extent that the experience is absolutely real to you. Within that experience, that play, the mental energy is real; but in reality it is not real. However, that experience, that fantasy, gives you the satisfaction of ejaculation—that is the total sum of your life.

The play of life is not real; but in your dream stage, you think it is totally real. This is because you do not understand the dimensions of it; therefore, you do not understand the success of it and you go by feelings. "In my heart, I feel…" "In my head, I feel…" "I feel, I think, I imagine…" All this is false. I don't want to tell you this. After all, you are mature people. But the great handicap, which keeps you from a successful life, is that you live—totally and absolutely—in that dream almost all the time. In the scriptures, it is called "mental masturbation."

Creative energy is the same. I am not discussing the physical level but the mental level—the creative level, the psyche— step by step. You must understand, thoroughly understand, one thing: this energy, this psyche, this creative energy, this sexual energy is totally yours and nobody can share it.

Kaam kaya ko tale, Kaam kaya ko gale.
"Lust makes the body weak."

Kaam means sexual excitement—horniness. *Kaya* means the physical body, *gale* means destroys. From time immemorial, some people have controlled their energy by masturbation. Others get this control from wet dreams and still others use anger. It is an ejaculation of energy; all of these practices are called outlets. In a simple sense, there is no such thing as anger. It is an outlet. Masturbation, the most common disease of the man, is an outlet and nobody gives it more importance than that. Both dreaming and wet dreams are nothing but subconscious outlets. And I'll tell you, in a wet dream, life is more real than in real life; and the performance in a wet dream is more real than the performance in real life.

To change this, you must start establishing contact with the subconscious psyche of your own personality. However this process doesn't begin until you are about 36. Your 30s are your years of maximum working capacity. You do your most creative work during these years. First you worry about which career you will choose, then you choose a career, then you think about that career and then you are actually in it, and you like it, then you have a middle-aged crises, all that. The whole drama is over by the time you're 36.

Until that time you are a vagabond. We call anybody under the age of 36 a psychic or spiritual vagabond. Here in the West, this person is called a 'Lone Ranger.' You may think, "I am great, I'm going to do this"; or you may experience the opposite, depression, a sense of inadequacy, feeling unfulfilled. This boasting or feeling inadequate, are the two things that bother people under 36 the most. If you do not make contact with the subconscious psyche and overcome it, if you do not compensate for your personality and combine your psyche, integrate it, with your own personality so that it works—so that you 'work'—life will not be successful for you.

What is a successful life? I agree that money "makes the world go 'round," but it does not mean a successful life. If you are married, marriage may bring you happiness, but that does not mean a successful marriage. Children may bring you fulfillment as a parent, but that doesn't make you a successful parent. The question is, "Who are you and what are you by the framework and flow of your mind?" In your framework and flow of mind you may not be successful at all.

I have known people who have reached the age of 80 or 90. They have large families, a lot of wealth, authority and respect but when the opportunity comes to speak to them, they deny their lives saying, "Oh my God, I wasted my life. I am miserable." This is because in the framework and flow of their minds, in the psyche of consciousness, they have not yet found their Self. The inner Self, the real Self, has to be found, has to be felt, has to be touched creatively before anything in life matters to us. Otherwise we are living like animals. We eat, we sleep, we marry, we have children, we go to work, we come home, we sleep in an air-conditioned room or a hot one, we are dopers, we are drug addicts, call it anything. But as long as you are not in touch with your inner Self, all the actions of the surrounding self are not your actions. You want to administrate the whole world around you but you do not want to administrate your own world within you. There is a very deep personality within you, much deeper [than most people seek]. If you do not find that depth, if you do not touch your dimensions, then your direction will never be complete. That is why some people start as doctors and end up as carpenters, or they start as carpenters and end up as an attorney.

Yogi Bhajan on **Legacy and Prosperity**

I don't want to see you without even a shirt while I go around in a silk gown. I don't believe in that. I believe that my pocket is your pocket, and these are all pockets of the same shirt. I don't believe in giving you God and a seven by seven space in heaven while you give me thirty thousand bucks. I don't believe in those kinds of numbers. I'm not into that kind of situation, and besides, our currency is not valid in the heavens, so let us not have any misunderstanding whatsoever.

I will tell you a story about a monk I once met. He was a celibate father who decided to leave the order. Then he started marrying. When I saw him last, he was on his nineteenth marriage. Just imagine! He asked me, "Why am I not successful in marriage?" I said "Why weren't you successful as a monk? There is no difference between being a monk and marrying 19 times in 5 years." These things happen because the inner psyche is not touched, not felt, not understood. It is not yet a part of you. You are just the shell, the shell of a human being, the shell of yourself.

You are not potent all the time. The psyche of the female affects you from her Third Eye, the *ajna*. Her psyche projects through her *ajna* to your *ajna*. In turn, your pituitary is affected, which stimulates the glandular system, then the circulatory system, then the brain and ultimately you begin to feel a certain hardness in your lingam [penis]. Then what happens? This is something I want to emphasize with you. What happens? You use the female to masturbate yourself. This is quite accurate. There is no other action. You use the female, and then you ejaculate. You are no more a part of the female in sex than your hand is a part of you in masturbation, even though it is attached to your body. You have no sensitivity. You have not understood the woman any more than a hand. That's why your marriages are unsuccessful, your children are crazy, you are crazy and the whole world is crazy around you. Basically and totally, you have not understood the whole thing more than your hand and that, too, only up to the elbow! I have to sit here and talk to you like this and you have to listen, because you don't want to see it, you don't want to listen to it and you don't want to understand it.

You marry a woman, you love her, you take care of her, you understand her, you go through all her ups and downs, you experience the whole situation. For what? Just for what your hand can do? You have an ego and you have a sexual ego, too. When your sexual ego is not satisfied by your woman, you want a divorce. Why do you want to divorce? Because actually that woman, that complete human being, which we have been trying to get you to respect, you won't. The Christians believe that God took the rib of Adam and created the woman from it. I don't believe that explanation is necessary because I don't think you can see anything above your elbow. That's all the woman is to you. The kissing, the intercourse, the whole paraphernalia, marrying, being with her, hugging her, is only that portion of you from your hand to your elbow. There's no feeling beyond that.

I am treating a man who likes to put yogurt on his wife. He massages her with yogurt; he finds it very stimulating. They have intercourse and then he sleeps. But his wife is sick and tired of sleeping in yogurt. She asked me, "What karma is this? You know God. Kindly meditate for me. Look into God and let me know about this strange relationship I have with yogurt." She doesn't feel that she is married to a man, instead she is married to yogurt. I told her, "You are lucky it is yogurt. Some people like rubber. They tune-in to the smell of rubber and they can't do a thing until they rubberize their wife."

Do you know what is actually happening? The man's pituitary is in tune with one particular smell. All smells are not yours. You are only tuned-in to one smell, the woman who provides you with that smell is the one who will satisfy you. Your hand cannot satisfy your attunement with that smell, so it cannot satisfy your sexual ego. That is why you seek a woman; otherwise you are all just masturbators. That is your basic instinct. It's what you do in your dreams, your waking life— that's where your basic satisfaction is. God built in the sense of smell as a safeguard, thinking, "If I make everybody a masturbator, there will be no child." So He has put this very powerful projection and condition within you—that you must relate to smell, this certain "creative smell."

I want to tell you about a very fascinating situation that took place in Tokyo. A business man I know went there to negotiate a contract. The day before the negotiations were to be finalized, he called his headquarters in the U.S. and said, "This contract will give us almost half a billion dollars loss and I don't think we should sign." The president told him, "You are our best negotiator. We need this contract badly so renegotiate it."

The next day, the man went to the meeting with his mind totally set on renegotiating the contract and saving his company the loss. When he arrived, he found that the negotiating party was accompanied by a woman. The other party was very apologetic, saying that the woman needed to be with him because his English was not adequate, which was a total ruse. Within three hours, to the complete amazement of this man, he had signed the original papers. Later, he learned that the smell of rose puts him in a state

The Creative Smell: **Mastering Your Pituitary**

I know a man who lives in an incredible mansion. When I arrived in this country in 1970, his home was valued at 10 million dollars. Prices were normal in those days—they have gone up since— and a good house could be purchased for as little as $40,000. I was taken there and I was very well entertained. During the evening, he asked me, very respectfully, if he could have a private session with me. Now the whole house was very normal, if not a little extravagant, with guest rooms and such; however, the master bedroom was just like a hayloft. Hay was spread everywhere and that is where he and his wife slept. The rest of the house was like a palace with silk everywhere, but his total, improvised psyche was absolutely fixated on hay. When he smelled hay, he became a man, very potent, very successful. Otherwise, he was totally impotent. He was the father of three children and they were all conceived in that hayloft. He told me he was sick of his fixation and he wanted to know if I could teach him some postures or give him any other yogic remedy for the situation.

I know you are interested in what I told him. (I know you were all imagining that big house and thinking that you should be there instead of him.) Now you will want to know the remedy. It is very common. Consider the hay. Who eats hay and who does not want to be in the hay? The cow eats hay

*and the snake will always try to avoid it. So, of course, he should do Cow Pose and Cobra Pose. I told him that doing these two postures along with Corpse Pose would cure him. Each of the postures is done for **11 minutes**, which effectively controls all sensitivity to smell and all creativity of the pituitary.*

There is another posture, simple enough in itself, which controls the whole olfactory system. It is called Peacock Pose. In this posture, the entire body is balanced in a horizontal position on the hands. The upper arms are brought together in front of the chest with the elbows touching each other and pushing into the Navel Point. The lower arms form a pedestal with the hands supporting the entire body, like a plank. This posture can be mastered in 30 or 40 days, or as few as 12. It is not a very difficult posture, and it will effectively cure all irregular sensitivity or insensitivity toward smell.

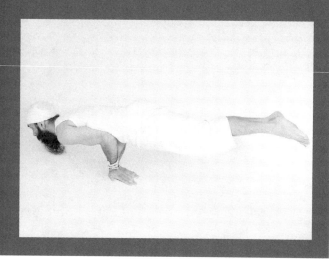

of absolute numbness. Not only was the woman wearing rose perfume, but also the man, and even the carpet had been scented with rose. His faculty to negotiate, to project, and to safeguard himself was gone. When your ego and sensitivity join together, you become totally defenseless; you can't protect yourself.

You are born to be successful. Success is yours and nobody can take it away from you. However, in your own framework, you have many effeciencies and deficiencies that undermine your life. All of your senses enter into this—smell, touch, sight, hearing, even your sense of creating a word are all creative senses. As we learned from this story, they are not insignificant. In fact, they actually control you because they overshadow your sensibility, your common sense.

Your success and your failure are based on your sexual creativity. Let us take the example of your projection to have a child. You think you want a child. Actually, you don't want a child, you don't love children. There is no such thing as a "child" within you, it's actually your own projection from start to end: it is your own sensitivity, your own creativity and your own projection from your own childhood that makes you want to create another childhood. But in fact, the child is nothing to you. That's why some people want children so badly and some people hate them.

Children are not a matter of sexual intercourse—no, not at all, there is no such thing. In the sensitivity of your own projection of your life, your future, your consciousness, you want to create a child, you want to raise a child, you want to make a child a man, what is that? What is this child business? Do you know? Superego—it is totally your subtle, superego. Whenever you go to a home where there is a child, the parents will present it to you. It makes no difference what your interest may be—you are not meeting the child. Do you understand? No man has a child. No man can create a child. No man gives birth to anybody. You are not meeting the child. You are meeting the subtle superego of the person you are visiting. That sexual creativity is a phenomenon in the personality and I want you to understand how it works.

Kriya to Create **Balance**
September 1981

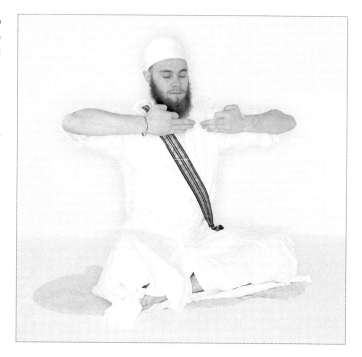

Posture: Sit with your spine straight. Bring your hands into Gyan Mudra and place them about six inches in front of the chest, about shoulder height, with the palms facing in and the three fingers straight and pointing toward one another, but not touching. The elbows are at shoulder level, pointing out to the sides.

Visualization: Stretch up and at the same time relax your lower back, your lower vertebrae. Now close your eyes, and become aware of your fourth lumbar vertebra. Project the entire power of all your thoughts to this area. Create a sensitivity in your lower back. Your breath rate will change if you feel it deeply. If you cannot create the feeling in your lower back, your breath rate will remain normal, as it was before you began.

Feel that you are getting lighter and lighter and lighter. Relax to the point of nap-sleep, and bring yourself to a dream stage. This is a million dollar therapy. Just hypnotize yourself. Get into a nap-sleep, feel your self as very light. Let all grossness go; feel that you are leaving the Earth; touch every dimension. Just think, "I am light, I am light, I am light…"

To End: After a few minutes of practice, stretch yourself up, stretch your back, and then relax.

Comments: If you can go into being light, then in life you can successfully communicate. Then you can succeed in achieving agreements, signing contracts, convincing people. This lightness of the self is the formula in which you are more refined than you think you are.

The fourth lumbar vertebra is a sexual point in the spine. By connecting with it in this way, you can control your impotency to the last day of your life, just by creating a balance between the upper body and the lower body at this fourth lumbar vertebra point. This kriya can be practiced sitting in a chair or on the floor. Anytime you find yourself very tired, your brain is very tired and not relaxed, try this posture.

Creative Sensitivity: **The Fundamental You**

The power to penetrate is the basic power that makes you male. Nature gave you the power to penetrate; Nature gave her the power to receive you and to relieve you.

Within each of us is a faculty to move our personality. It doesn't matter whether we are children, adults, or old men; we do move and we do project. We want to go. We want to project and conquer. The inborn attitude of man is to conquer. It is in his spermatozoa. To conquer is your basic natural faculty. But you forget the most beautiful aspect of it—your spermatozoa conquered the egg by entering it and becoming a part of it. It can never conquer the egg; it must *penetrate* it. The power to penetrate is the basic power that makes you male. In the male and female relationship, you do the same thing your sperm does. Nature gave you the power to penetrate; Nature gave her the power to receive you and to relieve you of that power through which you desire to penetrate. Therefore, there is a balance in the male/female relationship. You are motivated by your power to be hearty, to be projective, to be going in and penetrating. Then you move and you are relieved—you call this ejaculation. If you look at that basic human act, you can understand your total personality.

First it is mental: thought. Then comes the essence: heartiness. Projection follows in the movement back and forth, then ejaculation, then relaxation, completing, conquering. This is your basic, fundamental, rhythmic law. Anything you do against this law will be a disaster. It boils down to think, concentrate, project, penetrate, move, conquer. This is your fundamental base—the spermatozoa; you must understand this.

All action of the spermatozoa is caused by the movement of its tail. Your ego is your tail. Put your ego behind you where it can move you. Don't put it up front. That's the secret of success. Whoever puts his ego behind will penetrate. That is the primary lesson you need to learn as a male. The spermatozoa is the male seed. It moves forward by moving its tail. Put your ego behind you and go forward. If you put your ego in front you can never penetrate and you desire to penetrate. No man can relax without penetrating. But no man can enjoy without conception. When the female conceives, you are very joyful. Why? Because you have conquered; you have projected your subtle ego. Now, you feel you will not die; you have conquered death. You feel that you have come to be through the spermatozoa and through spermatozoa you are going to be again. Do you understand this about your subtle self?

You are moving from one meditative state to another meditative state, because you love yourself; it is not because you love children. Don't misunderstand that, for God's sake. You have been brainwashed. There is no such thing as the love of children. It is very common, in fact, for children to be molested and mistreated or wrongly treated because they are being raised by parents who are not loving. The child is your subtle projection of your own creativity, and your own love, into which you have projected yourself.

You are the seed. What can you do as a seed? Study the spermatozoa. It circles the egg eight times before penetrating it, before merging with it. So whenever you want to conquer anything—go around it. Normally that is not what you do. You go directly into it. We call it "male disaster." It doesn't matter what your faculty is, what intelligence you have, how rich you are, how poor you are; if you zoom directly in like an arrow, you will be broken in the middle. Is that clear? Is it understandable?

What you must learn is called "leaving the ego behind." You can go and conquer anybody by circling around and around and around them. In doing this, you totally stimulate the psyche of the person in ratio to your own proportion, and in this ratio and proportion, the other person becomes willing, becomes willing, becomes very willing to give in. But when you confront them and hit directly, you will never be effective. Confrontation is not your basic faculty and it never will be your basic faculty. If you want to merge with anything, go around it. You will be saved from destruction and you will save the other party from destruction. It is a principle of life that is unchangeable in its very nature.

You can sweat in life. You can work hard. You can work very hard to be successful. You want to be successful, you go out, you hit hard, you hit your head and then you faint. You use the same approach sexually and 40% of you fade sexually. That's the average; 40% fade and 60% are either too quick or too late. That makes 100%, and over that, you're lucky. Forty percent of the people are sexually inadequate because they are in a rush. They are not normal; within their sexual faculties, they are self-destructive, unloving and self-negating in this dimension of their lives.

Your basic rhythm, your basic foundation, your basic blueprint is determined by certain principles. You can't change it. It is your basic human faculty. To develop your psyche around a person, you must meet him. But meanwhile, you forget how to talk and you start 'wining and dining'. The feeling is that if you cannot reach the head then you will reach the stomach. Do you understand why people drink? When they drink, they get a little loose and they can talk. The booze offers a shelter. When people are sober, they realize that when they speak they need to speak wisely. Because they don't have much wisdom to speak of, they have to get a little high so that they can talk some foolishness.

But actually you are very sensitive. You are very sensitive and very penetrating. It is your faculty as a human being to penetrate. God gave you the basic, fundamental power to penetrate through anything. But you don't do it. You go and hit hard, you hit directly. You can understand the greatest secret of success by looking at the basic sexual act. Look at nature and look at your own creativity.

I want to share with you that your very fundamental self has been made in a very simple, mechanical way. Your basic sensitivity lies within your own sexual method of creating life. Everything is all right. You only need to study it. Here in the West, sex is either a sensitivity, a sensitive creativity, or a pleasure—no! Actually, sex is a study of the fundamental you.

Fit to **Act**?

It is an amazing thing, but the majority of people don't know that the sexual tract must be alkaline before ejaculation can be thought of. The prostate gland secretes and makes the pathway alkaline. Now it takes a while for this to take place. That is why all the lovemaking, the kissing and hugging and all that, is required. Between the time that your pituitary secretes and pulsates to give you an erection and the time you ejaculate, the urethra, the tract, must become alkaline. This is because your seminal fluid is acidic. If your tract is not properly alkaline before you ejaculate, you will not have your full capacity for the next full moon. Your magnetic field cannot be complete. Period.

If the seminal fluid is not properly balanced by the prostate secretion, the acidity of the ejaculation irritates the duct and in turn, the master gland, the pituitary, is affected. You lose two-thirds of your thinking, your projection, your intercourse, your creativity, and your success through this one simple mistake. You will work at one-third capacity. You will forget things while you are talking, you will be absentminded, you will not complete your work and your calls, and if there is too much irritation in your life, you will end up driving north when you want to go south.

If you are not hard you cannot have intercourse. If you try, you will have a time of it. Likewise, if you are not fit of mind and body, you should sit down, relax and sleep. You may be a grown male, five foot eight and your male organ is five inches. When that organ is not fit, then your performance will not be right. Realize what that represents and when your personality is not fit, don't act. When your personality is not fit, that's it. Don't act! "Those who use sex in a relaxed manner for deep relaxation are the princes. Others are animals." This is a saying of the masters. It is that simple.

Don't rush. That is a requirement. And don't put your ego in front of you. I want you to understand how powerfully strong you are, to know how much self-control you have.

Special Exercises for **Men**
September 1981

The following three exercises are very important. They are part of the man, and man is part of them.

Caution: After practicing these exercises, never just sit straight down. First stand up—and only then relax.

Exercise 1
Stand up and extend your right arm straight up toward the ceiling. Bend the left arm at the elbow and place the palm of the left hand on your right side, directly over your liver. Hold tightly at this spot. Keeping your chest and arm lifted, bend toward your left, extending your right side. Hold the posture.

Comments: Your liver will go through a lot of changes. Just watch it. Make sure you hold your liver tightly, bend as much as you can, and hold the arm in the air as straight as possible. Don't feel you have to do it a long time. (It was practiced for one minute during the course.) This posture develops your power of penetration.

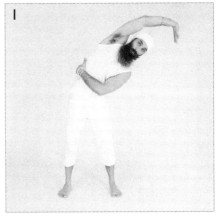

Exercise 2
Stand up. Bring your heels together and your toes apart, let you knees come apart as you squat down into a seated position. Your buttocks should go down, but not too much. Place your hands flat on your thighs and hold. Look forward. Sit balanced with your lower back in, your torso upright with chin in Neck Lock, and your spine straight.

Comments: If you want to develop your sexual potency, do this posture. This exercise should have been taught to you when you were a boy.

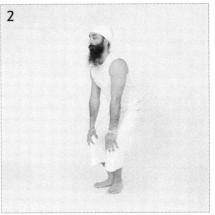

Exercise 3
Stand up. Stretch your arms overhead and form an arc over your head with your hands; the palms are facing down, directly above the shoulder area. Keeping the arms in this position, squat down as in Exercise 2. Try to sit down as deeply as possible in the posture while maintaining your balance.

Comments: This exercise is very good for relieving pressure from the lower back.

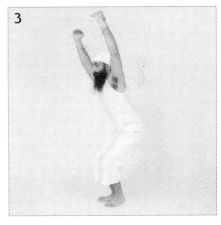

Sex and Your Life Span

The fundamental requirement of the human character is sex. Sex is a teacher. Creativity and creativeness come from the sexual act.

I know that these are very heavy subjects that I am discussing and they should be taken very politely—and lightly. The fundamental requirement of the human character is sex. Sex is a teacher. Creativity and creativeness come from the sexual act. Sex is the sixth sense, which contains all our dimensions, relative and irrelative. Sex is the part of your life that should give you success. I am not speaking of sex as you understand it in the Western world. That's not sex; that's a sexual sensitivity. It is performed with the attitude of just 'getting into it' and it is totally destructive. Sex, as I'm speaking of it, is a necessity, a biological necessity. It's a creativity, it's relaxing, it's very projective and expansive.

For each sexual act, when you get into the second phase, you re-create the other sexual act. It is called phase one of creativity. However, some of you are so sexual that you want sex 6 times during the night and 8 times a day—that's 14 times a day. Rabbits do the same thing. Someone once told me that his capacity was 18 times a day and his wife confirmed it. I asked him if he could reduce it to 12 times a day and he said, "No." I told him he could make a lot of money if he could teach people how to have sex 18 times a day and still walk. Now it has been two years and he is beginning to realize that it was too much.

There are creative years. Western people become sexually creative and have feelings of horniness by the age of 11. Actually, it is very dangerous for the man to have sex before the age of 25. Before that time, the pituitary and the testicles are out of synch. They come into rhythm in the 24th year. Understand that sexual intercourse is not to be performed before age 25, and if you stick to that law, then from age 25 to 75 to 100, whether you live or die, you will not be a paper man, nor insane, senile or weak. Your propensity of creative consciousness, your psyche of projection, will be very potent, smart and strong. You will walk tall.

Otherwise you pay the price after age 54. You start going downhill because you did not control yourself and you did not mature yourself to the point of full bloom, which happens in the 24th year. The woman should not indulge in sexual intercourse until she is 18.

Question and Answer

Q: *Does that include masturbation?*

Yogi Bhajan: Yes, and wet dreaming, too.

Q: *What can we do to correct the damage?*

Yogi Bhajan: Don't feel guilty if you have done it out of rhythm. There are two recipes you can use. First take chawan prash rolled in silver leaf every day with 8 oz. of milk either for your breakfast or along with whatever else you want to eat for breakfast. Secondly, eat two pistachio paranthas for your food one day of each week.

Q: *How long should we take the chawan prash?*

Yogi Bhajan: You have to take it for a long time. It is an Ayurvedic remedy and Ayurveda is a building system. It will keep you going and build you up gradually and slowly. Both allopathy and homeopathy are wonderful systems, which hit right on the spot, but Ayurveda builds.

Currently we are creating a formula to build potency. I am going to test it myself. It is part of an herbal remedy series we are producing. We call it the "R" series and it is based on the ancient herbal formulas from the old, old times when those wise, non-mechanical people cared for themselves. The male potency is called "17-R." There is another with a chili base called "14-R."[1]

Q: *How do we go about teaching our children not to have intercourse before they are the proper age?*

Yogi Bhajan: My grandfather sat me down and talked to me exactly as I am talking to you. It took him three days to explain everything to me. He told me about maturity and how the organ develops. He told me about semen and about blood. He explained the amount of pressure intercourse has on the thyroid and parathyroid. He told me everything.

In my life, I experimented and found that he was absolutely accurate. Don't think I didn't do anything wrong. Left to my own recourse, I would have made many blunders. I am a rebel. But, thank God, I was taught in time. Unfortunately, I didn't realize that I was going to have to come to the United States. If I had known that I would not have married until I was 50. With your own children, you have to be very friendly, very honest and very straightforward; let them understand what's going on in the world.

Q: *What causes wet dreams and what preventive measures can be taken so that you don't develop them?*

Yogi Bhajan: Heavy exercise and meditation are the best ways to control this. One student told me, "I just want to live a celibate lifestyle." And she gave me her past history. There was no exercise facility available to her, but there was a very large courtyard where she lived. It was about 90 feet by 90 feet.

---

[1] These formulas are available from Herbal Gems and can be purchased through Ancient Healing Ways: www.a-healing.com or through your local health food store.

I advised her to buy a soccer ball and use that. She bought the ball and she plays with it for an hour or two until she sweats. Then she bathes, goes to bed and sleeps. She never has any problems.

She used to have horrible dreams. Not just wet dreams, but sweat-wet dreams. Her dreams were very peculiar, incredible dreams. She would dream that someone would come and rape her, cut her neck and drink her blood and then cut off her foot and eat it. She would dream these dreams night after night after night. Now—nothing.

Meditation is also very wonderful for getting rid of the garbage—mental as well as physical. It is very potent.

Q: *Why is it that girls begin menstruating three or four years earlier than those of a decade ago?*

Yogi Bhajan: This is due to the influence of television. Our lives are in great jeopardy because of TV and the media. We are being mistreated. You have no idea how deeply horror movies and that type of programming affect our children.

Once I walked into a house where a group of children were watching TV. There were at least five children in the group. In four minutes, I was upside down because the program was so horrible, so horrible! A man cut off a woman's leg, then he had intercourse with her while she was bleeding to death. And, there were the children, watching it! What do you expect?

Q: *You once said in a lecture that if a person had ever done cocaine, he could never experience God. Is there any way we can compensate for this behavior?*

Yogi Bhajan: Yes. Breath of Fire and Sa-Ta-Na-Ma meditation are the fundamental techniques which can correct and cure any situation. Half an hour of Breath of Fire will help those who have sniffed cocaine even to the point of bursting their noses and it will also help those who have done much worse things than cocaine.

It's no big deal. It is based on simple logic. I don't believe in making it complicated, where you have to be shrouded in mystery.

Q: *Is there any particular mudra or posture we should use for Sa-Ta-Na-Ma's and the Breath of Fire?*

Yogi Bhajan: We have given all this and it is very commonly available to you. This course is not to discuss Sa-Ta-Na-Ma meditation. *[Editor's Note: Yogi Bhajan is referring to Kirtan Kriya.]*

Q: *What negative effect, if any, occurs if one gets stimulated and doesn't ejaculate?*

Yogi Bhajan: Oh, it's very boring and it's very painful, isn't it? In the scriptures the woman who does that is called a "pig woman," *soorneeaa*. In the orient calling someone a

Two Techniques to **Save the Day**

Breath of Fire and Sa-Ta-Na-Ma meditation [Kirtan Kriya] are the fundamental techniques which can correct and cure any situation: 31 minutes of Breath of Fire and 31 minutes of Sa-Ta-Na-Ma are the most effective tools we can apply. We state publically that we know the results are 100% effective—100%. There's no duality in our mind about it and there shouldn't be any duality in any mind. There's nothing more than that. Everything else is just talking.

If a person wants to declare himself a god or a guru, God bless him. I'm not going to be down on anybody. But all meditation stops at Sa-Ta-Na-Ma. There's nothing beyond it. All pranayam stops at Breath of Fire. There's no pranayam beyond that. If your pranic body can overtake all the bodies, then you will be hale, healthy and perfect.

Breath of Fire

This breath is used consistently throughout Kundalini Yoga kriyas. It is very important that Breath of Fire be practiced and mastered by the student. In Breath of Fire, the focus of the energy is at the Navel Point. The breath is fairly rapid (2 to 3 breaths per second), continuous and powerful with no pause between the inhale and exhale. As you exhale, the air is pushed out by pulling the Navel Point and abdomen toward the spine. In this motion, the chest area remains fairly relaxed. The inhalation will occur naturally from the vacuum created by the exhale. This is a very balanced breath with no emphasis on either the exhale or the inhale, but rather equal power given to both. The inhale will feel easier than the exhale because the natural force of the diaphragm relaxing helps it.

Breath of Fire is a cleansing breath, renewing the blood and releasing old toxins from the lungs, mucous lining, blood vessels, and cells. It is a powerful way to adjust your autonomic nervous system and get rid of stress. Regular practice expands the lungs quickly. You can start with **3 minutes** *of Breath of Fire and build to* **31 minutes**.

Kirtan Kriya

Sa-Ta-Na-Ma, the Panj Shabd, is used in dozens of kriyas and meditations that Yogi Bhajan gave over the years. Kirtan Kriya is the foundation meditation using this sound current. It clears the subconscious and the arcline. It can be done for 11 minutes to 2 ½ hours, but 31 minutes is the most common discipline.

Kirtan Kriya

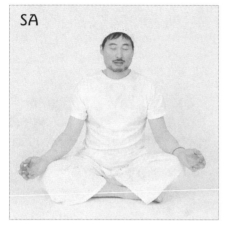
SA

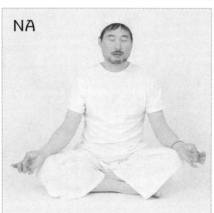
TA

NA

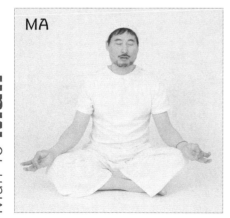
MA

This kriya is one of three that Yogi Bhajan mentioned would carry us through the Aquarian Age, even if all other teachings were lost. There are four principle components to practicing Kirtan Kriya correctly: Mantra, Mudra, Voice, and Visualization.

Mantra
This kriya uses the five primal sounds, or the *Panj Shabd*— S, T, N, M, A— in the original *bij* form of the word Sat Nam:

SA — infinity, cosmos, beginning
TA — life, existence
NA — death
MA — birth

This is the cycle of creation. From the Infinite comes life and individual existence. From life comes death or change. From death comes the rebirth of consciousness. From rebirth comes the joy of the Infinite through which compassion leads back to life. Chant the 'A' as if you were pronouncing 'mom,' in the following manner:

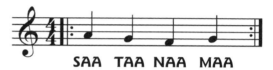
SAA TAA NAA MAA

Mudra
Each repetition of the entire mantra takes 3 to 4 seconds. The elbows are straight while chanting, and each finger touches, in turn, the tip of the thumb with a firm but gentle pressure.

Sa — the index or Jupiter finger touches the thumb;
Ta — the middle or Saturn finger and thumb;
Na — the ring or Sun finger and thumb;
Ma— the pinkie or Mercury finger and thumb; then begin again with the index finger.

Visualization
You must meditate on the primal sounds in the "L" form. This means that when you meditate you feel there is a constant inflow of cosmic energy into your solar center, or Tenth Gate (the Crown Chakra). As the energy enters the top of the head, you place **Sa**, **Ta**, **Na**, or **Ma** there.

As you chant **Sa**, for example, the "S" starts at the top of your head and the "A" moves down and out through the Brow Point, projected to Infinity. This energy flow follows the energy pathway called the golden cord—the connection between the pineal and pituitary gland. Some people may occasionally experience headaches from practicing Kirtan Kriya if they do not use this "L" form. The most common reason for this is improper circulation of prana in the solar centers.

Voice
We chant the mantra in the three languages of consciousness:

Aloud	the voice of the human	awareness of the things of the world
Whisper	the voice of the lover	experiencing the longing to belong
Silent	the voice of the divine	meditate on Infinity or mentally vibrate

To Begin the Practice
Sit straight in Easy Pose and meditate at the Brow Point.

Chant aloud for **5 minutes**, then whisper for **5 minutes** and then go deeply into silence, mentally vibrating the sound. Vibrate in silence for **10 minutes**, then whisper for **5 minutes,** then chant aloud for **5 minutes**.

Close the meditation with a deep inhale and suspend the breath as long as comfortable—up to a minute—relaxing it smoothly to complete **1 minute** of absolute stillness and silence.

To end: Stretch the hands up as far as possible and spread the fingers wide. Stretch the spine and take several deep breaths. Relax.

Comments:

Each time you close a mudra by joining the thumb with a finger, your ego seals the effect of that mudra in your consciousness. The effects are as follows:

SIGN	FINGER	NAME	EFFECT
Jupiter	Index	Gyan Mudra	Knowledge
Saturn	Middle	Shuni Mudra	Wisdom, intelligence, patience
Sun	Ring	Surya Mudra	Vitality, energy of life
Mercury	Pinkie	Buddhi Mudra	Ability to communicate

Practicing this chant brings a total mental balance to the individual psyche. As you vibrate on each fingertip, you alternate your electrical polarities. The index and ring fingers are electrically negative, relative to the other fingers. This causes a balance in the electro-magnetic projection of the aura. If during the silent part of the meditation your mind wanders uncontrollably, go back to a whisper, to a loud voice, to a whisper and back into silence. Do this as often as necessary to stay alert.

Practicing this meditation is both a science and an art. It is an art in the way it molds consciousness and the refinement of sensation and insight it produces. It is a science in the tested certainty of the results it produces. Each meditation is based on the tested experience of many people, in many conditions, over many years. It is based on the structure of the psyche and the laws of action and reaction that accompany each sound, movement and posture. The meditations as kriyas code this science into specific formulas we can practice to get specific results. Because it is so effective and exact, it can also lead to problems if not done properly.

Chanting the *Panj Shabd*—the primal or nuclear form of *Sat Nam*—has profound energy within it because we are breaking the *bij* (seed or atom) of the sound, *Sat Nam*, into its primary elements. You may use this chant in any position as long as you adhere to the following requirements:

1. Keep the spine straight.
2. Focus at the Brow Point.
3. Use the "L" form of meditation.
4. Vibrate the *Panj Shabd* in all three languages— human, lover, and divine.
5. Use common sense without fanaticism.

The timing can be decreased or increased as long as you maintain the ratio of spoken, whispered, and silent chanting—always end with **1 minute** of complete stillness and silence. Yogi Bhajan said, at the Winter Solstice of 1972, that a person who wears pure white and meditates on this sound current for 2½ hours a day for one year, will know the unknown and see the unseen. Through this constant practice, the mind awakens to the infinite capacity of the soul for sacrifice, service, and creation.

soor, pig, is the worst of all abuse. It means that you have no sensitivity to what is going on. Mud and silk are the same to you. You know how pigs are. You clean them and do everything to educate them and when they graduate, they go into pig shit and do their thing. It is a very sad experience to be stimulated and not ejaculate. It's very boring. Avoid the company of people who will put you in that situation.

Q: *You mentioned that sex should only take place in a relaxed manner. At the same time, a lot of people have phobias and fears about sex. Should you resolve your sexual phobias before engaging in sex?*

Yogi Bhajan: I understand the phobias and I understand that impotency comes from phobias. There are internal blocks and external blocks. The external blocks are triggered by the female and the internal blocks are from the male, his own force. Eventually I have to discuss that, too. I don't think that we should hold more than two courses per year but gradually we are covering a lot of areas, slowly and efficiently.

I want to talk to you about using your subconscious energy to penetrate through your fears and phobias. During these courses we have been emphasizing basic information and philosophy, not the practical aspects. I think that in the next course I will arrange one day as a workshop and I will demonstrate techniques for renewing yourself and I will get into the practical applications of all these teachings.

Q: *Previously you spoke to us about the necessity of the glands to secrete sufficiently so that the urethra will have the proper alkaline levels and not become irritated by the seminal fluid during ejaculation. How much time does it normally take for that to occur?*

Yogi Bhajan: Because you asked the question, I am obliged to reply correctly; the minimum maturity time is ten days. If you decide you would like to have intercourse on Friday, then you must begin to prepare for it on Wednesday, a week before that Friday.

Sex starts in the living room. It starts with certain notions. It starts in the imagination with certain mental masturbations, thought extensions and thought projections, and then it has to be developed. True human intercourse is like a long, long love story. It matures. It matures like something that develops slowly and gradually. It's just like growing and graduating. What you do cannot be called intercourse. It is a very great insult to call it intercourse. Don't call it intercourse; it is called "pistoning." Get up, get in, get out. Thank you. That's all it is. I think you must have been steam engines in your last lives.

Also understand, you must not feel guilty about it. There are some metabolisms that are very strong, which can and need to be satisfied. I remember a case of a gentleman that could not digest his food if he did not have intercourse two times a day. His doctor prescribed it. I had to counsel his wife to accommodate him. One day she said, "Well, you are not going to eat today." He said, "Why?" She said, "I am not going to be responsible for your indigestion and I'm not available."

You must understand that each human being has a different metabolism, a difference in need. We are discussing the central line of it, the mean, and we are presenting one extreme to the other. I have seen people who are very sexual, into it too much and in their maturity, their metabolism changes and they become subnormal in their sexual drive.

Q: *In some of the ancient books, the sex act is called the "holy of holies." Why is that?*

Yogi Bhajan: Because it is the holy of holies. If it had not been performed, you would not be sitting in this room. It is your fundamental act. If it is performed totally as it should be, it is very holy, very meditative, and very excellent. It is a most beautiful thing. It is very, very calming. The idea of it, entering into that idea, and getting into it, thinking about it, preparing for it, and having her prepare for it, too, and then having it; it's a lovey-dovey thing.

I'm not talking about this pistoning—stand up, kick the tree, 'just shake the tree' a little bit, and shake yourself and shake her and it's all over. That's love American style. I'm not a part of it. In reality, there's a human grace and both graces join their hands together.

Q: *Is all creativity based on sexuality?*

Yogi Bhajan: Yes. All creativity is based on your sexual potency and the direction of it. There are no two ways about it. That direction determines how you control your sex, how you control your temper, how you control your tempo, how you control yourself. How you control yourself affects how you control your environments; how you control your environments is how you project what your environments will be and what they will produce for you. That is the law of creativity. It is totally rhythmic and there is no gap in it.

Q: *You talked about frequency of intercourse. What practices can the man use during his wife's pregnancy to curb his sexual appetite?*

Yogi Bhajan: Actually the man has no real problem. He can be as sexual or as celibate as he wants. You can use Breath of Fire to totally regulate your urgencies. I will give you the details of this in the next course.

Q: *What do you think about having sex without ejaculating? In a book that is not commonly available,* *the author says that it doesn't matter what the frequency of intercourse is, as long as the man doesn't ejaculate, but controls his sexual energy. The book is supposedly based on an ancient Chinese text.*

Yogi Bhajan: Yes, there is one very beautiful group who preach that you should never ejaculate but transmute the energy upward. Their leader died of cancer of the prostate.

I want you to understand. God is never wrong. Please, if you ever have intercourse, you must ejaculate—if not into the woman, then in the bathroom. Don't carry it. That is ridiculous. Who taught you those things? Those ideas are inhuman.

One day when I was out at my ranch, I was talking with that stallion, Mantequilla. I said, "Mantequilla, whenever people come around you, you get horny." That beautiful horse looked at me and he ejaculated right there! I thought to myself, he understood the whole thing. I was very glad that although he was a Spanish horse, he understood English. Then while I was looking at him, he did that little whinny that horses do with their lips. I did it back to him; we were thanking each other.

Are you less intelligent than Mantequilla? That horse understood it. These things like holding your ejaculation are crazy. Go by God's way. Get to God by God's way. Don't create your own nonsense.

Once I met a yogi who was prolonging his life. He was doing a very particular pranayam with honey, which I knew. The honey was in a container, which allowed it to ooze out very slowly, drop by drop. He correlated his breath with the drops so that he savoured each drop, constricting his breath until the drop had permeated his whole body.
I said, "Why are you doing this?"
He said, "I want to expand and extend my life."
I said, "Are you crazy? It is so costly to get all this honey. Then putting all the honey in your body is too much, plus doing all this pranayam business is just too heavy. I don't think you are supposed to do it." But he wouldn't listen to me. He might have extended his life if he had, but he died of lung cancer, which was ridiculous.

I think all of these people who are doing these weird things are very self-destructive and very un-Godly. I only share God's way with you. If you believe in sex, fine. If you don't believe in sex, and you don't want to have sex, then God will make you impotent anyway, so what's the big deal?

You never see a man being very sexy when he is 92. His whole body will shake. If you don't want your body to shake, then try to control and proportion your sexual energy. Plan it. It is the same thing that I have said to you. You have "X" amount of energy. It is yours and it cannot be anyone else's. It is your free choice to use it the way you want. You can control it, you can proportion it, you can dish it, you can destroy it. But with the same energy, you can create an empire, you can create a heaven or you can create a hell.

Q: *Is there any way to tell when the urethra has the proper alkaline balance?*

Yogi Bhajan: Yes. Just press the tip of the penis and you will find something coming out of it.

Q: *After strenuous exercise, like working up a lot of body heat playing soccer, is there a proper way to cool down?*

Yogi Bhajan: I can tell you what we did when I was young. We used to play soccer for about three hours and work up such a sweat that we were absolutely wet as hell. Then we would eat. We would sit on the ground and eat and fall asleep on the spot, some of us into our own plates. That's the truth. We would sleep for about an hour and then we would work out again for about three hours.

We would get home late at night and immediately lay out on our beds. Our servants would remove our clothes, and we would go straight into a beautiful hot tub of water. We would lie there for 10-15 minutes, come out, towel off, relax for a few minutes, and then get back in for a beautiful cold shower. We would dry off again, put on our night clothes and go to the kitchen and eat—maybe 30 chapatis, something like that. Then some people would regularly be carried from the kitchen to their beds. I never suffered any injury whatsoever.

Now at my age, 52, I am not supposed to eat butter, and I'm not supposed to eat this, and I'm not supposed to do anything. I'm not even supposed to breathe. But in those days, 12 chapatis made with cauliflower and two pounds of butter and eaten straight with four kilos of yogurt used to be an ordinary breakfast, plus a couple of quarts of buttermilk. Furthermore, the body was so skinny that every pair of knickers I wore would fall off. I was never naked, thanks to our underwear.

Then I came to America. I think the air here is very bad and the water is terrible. I have no complaint about America except that the water has no minerals and it is not healthy water. Healthy water can take care of a lot of problems for you.

Q: *When you were playing in those days, did you do anything to protect your sexual organs? Like a jockstrap?*

Yogi Bhajan: Yes. We wore a loin cloth; the jockstrap does the same thing. You need to do it. Hanging testicles are the gateway to impotency. Wearing tight underwear is very healthy and very required. Some of you don't mind being loose and you don't take care of yourself. The result of that is terrible. All of this is because the length of the testes varies greatly. The phenomena is called "rotation of the testicle." You know it even changes when you bathe. For this reason, some people never remove their underwear all at once, but remove one leg, then put the other one on. They are very particular that this won't happen.

This is the only country where nobody cares. They think the scrotum is just something extra hanging there. But I think that in the realms of consciousness, the testicles are very important. They are always a couple of degrees lower than the body and that temperature should be maintained. Everything should be done to insure that.

Q: *I couldn't understand your grave message about mental masturbation.*

Yogi Bhajan: I am saying that your projections are mainly mental and what brings you to wet dreams is totally mental. You work through mind and body but the body is subjected to the mind.

Q: *Should the testicles be held in place at all times?*

Yogi Bhajan: Yes. This is required.

Q: *Two questions: first, how do people become fixated on a scent; and secondly, what other exercises can one do for the other senses that will have the effect that Peacock Pose has on regulating the sense of smell?*

Yogi Bhajan: Basically the sense of smell is related to the pituitary. This connection is enjoined in many books and many sutras where it is related to the Third Eye Point which is nothing but the pituitary gland. The sensitivity which the body has is to its own odor. Each body emits a certain odor and desires an odor in return. Some people are fixated on a certain flower, some on wood, some on hair, some on rain. Some people are very horny on hot days. Sometimes on that very hot day, it will rain and the earth smell will come out. There are some people who cannot control themselves at all under those circumstances.

If you do Breath of Fire regularly, everything will normalize. That is why Breath of Fire is called Breath of Fire. It burns all inadequacies.

Q: *Should Long Deep Breathing or Breath of Fire be done with Peacock Pose? And, how long should we hold the posture?*

Yogi Bhajan: A long, slow breath would be best and hold the posture from 11 to 22 minutes. Try it.

The Tip System

What should you drink after intercourse? Warm milk? Ginger milk? Yogi tea? Coke? No, Coke will soak you to death and you'll pay a heavy dividend for it.

Take hot milk with a tablespoon of sesame oil in it. You may not have your birth control things around, but if you want to keep going in your life, keep a glass of milk and sesame oil handy. Take it after you have finished your sexual indulgence and activity.

Have you ever watched the horses or the elephants at the circus? After they finish their performance, they are given a little something, a reward, a tip. We call it the "tip system." That tip says, "You have done well, boy," and that little boy of yours needs a little tip. Don't treat it lightly. It can put you to shame if it won't perform what you want it to perform, so giving it a little glass of milk and a tablespoon of sesame oil is not a bad idea at all.

■ ■ ■

Sex Is a Natural **Thing**

Does the spermatozoa control the egg? Does the egg control the spermatozoa? No. They totally merge, they totally get lost in each other.

When sex is without worship, it is rape. God never intended people to have sex with those rapist tendencies; it's damaging. When it is done with a kind of worship, it's advantageous.

In the old civilizations, I am not talking about the barbarian civilization in which we Westerners live, but in the true civilizations, people understood things, which we can understand today. People added certain rituals to sex, a kind of worship, and it had qualifying attitudes and attributes. For example, no man, no matter how idiotic he may have been, would indulge in sex within three hours of having eaten.

If the stomach is full, sex is out, like the tide. If sex is in, the stomach should be empty. This rule, this proportion between sex and stomach, is so essential to your life—you cannot live without it. Full stomach and full sex, you are dead. This combination will bring you every trouble, known and unknown, and there's nothing I can do. There's no prayer, no meditation which can prevent the damage. So don't think that the cause and effect will not take place.

Take what used to be a very simple Western system: go out and have dinner and dance. Come midnight, they would wind up the evening. They would wait a while and then maybe indulge in sex. These days, you take somebody out, give that girl a sandwich or something, pull her off somewhere and just do it, and that's it. If he's really trying to impress her, he may take her to the falafel stand. I call it "sandwich sex." There is no system, there's no rhythm, there's no understanding that if you are putting something in and you are taking something out, the procedure cannot be that fast.

Your whole personality is based on this area called *agna granthi*, your stomach. It involves your circulation, your digestive fire, your blood and body heat, your metabolism, and your entire digestive system including the intestines and the colon. Please take note: When above the navel is busy, below the navel should be nonfunctional. Do you understand? Never indulge in any sexual activity with a full stomach.

A Vitality Formula: **Parsley Pilau**

If you have a beloved, or a partner, or a wife, whatever sex scandal you are in . . . ask her to cook this for you. If you want to live, and live light, if you want to be very brainy, very intelligent, very successful, if you don't want to be pushy or feel agitated or eaten up, it's a very simple thing.

PARSLEY PILAU
1 cup rice (uncooked)
1 cup parsley leaves, dried
2 cups of unskinned potatoes
Onions
Masala: Ajwan seeds, Red pepper, Turmeric, Black pepper, & Bay leaves
Ghee (Clarified butter)

Saute onions in ghee, adding spices to create a masala. Then add rice to that sauteed onion dish, add potatoes and parsley and then stir for a while. Add water to the dish. Cook everything for 10-15 minutes.

When you get headaches and heaviness and you feel very sleepy and fatigued, eat this very human food. We call it very human male food; male food in the sense that males are very aggressive. One thing you experience as a man, which you do not understand, is that sometimes, your skin feels small and you feel big. You feel that you are going to burst out of your skin; you feel like you are being suffocated, stitched into your skin. You understand that irritation? It is an irritation of the capillaries. It happens to lot of people who feel handicapped or inadequate.

It is a mono diet: not more than three days. If you are a hardworking man who may need more energy to get through your work day, you can take it with yogurt. It's very delicious. The only danger is, don't overeat it. You can serve it once in a while to your friends, whatever you want to do, but it's very good for the brain. It's very good for you.

Further, I am worried about people who eat meat, not because I'm against it. If you want to sleep with a pig at night and eat him first thing in the morning, it won't bother me if that is your bacon. The real thing I am worried about is the food that doesn't come *out* of your body within 24 hours; it is very damaging to sex, to creativity and to maintaining what is called the "grit" of the man, the real man. The real man is the man that stands within your Self.

You will find that people who eat meat throughout their lives, become bulky after the age of 54. They are bulky in their face and their body; they even become bulky in their behavior. They lose their sophistication, their delicacy. Their behavior will become very itchy, and sexually, they will have as many diseases as you can list.

I talked to a man who came to me in tears, and I could understand why. The guy was 39 years old and totally impotent. Totally impotent at age 39! It was a shock even to me. I asked him if there was any time in his life that he ate too much of any particular food over a sustained period of time. I found that while he was in college, which is known as a time for shoving food into our systems just for convenience, he would eat six raw eggs blended in milk with a shot of brandy every day. I couldn't believe it. I told him that the only effective treatment would be a tablet of potassium cyanide! There is no treatment, that is, no allopathic or homeopathic treatment. Fortunately, there is treatment and there is treatment: three foods from India can be made into a juice that will help. So I called a friend of mine who sent it over here, and by Guru's grace, he is all right now. But who wants to go through that?

Now I am going to tell you something that you don't understand and don't want to understand. You are going to experience failure. Have you ever known a child to be born without a pregnancy? Is there any way for you to have intercourse today and three hours later, push, a child emerges? No. What happens? You get hot, you get horny, you have intercourse, and out of a lot of intercourses—you miss so many shots you wouldn't believe it—there is one pregnancy.

Sometimes you say, "A-ha, I'm a great man!" Other times, it's "Aye aye aye." I mean, that is life, isn't it? You fail every day. Are you crazy? It is a part of life. You must understand—it's the price we pay for pregnancy. But when you fail, you say, "I'm inadequate. I can't do anything." Once someone came to see me who was very crazy; he had failed at something and his rage was such that he had scratched his cheeks until they bled. He came to me and I said, "Can you believe what you are doing to yourself?" And I sent him to get first aid. They treated him, gave him a tetanus shot, and charged him $39. It is ridiculous. A part of the natural, sexual indulgence, which is given by God, is that out of many intercourses, many chances, there is one pregnancy. This is the fundamental creative law of success. It must be accepted. All of you who want to get in and then out and be done, that's it. You're crazy. That's not the natural path. The natural path is indulgence, intercourse, penetrate, indulgence, intercourse, penetrate, and so on. Remember it. It is a natural law. Nobody else will teach it to you and then I'll be gone.

You Americans think you are very sexy, but I find you very dumb. You don't know anything about sex. It's ridiculous. Sex is penetrate, indulge, and intercourse. Keep on doing that until you feel the situation, the object, is pregnant. From the pregnancy starts the attitude of success. In pregnancy,

The Reaction of the Male **Organ**

If through overindulgence or masturbation or some other circumstance, your organ becomes bent —this normally happens to most people—or if you find that your erection doesn't catch up from the base, which is a problem shared by 80% of all men, then you are going to have trouble. Immediately after intercourse, your organ should begin to shrink back, but due to these problems, you will find it is just slumped down like a broken tree branch. You do not understand how damaging this is. It irritates the entire system in the brain.

Not only is it very irritating but it is a slow irritation. It takes 72 hours for the reaction to occur, then when you get up, you will feel very heavy headed and your body will feel sluggish. It gives you a feeling of having sinned. That is the physical origin of the idea of sex as a sin. The Catholics didn't dream it up, they just propagated it. It is called the "reaction of the male organ."

This pistachio chapati, which is very costly and very good, can put you back into gear. Do you understand what I am saying? I am a holy man and I must stay within the boundary of the law so that what I say does not appear sexual, but I have to teach you God's laws. If you break manmade laws, you go to jail and get out on parole. If you break natural laws, there's no parole. I am concerned about this and believe that no man should break a natural law.

the attitude of success is nursing. Be it a marriage, a business, a relationship, a church, God, whatever it is, the most sophisticated thing you can do as a human being on this Earth is called nursing. Nurse friendship, nurse relationship, nurse everything!

The greatest phenomenon of sex and success is totally qualified in one word, one dimension, one thing: the art of nursing. You can learn it from the woman. She turns her blood into milk. You turn your anger into *seva*, service. Do you understand what I am saying? Just as a woman turns her blood into milk to nurse a child, you can turn your anger into service. No matter how dumb a man may be, if he serves, he'll be successful, because this simple law—*seva*—is the secret of success.

Why do we want to do our thing? Why don't we just do what God does? Don't you want to be successful? Is there anybody on Earth who doesn't want to be successful? Success comes from nursing. That is how God laid the law of success. Nursing means tenderness, handling it right, letting it suck on you. You Americans abuse that word, "Ah, he's a sucker." I don't like it when you abuse it that way. It's not right. If you can afford it, let it suck. People will want to lean on you, to leech off you, to get things out of you. But remember, it is the law of nursing. When somebody comes and uses my telephone to make a drunken call, I know it is a drunken call. It is not going to be a local call and I'm going to pay the bill. I know that. There's nothing to be mad about. Why? I know that he is sucking. It is the law of nursing. I say, "Hail, hail to Guru Ram Das that I am competent enough to tolerate this." You've got to hail.

I had a very beautiful friend. After many years, he came to me with a request. He said, "I want to do something."
I said, "What?"
He said, "You know, I want somebody to take me around, drive me around, and I want you to give me the car."
I said, "All right, I'll give you the car. What else?"
"Get it gassed up for me."
"What else?"
"I want that plastic card so that if I need more gas, I can get it filled."
"All right, what else?"
He said, "Then give me $500 also."
"What else?"
"Well, if you can afford to give $500 to the person who is going with me."
I said, "Wait a minute."
I got the whole idea. I made a call. I said, "Rent him a car and go with him if he wants you to. If he wants to go by himself, it is all right. Let him have his fun."
He did that for one day and then he came to me and said,

"I didn't enjoy a thing."
I said, "You must understand a simple law, if you overeat, you vomit—even when it's milk from the mother."

That's called the law of vomiting. You vomit sexually when you overindulge, especially when you are young, the simple years. But the most dangerous vomiting is done by those between the ages of 36 and 54; because when you overindulge in sexual activity at this age, it means you're not preparing for your creative activity, your creative years. At that time, one wrong intercourse will not let you think right for seven days. I repeat: one wrong sexual intercourse will not let you think for one week—four of them and you are out for a month.

What is more, sexual intercourse, from the point of penetration, indulgence and ejaculation, must be done tenderly, completely. If not, it will give you indirect anger. Indirect anger results in a hot temperament, and a hot temperament comes from unsatisfied sexual relationships. This means the sexual relationship is done without Ram–Lila. We call it Ram–Lila love, Krishna–Lila love. Lila means play, playfulness. Many games must be played in love making. Watch what happens, watch animals or a healthy child, when it is taking milk from its mother, it will use its hands and you will see the play there. There must be a play from the beginning to the end, just to be normal.

The beauty of the woman is not her eyes, or her lips, or her nose, or whether she is young or old, and all that, her beauty is her playfulness.

This indirect anger—hot temperament—is called "shadow anger." It is a sexual disease that has not yet been discovered by medical science. Shadow anger is the disease of people who are sexually dissatisfied or unsatisfied. Their sexual relationship is not normal, it is not complete, it is not properly nursed. It can result from sexual intercourse with a full stomach, an upset stomach; it can also result from not having cozy environments, or a rhythmical system, or a playful woman; it's quite a tragedy.

A woman who is not playful, who says, "Touch me not, touch me not," is not even as good as a pillow! You are better off to go to a good department store, buy a big pillow and marry that. It is soft, it is cozy, it won't answer back, it won't tell you, "Go away," and it won't cost much. A big, long pillow will cost you about $20 and you can put it between your legs and sleep nicely. A woman who is not playful is not worthwhile. The beauty of the woman is not her eyes, or her lips, or her nose, or whether she is young or old, and all that, her beauty is her playfulness. A woman who is not playful is dreadful.

Understand the system. Sex is a natural phenomenon—sex as it is, is a totally natural phenomenon. Don't associate sex with guilt. Thanks to Catholicism, sex is a guilt, sex is a bad thing. Sex is neither. I have said many times, there is nothing in sex and there is nothing without sex. If sex is wrong, there is nothing in it; yet without sex, none of you would be here. Somebody, somewhere, has indulged sexually in order to produce each one of you.

So kio mandaa aakhi-eh jit jameh raajaan.
"Why call that thing bad from which kings are born?"
—Guru Nanak, Siri Guru Granth Sahib, p. 413

The greatest wrong Jimmy Carter ever did was going to Sunday school on Sunday instead of having good sex. When he wanted to be the President the first time, he was very relaxed. But when he ran the second time, his face was very tense. His life was not normal. When life is not normal, then the sex life is not normal. Vitamin deficiency, protein deficiency, this deficiency, that deficiency—all these deficiencies mean inadequate sexual efficiency. Wrong sexual indulgence, wrong sexual life, wrong sexual projection, all these wrong sexual situations are anti-self, anti-success. They give you shadow anger and that shadow anger is such an irritant that it won't let you have completion in your life. Do you understand?

There is a very delicate concept that I want to express to you here. Try to understand. Each physical intercourse between male and female is a psychological action, a psychological action of your own psyche of success. Feeling successful, that's all. When you feel successful then you feel successful in everything. When you don't feel successful at this, you feel defeated in everything. It is as simple as that. The total dimension of success is relevant to your sexual behavior. We have to learn from the spermatozoa and we have to learn from the egg. The egg teaches us a beautiful lesson. The spermatozoa completely enters the egg and never comes out. This is pregnancy. You see that a relationship must be total, complete and everlasting. It is called "absolute harmony." For any creativity there is a success and for any success, there must be absolute harmony. Absolute.

You ego keeps you from harmony. Does the spermatozoa control the egg? Does the egg control the spermatozoa? No. They totally merge, they totally get lost in each other. That is called pregnancy. From pregnancy to delivery, from delivery to nursing, from nursing to childhood, childhood to adulthood, adulthood to old age; take every project of life and just apply the same formula.

The Origins of Sexual **Neuroses**

An Interview with Michael Ebner, PhD[1]

Yogi Bhajan: Michael is our family friend. He is able to read faces. Michael, what are the facial characteristics of an impotent man? Imagine the picture and features of an impotent man.

Michael Ebner: I get two types. One is an individual who feels powerless and shows it. His eyebrows droop, the face muscles droop and there is a sort of softness and downward turn about the mouth. He feels that he can't impact the world. All this comes from a message in his earlier experience, especially from his mother, that he's a wimp and he buys the message.

The second type has a lantern jaw—very square jaw. He's super-macho, the powerhouse trip. He received the same original message, but when this person was confronted with "You're a wimp," he bent over backwards to express, "I am not." However, when he gets involved in a close relationship with women. . . .

Yogi Bhajan: Close contact . . .

Michael Ebner: Yes. When he gets into close contact with a woman, his jaw goes up and his penis goes down.

Yogi Bhajan: Can you tell us about the moderate man? Someone who is neither impotent nor the most potent?

Michael Ebner: This is an individual who is at home with the world and with people. He is able to be tender, expressive and vulnerable in close relationships; but at the same time, he is able to be assertive and protective if need be, and to be potent and powerful.

He has a muscular firmness about the face, not tautness or gauntness or a jutting type of face. There is a flexibility in the face. The eyes are rather open, the mouth is full but not the super-full mouth and the face tends to be rather oval in form. The body musculature is broad shouldered, relaxed and supple.

Yogi Bhajan: What do you see about the tendency of people who are sexually like rabbits?

Michael Ebner: Do you mean wimps?

Yogi Bhajan: No, rabbits.

Michael Ebner: Studs.

Yogi Bhajan: No, not studs. The stud takes time. These people don't take any time. They are in and out. "Touch me and I'm done."

Michael Ebner: The premature ejaculator.

Yogi Bhajan: Well, just at the gate, at any rate they cannot get further than the gate.

Michael Ebner: I call that the running-everything-through-the-penis trip. This is an emotional situation. In this culture men are not allowed to express emotion for the most part. They can express anger but certainly not tender emotions. Because of this, they sit on their emotions and eventually, they channel them through sex, which is the only emotional outlet allowed by their families. Whenever they begin to become sexually aroused, then the power of all those unexpressed emotions wells up within them and they go off. They can't control it because they've got all that other emotional stuff coming through the penis.

Yogi Bhajan: You know all these things I am discussing with you, I learned at the completion of my sixth year of life. I am just introducing you to my childhood. We were given this training. We were taught what personality is, what a man is, what his features are, what his motivation is, how he deals, and why he deals the way he deals.

So Michael, what about the sexual acrobats?

Michael Ebner: There are two aspects to this phenomenon. One I call the perennial child. That's the individual who is into having a good time and making a lifestyle out of living for the moment, in the moment, and doing nothing but that. If it doesn't feel good, he doesn't do it, and if it does feel good, he does it continuously.

The other aspect is the selection of sexual skills as the basis of personal identity. As far as this person is concerned, sexual competency is the only thing that matters. Some base this skill on physical strength, others on technical skills and still others create a sort of sexual service situation. The basis of this individual is his extreme finesse as a sexual organism.

When these aspects are merged, you get an individual who is just a walking ego trip, trying to prove he is the world's greatest lover. At the same time, he is a total pig, using his sexual acrobatics to give himself a good time. He is only concerned about his partner's experience to the extent that he can get some ego strokes from it.

Yogi Bhajan: There is a kind of man that we call good-for-nothing. He cannot sustain a relationship. He doesn't know how to give in to a woman. At first he will kind of barter, then he begins to sell out and ultimately, he is gone. Can you feel the features of that man and analyze the personality, the basic root of it?

[1] Michael Ebner was also known as Dr. Narayan Singh Khalsa.

Michael Ebner: The basic root of that personality is the perennial child that I just mentioned. This man's mother, who is programmed by her own experience as a child, primarily by her father, by his withholding and self-involvement, has a lot of anger toward men. At the same time, she is vulnerable to men who are like her dad, so she marries one like him. She becomes highly dissatisfied with him and then turns to the son as a substitute lover, so to speak. Of course, she programs the son to be just like the father.

Yogi Bhajan: I want you to go into full detail about this "substitute lover" business. I can't go into it in detail because I am a holy man. Ninety-nine percent of all women do that, and in America, I have seen almost 90%, which means that 90% of all men are impotent because of their mother's trip. I call it the mother's day gift. I want you to give the details of it.

Michael Ebner: This is basically where the child has been told by the mother, "Don't sit under the apple tree with anyone else but me . . . or I'll kill you." That message comes from programming in early infancy, when the mother can withdraw basic life support from the infant. The moment the child starts to show an interest in anything besides being the mother's basic support system, she engages in abandonment behavior, which builds a fundamental panic in the child. All she has to do to subsequently control behavior is purse her mouth or tighten up a little bit and the child/man responds with total panic.

She uses her polarity to tie him into her so that she becomes, virtually, the most important person in the world to him. Simultaneously, she shapes him, through this very subtle behavior, to become a specialized support system for her. As a result, he is unable to separate from her, afraid to do so, and terrified of her. Underlying all this is that shadow anger you spoke of. The more intense the pattern gets, the heavier the shadow anger gets; it can even reach homicidal proportions.

A lot of men who have been really engulfed by their mothers have an enormous rage at having been, in essence, castrated by the woman. They have not been allowed to become persons in their own right, to have personal power, or personal potency, or to form relationships anywhere else. Many have not even been allowed to pursue their own careers because the mothers are so hell-bent on keeping them around. As the man gets older, the sexual deprivation the mother feels from the alienated relationship with her husband (who is her father whom she married, and who she is now creating in her son) turns into a subtle sexualizing of the son. This is all on the subconscious level, you understand. But the mother develops a situation of …

Yogi Bhajan: "Unseen intercourse."
Michael Ebner: Exactly, that's beautiful. I'll use that.

Yogi Bhajan: Unseen intercourse is responsible for bringing a lot of impotency to all men. The result is that the man grows to an adult and either cannot get enough sex to satisfy that unseen sex, or he's undersexed and even rejects his legitimate mate. Could you explain the origins of that?

Michael Ebner: There are three parts of it. One of them is the fear of engulfment that comes with closeness. Another is the incest taboo reaction that comes when the man starts to become turned on sexually to his wife. That stimulus activates the memory of the mother's sexualizing of the son and an incest impotence results. The third part is that rage—that shadow anger.

Those three aspects, the two anxieties and the anger, are effective anti-aphrodisiacs and they literally cut sex off at the pass. That man has a triad of very powerful negative emotions that are activated every time he starts to get close to a woman.

Yogi Bhajan: Do you understand that parenting style in which the child is taught to "be a pimp, not a man" and "be a prostitute, not a woman"?

I want you to discuss the hierarchy of the man, the producer. Why do the producers subconsciously produce the prostitutes and pimps that we say have shadow sexuality? Freud never used that word because he was afraid the people in his time would eat him alive, but the ancient scriptures use the words, "shadow sexuality." Shadow sexuality is the result of the children being influenced by the deficiencies and efficiencies between the parents themselves.

Michael Ebner: We need to see the nuclear family as a backdrop to this situation. Originally the family evolved as an extended group in the midst of a community that was pretty much committed to the individual. For the most part, child-rearing practices were shared among the community. Now we have set up an industrial-technical society where the male, by design anyway, is pulled away from the family and the female is kept at home. All the major support systems for the child-rearing procedure are gone and only one individual has to handle the whole damn thing. This is virtually impossible. The wife can't be all things to one person, the husband, much less be all things to one person and to the kids.

Those are the kinds of dire straits we find in the nuclear family. It is like an octopus with its tentacles cut off, who is then told, "Now go out there and survive." The result is that the family sees itself as a sinking ship, and the kids are put into the position of bailing, right along with the parents, to keep the ship afloat. That becomes a bottom-line demand on the nuclear family as we find it at this point.

Over several generations, the children are trained from

early infancy to the job they must do to keep the ship afloat. Very frequently, even the choice of the child's name is indicative of the role they will be forced to play in the survival of the family. In this situation, the children are shoved into these roles to help the ship, which has the effect of literally cutting off parts of their personalities, parts of their potential, forcing them into lifelong patterns of surviving and functioning. When they grow up, what they get to do is choose a mate.

Now in a society where many adults are involved in the child-rearing process, the kid is able to turn on to virtually any kind of person. This is why arranged marriages work. But in this culture, the child was only turned on to one person, and possibly a shadow person, the father, during the early formative years. So this child ends up with nobody to select from except someone just like mom and dad, and the typical result is that they do just that.

There is a combination of the children's personal limitations, which have been created by the crisis in the family situation, and the selection of "nemesis" figures, somebody just like mom and dad, which draws the person involved as a spouse to think, "Oh boy, this time it is going to be different. I'm going to be able to make mom (or dad) love me like they never did the first time." This is quickly followed by disillusionment, disengagement and an enragement process wherein the person, who is not the parent, turns to his kids as substitutes (and bailers) and the whole thing moves on, getting worse from generation to generation.

Yogi Bhajan: Michael, there is a situation that gives the ordinary man the feeling of being hollow inside. It is called "empty sexual erection." Could you give the basis of that?

Michael Ebner: This is the whole business of sex without love. As you know, in a lot of families, love means engulfment, love means becoming a specialized machine, love means cutting your own balls off and becoming an impotent eunuch. At the same time, sexuality means disengagement and distance, the closest thing you can get to love without being involved. Love implies vulnerability, and with the family system we've been discussing, vulnerability is potentially lethal. Consequently, you don't get love; you don't get near it for that matter. Through our present cultural and parental set up, love has become attached to annihilation in one way or another, so we avoid love like the plague. Sexuality is what we use to stay alive, to keep those cards and letters coming in. Because of this situation, we engage in sexuality without love.

In some cases, the opposite exists: love without sexuality. This is an individual who has been shaped by the parents to be a parent, a substitute parent for the parent, and the individual becomes a constant caretaker. Love without sex. This individual enters the marriage relationship in a parental role, unable to be sexual because he doesn't conceptualize it as part of the love relationship.

Yogi Bhajan: Isn't that how the button system developed? The man has an imaginary woman and the woman, an imaginary man, who have certain buttons, like those mechanical games we play for a quarter. When the man touches a certain place, presses the button, then the woman should respond with a long kiss; when he touches her thigh three inches down, then she should come up four feet. Please explain that.

Michael Ebner: Here we see the person shifting out of commitment, connection and contribution, which is the major function of our lives as human beings, into sensuous substitution as a lifestyle. This is the sexual acrobat you were speaking of, the person who has become highly specialized in his sexual performance.

Yogi Bhajan: The person doesn't care about gratifying his partner. They want mechanical sex, the push-button system.

Michael Ebner: The performance—"How am I doing?"—is ego-based. The degree to which that person is concerned about the partner's reaction is the degree to which he himself is receiving strokes for his competency: "Was I good?" that sort of thing. The other part of his concern is "Are you coming through for me?" Is the partner performing to this person's specifications? The whole idea is sex as a stimulation, the empty stroke, as opposed to the tantric idea of sex as the expression of universal, dyadic, and physical all in one, a connecting cycle, a circle of energy. What we've done is to disconnect sexuality from what is real.

From this it is very easy to get into self-blame or into putting the responsibility onto the parents. The best approach is to simply be aware of the situation and to begin healing it. Accept that it just is, or was.

Yogi Bhajan: There is something that happens in all marriages in the Western world whether they are performed in Chicago, Miami Beach, St. Louis or anywhere on this continent, or in Europe. It is an attitude that develops within the male and female. It starts from the first with a lovey-dovey scratch, "I eat you, you eat me." From that point it becomes "Touch me not." Could you explore the parental guilt and the whole background of it?

Michael Ebner: That one has three sources. The first one is most common to women. They feel sexually exploited by the man, by his predatory pawing, and that eventually creates revulsion.

The second part is the parental guilt you mentioned. Again this is the situation where sexual arousal is a form of pleasure that is forbidden within the family context because of its erotic overtones and implications. In addition, the man carries the message, "You, kid, are here for me," not the other way around.

The third source is parents who are intensely self-involved. The child finds out very early in life, within the first few weeks, that when he looks for support and sustenance in the environment, the environment is out of synch. This may not be in the form of gross neglect or abuse; scheduled feeding is a better example. The message is, "Mama knows best what you really want," and she reinterprets your desires or needs to hers. The family is simply not dancing the life support dance with the kid.

This child has to seal over his emotional openness and shut down his vulnerability because to be vulnerable is to have to depend on these undependable systems. The individual concludes that he is alone in the world, taking care of himself and raising himself by his own bootstraps. The net effect is that the individual becomes hypersexual, using sex as the nearest thing to love that he can get and still be in control, without getting caught up in any issues of vulnerability.

Simultaneously, because the child is only about three months old when he reaches this conclusion, there is the issue of physical vulnerability. Consequently, you have a person who is at risk in the world and who must be in charge of his body, his environment and his circumstances constantly. He becomes very vigilant about it and we see the emergence of the mottos, "I need my space," "Don't tread on me," "I need to run my show," "Your entrance into my life is on my terms."

This is not a paranoid stance. The paranoid is an individual who has been systematically attacked by his parents in a violent and negative way. The parents responded to the kid as though he was an undercover agent from an enemy government. The child concludes that the environment is out to get him and he had better get the environment first. It is a relatively rare disorder in this culture at this time. The bootstrap neurosis is much more common. It is the delusion of indifference in which the deluded person feels that the world is full of people who back out of driveways without looking. Not that the world is malevolent and out to get him, but that the world just doesn't care and "I've got to take care of myself because nobody else will."

Yogi Bhajan: Their basic motto is, "Nobody is nobody." So for them, everybody becomes nobody.

Michael Ebner: Right. These people have a basic sense that they have to take care of themselves and they have to control everything that they experience. As a result the, "Don't touch me," attitude comes out in terms of, "I didn't initiate this. Get out of my space." They will get quite defensive about this because they are afraid that if another person or other people really start to encroach on them, their survival will be jeopardized.

Yogi Bhajan: Michael, give us an image of a person who is real, patient, continuous, flowing, merging, surging, being, to be.

Michael Ebner: Physical?

Yogi Bhajan: Physical as well as qualitative, and also the source of such a person.

Michael Ebner: The source for this kind of development is in the early period, especially during the first two and a half years. The parents demonstrate to the child that they are really there for him. Plus, the right environment is there for the parents. That is one of the key elements for the positive development of the child. It is damn near impossible to provide all the child's needs by yourself. The parents need support for themselves as adults, as well. It comes down to this: when the child has needs, the parent is there; when the parent has needs, their needs are met. This parent is able to communicate with the child that sometimes the parents' needs may take priority. All needs are taken care of in a balanced, dancing kind of way.

It's a combination of reality enforcement, that there are pragmatic things that exist in the real world. It is a reality that parallels the reality of the young infant whose needs are his world at this point and this must be respected. The basic process is to integrate and coordinate the personal and pragmatic needs in a lifelong synchronized dance.

The successful process results in a person who is highly competent and well-developed physically, mentally and spiritually. This person has capable responses to almost anything that comes his way. He wants to express his love both in the form of contribution and in the form of receptiveness and sensitivity to other people's needs. This is an individual who moves in response to the demands of the situation rather than to a bunch of principles. He can be concerned about his impact on another's environment without becoming entrapped with either, "What will they think of me," or, "I don't deserve anything nice."

Yogi Bhajan: Now, Michael, tell us about the person who looks for sympathy out of disaster, the person who takes the air out of his own tires and then waylays others to help him, asking for a jack or a spare, or what have you.

Michael Ebner: I call that person the professional victim. There are three or four different causes for that. One of them is the overt hostility of the parent toward the child. The parent is an extremely angry individual who systematically and consistently acts sadistically toward the child, "If you don't like this, kid, just try objecting and you'll find out what pain is." These parents also engage in overt threats of physical annihilation, either by actual physical assault or the constant threat of it. The message the child gets is, "All right, kid, your job is to sit there and take it and not give me any lip." He also learns from the family that some targets are acceptable for the rage that ensues from this treatment, while others are not. The result is an individual who will sit there and take it and then take it out on everybody else. This person sets himself up to be a victim of circumstance in certain situations. He will also ensnare another person into the process, through the rescue operation, and then tell that person that the job isn't being done right. He becomes highly passive-aggressive and does a subtle, sneaky, sadistic persecution of the helping person.

Secondly, there is the professional victim that can be seen most clearly in the alcoholic script; but can originate from any situation where the parents systematically withhold support, affection, attention, etc., unless the individual is in dire straits, unless he is hurting himself in some way. Here the message is that the only way to get strokes, to get life support, is to hurt yourself and so a self-destructive lifestyle emerges.

Another is the man-who-came-to-dinner. This is the hedonist who uses the victim-of-circumstance ploy to get his foot in the door, and then never leaves. If you haven't heard of "The Man Who Came to Dinner," this was a fellow who came to dinner and fell down the stairs, breaking his leg. He ends up spending the rest of his life living upstairs, an absolute asshole.

There are a few others. There is the individual who is the chronic parent, whose own parents have become so dependent on him that they have trained him to what I call "Quasimoto" behavior. (Quasimoto was the hunchback of Notre Dame.) This guarantees that the child will be such a gross yuck that nobody in the world will be able to stand him. The child perpetuates his yuck reputation by setting up such awful situations that the other people involved are crying, "Oh my God, get out of my life," which forces the kid back into the family per the parents' original plan. This is an individual who appears to be a total monster on the surface, but who is actually a very nurturing, supporting person to everyone but himself.

Yogi Bhajan: What about the "Ma, ma, ma, I'm back"?

Michael Ebner: Oh, yes, the mom-addict. That one is created by the parent, the mother in particular, engaging in a couple of behaviors. One is overindulgence. She is always there, giving him whatever he wants, whenever he wants it, spoiling him. Secondly, she makes sure that in the kid's life and experience, everything and everybody else is put down as a piece of shit so that the child becomes convinced that mama is the only thing in the world that offers him anything relevant. Plus, sonny has got to have his goodies and mom is the only one who can provide them. This is a hand-to-mouth addictive lifestyle combined with a total dependency on mom. If he tries to leave, he ends up coming back because nobody does it like mom.

Yogi Bhajan: Last of all, tell us about the person who says, "I hope so, I cannot commit."

Michael Ebner: Oh yes, the will-of-the-wisp. A real will-of-the-wisp is the head of the dandelion that has gone to seed. It is grey and fluffy. When they float by, they look very attractive so you reach for them, but with the mere pressure of your hand, swoosh, they are gone. You go for it again and the same damn thing happens. There is no substance there.

The parent of this child developed a very special relationship with him in the form of a "dance away" parent. "One of these days, kids, I'm going to really connect with you, and really be there for you, but right now I've got these other things I've got to do. Oh, don't go away, I want you there, but I've got these other things to do." This is the carrot-dangle, carrot-yank phenomena. As a result, the child invests all his eggs in the basket of getting that mother or dad to come through, and he is unable to commit anywhere outside the family, or even to himself, because he is so hung up on the parent he sees dangling before his eyes. It produces a lifestyle of systematic commitment avoidance. He can't commit to anything. He'll start to commit, and then he'll withdraw just like the parent. These folks do the same carrot-dangle, carrot-yank play that was done to them.

Yogi Bhajan: I am really very grateful that you are very committed and that I am very committed to the essence of life.

I am grateful today that when I was very young, very innocent, and very unknowing of myself, I had very heavy environments, pressures and circumstances. I am grateful that one fine day, through the grace of God and Guru, I touched the lotus feet of my spiritual teacher who kindly, gracefully, slowly and graciously, in spite of my rejections, my obstructions, my cries, my faith and my lack of faith, took me to the Word of the Guru, which took me to God. When I look back at that procedure, I feel, that without that touch, I would have been very neurotic, a human product of my environments and the pressures of circumstance. I might have been cooked or I might have been left raw, I might have been accepted or rejected. But my very inner Self, which came through my commitment, brought happiness, balance, integrity, dignity, service, giving and grace.

In your life and in your virtue, you can have as many things as you want, but you cannot buy grace and you cannot sell it. In reality, if you look to the best of your life, you cannot live by your body—don't speak of money or anything material; you cannot live by your mind—don't speak of your intellectual and intelligence trips; and you cannot live by your soul—don't speak of your God-given gift of the ever-enlightening self. You can only live by the experience of your wisdom—and that comes from following a wise man.

The company of the holy is the whole trip of life. This is to say, and I conclude with this line, if you ever want to be a great man, use your entire intellectual intelligence to follow a great man because all greatness ends with great practical experience.

Thank you for being here. With true love and affection, I thank you for being here. I am very grateful that you all came and I am grateful to God and to each one of you who takes so much interest in your own improvement and in your own self. I am very grateful that Michael flew all the way here to do this hypnotic, on-the-spot, personality behavior analysis and description for me. I am also grateful to those beautiful sons of mine who covered different aspects of life each morning of the course.

We have a tendency to grow and we have a capacity to grow. With the outside world becoming very costly and very heavy, we need to join together and increase our business acumen and our success. We all need to grow at a fair speed and to understand that success is material as well as nonmaterial. If the material and nonmaterial are combined in equilibrium and the person is totally administratively an administrator and totally meditatively human, then we are surrounded with the possibility of overcoming our handicaps, our images, our imaginations and our tendency to pull the rug out from under our own feet. We are all haunted, we are haunted homes, we are haunted by our handicaps. Instead of being haunted human beings, we can become beautiful, graceful, radiant human beings.

My only effort is to improve your lives so that you can enjoy your full potential. I am a servant, not a controller, and I enjoy my services and the benefits I receive in return for that. I can deal with egos; I can deal with handicaps; I can deal with a lot of situations, the best and the worst, because there is one thing I will get in return: One day I'll be gone, physically, and I'll leave behind enough teachings for you to follow, and to be proud of, as I am proud of them today.

One day I touched the feet of my master and I became a master. You touch the feet of your master and you will become a master because all life is dedicated to the mastery of life itself.

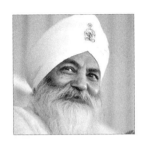

Man to **Man** 7

The Successful Man

Circa 1982

*In the garden of God, you are His one and only rose.
Carry your own smell with your own deeds.*

- Aspects of **Success**
- Physical **Aspects**
- Mental **Aspects**

Aspects of **Success**

The first rule of success is to go slowly.

I have wanted to teach you these next principles for 14 years. Now I think you are ready. There is much to cover. The idea is to educate you, to go slowly so that you can learn.

The first rule of success is to go slowly. The body has a certain temperament, which has its own speed requirement. As an example, the walking speed of the body temperament is four miles per hour. Any person walking faster than that is moving more quickly than the body is built for and that person will mess up. There are also temperamental requirements for talking and hearing. When you talk fast, you mess up. It doesn't matter what you are trying to achieve, you will not achieve anything. This is because the ears are designed to hear at a certain wavelength. When you talk, you talk to be heard by somebody. You don't talk for yourself. So you must tune-in to the wavelength of the listener.

Success has many aspects and you must be successful in all of them to be totally successful. These aspects include physical, mental, social, personal, spiritual, business/professional, financial, political, matrimonial, family, and general. Besides these 11 there are 5 more: sexual, behavioral, self-confidence, self-recognition, and the hearing habit. These 5 are very important. We will discuss them before beginning on the physical and mental aspects, which are more complex in their function.

You must clearly understand that sexual success and matrimonial success are *not* the same thing. This difference must be known by you. There is no success if your behavior is not successfully approved in all the dimensions of your life—that's why we succeed only temporarily, but fail permanently. The key to your life is your behavior and successful behavior is wonderful; however, if you have successful behavior and you have no self-confidence, you have no roots. No roots at all. Ultimately, nothing means anything to you.

When your self-confidence has not been successfully developed, you reach the top but you go berserk. When you are truly confident, death only stops the existence of your personality. Others will pick up the example of your life and keep it going. That is called self-confidence. Self-recognition is just that, recognizing the Self. The hearing habit is the final aspect. It is most important to your success that you be able to communicate to others that you hear them. You have the capacity and the willingness to hear them. This is a most winning aspect. People want to be heard.

All these 16 aspects are the 16 fingers that will make the fist of success. When you make a fist with these 16 and you punch, time and space will give you the space. The problem in this country is that no one teaches you about success. How can you be successful when you are not told what success is, what its elements are, what its projections are? I was exactly four years old when I was given a lecture on successful living. Tell me, how many of you got it?

■ ■ ■

Physical **Aspects**

When you start out—look good. Look in your mirror, look in your consciousness, look in your intelligence, look at yourself—body, mind and soul—and ask one question: "Can I win the trust?"

Now let us deal with the physical aspect of success. This aspect has eight parts: look good, smell good, speak well, socialize, use kind language, good manners, good etiquette, and projection. Projection is the most important of all self-behavior. Your projection is how you do anything you do and how that doing is perceived by others. Why do you want a good projection? For success.

Look good for success. Don't dress so that you look common. Don't look common. Project your special image. Present your special image with a special personality, a special being-ness. God has not made anybody equal. We are not the same in size, shape or dimension. That's the law. Each one is individual, and each one must appear as himself. Clothes don't mean anything. Beggars have commanded the respect of kings. One of the sickest things you can do is to follow the general trend in your dress. Today everybody has to wear a three-piece suit and a tie. You don't even have the guts to break away from the conventional situation.

I went to a party. The waiters were wearing those flowery dress shirts, tuxedo shirts. The host and the guests were also wearing them. There was absolutely no difference, no way to tell who was who. Actually the waiters were prettier because they were professional and they knew how to wear those clothes. The others were in bad shape. They had to rent the clothes for the occasion; and they didn't know how to deal with them.

What we mean by looking good is looking like you can be trusted. Give the person you are relating to a break, give him a saintly look. You know that when you see a guy coming in a three-piece suit, he's going to want to make a buck off you. Your first impression is to be careful of this clever guy, you ooze. If a girl comes along, oozing, just like that you know she's going to do you in. She may be very saintly, who cares? You have been taught, according to your American civilization, to ooze, to be smooth. Your personal look is oozing, but there is only one word that defines you in the mind of another person, "Oh, God, S-H-I-T." That's it. It's an automatic reaction. Don't misunderstand me, I'm not trying to put you off; but at that moment, you are oozing, just like a pimple oozes out. The feeling of pus is there, and then there is relief when the pus is out. In every appearance where I can see that it is good, fashionable, but where my mind understands that it is not good, that there is a split, some duality, I will be cautious.

To get past that cautiousness, people say, "Come on, let's have a drink." First they freak out, then they pass out, and then they negotiate. This is because they realize everybody has a wall. When you have the appearance that you are out to get something, you actually give the other person a clue, to be cautious of you and not trust you. So then you must get past those barriers of distrust. Look good and win the trust. I dress like this all the time. It's nice. Somebody may not trust me immediately, but they will in the end. There is no hurry to win the trust. Don't hurry, just look good and win it. How many of you knew that you should look trustworthy? In your life did anyone teach you about it?

You may be very well-dressed, well-mannered, well-positioned, well-equipped, well, well, well, in everything, but if you do not win trust, you have not arrived. There is no point in corresponding, in traveling miles and miles, in hugging, kissing and all that when you have not reached the other person at all. When you start out, look good, look in your mirror, look in your consciousness, look in your intelligence, look at yourself—body, mind and soul—and ask one question: "Can I win the trust?" Then, after winning the trust, can you keep it?

I never react to anybody, because all of you have given your trust to me and I have to keep it. There's one more thing you have to do: You must give it back. You must deliver it. When you were born, it was called delivery. Trust is no good if you can't keep it. Keeping it is no good if you can't deliver. Why should you win the trust to begin with? For success! There is no success without it. We are not here to learn to be failures. We are here to learn to be successful. I am teaching you how God has planned human success. This is not my personal lecture; I'm no party to it.

Americans think they are successful. Let me tell you, Americans are the biggest failures in the world. Every American is a failure. In 200 years, we have exploited this great country and we have brought it to the brink of failure. No other nation in human history has done that to a piece of land that it has called "country." So what you call success, I call failure. We give billions of dollars to other countries, we create friendships, and yet nobody trusts us. Sometimes we win the trust in our foreign policy, but we cannot keep it. Why? Because we cannot deliver it. Why should we personally win the trust? Because it is the first step of success.

We win trust by looking good. By looking good to whom? To whom do we want to look good? We want to look good to the memory of the other person. Try to understand. We don't need to look good to the eyes of the other person, not that you don't want to look good as you are, but it is their memory that you want to impress. When your name is Yogi Bhajan, what is the memory? That he is good, compassionate, nice, kind, so many things. Look good to the memory of the other person—to their memory, memory, memory, memory, memory. Get to the bottom of it.

Your remembrance must be good. That person must remember you looking good to him. Look good to the memory. That is where you establish confidence. Whenever you are remembered by the person the memory must create a good feeling. The pineal, the pituitary, and the hypothalamus must secrete accordingly. When you win the memory, you win the glandular system. The good feeling comes from the accompanying glandular secretions. If you don't win the glandular system of the person and his glands secrete negatively, it doesn't matter what you say, it doesn't matter what you do, you are a _____. I am not going to speak the word, but it's the opposite of success.

Sometimes you will appear before someone and actually make him nauseous. He will think, "I can't take it." Then he pulls himself together and takes care of business. He says, "Yes, yes, I will do it. Thank you, thank you, thank you. Go." This all happens because your relationship is not good with the glands. Your presence, your look, your talk, your manner, your projection must win the glands. They must make them secrete in your favor. Make-up, perfume, all that stuff, that bizarre situation, which convinces you that you need it to win the memory of the other person, to win the memory of their glands. It is brainwashing! It will never work.

There is another sick thing that you do when you want to make a space in the memory of the other person. Instead of making a memory of being successful, cheerful, bright and beautiful, you go for sympathy. It is so silly, so neurotic, so pathetic. Do you know where you learned that babyish behavior? From your parents. It's the sickest thing that you have learned from them, acting pathetic to get sympathy, to get their forgiveness, to get their love, to get their anything. Do you know what you look like when you do that? You look like a cornered cat. It is called the "cornered cat personality." Shame on you for learning that! It's ridiculous. When I look at that behavior, I think, "Where is the soul, where is the spirit, where is the godliness? The guy is so great and he uses that pathetic behavior." It is called "the dead look." Who can trust a person who has that look? When you get that feeling, that look, that projection from a person, do you want to trust him?

Don't act that way. Don't look for sympathy. When you come home, come home. If you are tired, be tired. It's okay. Announce, "I'm dead tired. Do something, please; bring me back." That's the honest look, the bright look of a dead tired person. But you don't do that; no, you say, "Leave me alone." Then you run toward the other room with your shoulders slumped—that's the dead look. You say, "I'm all right, I'm all right. Don't worry. I'll be with you in two hours." You rabbits, what are you trying to do? You call yourself men. Is that manly? Call her out. "Hey, wife, I am sick to death. Do something!" Then lie down flat. Break 3 glasses, 20 cups, who cares? But speak, announce.

When you say, "Don't worry; I know I have to go to dinner with you. I'll be all right in two hours," your behavior is sheepish and nobody likes it. As an animal, the sheep is good; it gives wool, the lambs are pretty, but it doesn't become you. I have some students who are always afraid of me. When I address them, they have a scared look, as if I'm going to eat them alive. Their knees bend, they become one inch shorter. At the very idea of fear, the shoulders drop, the legs drop. They look like Charlie Chaplin. Charlie Chaplin. That's your image of a successful man. That's why somebody stole him from the graveyard. Your feet go wide to the sides, your shoulders drop and you start walking like that. Why was Charlie Chaplin so successful? Because he related to that sheepish look and there are so many sheep that he really made the bucks. It's the same reason pornography sells so much; because it is all in our heads, too, just like Charlie.

But remember, that kind of success is not everlasting and success that is not everlasting is a failure. Please remember it: First, success which is not everlasting is failure. Second, success is only success when neither time nor space can take it away.

Nobody can take away the success of Mohandas Karamchand Ghandi. His was the success of peace. Nobody can take away the success of Guru Gobind Singh who stood for the weak and poor, for truth and justice. Nobody can take away the love and humility of Christ Jesus. Nobody can take away

Please remember it: First, success which is not everlasting is failure. Second, success is only success when neither time nor space can take it away.

Keep the trust. That is what I mean when I say, "Keep up." Keep up means keep the trust flowing, keep the trust going, keep the trust living, keep the trust accelerating.

the wisdom of the oneness of God through the Gita. Truth is the base, the beginning and the end of Buddha. Nobody can take it. Nobody can take away the ability of Elijah Mohammed to be humble and eat the evil. Guru Nanak praised God as all in one and one in all. Nobody can take it away. Nobody can take away the truth of Guru Ram Das who said that love is eternal and love is all that God is. Service can win the God of Guru Amar Das and nobody can deny it. Nobody can beat the success of William Shakespeare to project and encounter human neurosis. Nobody can beat the success of Sir Isaac Newton in finding the truth about the force of Earth and God.

Success is success. It has no time and no space, so don't, don't, don't be in a hurry. Don't worry and don't hurry. Worry and hurry are the two enemies of success. Keep the trust. That is what I mean when I say, "Keep up." Keep up means keep the trust flowing, keep the trust going, keep the trust living, keep the trust accelerating. Keep the trust in the memory of the other person forever and ever, and ever and ever, and ever and ever. Then, ultimately, you'll become God. I'll give you the secret of how to become God. When you are called in the name of trust by another person, and you come through and you deliver it, you are the God. When God is called upon in the name of justice and truth, God delivers it. Simple.

Har bolo mere gursikh bhaa-ee.
Bar bolo sabh paap lai jaa-e.

"Speak the word, *Har*, my Gursikh brothers. By speaking the word, *Har*, all sins shall depart."

One sound of the word *Har* takes away all sins, but we must know how to speak it. *Har* means call on God for redemption. Call. Learn to call, learn to call, learn to call. Call your friend, call your son, call your mother, call your father, call your teacher—call, call, call, call, call. Call on your wife. Call on that little stuff hanging between your legs. Don't you have to call on it, too? Does it work automatically? Nothing works without a call. Whatever you have to solve, call.

When you call a name, it is a bad thing. When you call on God, it is a good thing. Don't call a person a name, call the name of God. See how the polarity works? The worst thing I have seen in Western countries is that you don't call and you don't answer. It is creating a mess in your lives. It is making you unsuccessful. It is your hidden agenda. You don't call and you don't answer. You are afraid to call because you are afraid to answer. The rule is: when you call, you are bound to answer the call.

Call: *Jo bole so nihaal.*
Answer: *Sat siree akaal.*[1]

It is a simple formula. You follow it every day. *Jo bole so nihaal*, whoever shall speak shall be blessed. It is a simple law of life that is being taught to you every day—and you don't remember it. You don't understand it. You don't go into the depth of it. The law of success is, call and answer the call. *Sat siree akaal* means that the Great Deathless is Truth. Deathlessness is Truth and Truth is Deathless. Therefore, success cannot be eaten by time and space.

Do you think I am crazy or do you think Guru was crazy telling you, *Jo bole so nihaal, sat siree akaal*? Everything in your life is solved when you call. Christ says, "Open your mouth. Speak. It will be." It will be answered. Let it be the same with you. When anybody calls, answer the call. Whenever you are called upon to deliver the faith, to deliver the trust, to deliver the confidence, what should you do? Answer. Come through. If you fail another person, God shall fail you. There's no other way that you can succeed. Do you understand? Do you have any questions?

I'll give you the secret of how to become God. When you are called in the name of trust by another person, and you come through and you deliver it, you are the God. When God is called upon in the name of justice and truth, God delivers it. Simple.

Question and **Answer**

Q: You said clothes don't mean anything but what is bana?

Yogi Bhajan: I didn't mean clothes don't mean anything as you have understood. If you follow the fashion trends in clothes and think that because you wear a three-piece suit, you will be successful, you are wrong. It doesn't matter at all. I'll tell you what *bana* does. *Bana* has a message. *Bana* tells another person, "I am a committed individual of God and I shall not betray it come what may." That's what it is. It is a ministry of trusted individuals. In most cases it will provoke a first query, "Who are you?" Then you will answer the call. *Bana* creates the call. It has that one virtue. Even your own wife who lives with you will ask what you are up to when you appear out of *bana*. Any day your turban is off, your neighbors will ask what is wrong with you. That is the power of *bana*. *Bana* creates the call. In every mind, no matter how blind that mind may be, that is what *bana* does.

We wear white, do you understand? White. White. White. It increases the projection and it increases the confidence and it cleans our power to deliver. Most people love to

---

[1] A traditional call and response in the Sikh path.

wear colored clothes. They want to be anonymous, synonymous, simple—one of the crowd. This is because in their minds, they have already accepted that it is difficult to deliver.

Q: *If you have a negative projection, will white increase your negative projection?*

Yogi Bhajan: If you have a negative projection, the moment you look at yourself in the mirror and see the white reflected, automatically, subconsciously, you are giving yourself the message, "I've got to be nice now." That's what it does.

Q: *You mentioned the hidden agenda and gave a meditation² for it at Ladies' Camp. What's the time on it and will it work for men?*

Yogi Bhajan: At that time I was only addressing the women. That's the only difference. I knew they would come home and share it.

Do you understand this one thing? Look good and win the trust, keep it and deliver it. What will that give you?

Students: Success.

Yogi Bhajan: With what?

Students: Memory.

Yogi Bhajan: Memory. The glands shall secrete in your favor. You have seen the rooster and the pigeon. They make their necks swell and puff up Boom, boom, boom. They speak good, they look good, and they dance so that the creative sexuality of the hen shall come through. Do you see how natural that is? They lie low and they dance to win the trust. The male could just pounce and get it over with, but he knows that raping is not the creative act. It is the destroying act. Don't rape the privacy, the confidence, the coziness of anyone.

When people yell and scream and throw tantrums and create traumas and do all that, they rape the decency of the other people involved. When you hurt somebody that way, how can they love you? All that yelling and screaming and being neurotic and being emotional and being negative with somebody, and this body and that body—all that trauma—doesn't mean a thing. To himself, every person is a decent individual. When you break the barriers and rape the decency of that individual, his memory hates you. What is animosity? Habitual hatred. What is love? Habitual longing. Habitual rejection is hatred. God created no threat to you. God created you, so don't be hateful to anybody.

There are three rules of success: Never speak ill of anyone; never act ill toward anyone; never listen to anyone speaking ill of anyone. Some people enjoy that gossip. It will make you ill. Those gossipers will say, "No, no, no. Don't mind. I'm just telling you my opinion about so-and-so." Tell him, "Very good, very good opinion. Keep it with you."

There are three rules of success: never speak ill of anyone; never act ill toward anyone; never listen to anyone speaking ill of anyone.

You are going to have to be successful with the most rotten stuff. What is success? Succeeding with *adversity*. You have to succeed with every failure. To succeed with failure is living—it's called life. To succeed with the successful and to succeed with the normal is a common idiot's job. Classified common idiots succeed. When the time comes, every ship goes into the harbor. When the tide is normal, everybody can be guided in. When the tide is phenomenal, and still you make it, then you have made it. The joy of that is called ecstasy.

Succeed with every failure. You understand? It isn't the life that matters, it is the courage you bring to it. *Fortitude*.³ Read that novel. Make up your mind. Make up yourself. Make up your projection. Make up your look—and what should that look be? You should look like a man who succeeds against every odd, a ship that can go with every tide. You'll never be burned out. Your profession is not to burn out; instead your profession should burn out the failures and make the path. "If one falls, ten should come in his place." "When things are down and darkest . . .

Your breakfast should be failures. Your lunch should be adversity. Your tea should be misery and your supper should be disaster.

Students: . . . that's when we stand tallest."⁴

Yogi Bhajan: Ah, that's one line to write in your heart. "When things are down and darkest, that's when we stand tallest." That is the character, the personality, the being, the image of a successful man. That is the look. Look good. Got the idea? Your breakfast should be failures. Your lunch should be adversity. Your tea should be misery and your supper should be disaster. Then you follow me, right? My trouble is that sometimes I overeat them. Count your meals and you should come out successful.

I will tell you another thing. There is no such thing as a failure. Life is a flow, sometimes quick, sometimes it doesn't go. This word failure is the language of paranoia.

---

² See Appendix A
³ A 19th century novel by Hugh Walpole that was very influential in Yogi Bhajan's early life.
⁴ From *Song of the Khalsa* by Livtar Singh Khalsa

Paranoia comes from guilt-consciousness. It comes from the devil and there isn't any devil. Man rebelled against God and created an imaginary god, which he called the devil. It is normal to be sick. It is normal to be weak. It is normal to be crazy. It is sometimes normal to be oversleepy. Sometimes it's normal to be downhill. Cars break down. Computers shut down. Everything does it and it is a normal thing. However, we allow other people to judge us; and those who rebel against God judge us and they judge us as bad. They want to make us feel bad. It is so sickening. When I explain to somebody what is right and what is wrong and when I explain what that wrong action will lead to, they say, "You are pressuring us." No, no, no! There is no pressure. It is just explaining.

So actually there's no failure. But if there's any eating, you'll have to eat your own failures and you'll be surprised how hungry you'll get—because there are none. The cycle of time and space shall continue. It is how you can guide yourself. Do you understand that? Then what are you afraid of? What is anybody afraid of? Where can you fail?

Life is just a switch on and a switch off. Is that true or not? So when the switch is off up there, why are you worried? When it is on, why are you upset? As long as you are on, why don't you enjoy it? When it is off, you won't be there to judge and nobody will be judging. It is the judgment of other people that makes the normal flow of life abnormal. Therefore, if others are going to judge you, you had better judge yourself.

The Sweet Smell of **Success**

In the garden of God, you are His one and only rose. Carry your own smell with your own deeds. Create your own smell through your deeds. The successful smell in life is your own good, great deeds. Helping is a deed, giving is a deed, answering the call of faith is a deed, carrying somebody's trust is a deed.

What is a rose? A rose as you see it? Here is a rose. You can't smell the rose but at the sight of it, the thought of it, you smell it, too. Is that true or not? As it comes nearer and nearer and nearer, you become happier and happier and happier. When it reaches you, you say, "Wha! Good." That is called effectiveness. Smelling good is more effective than looking good. Judge yourself and project goodness to others. That's the good smell. That's the secret of success.

Be your own judge. You'll smell good. I say, "be your own judge and you'll smell good." What is good about smell? Looks cannot go beyond certain boundaries. Smell goes. Smell goes into the enemy's kitchen. Make a feast in your house. All the neighbors will smell it. Do you know how rude it is to make a feast in your house and every neighbor smells it and you don't invite them? Do you know what animosity you can create? It's a normal reaction. Whatever looks can do, looks can do; but what smell can do is far out. Smell fits right in with memory.

Smell good. How? Judge your soul. Be your own judge. There'll be no fear and no failure within you—and then you will smell good. Do you understand that? You think that by spending $10, you will smell good. No. They are selling you smell to get your money. Smell has the power to project beyond all obstructions, and if you don't smell good, you won't smell good. Smell is so powerful that we can make a special fire with fragrant woods and incense and the smell will attract the angels to come to our aid. Good spirits help us when we smell good. Judge yourself and be so judged that you will smell good.

Q: *If we judge ourselves as right or wrong, then we will smell good. Do you mean that literally?*

Yogi Bhajan: Oh, yes. Literally, quite literally. Judge yourself literally. If you look good and someone talks to you and you cannot talk good, then you ruin the impression, right? But if you judge yourself, you can tell the person, "I cannot speak well with you at this time."

You have prejudged yourself and you know yourself. Smell. Good smell and bad smell. It is a common phenomenon of life. If you have judged yourself, and judged yourself, and judged yourself—personality-wise—then you are ready to spread your fragrance. What is this word fragrance? This is the good smell of your deed. The fragrance of your deed is the by-product of your self-judged activity.

I'll give you an example. "Okay, my friend, you stay in town. I have to go somewhere." "Why? I want to go with you." "No, I have to do a creepy thing and I don't want you to come and share it with me. It is my personal affair." Then you go and do your creepy thing. You come back and you tell the story of the result to your friend. The next time that you need to go and you say, "My friend, this is it. I have to go," the person will let you go, no questions asked. He will honor your decision not to indulge others in your miseries.

When you smell good, you smell good and you do not involve other people in your miseries. I won't ask you not to involve yourself in doing wrong things—yet. If you do wrong things, good for you but don't involve others in your wrong doings. Wrong risks, uncalculated mental phenomenon, outrageous daydreams and ridiculous hopes are called mental pimping. Do you know what a pimp is?

It is one who solicits sexual activities in a negative way. That kind of mental activity I described is called mental pimping. When you involve yourself in mental pimping, you will never smell good. You will not smell good to the memory of that very person you were thinking about. When some people walk into my room, I say, "Uh, oh," because I know what I'm going to be up against. My memory, my tape tells me. Don't let anybody's tape recorder recall a warning about you. When you walk in, let somebody say, "Hah, hah, hah—yes."

What is a rose? A rose as you see it? Here is a rose. You can't smell the rose but at the sight of it, the thought of it, you smell it, too. Is that true or not? As it comes nearer and nearer and nearer, you become happier and happier and happier. When it reaches you, you say, "Wha! Good." That is called effectiveness. Smelling good is more effective than looking good. Judge yourself and project goodness to others. That's the good smell. That's the secret of success.

Don't make a partnership of your own miseries. Deeds smell. Have a radiant look; your deeds should smell good, because from a mortal you have become immortal. That's the purpose of life. Don't do cheap things, temporary things, circumstantial things. Don't con people or do that cheap kind of stuff. Don't make your personality out of plastic.

When I came to you, I said, "I have not come to collect students." Do you remember that? I have come here to build teachers. I may succeed or I may not, but at least I am trying. I have a goal. Why do gimmicks? Never, ever smell of gimmicks. You know, people wear that sexy smell and their woman says, "What are you up to?" You have been given a sovereign personality but you prostitute it because you don't know how to smell good. Just remember, for sexual purposes, also, there is only one smell in the world that is good for you—and that is your own smell. Don't interfere with the body's smell. Some people wash with soap every day; every day they soap their bodies. Every day they soap themselves up and put lavender on their clothes. What are you doing? [Your smell] is natural. Once in a while, soap your body. The rose is not the jasmine and the jasmine is not the gardenia, so why do you want to put gardenia on the rose? In the garden of God, you are His one and only rose. Carry your own smell with your own deeds.

Do you know what your greatest failure is? When you are a piece of junk, you want to look pretty; and when you are pretty, you want to look like a piece of junk. Have you seen these punk people? Do you understand their psychology? They are indifferent to everything in life. That is their religion. There is nothing bad in it. The worst is that someday they are going to become indifferent to themselves. That's where the danger lies.

In the garden of God, you are His one and only rose. Carry your own smell with your own deeds.

Create your own smell through your deeds. The successful smell in life is your own good, great deeds. Helping is a deed, giving is a deed, answering the call of faith is a deed, carrying somebody's trust is a deed. Do you understand how many deeds there are? One girl said to another, "Oh, so-and-so is coming. Let's get away." The other girl said, "No, no, no. Let's talk to him. He smells so good and once you smell him you're dead." What was she referring to? The deeds. A great sign of success is keeping your failures and your miseries to yourself. Don't ever share your failures and never allow anybody to participate in your miseries—nothing doing. Your failures and your miseries are just food for you. Eat it. Digest it. Let your deeds prove your majesty, and let your deeds prove your grace. Don't think that thirty cents worth of that stuff you put around your ears and neck will cover up your dirty smell. Got the idea? Now you understand smell better than you did before.

Yogi Bhajan on **Polarity**

None fly high without the opposing winds. The moment you become spiritual, character assassination is a must. The moment you become rich, the eye of the thieves is always on you. If you are pretty, somebody will want to use you, whether you like it or not. If you are young, somebody will want to exploit you. This is the law of polarity. It will always happen. It has always happened, so why worry? Don't worry and don't hurry.

Q: What about sandalwood oil?

Yogi Bhajan: Sandalwood oil is all right for the skin, but you are not the skin. You are not the body. I am talking about the scent of you. You are a tenant in your body. You are not the body. Your smell is your deeds. Your skin will smell good if you wear sandalwood oil, with that I agree, even jasmine will do. Our oil business wants money and your skin will smell fine, but that is a very limited view.

Q: One question more. When you make contact with someone that you perceive as smelling good, can you experience that at all?

Yogi Bhajan: You experience it immediately. Your glandular system will do it. You feel goodness or badness right away. If you want to be phony, that's your problem.

Now we will discuss how to speak. Speak good. What does that mean? Sometimes there is that occasional rascal person who does not understand your good night story. You've got to speak good to him. The word is "speak good."

Students: Do the job.

Yogi Bhajan: Hail! Do the job. Your language should be effective, direct and exact. That is called speak good. Speak good and don't hide under the good.

Don't cover your personality when you are speaking. Speak with authority, with your majesty, with your grace. But when you speak, speak exact. Don't worry about right and wrong. That comes later. When you have already judged yourself, you won't speak wrongly. Monitor what you are speaking; your speaking must represent you: not your emotions, not your commotions, not your neuroses, and not time and not space. Is all this clear to you?

You must socialize, socialize, socialize. You are a part of the universe and the universe is a part of you. Create harmony. Take the initiative. Say hello, say hi, greet people. Socialize means greet people. But don't be phony. When you greet people, your body, mind and soul should be in it.

Q: I work in a health food store, how do I put my body, mind and soul in it, when I see hundreds and hundreds of people every day?

Yogi Bhajan: Serve those people. Sell them good food. That's why you are there. Socialize with them. You're making a sale, put on a smile.

Q: Is there a way I can really get myself into it? It gets so repetitious after awhile.

Yogi Bhajan: No, no, no. It is not repetitious. It should make you happy that a lot of people come into your store. Think of those whose stores are barren, who are going under. You must understand that your living is involved in those visits. Each of those faces who come into your store and smile at you is giving you something, not taking from you. It is called profit, and if profit is bothering you, you must be going through a mental holiday, or otherwise, you must be a lunatic. Who? Who doesn't want profit? What is commercial about it? What is routine about it?

Q: Then it's a matter of constantly calling on your creativity?

Yogi Bhajan: No, no, no, no, no. Each moment is new. Smile, it doesn't cost you anything. Do you have a coin slot in your body? Do you only smile when someone puts in a dime? Why not smile all the time? Why not be a smiling Sikh? A smile will give you something, but each frown will cost you something. Each frown, each trauma, each commotional act will cost you something. Each sincere act, each help, each goodness, each smile will give you something.

You've got to balance your life on the profit side. Credibility. Create a credit. Life is a credit. Each moment you have to create that credit. If a thousand people visit your store, make it possible that two thousand will visit tomorrow. Why do you display things in your store?

Why do you put up signs? Why do you decorate? You do all of this to encourage people to come into your store. You do everything to invite them in and then you are bitchy. Do you realize what a disaster that is?

Because you are a part of society and society is a part of you, you must socialize. This doesn't mean you barter your values, or exchange your values. Just socialize. The law of socialization is: to be, to be. To be, to be. I am, I am. It is very important. Greet people with an open heart, with open hands, with a big smile. Open heart, open hands and a big smile.

Now we cover number five, kind language. Suppose somebody calls you a son of a bitch, what should you do?

Students: Say, thank you very much.

Yogi Bhajan: No. You say, "Ouch." The guy will say, "What for?" You say, "God, it has hurt you, not me." Don't accept names other than God's Name, and then return it spontaneously. That is kind language. That way you won't hold a grudge and you won't be mad. You'll get even. Once somebody said to me, "Hey, you are a fake." I said, "Oh, my God, that is fantastic." He said, "What is fantastic? I just said you are a fake." I said, "Yeah, it is fantastic that you have realized your real self." He didn't know what to do next, and meanwhile I was ready for his reply.

Use kind language against the crudest environment, the crudest circumstances, the crudest provocation; but don't give it a place in your heart. If you do, it will hit you so hard on the physical level that you will develop a disease. Don't take it to heart. You will want to say, "Oh, somebody has done this to me." Nobody has done anything to you. Just return it. We don't take home what we don't need. There's a law about kind language: "Return the garbage duly covered." Learn this language, kind language, and return the garbage duly covered.

Now I'd like to have a volunteer who can make the most rude comment to me and I'll return it kindly. Listen and see how I do this. Normally you don't see that side of me. Come on, speak.

Student: *[Makes a comment about Yogi Bhajan's genitals. Terrific laughter.]*

Yogi Bhajan: Far out. You see that wonderful thing. I doubted your eyes before. Thank you for the insight. *[more laughter]*

Do you see? You can return anything with very kind language. It will keep your blood pressure in good shape, your mind in good equilibrium and the other person will learn out of the grace of your kindness. Some people love to spread garbage. But if you are kind enough to return it, they will understand the load of it and that will save you a lot.

Q: *What do we do when somebody rides by in a car and yells out an insult to us?*
Yogi Bhajan: You mean like, "Hey, you white-turbaned pig!"?

Give that person a big smile. When people yell and honk at you, you all know the stuff they do, put your hand out and give him a big wave. That's what I do and it's very effective. They don't know what to do.

Q: *In other words, they give you one finger and you give them all five.*
Yogi Bhajan: No, no, you just wave at him. Don't interpret your behavior. That's where you fall. A sacred secret should be left a sacred secret. That's it. The interpretation will be yours. Let him enjoy his interpretation and your act. Don't try to interpret others. If you are interested, ask them to explain. If you really want to get even with somebody who calls you a name, just ask that person to explain. Somebody once abused somebody over their mother.

"You are a so-and-so."
"Prove it to me."
"I can't prove it to you."
"The proof is what you are when you do it to your mother."
"What did you say to me?"
"It's the same thing that you said to me. Prove it."

It is called gap language. Give a person one wonderful word and then return his materials in the original back to him. Self-defense is not bad, just learn to change the frequency. Somebody will always use language to hit at you. Put it in reverse gear with kind language. It's more effective. When your frequency and the other frequency become more and more intense, and more and more negative, then the situation will end in a big spark—Boom! That's not what you want.

Remember, never try to be mean to anybody. Speak good about the enemy. "He's my number one enemy. God bless him and may he get to heavens fast." Why say that you want him dead? There's no need to say that. "My friend, my prayers are with you. May you be ahead of me in heavens soon." Do you get the idea? One person once said to another, "May your children roam all around the north and south poles." Always, even in the first flush of anger, language should be kind—both spoken language and body language. Even slang language should be kind. Use very kind slang and be careful about using it. Slang changes its meaning every 12 miles. Speaking manners, dialect, changes every 250 miles.

Manners is something else we need to cover here. By manners I don't mean being polite. No. I'm going to say the heaviest thing. Success is to have your manners and introduce them. First, you have your manners; then introduce them. As an example, you should not walk one way in one place and differently in another.

Q: *Are these mannerisms as opposed to etiquette?*
Yogi Bhajan: Mannerism is the combination of your personality and your projection and your feelings and your dealings in a situation. Manners are your projection with the time and space you are in. That's manners. Some people have different manners in different situations. They always end up in failure. The main cause of failure is no manners.

Failure doesn't come from the heavens, we create it. Success is our birthright, but when we aren't consistent in our manners, we create a big mess. For example, we go to a rich man's house and we start doing very shallow things. Then we go to a poor man's house and we get very uptight.

People come to see me and they cower. When they do this, I understand. "Come sit down properly. Now what do you want to say?" "I just did something." I say, "Look, it doesn't mean I'm going to forgive you. Just tell me what you did. Speak clearly to me." What is this habit you have of putting your tail between your legs? I say this doesn't work. That person wants to relate to me as his father instead of relating to me as his Teacher. I don't buy it. When I'm a Teacher, I'm a Teacher; when I'm a father, I'm a father; when I'm a man, I'm a man. There's no getting in and talking to me in that cowering way. It's baby talk and it won't serve the purpose. Be like a man and speak like a man. Wrong is wrong.

"Uh, yes. I've done wrong, sir. I'm sorry. It didn't work out right. I couldn't call you. The situation is grave. Please tell me what to do." It is a simple thing. Keep your manners simple.

Now we come to etiquette. The greatest etiquette is to deal kindly with every person or thing, living or dead. Deal kindly, gracefully, kindly, gracefully, kindly, gracefully. And, what is the third?

Students: Respectfully.

Yogi Bhajan: Respectfully. It's very important. This mannerism of respectfulness can bring you huge dividends. There's a very common saying, "Flattery works even with God." It is a very shallow expression, but if you are respectful that will make you God. If you respect the creation of God, you will become God.

You are very disrespectful with your cars. Deal with your cars and don't bang them up. You put your car in reverse gear and back it into a pole. The pole cries, "Aaaaaaaah... 3HO." Within the entire parking lot you can recognize the 3HO cars by their dents. Those cars are silent servants. They augment your capacity.

Be respectful to those who direct you and those who serve you. That is the secret of success. Be respectful. Be respectful. I didn't say obey them or do everything right. Try to understand.

Now we come to the last item to be covered under physical success. It's called projection. Projection means penetration, going forward, getting into something. It can be defined in many ways. What does projection mean to you?

Students: To take a representation of the self and put it outward, forward into the world. It means creation of an image, creation of your image in other people's eyes. To be a pipe or clear water. Radiance. Exercise of my sensitivity. The clarity with which you can project yourself out. Your well-being. Presentation of yourself.

Yogi Bhajan: Bunch of fools! Projection is you, nothing else. Speak it.

Students: You, nothing else. **Yogi Bhajan:** Speak it again.
Students: You, nothing else. **Yogi Bhajan:** Speak it again.
Students: You, nothing else. **Yogi Bhajan:** Speak it again.
Students: You, nothing else. **Yogi Bhajan:** Speak it again.
Students: You, nothing else. **Yogi Bhajan:** Speak it again, everybody.
Students: (emphatically) You, nothing else!

Yogi Bhajan: You know simple things. Life is a very simple thing. Don't try to make it complicated. Projection is?

Students: You, nothing else.
Yogi Bhajan: Now, who will remember this?
Students: You, nothing else.
Yogi Bhajan: You're right, I will remember it. [laughter] Yes, I will remember it. In America, the best thing for a teacher to do is to remember the teaching and nothing else. Do not project your emotions, nor your commotions, nor your dividends, nor your profits, nor your losses, nor your defeats, nor your badness, goodness, helplessness, power, nor might. Only project, very gracefully, very kindly, very respectfully, you—the self. The day you can project you and nothing else, that day you have succeeded.

Mental Aspects

What is meditation? It is a conscious effort to clean the mind, to control the mind. It is so simple.

Today we are talking about the mental aspect of success. If you understand the mental aspect, there is no way that you can even *touch* failure, forget about failing or being failed by this or that. You have the Negative Mind, you have the Positive Mind, and you have the Neutral Mind. On the axis of x and the axis of y, M- is the initial area of the mind, M+ is projection area of mind and M (neutral) is your initial area. Divide your mind into four parts: initial basic, elementary negative, elementary positive, projection. (See Figure 7.1 Thought/Metabolism)

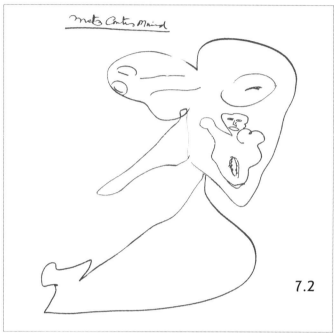

7.2

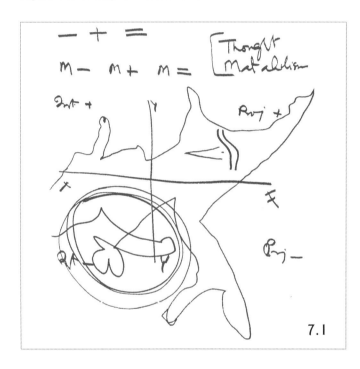

7.1

I'm being honest with you. There is nothing in this world at all. This world is all a joke. It's the biggest joke! All spirituality is the biggest joke and any spiritual teacher who doesn't know this basic information is the biggest crook. I'll state it clearly: All this paraphernalia, this and that, is just straightforward Detroit junk. Everything—yoga, religion, new techniques, old techniques, philosophy—it's all junk. It doesn't make sense.

What is the power of the mind? Everyone believes it is thought. No, it is not thought. When thought joins with metabolism, you feel like a human being. Nobody will tell you that. It's a great secret. This idiotic, foolish human being has kept the secret from himself, and no human wants to admit it. But it is a metabolic necessity. For example, in Figure 7.2, your metabolism is putting pressure on the mind.

Actually the mind should be putting pressure on the metabolism. (See Figure 7.3)

That is the power of the mind. It's all in the brain—there's nothing to it. The whole thing is either sick or Sikh.

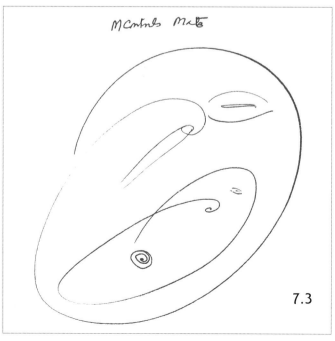

7.3

If thought form is governed by the mind and the mind is under the pressure of metabolism, you will be a freak. You do things and you pretend you are not doing them. In the end you will be empty—hitting the wall. But if your mind controls your metabolism, you are divine. There are two ways to look at it: either you're divided or you are divine.

Q: *What do you mean by divided?*

Yogi Bhajan: Jekyll and Hyde. In the morning you look like a saint and at night, you sneak into clubs. Split. Two men living in one, like vanilla and chocolate ice cream. It's a very sick life, it is the sickest life.

Life goes like this. This (Figure 7.1) is a drawing of the male sex organ. It is divided in four ways so that you can study it very well. The shaft is the danger area. It's called the "horniness initial". You are a total being and your metabolism has a barometer, which is a piece of meat 6 to 18 inches long, hanging between your legs. That's all it is. Your entire metabolism is located in the shaft of your sex organ. What do you call it? Your "dick" or penis? That's your God. You are totally pretending that you love God. It is totally bullshit. There is absolutely no truth to it. You lie day in and day out. You're the biggest confirmed liars. This is true of all kinds of men, including yogis, swamis, priests, fathers. Every religious person is basically lying through his teeth. That's why God hates you all. Actually your God is called Penis. It goes up, you go up; it goes down, you go down. That is your barometer. It also controls your metabolism, it controls your glandular system, it controls your environments, it controls everything around it, with it, under it, and over it. Are you willing to face that truth or not? No, you are not. You can't. You don't even experience that this six-foot-long human being is being controlled by those six inches of meat. However, if you really watch your mental capacity, you'll find that it doesn't go beyond that. In 500,000 centuries, it never has. Your wars, your territory, your country, your production, your discovery, your creativity all depends on that one thing.

What about that blonde actress, Marilyn Monroe. Everyone wanted her. Why? Because she was a sex symbol? She was a stinking old bitch, a habitual neurotic, and a flop. She started with nothing and ended with nothing. But when we look at where she was, what she was doing, we must ask how she could achieve so much fame. She could create a thought in every metabolism. Every mental thought could coordinate sensually and sexually with the metabolism because of her. Do you understand? It is this mental/metabolic, sensual/sexual energy that produces a need for six million young white bodies to cater to the sales force of the United States of America. Every salesman is bribed, wined, dined and sexed. It is a complete industry.

That's why we rise and we fall, and we fall and we rise. It is a rhythm, a biorhythm. But *you* are not a biorhythm; it is your biorhythm. You are not the horniness; it is your horniness. Separate your Self from the environment. You are the master and the environment is the slave. As long as you experience yourself as the slave and the environment as the master, how can you be successful? There's no end to the playboy. All of you are either a crude playboy, a rude playboy, or you are a little sophisticated and soft. Look deeply into it, don't just accept it superficially. All of this makes you unable to deal with failure. When you meet failure, it becomes a disaster

---

Meditation for Mental Control of the **Metabolism**
September 25, 1982

Posture: Sit in Easy Pose or Rock Pose.

Eyes: Closed.

Mudra: Put the right arm straight out in front of you, 45° to 60° above the horizontal, with the fingers straight. Place the palm of the left hand, with the fingers straight, onto the right arm about midway between the shoulder and the elbow. Keep the left elbow up and the head straight forward, as though you are looking at something.

Mantra: Chant Har Har Har Har Har Har Hari with the tip of the tongue, without moving the mouth, in a monotone.

Time: 11 Minutes

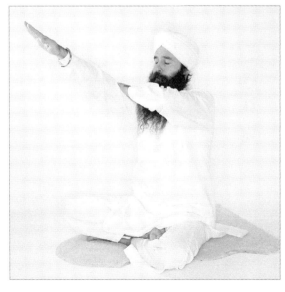

because you don't have good brakes and what car can stop without good brakes?

Your thoughts are your good brakes. You must project your Self. Your thoughts must control your metabolism. Your metabolism must not create your thoughts. When you get thoughts, they multiply with the metabolism and then they become your traumas. So you must separate your self from your metabolism. You have rented this body. You live in this body. You are not the body.

Q: *Do you dream if your metabolism is in control?*

Yogi Bhajan: I don't know. I can't talk on that subject because I have never dreamt. I don't know what a dream is. I have no experience on the subject at all. I sleep. I put my head down and I take my head off. Sometimes I go to sleep on the right ear and I wake up on the left. That's all.

Normally dreams are just an outlet for the subconscious. There is a network between the conscious, the supreme conscious, and the subconscious—like arteries. The conscious mind relates to the supreme conscious and the supreme conscious relates to the conscious, but sometimes the pathway gets blocked in the subconscious. We call these blocks metabolic temporal obstructions, MTOs. (See Figure 7.4.) We burn MTOs in White Tantric Yoga[5].

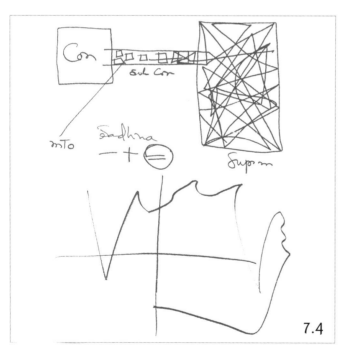

7.4

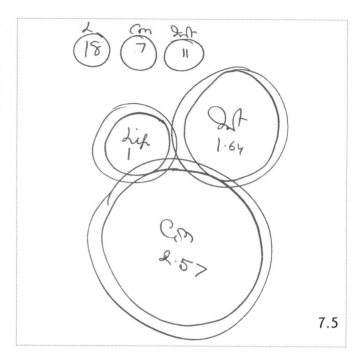

7.5

Looking at the figure you can see how terrible it looks. It's a glowing powerful thing. When this block exists, you can't get to your supreme conscious through your conscious, and your supreme conscious can't get to you. The release of the subconscious is done in sadhana. That's what sadhana is. In sadhana we get up in the morning, before we do anything else, and work on our mind and metabolism. Through sadhana, you calm down the metabolism, you calm down the mind, and you create a harmony. Sadhana belongs to the Neutral Mind. In sadhana the Negative and Positive Minds become the Neutral Mind. Without the Neutral Mind, success can only be temporary. It will not be everlasting.

The cycle of life is 18 years. Consciousness is 7 years and intelligence is 11 years. At 18 years, one cycle of life is complete. The life cycle is in proportion to both the consciousness and intelligence cycles. This is accurate to one-tenth. So the proportion of 18:11 is 1.64 and 18:7 is 2.57. (See Figure 7.5.) These proportional cycles form the circle of life, the circle of power. It is within these proportions that a successful individual will proceed. These are called rings of success, proportionate rings of success. If they are in harmony, success is guaranteed. If they are in disharmony, there shall be pain in life. This wheel is your friend and this friendship should be mutual. Every other relationship is false. Every other relationship is time and space. The relationship in your life is between your intelligence, your consciousness and you, the life cycle.

Q: *Can you give an example of how you would know if you are in balance?*

Yogi Bhajan: Yes. When I am 18 years old, I should be 2 ½ times more conscious and 1 ½ times more intelligent than I was at birth. But what happens to me? I grow old physically and I am dumb intelligently and my consciousness is very poor.

---

[5] White Tantric Yoga is a full-day meditation done with partners. For more information see: www.whitetantricyoga.com.

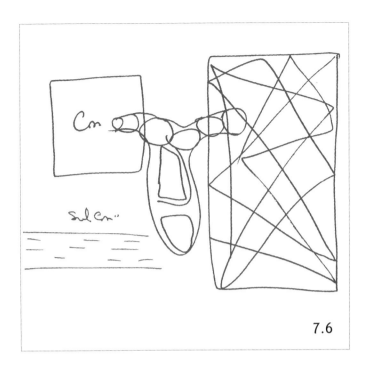

7.6

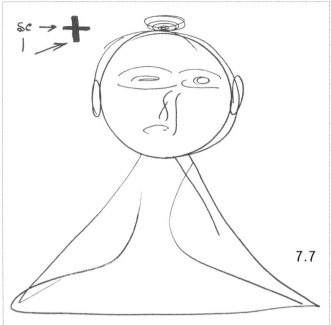

7.7

Q: *In other words, you should grow in proportion so that at 36, you are that much further developed than at 18, etc. So if I was 18 years old, how would I know if my life was correct at that point?*

Yogi Bhajan: You don't need to know, it happens. That is the baseline. Life, your bag, will remain the same but your balloon will change, and your being will enter a different dimension.

Q: *What happens to the subconscious mind when a man becomes 36?*

Yogi Bhajan: There can be an overload of obstructions, MTOs. Too much overloading is not permissible. The supreme conscious is always divided into 40 triangles. The conscious is always kept clean. The subconscious consists of two connecting lines like a roadway and lanes. (See Figure 7.6) You can see the subconscious railroad. That is the way the subconscious is supposed to be. The penis-like structure is the overload.

Q: *Does the body actually move away from the soul as death approaches?*

Yogi Bhajan: Yes. The soul has to get out of the body when the lease is up.

Q: *Does that mean that meditation is automatically easier as you approach old age?*

Yogi Bhajan: No, it means life is easier if you meditate. If you have a habit of meditating, life becomes easier because you can balance your combination of minds and consciousness.

What is meditation? It is a conscious effort to clean the mind, to control the mind. It is so simple. When you meditate your subconscious releases thought and all you release is the tongue. See this guy, Figure 7.7. The subconsious releases negative thought, while the "I" releases positive thought. Perpendicular energy and parallel energy cross each other, and the net result is that life becomes a plus.

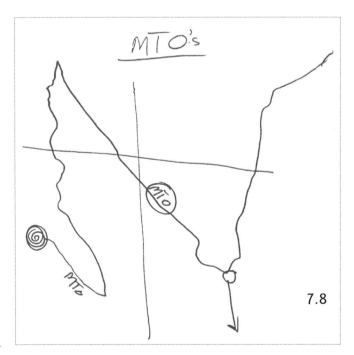

7.8

Q: *I still don't understand MTOs.*

Yogi Bhajan: Let me explain it. Between axis *x* and axis *y*, life—your life—started. (See Figure 7.8.) It started at initial negative and then went out of initial negative. Then one day you got up and you wanted to start working up and you did start working up. Then you were made. This gave you the initiative to prove to yourself that you were playing a fair game. Repeat after me, "We are playing a fair game."

Students: *We are playing a fair game.*

Yogi Bhajan: Always remember, nothing succeeds unless it is fair. It should be fair to me, it should be fair to you and it should be fair to . . .

Students: *Us.*

Yogi Bhajan: That is the secret to *all* 16 aspects of success: I should be fair to me, I should be fair to you and I should be fair to us. That is the mental game you should always play. Make it a habit.

Q: What if you are counseling somebody and you know they don't think you are being fair but you know your advice is best for them?

Yogi Bhajan: Counseling does not mean telling someone what is fair to them or to you. Counseling is putting people back on the rails. Whenever a human mind or a human body or a human projection gets off the track, counseling is used to put it back on. It is always fair but sometimes the disaster is so bad and someone may be off the tracks so much that it is very difficult to put him back on. That will bother you. Some people are so sick that you don't want to deal with them. But if you have a lot of compassion and a lot of health and a lot of life, you will like bringing them back onto the track. Talking, counseling, consoling, advising, all of that is the track. But God, if you don't know the track, and you try to put someone on the track, and there's no track, you've got hot stuff on your hands. You had better know the track.

The mind must play and you must play. The game of life is "I, you and us." Whenever you mess up something in the game, life will bring you pain. Play fairly, play justly, and play gracefully.

Q: Should that be like pratyahar, *while we're doing the do, we meditate on not doing the don't?*

Yogi Bhajan: No, no. You don't understand. Do the do's and do the don'ts. The don'ts have to be done, too. You act out what you're not supposed to, that's why the don'ts

The game of life is "I, you and us." Play fairly, play justly, and play gracefully.

aren't done. It is a total mental problem with all you Western people. I have seen it for 14 years. You are oriented just to do the do's.

Q: You mean if the don'ts occur to you, you should do them?

Yogi Bhajan: Speak the truth. That is a do. Don't tell a lie. That is a don't.

Q: So if it occurs to me to tell a lie, what should I do?

Yogi Bhajan: Don't do it because that is doing the don't. It only works that way. Doing is your nature. It is your nature to flow with life. You keep flowing, you keep doing. It is what you want to do. You want to do everything, including the don'ts.

"Thou shalt not kill." It is a commandment, so why do you kill? Because you don't do the don'ts. "Thou shalt not kill." In that case, no Christian or Jew shall eat meat, right? That is not practicing the don't. The main problem, the main mental problem of this world is that we don't do the don'ts.

Q: Is not doing the don'ts like avoiding the issue, not confronting?

Yogi Bhajan: It's avoiding the happiness of life. It's avoiding success. A Sikh shall do sadhana. A Sikh shall not miss sadhana. When both the do's and the don'ts are done, then you will have a posture. The posture of your personality is essential for life. Project your posture, not you.

Q: Sir, earlier you said project you and nothing else. How is that different from projecting your posture?

Yogi Bhajan: You have to become the posture. Your posture is that which everybody understands you to be. You will have a posture when everybody in the world knows that you do the don'ts and you do the do's. If people come to know that you only do the do's and don't do the don'ts, you won't have a posture. You are not confirmed.

When you study to be a doctor, you must pass an examination. When you pass, you are confirmed to be a doctor; you are examined and confirmed to practice. Then what is your posture? Dr. So-and-So, or So-and-So, D.C. This is called posture. Posture gives people general trust in you. It gives people a general public relation about you. It can tell people what you can do and what you can't do. It gives people trust in you. You carry the trust and you deliver. Nothing else.

Don't forget to remember: you need "you" and "us". We forget it all the time. We push the "I" to the point that we create our own disasters. "I" needs "you" and "us." That is the name of the game. Play the game fairly.

The Yamas and the **Niyamas**

People will tell you, "I'll give you happiness." But they will not give you discipline. The law is **yam** *and* **niyam**, *do's and don'ts. When you practice do's, you have to know the don'ts. Every do has a don't, and every don't has a do. It's a law. You have to have the do's and you have to have the don'ts. Your problem is that you do the do's but you don't do the don'ts. Do's without the don'ts and don'ts without do's do not work.*

The mental game. The mental reach. What is mental reach? It is reaching everybody mentally to create a relationship, to create mental understanding. The mental reach should be to create a mental understanding: "He's fair." "He's my friend." "He can do this." "No, it is not to be expected of him. Impossible, forget it. I will bet on it." Why do people do this for you? Because you have created a mental reach. Let your mental game be known. Let it be known that your mental game is fair, that it excels. Your mental reach should be genuine, and it must create an understanding. You mental profile should be just, fair and neutral. Think these words, "He is just, fair and neutral." How does it sound? "He's just, fair and neutral." It's a mental attitude. "He's kind and he listens." Not listening is the biggest crime in the mental game. Listen more. Speak less.

Now, I'll tell you the secret. If you put the physical and the mental together, what does it give you? Professional success, everlasting professional success in every field. You didn't believe that I could cover the subject so quickly, did you?

Next time, we'll go totally into the professional foundations, such as balance sheets and how to balance them, how to balance activities, how to differentiate between sales and supply and demand, their effects, and all those kinds of topics. Then we'll talk about economic vigilance. That's very important. Professionally, we fail primarily because we don't create economic vigilance. It is a technical area but it is essential to go through these basics.

Q: *Although we only covered two topics in a list of 16, you summed it all up in the end. However, I wanted to hear more about hearing habits, number 16.*

Yogi Bhajan: We'll cover that. We'll go slowly, slowly, slowly to the subject because it is not professionally right to overdose you and then try to get results. The idea is to keep a successful human being. The idea is not to teach the subject. Do you see this? (See Figure 7.9) If the filament is surrounded by a vacuum, we have light. That vacuum is the vacuum of ego. Whether or not to surround your ego with a vacuum is your choice, my friends. But when there's no vacuum, we have a heater; a heater gives off very little light.

Q: *Is the vacuum of ego self-control?*
Yogi Bhajan: Self-illumination.

Q: *How is the vacuum created?*
Yogi Bhajan: When you eat up your own ego. Now, there's one exercise for success that I would like you to do. Reach the point where you can perfect it, and then let me know how great you are.

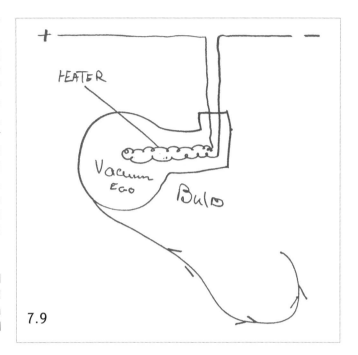

7.9

Q: *Is there a correct and incorrect way to clear the monkey glands?*

Yogi Bhajan: The correct way is to take your toothbrush, brush your teeth and the back of your tongue; rub the back of the tongue properly and you'll throw up. The whole congestion around the monkey glands will come out. It is there.

Meditation for **Success**
September 25, 1982

Posture: Sit down in a yogic posture, chin in, chest out.

Mudra: Put your right hand over your left, palms down, just in front of the Heart Center. Keep the elbows up and balanced. Lock your hands in place. Don't shift your hands or your posture throughout the meditation.

Mantra: Inhale deep, look at the tip of your nose, and chant very rapidly, 12 times per breath:

Wha-hay Guroo, Wha-hay Guroo, Wha-hay Guroo, Wha-hay Jee-o

Jio should be loud and clear no matter how fast you may go.

Time: 31 Minutes

Comments: Practice it early in the morning when you have eaten nothing. Clear your monkey glands, then take a glass of warm water with vinegar and honey in it. (I use about half an ounce of vinegar, malt vinegar, and about a teaspoon of honey. It is about 4:1, vinegar to honey, mixed into the warm water.) Then do this exercise.

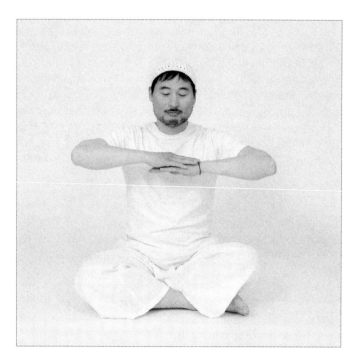

Q: With the meditation does it matter whether it's before or after sadhana?

Yogi Bhajan: No, it's your personal choice, but you can't have eaten.

Q: Is there any pressure on the hands, up or down?

Yogi Bhajan: Nothing.

Q: If your mind is totally meditative, you've done this and you've done that and your pratyahar is good . . .

Yogi Bhajan: What is *pratyahar*? I'll tell you what it is since you want to know. In *pranayam*, it is from you to God outward. In *pratyahar*, it is from you to God inward. (See Figure 7.10)

Q: When I do pratyahar, I take whatever emotion I'm feeling and just attach it to the mantra. If I'm angry, I start doing Wahe Guru Wahe Guru, pretty soon the mantra neutralizes my anger and I'm gone. Is that the way I should live my whole life?

Yogi Bhajan: Well, ultimately you don't have to bother. You don't have to do things to create that neutrality. Ultimately, you'll start doing it. Habit. Habit does it. Create a habit. *Pranayam, pratyahar* are habits.

Q: Sir, is silence silence?

Yogi Bhajan: Silence is not the outside silence but the inside.

Q: What about an expression of a sound, like singing out loud or doing a mantra internally.

Yogi Bhajan: That's very silent. Singing gurbani kirtan is very silent. You have to cut down everything to create the music and the words and the sound. Kirtan is the absolute experience of silence because nothing is yours.

> *Singing gurbani kirtan is very silent. You have to cut down everything to create the music and the words and the sound. Kirtan is the absolute experience of silence because nothing is yours.*

Q: Then there's no such thing as silence? There's only cutting down all the noise so you can hear the sound of life?

Yogi Bhajan: You are crazy. Your life atom is vibrant. (See Figure 7.11) How can it be silent? Silence happens when there is nothing that is yours.

Q: Sir, did Gurmukhi develop in trying to communicate that experience of silence?

Yogi Bhajan: Guru Angad brought it directly from God. He became a part of Guru Nanak and he manifested that as Gurmukhi. He knew what he was talking about.

Q: Sir, how did Guru Nanak pass on his essence? The gurus are all one, they're all Nanak, but what does that mean? How did Guru Nanak pass into Guru Angad, Guru Amar Das, etc.? What happens?

Yogi Bhajan: Hey, fool! A part of me lives in you. You don't accept the whole, that's why you cheat on me. I have passed into many. What's the difficulty?

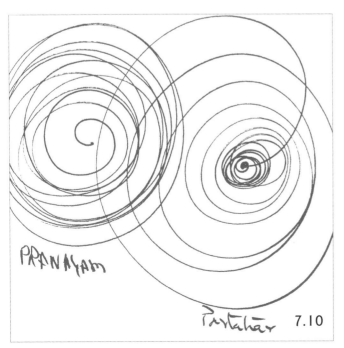

7.10

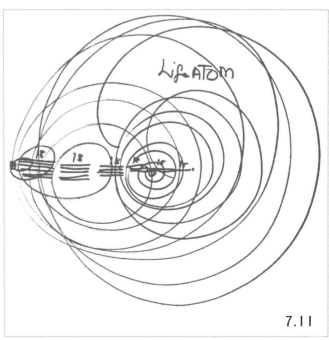

7.11

Pratyahar–Pranayam Sank Chalnee **Kriya**
September 25, 1982

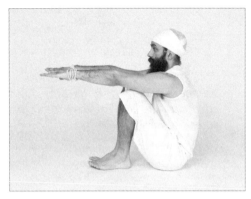

Posture: Sit down, putting your weight on your feet, try to stand up. Slowly, slowly, there's no hurry. Come all the way up **onto your toes**, and try to fly. Then come back down into the starting position.

Eyes: Keep your eyes open.

Time: It should take you **one minute** to get up and **one minute** to get back down.

Comments: Don't do more than 52 repetitions per day. You will be flying yogis. Your breathing will be automatic after the first few minutes and then you will breathe through every pore of your skin. The breath is a very special pranic breath. It's a man's challenge, and it is a very, very sacred exercise. If you really want to experience life, then do it sometime.

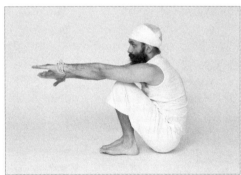

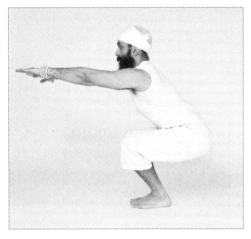

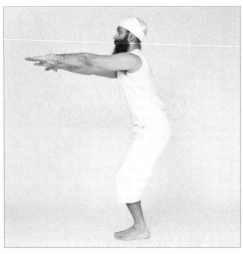
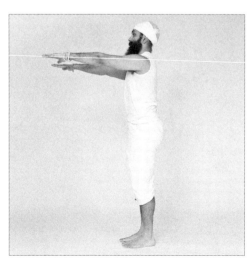

Note: This photo doesn't show the final pose—up on your toes, flying. Arms are suggestive only; you can interpret flying as you like.

Q: *Sir, if every atom has a soul and we as human beings have one soul to relate to . . .*
Yogi Bhajan: Every part of you is a part of that soul.

Q: *Where is God?*
Yogi Bhajan: I don't know where. Somewhere. Do you want to do a *pratyahar–pranayam* exercise? It will make you feel good.

Q: *Can you cross your ankles when you get up or do you have to keep them straight?*
Yogi Bhajan: Either way. It suits each metabolism, each height and each weight differently. *Sank chalnee: Sank* means conch and conch is the Navel Point. *Chalnee* means "starts it." It is a meditation and a pranayam complete within itself.

I want to conclude this course by lecturing to you about the most important part of the mental aspect. It is called mental play. Mental play is playing, mentally, that you are you; that you should be successful, you should be powerful, you should be grabbing, you should be in control, you should be known, you should be understood, you should be loved, you should be this, you should be that. Actually that is self-defeat. Why? Because you are "I," and "I" has to have a "you," and "you" has to have something to play with. I must have you to play with, and you must have I to play with, and you and I must play, and somebody must watch the play. In that way, we are always I, you and us. If you understand this, you understand the whole thing.

I need you. You need me. And there is somebody who understands what this need is about and that is us. Therefore it is I, you and us. Anyone who lives only by "I" will live in pain and frustration. Anyone who lives by "you and I" will live in disappointment. But anyone who will live in "I, you and us" will live fulfilled, happy and groovy. Mental play is I, you and . . .

Q: *Us.*
Yogi Bhajan: Us. That's the keynote.

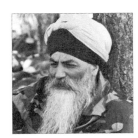

Man to **Man** 8
The Invincible Man

Circa 1983

You must realize that the strength in you is you. The material world around you is to supplement your strength or to complement your strength; it is not your strength.

- Evergreen **Exercises**
- The Flow of **Life**
- Communication Is **Personality**
- Health Is **Flexibility**
- **Who** Are You Subject To?

Evergreen **Exercises**

A man can become invincible and evergreen if he wants to. Through certain exercises, which call upon you to command your own self and your environments, you can recuperate yourself.

Recently I celebrated my 54th birthday. At that time I realized that since coming to the United States 14 years ago, I have travelled more miles than a flight attendant. By this time I should have all the symptoms and sicknesses that they get, plus I should have become weak and contracted some complicated diseases. Eighteen hours a day I have taken work and abuse on my body by dealing with negativity, filling a role of leadership, motivating people, inspiring them, directing them. It isn't to be expected that I should look very young and enthusiastic by now. In fact, all of this should have led to burnout.

Before coming here, I sat down and reviewed my situation. I asked myself, "What is the secret?" After all that I have survived during 14 hard, intense years in this country and 18 previous years of government work in India—the answer came: A man can become invincible and evergreen if he wants to. Through certain exercises, which call upon you to command your own self and your environments, you can recuperate yourself. It doesn't matter how difficult your life is.

God has given us the power of self-recuperation, which is much stronger and much better than we expect. It is far greater than we know or feel it to be. It is through this power that this delicate man, called a human being, is competent to be male. I am going to cover the psychological, sociological and other weaknesses that you've created; because God never made you weak. You should have nothing to do with weakness.

Everywhere, we see that with time men get weaker. They get mildly impotent earlier, they aren't honestly impressive, and they die younger than women. Temperamentally, every strong man slowly loses ground and this is true internationally. We get eroded before we even know that we are gone. When we are very young—from our teens to our late twenties—we perform well sexually, but in reality we become very weak sexually. I don't understand it. You should be as good as an 18-year-old person until you are 90. After all, you don't get stretched out or shortened or anything like that. As a man you have the capacity to recuperate yourself within 72 hours. This is the real secret of a healthy life.

Your real strength is in your blood chemistry. Is your blood young or not? That is what decides it—not you. You feel that you are either young or old based on your years; I believe that is a total diversion from reality. I believe that you are neither young nor old, but if your blood is hot and young, you are young, and if your blood is cold and weird, then you are old. We are going to work to find out how healthy you are and then we'll talk.

Evergreen **Exercises**
September 10, 1983

1. Stand up and stretch your arms out to your sides from your shoulders, lock your pinkies under your thumbs and lean back. Go to the maximum without losing your balance. **3 Minutes**

Comments: Don't think you are a great hero. You are assaying the final flexibility and conception of your body. Your blood chemistry will change under this pressure. If you get dizzy, straighten your body. Any kind of dizziness in this posture means that your brain and your circulatory system are not corresponding. This indicates that you have the potential to develop problems with your blood, or worse, to develop a terminal disease at an early age.

I am warning you. Give yourself a proper test. Get into the posture and hold it. This posture is equal to thousands of capsules of Vitamin E and Vitamin C, B12 and B6, and everything else. The last 60 seconds of this exercise are worth 60 years each. If you sweat, you are okay.

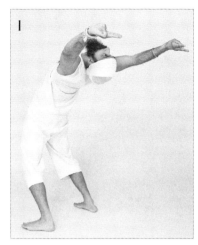

2. Immediately take your left foot in your hands and straighten out your leg, standing on your right leg. Don't let your left leg bend. Your sense of balance is in your ears. Use it and balance steady. **4 Minutes**

Comments: This posture balances your brain. To get the same effect with yoga you would have to do Tree Pose for years and years and years. If you do this exercise, you can always win a debate, no matter how dumb you are. That man who cannot talk to a woman is impotent to start with, so keep your leg straight. What else can you keep straight if you can't even hold your leg straight? Your performance has nothing to do with how religious you are. I promise that no woman has been born on this Earth who can shake you off your feet with her conversation if you dance this simple dance. Do it by the will of your brain, not by your physical will.

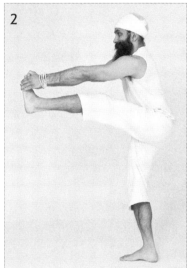

3. Now stand on your left leg, and hold your right foot with both hands. Bring it in toward your buttock. From this position, bend forward from the waist and come back up. Continue going forward and back, forward and back. **1 Minute**

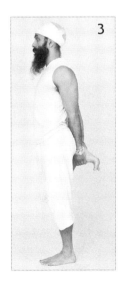
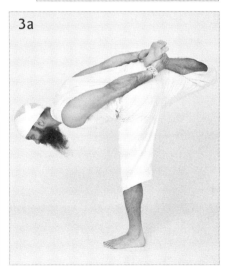

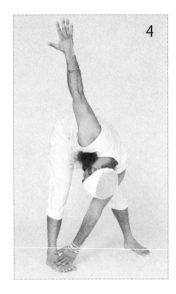

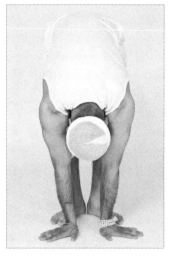

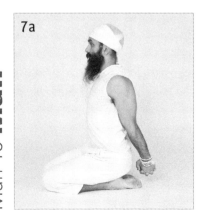

4. Stand with your legs spread wide. We are going to repair the liver. Put your arms out to the sides, parallel with the floor. Twist your body to the right as you bend down and touch your right foot with your left hand. Relax your head and stay in this posture, keeping a straight line between your left and right hands. A fantastic pressure will develop. We are not here to harass our bodies but to repair them. **2 Minutes**

5. In a standing posture, put your heels together and spread your toes to 60 degrees. Bring your palms to the floor, stretch and hold the posture. Inhale through the mouth, and exhale through the nose. Use a powerful breath. Put equal pressure on the hands and feet. Press with the hands. This is the secret. **5 Minutes**

Comments: This exercise is very unique and very advantageous. Don't feel it as a person. Don't feel anything as a person. Experience it as a man. This exercise can give you that experience. If you find yourself becoming dizzy while you are doing this exercise, stop and get yourself checked out by a heart specialist.

6. Bring your left foot up into your buttock and hold it with your left hand. Stretch your right hand up into the air and keep it straight. Now open your mouth wide and begin to breathe in and out through the mouth, pumping the belly like a bellows. When you exhale, your belly must contract as if you have received a blow. This exercise is the best thing for impotency or partial impotency. Get rid of it now. **3 Minutes**

7. Sit on your heels. Bring your arms behind you and lock the hands in Venus Lock. When you bring your forehead to the floor, lift your arms up behind you. Done to the musical version of *Jaap Sahib*. **31 Minutes**

Comments: We will do a special kriya to Guru Gobind Singh's prayer, *Jaap Sahib*. You will bow and come up to the rhythm of it, one complete bow to each line.

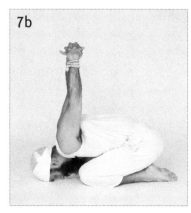

8. Sit in Easy Pose. Extend your arms straight out in front of your body from your shoulders parallel with the ground. Your right arm will move up and down 90 degrees. Nothing else will move, and that arm will move faster than you think. There is no bend in the elbow. The left arm is totally balanced with the earth, while the right is in total movement. **5 Minutes**

Comments: Let us go through this psychological test. It will create a balance in your nerves. That balance lies within total stillness and total movement. You don't want to have to go home to your wife and apologize, "Sorry, honey. I'm too tired tonight," If that's the case you should be at Jane Fonda's Workout, you are not supposed to be a man. Keep up. I am convinced that you can make yourself into a man of steel.

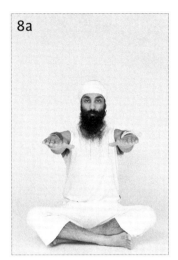

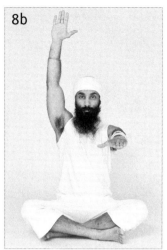

9. Stand up. Come into Half Chair Pose by spreading your feet about 18 inches and bend your knees as though you were sitting on the edge of a high stool. Put your right hand into your left and cup them just in front of the pelvis. Now open your mouth and begin pulling your tongue in and out. Move it. Pull it in and out quickly. Breath has nothing to do with it. **2 Minutes**

Comments: It will give you an experience that you have never had before. If you want intelligence, this exercise will do it. It is very intelligent to control your tongue.

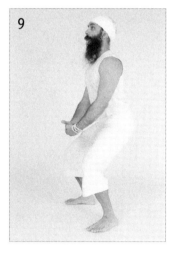

10. Lie down on your back. Relax with your legs straight and put both your hands beneath your lower back. Listen to *Ardas Bhaee*. **20 Minutes**

Comments: Come out of your relaxation. Check your muscles and feel how you feel. You must understand plainly and clearly that these are the exercises you must do. Within 72 hours your body and your blood cells have to change your physical body, your tissues, your total metabolism. With each hour of delay, you become more aged, nervous, and unintelligent. Five thousand years ago human beings knew that the man's success was in the chemistry of the blood. These are very powerful exercises. They are not very strenuous, but they will bring an unbelievable change in you.

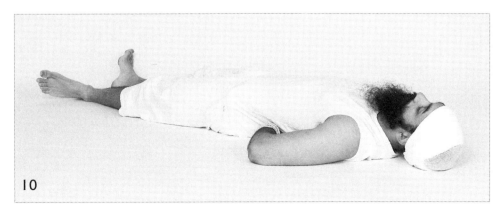

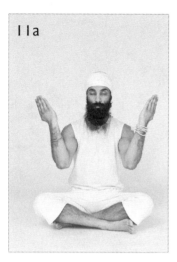
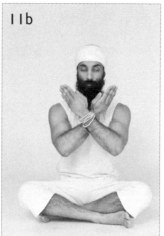

11. Come sitting in Easy Pose. Bring both hands up with your palms flat, facing the body. Now keeping the hands very hard, like the male organ, begin to cross the hands in front of the face, right hand close to the body, left hand away. The movement is from the elbow. Concentrate on the movement. It is a very male action. **2 Minutes**

Now begin to criss-cross the hands, alternating them, left in front, right in front, left in front, right in front. Move fast. Move like a weaving machine. Weave in and out. Weave your magnetic energy. Work both hands, both sides. The frequency you must build allows you to move faster than you think you can. Go beyond your capacity. Be virtuous. There is nothing more important than you. Move faster than your capacity and your thought. If you think you can move 10 times a second, then try to move 20 times a second. Keep going and close your eyes.

Visualization: As you sit there, imagine that flowers are coming out of you. Flowers, roses, marigolds, think of all the flowers you know. Every time the hands criss-cross, you create flowers. Bunches of flowers are coming out of you. Tons of them. A heap of flowers is building around you, and you are totally merged in them.
6 Minutes

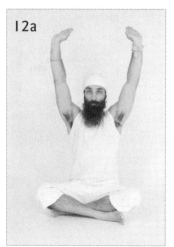
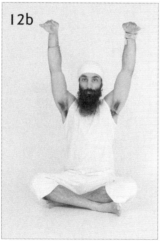

12. Open your eyes and lift your hands straight up over your head and wave them from the wrist only. Imagine that a ship filled with your relatives is leaving the dock. You are waving to each one very affectionately. They are going to a very joyful place, a place that is beyond death. You are not going to see them again. Wave to them and give them as much love as you can. Wave your hands to all your ancestors and your ancestors' ancestors. All of those people. Imagine a beautiful gold and silver ship. Every relative you have is boarding and you are waving goodbye to them. "Bye-bye. Love you. I'll be coming there one day too." **2 Minutes**

Comments: Those of you who have a fear of death can get rid of it with this exercise. This is a brain exercise. We have to bring a permanent change to your computerized material. That fluid which carries the messages from one part of the brain to another has to be recaptured completely and made absolutely new.

13. Lock your hands in an inverted Venus and extend them straight out in front of you parallel to the ground. Close your eyes and imagine that you are flying through time and space. Feel you are going through time and space. Bend forward slowly as you imagine that. Just move slowly; you are penetrating through space millimeter by millimeter. You can transform a person by changing the blood chemistry, and the nearest and dearest person to you is you.

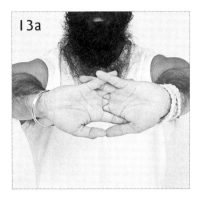

Let the power come from your spine and let yourself penetrate through space. Penetrate through space. You are the bravest, you are the most powerful, you are the most positive, you are intelligent, you know all, God made you special, you are special. "I am a beautiful being. I am beautifully a beautiful being. I am beautifully a beautiful being." Hold that thought, that projection. Keep steady. Hands stretched out, perfectly extended. The Kundalini awakens and the man becomes super-intelligent. There are simple ways to do it. Energy is coming from afar. It is fresh. It is going through all of you. It is the most energetic time for you. Use it.

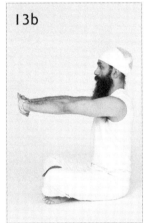 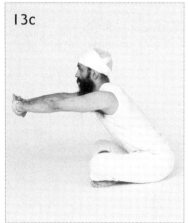

Inhale very deeply. Hold the breath, and project that you are beautiful, the most beautiful. Hold the breath and project "I am the most beautiful, I am the most beautiful, I am the most beautiful. Everything is happy and perfect. Everything is happy and perfect. Everything is happy and perfect." You have to do it right. Project out that you are perfect, you are penetrating, you are invincible, you are great. Keep on holding the breath to the maximum capacity and penetrate. Relax. **5 Minutes**

14. Lie on your back, pull your knees into your chest and roll up and back on your spine. Roar, roar like a lion. Roll and roar. **1 Minute**

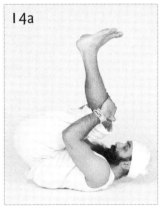 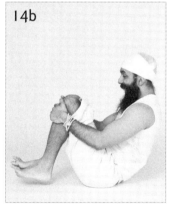

You have initially set yourself and now you are ready for the lecture. We will discuss the philosophy of reading beyond time and space. That's where the power of the invincible man lies. These exercises were a physical stimulation I wanted to share with you. I will be very, very grateful if you express your joy in a very controlled manner. Just imagine for yourself how you can express your happiness. Imagine the power of the man. You may think man is just useless and a sinner. But I would like to share this with you: Man can experience God and prove God's existence to all other men. How beautiful that is! Sometime in your life you may feel difficulties. But difficulties are not what they seem. They come to you only because God thinks you have the capacity to take on the challenge. We will speak more of this and magnetic vibrations and penetrations.

■ ■ ■

Guru Gobind Singh's *Bowing Jaap Sahib*

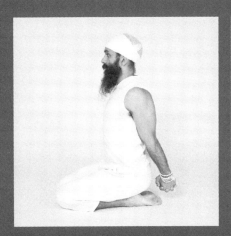
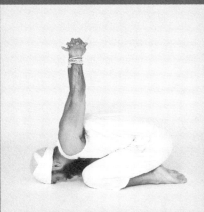

Guru Gobind Singh never did miracles. He made his people run with their horses chanting *Jaap Sahib*.

One percent could stand with only their grit against 125,000 people and not lose. This is something which happened a few hundred years ago. This is not a legend from the ancients. If it could be valid any place, in any community, it can be valid here.

Yoga Mudra is the redeemer of all diseases in the body—on the spot. The rhythm of *naad* is provided by the Guru's *Jaap Sahib*. Through this exercise you will understand the power of the *banis*, the Sikh prayers. You cannot be unhealthy if you do it every morning. Do it honestly. Even if someone breaks a stone on your thigh, just keep doing it. You have a right to be healthy.

Exercising to the rhythm of the Guru's word is the one way to understand it. It is the one way to become the Self. It is the one way because "in the beginning was the Word, the Word was with God, and the Word was God."[1] This Word from the Guru inspires you and it can inspire the Word in you. Plus, if the body can get into the rhythm of the *naad*, anything that could kill you, make you weak, make you diseased, make you poor, or make you totally naive will leave you right then and there. Remember the Word is a beginning, so it grants you a beginning each time. There's no reason for any man to say, "I am burned out" or "I don't know what to do." You get burned out when the blood does not feed your brain properly and when the quality of the blood is impure. It isn't that you don't know.

Intelligence is not taught in a university. Intelligence is a personal thing. To not be intelligent is to be dumb. Wasting time, getting involved in worthless conversations, getting totally bogged down, being told that you are good for nothing, accepting that you are hopeless, useless, "blah, blah, blah," is the story of unintelligent idiots. Whether you are 50 years old, a 100 years old, or 2 years old, intelligence and you can interact all the time. Intelligence is the name of the guardian angel. The Guru can give it to you but you've got to take it. It's all in you. Only you can invoke in you the power to be you. Everything else is false. You are a reality living in a non-reality. If you invoke the realization of that non-reality within yourself, the non-reality of the outside can never bother you. You need within you, inside you, the realization of what non-reality and reality are.

No man is born to suffer. It is only through your wrong acts—without your own intelligence, without your own confidence, without your own success—that you suffer. Then you go to religious people, you go to astrologers, you go to numerologists, you go to doctors, you go to consultants. You go, and go, and go. You go for one thing, one simple thing: just to live. Just to live you become a slave to so many professions and professionals and situations. You become such a slave to your emotions, your commotions, and your trauma that your life becomes a drama.

Don't let your life become a drama. Don't. Life will not be worth anything to you. You will be acting, and acting, and acting until finally you will get tired of acting and you will never know why you were acting. You have come to live, not to act. You have come to be because you are—you are. Everything comes from you. You think you can get something from the outside. It is not true. Nothing comes from the outside. It has been proven time and again. Getting everything from the inside is what Kundalini Yoga is all about. Uncoil yourself. Let the world know. That is the way to live.

Nothing can happen to you. You have the right to live. You can live. If you can't, you can die. The most important thing in your life is to live honorably and to die honorably. Materially, you can lose everything and you can gain everything, but if you lose your reputation, you cannot gain it back. Lose the whole world, but not your reputation. You are a man forever, so be a man to yourself.

[1] John 1.1, a favorite biblical verse, often quoted by Yogi Bhajan.

The Flow of Life

Life is a continuous factor. Earth is a flow of that life. You come to Earth to flow.

Occasionally, you may be surprised to see me walking with a walking stick. It is only an indication of the conditions of law and order in the United States. It is not an indication of my health. I think all of us should have very fashionable, very strong, very beautiful walking sticks. A walking stick will keep a knife at least four feet away from your ribs. In Germany I saw a very fine walking stick. It had a handle of horn that was very beautifully done. It was called a hunter's stick. I think that if you have that stick and the other person has a gun, chances are you will win and he will lose. In spite of the fact that we don't understand it ourselves, we are soon to enter 1984. The years 1984 to 1988 are a very special time. You may need that stick.

We have come to talk about that reality, about that beauty, about that truth that you have never believed. You realize that nobody can create anybody like you. Forget about creating you. If you get damaged, you cannot even be repaired perfectly. You are who you are. Ultimately it gives you a chance to prove that you are created by the Perfect God, the Infinite God. We coined the word God because as we started looking into the depth of our own self, we started feeling, very honestly, that each one of us is special in his own right. However, you don't believe it. You know it. But you don't believe it. Your behavior doesn't reflect your knowledge. You know it but you don't behave as if you believe it.

Your creative nature is known to you. Your destructive nature is known to you. Your weaknesses are known to you. Your strengths are known to you. You want to win but you lose. Your only problem on this planet is boredom. If you learn how to conquer your boredom, you can conquer all the environments of your life and life will be very pleasant.

Let us take a closer look at this boredom. You know so much about yourself that you think you are the world's wisest person. If anyone tells you anything about wisdom, you say, "Well, wait a minute. I already know that." I agree with you that you are wise. You are very wise. I have no doubt about it. However, you are not wise in following your intuition. You use that very wisdom to follow your emotions. You insist on following your commotions.

Some time in your life, you must have met a person with whom you simply could not communicate. It's like talking to a wall. The person is so rough that you feel he is a super idiot. Emotional trauma has taken over the personal personality of that person. Intuition, logic, and reason have no place in him. When this happens to you, you think that you cannot be rich, you cannot be happy, you cannot be great. Forget it. I am telling you that you are born to succeed. You are born to enjoy.

You grow, you have been growing and you shall continue to grow. Nobody can take that away from you. It is true even to the extent that when this body dies, you will still grow out of it. There is no such thing as death. You were alive before this body. You will be alive after this body. Something came into a cylinder and something will go out of that cylinder. Within the time that you are in the cylinder called body, you will experience a lot of emotions and a lot of intuitions. Often you go toward your emotions and commotions. But your system of intuition is the source of your happiness. It is the source of your victory. It is the source that can make you invincible.

One thing always surprises me. You always want to look beautiful but never to yourself. That is an amazing phenomenon. You never want to look beautiful to yourself. You never want to look intelligent to yourself. You never want to look confident to yourself. You never want to look powerful to yourself. It is important to you that you make impressions on others. Yet there is nothing which you yourself choose to relate to within yourself; but you need to relate to everything about you to yourself.

Somebody once said to me, "You've got a lot of students."
I said, "Not a lot. I could have had many, many students. I could have had a lot of students."
"What went wrong?"
I said, "The problem is that I teach people to be teachers; therefore, I couldn't get students. I make teachers. I can get people. Spiritual masters can attract people. Saints and holy men can do this too. It's very easy, but I make teachers. It's a workshop, a factory. When the goods in a factory are completed, they are ready to go out. That is my approach."

Each one of you, being the creativity of God, and having the faculty of intuition, must be wonderful. Otherwise you cannot live. But there is something you do not realize. I am going to tell you what it is. I will proceed very slowly because I want you to take the information inside and believe it. You are not here to experience life. Earth is not the experience of life. Earth is the experience of death. You will be shocked to know that. You have been told differently. You have been told that Earth is the experience of life—that is wrong from the beginning. Life is a continuous factor. Earth is a flow of that life. You come to Earth to flow.

The mistake you commit, the brainwashing that you received (and you have been damaged from the beginning) is that you don't use your intuition. You have a memory so you remember yesterday. You have strength so you act today. But because you don't use your intuition, you cannot compute tomorrow. This is your behavior:

"Hey, who are you?"
"What do you mean. 'Hey, who are you?' Why don't you speak politely to me?"
"I'll speak to you however I want."
"Why you idiot, you so-and-so . . ."

In the end, you fight it out because today is to act. When you use your intuition, you are aware that tomorrow is another day. Tomorrow we will meet again. Be polite today so that as you look to tomorrow you may smile at each other. Intuition will never let you have a war. It can never allow you to fight. You don't need quarrels. I want you to understand how foolish it is. If I feel, "I'm going to grab from him," and I grab from him, then somebody will grab from me. Eventually this whole world will become a grabbing world.

You are not here to experience life. Earth is not the experience of life. Earth is the experience of death. You will be shocked to know that. You have been told differently. You have been told that Earth is the experience of life—that is wrong from the beginning. Life is a continuous factor. Earth is a flow of that life. You come to Earth to flow.

You are involved in passion. You believe in victory through passion. There's no such thing as victory through passion. Victory is through intuition. You are mortal, but there is an immortal in you. You are immortal, but the body is mortal. Every one of you has a given intelligence. If the given intelligence is combined with developed intuition, given intelligence and given intuition are developed together. If intuition is developed, intelligence is there. You are victorious. You are successful. Nobody can ever do any harm to you.

Gurmat is the Guru's way. *Gurmat* means "the churned out, classified as known, everlasting, Infinite Truth." In the West we say patience pays and that tolerance is a virtue, but in the oriental language of spirituality it is called *santokh*—satisfaction, eternal satisfaction. I know that there are some things that you are impatient about that are bothering you. You have a career and you are worried because the economic unemployment of America is affecting certain areas. Certain shifting and certain changes have to take place. Have patience and you will have *santokh*.

I have guided people who are here and who have worked for 3HO into certain industries that will be the last to be hit. That's why there is so little unemployment in the 3HO family relative to the nation at large. Unemployment has not hit us because we are very flexible, because we are a very special type of people. We believe in our intelligence and our intuition. When we put intelligence and intuition together, two and two made four to us, and we decided to go into those industries that would give us self-respect—productivity through self-respect. With this approach we can never be unemployed.

If somebody is a carpenter, somebody is a carpenter. If he is a building contractor, he is a building contractor. But if you are a building contractor and times get hard, you can work, you can work as a carpenter. If you are a carpenter, you do something else. In this world, the honorable thing is to work for the honor of doing the labor, not doing the labor to achieve status and honor. All work is honorable, *keerth karni*.

The quality of a man who invests fast and wants to become rich fast is very shallow. Do you build goodwill or do you build greed? You build your insecurity. You should be deep-rooted, not emotional. You should be intelligent. A major problem is that you are not what you think you are. Some of you actually feel that your profession determines your status. You are never judged by your profession. You are judged by your intuition. You are judged by how intuitively intelligent you are. Your profession, your money, your cars, your home, your everything, only gives you a very temporary, shallow edge. There is no depth in it. The greatest weakness that men have is that they do not intuitively work for their tomorrow.

A woman can be emotional because she has 16 times greater intelligence than you have. She has this God-given intelligence because she is to bear children; plus she has to raise them. Woman, as an institution, is prepared to bear four children. Four times four is 16, so she has 16 times your intelligence.

Your goal is to be successful as you. This establishes your character and your victory. A career is part of it, money is part of it, a home is part of it, but if you are not you, you will have only parts. You will never be whole. It is like a wonderful body without a brain. The muscles are strong, the fingers are lovely, the nails are marvelous, body is like a crystal; but if there is no brain what are you going to do with that body? Or consider the person who is beautiful, intelligent, and perfect, but obnoxious. Tell me, how long can you deal with an obnoxious person? Or, so-and-so is great, but, my God, is he shaky. Think about it.

Life is a flow of life is a flow of life is a flow of life. You know this is reality. You know that you have not created yourself. You have been created by God and everything is totally, confirmedly, positively yours. You don't believe in that reality because you are not using your intuition. You are totally emotional. God wants you to have a career where you can be penetrating, where you have a domain, where you can give people more than what they have.

It is not possible for people of intelligence, normal intelligence who have normal intuition, too, to live in isolation. How many of you would like to live by yourselves? Have your little home, little wife, little children, little sports car, little boat, little airplane? There are so many little things: little television, little walkie-talkie, little workshop, little tool shop, little machine shop by the side, little garden and gardener, chauffeur and all that stuff. You all have it.

You must realize that the strength in you is you. The material world around you is to supplement your strength or to complement your strength; it is not your strength. You will say, "I know it"; you will say, "That is right," but you don't believe it. You don't believe this earth is Earth. You do not believe this earth is Earth and you are you. They are fundamentally wrong interactions. That's why your life sometimes becomes miserable. That's why there is boredom in your life.

There's boredom in people's lives because they don't have purpose. It is a very simple, psychological answer. The root cause of boredom is lack of motivation. Plus the boredom in your lives is a lack of your own intuition to share with others. You don't trust your own soul. Fortunately, the soul doesn't need your trust to go on. When you do not use your intuition to serve others, to be with others, to establish relationships with others, it doesn't matter how much wealth or security you have, you'll be bored to death.

Besides boredom, you claim to get burned out. You never get burned out; your ego gets burned out. Your problem is that you want to achieve, and then, when you do achieve, you do not know what to achieve next. When you do not become a part of the flow of life and life does not become a part of your flow, you split yourself and separation takes place.

When I came to the United States, I said that I didn't want students. I wanted teachers. I have to produce teachers. It's an endless job. I'll never be bored. I'll never be burned out either. I'm very intelligent. I said, I'll create teachers. If I get students, then I've got students. Then what? Do I sit down, close my eyes, and say, "Bless you. Everything is going to be all right. Meditate. Pray for you. Thank you"? You'll be bored to death. Besides, you yourself could sit on a chair and say, "Bless you. Pray for you. It's going to work out fine. Meditate." Why would you need me?

Do you know why you need me? Many of you love me very much. I know that. Many of you need me very badly. Have you ever considered the reason? It is because I have one wonderful attribute. You may do many wonderful things for me, but you can never satisfy me. My appetite has no bottom. If the word challenge exists, then my name should have been Siri Singh Sahib Bhai Sahib Challenge Singh Khalsa. People sometimes write letters to me. They claim that they don't find any challenge in life. I say that it is a challenge not to find a challenge. There is a challenge in everything. Are you so worthless that there is no challenge for you? No. The problem of boredom is that you do not use your intuition. You use your ego. The ego is very confining and the ego will limit you. However, you can shape your ego very well.

Richness is how much of yourself you achieve. Richness is not how much you have amassed around you—that's a weight.

Whether you are rich or poor neither involves nor solves who you are. You think that if you are rich, everybody will respect you. You think that if you drive a Cadillac, people will think you are rich. When I take an evening walk, I think I am very rich. Everybody drives Cadillacs, but very few people take a brisk walk. Very few people go on a picnic and don't get drunk. When I go on a picnic and don't get drunk, I think I am very rich. Richness is how much of yourself you achieve. Richness is not how much you have amassed around you—that's a weight.

Once there was a king who slept on a bed of flowers. Each day about a hundred pounds of flowers of different colors and kinds would be made into a bed for him. He had a very special maid who would make that bed and decorate it every day. One day, she thought, "The king sleeps on a bed of flowers every day. I wonder how it feels." That day, after finishing the basic decoration perfectly, she just got onto it and closed her eyes. The breeze came and the fragrance of the flowers came, and she went deeply to sleep. She slept for a long time. The king came into his chamber and was outraged to see his maid sleeping on his bed. He picked up a stick and started beating her left and right.

Although she was beaten mercilessly, the maid began to laugh among her cries of pain. When his rage was spent and he had calmed himself to an ordinary anger, the king said, "Tell me why you were laughing or I'll behead you." She began to laugh and he picked up his cane again. She muffled her laughter and said, "Do you want to know the truth?" He said, "Yes." She said, "I slept for a few hours on this bed of roses and you beat the heck out of me. Now I am wondering about the one who sleeps here every day. What will happen to him? Although I am in pain, I am trying to understand what kind of cursed situation is this? I know that I intruded on your privacy and that I didn't do my job properly, but what a punishment! Since you have been sleeping on this bed for many years and since I have been making it every day for you, I wonder what will happen to you?"

I know what kind of thoughts of vengeance and negativity come to me when I become emotional and experience the pain of that, but I am asking those of you who live by the emotional self, where are you going? The credibility within you is your credibility as a man. What you want on the Earth, what you want as a man, is to be recognized as a man. Understand that. The purpose behind all the wealth you are using, all the status you are using, all the emotions you are using, all the commotions you are using is that you want to be recognized as a man. Basically, if people don't trust you, doesn't matter who you are, you have no value and no influence. Do you understand? As a male you have to understand that you will only be recognized as a man if you are trusted. If you don't gain the trust of the people to whom you relate, it doesn't matter who you are, or what you possess, or what you think you can influence, you have nothing to commend you as a man. So how can you be trusted? Your word must be everlasting, for your word to be final, you must be in touch with your intuition. Your virtue is in your intuition, not in your emotion.

Sometimes people ask me, "What about your feelings?" Those feelings are waves; they are not trade winds. A ship does not move because of the waves; a ship moves because of the trade winds. Intuition is your trade wind. You don't understand intuition; that is why you are unable to see opportunities and that is why you always feel that you are at fault in your own life, in your own realm of flow. Intuition is the knowledge of tomorrow, of the next minute, the next hour, the next day, next year, next life. Intuitively you should be able to identify your next life. Not only are you unable to do this, you have not even thought about it.

Religion has been on this Earth for thousands of years, and I am one of the religious persons, yet here, among our congregation, there is not one who has a thought about his tomorrow—what a failure. Yesterday has gone to memory. Today is acting. Today also invites tomorrow. The tomorrow comes from your life's flow. Yesterday is a part of your life's flow, today your life is flowing, and tomorrow comes from your life's flow today. Basically there is nothing beyond life's flow. Your life's flow on Earth comes from Infinity and goes into Infinity.

Never multiply yourself with time and space. That is the secret of happiness. You will always change. I am depressed now. I was not depressed yesterday and I shall not be depressed tomorrow. Today's depression is not mine, it just came. It's like saying, Today it rained. You let your emotions get in the way of intuition. Emotions and commotions are caught by the ego, and whatever is caught by the ego, in that moment, is perceived by you to be the reality forever. There is no such thing as a reality forever. There is only the reality of that particular time, the reality of that particular space. Whatever the reality of that time and that space may be, it is on you but it is not you. Can you separate it?

You are not time and you are not space. You are passing through time and space. Time and space are not reality, they are an orbit. Time and space provide an orbit.

The power of poverty is not you. The power of poverty may be on you like a cloud, like a storm, like a twister. Basically you have to understand one fundamental thing: You are not time and you are not space. You are passing through time and space. Time and space are not reality, they are an orbit. Time and space provide an orbit. It is like a railway through which your brain goes. All those curvatures, those highs and lows are part of the track. The railroad track is a part of the railroad company, but it is not the company. Time and space are not life. If you understand this, I can bet that tomorrow, the day after tomorrow and thereafter, you'll be healthy, happy, holy and prosperous. You will start using automatic intuition, other people's intelligence (OPI) and other people's money (OPM). You will start growing and growing and growing. You are not going to experience death. The word death has connotations that confuse what it really is. The word death represents a fearful end to us. It does not represent an exit, which is what it really is.

I want to give you another lift. I want you to know that depression is an emotional lull. You can get out of depression right on the spot. If you are depressed, think of the evening star. I will teach you a kriya for meditating on the evening star.

Meditation on the Evening Star

September 10, 1983

Posture: Sit in Easy Pose.

Mudra: The mudra involves exact angles. Bring the left elbow directly back into the ribcage. The forearm is at a 45-degree angle and the hand is in Gyan Mudra with the palm up. The right arm is parallel with the left but extended further forward, so that the elbow of the right arm is adjacent to the left wrist. The right hand is in Gyan Mudra also, palm up. Lock yourself into this posture.

Eyes: Closed.

Visualization: I want you to experience how you are connected with the entire universe. As you sit there, bring before you a blue sky and a bright evening star. Create that image and concentrate on it. Imagine an evening sky, the bright deep blue of the evening sky, and imagine a huge evening star. Create this scene with the intuitive mind. Keep it perfectly before your closed eyes, and hold your concentration. Concentrate.

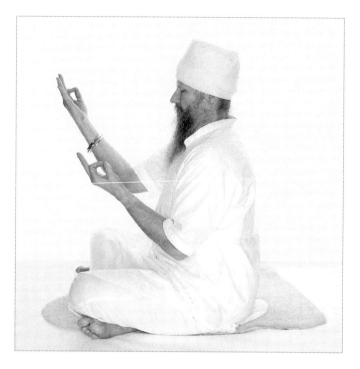

You have seen the evening star. It is called Venus. Imagine that a beam of light is coming from this star. It is making a pathway directly to your Heart Center. You can walk on the pathway. You can walk to the star. Try walking continuously on that beam of light.

This is imagery. We dream, daydream, fantasize, do all those things, every day. Imagery is a reality and reality is an imagery. Do this imagery. Just go through it and you will go through the experience of it. Walking toward the evening star, you see the beam of light coming and making a pathway for you, beaming from the star right to your Heart Center.

Anything that is higher than we are, any light that we can walk toward, calls upon our character and our faith. That's why we need character, that's why we need God, that's why we need meditation. That's why we need to be good. Light gives us purification and character gives us a pure, clean self. We have character when our acts are pure and clean. When we become an institution which acts purely, cleanly, and truthfully, we are people of character.

Walk unto the star. Hold it in your mind and keep going. Make it a reality and give yourself an experience of walking on a beam of light. We will do it in the space age. We are going to develop a technology through which we can be transported through the beam of light. You are walking toward the beam of light, toward the evening star, which is shining brightly on the blue evening sky.

You are sitting in a posture that locks you to the magnetic field of your body. This gives you the power to transfer yourself into the subtle body and the subtle body gives you the power to walk on the beam of light. It is possible that your body may go through certain changes because you are getting lighter and lighter. Don't move your body. Let your nervous system balance out. Bring your body to a calm stillness, keep a firm attitude and keep the imagery going.

See that beautiful bright evening light shining in the middle of the evening sky. Because this evening star is Venus which represents love and the heart, the huge beam of light that comes from it hits your heart, making a pathway like a road on which you can walk to the star.

Now as you walk step by step and you see the bright light, intersect that light with this mantra, "**I am beautiful. I am light**." Beauty and light connect. Connect beauty and light. The only way to get rid of depression permanently is to connect beauty and light. Chant aloud. Pronounce. Hold the image and connect that light. Chant aloud. Pronounce. Hold the image and connect that light. Don't let go of the imagery of that blue sky and that bright star. Don't forget to walk up the beam of light.

Please do all these complicated things in a very simple way. Then pronounce, as though you were announcing to the whole world, "I am beautiful, I am light."

To End: Inhale deep. This is the time you can experience oneness with that beautiful bright blue light in the beautiful blue sky. You have oneness with it. Experience that oneness. Slowly exhale. Slowly inhale very deeply. Hold that breath of life and feel all the energy coming from the beam of that star at your Heart Center. Slowly exhale. Breathe in deep each time, hold the breath and feel it as a part of your soul. Feel the breath as a part of your soul. Connect your life, your soul, and your life breath, making them into one. Breathe in and breathe out but hold it to the maximum.

Victory is your birthright. Hold the breath of life in your Heart Center, mix it with the beam of light of the beautiful evening star, and experience, experience the oneness. Not only will the idea of depression go away, the whole brain structure will change. Your real value in living is living as soul, as the breath of life. Feel it. Inhale it. Hold it to the maximum and don't let it go. Exercise it effectively and mix it with light. Let the concept of "I am beautiful, I am light" surround you mentally.

We are trying to change your brain patterns, to change the quality of the gray matter. Keep on holding the breath, mixing it to the maximum with the light of the evening star, and feeling it in the Heart Center as part of your soul. If you really feel that you are bright and beautiful and you feel it in the Heart Center, then speak the mantra honestly. If you do not, continue the breath and the concentration.

Inhale. Relax.

Effects: We are dealing with the total magnetic field of this human body. This kriya provides a basic one-sided projection. The body is in a perfect magnetic field. Understand that this kriya will take away depression. Depression takes away your happiness; it takes away your power to succeed. It makes you poor.

Timing: This meditation was as long as the guided visualization. It may be 11, 31, or even 62 Minutes as you guide yourself.

Communication Is Personality: The Art of **Suggestion**

Learn this—this is all you have to practice and understand: when you communicate, you communicate your personality.

To create success as a human being, you must know how you talk, why you talk, when you talk, and what you talk. You must know what you are conveying. You believe that you can say things and get away with it. If you are angry, you want to talk angrily. If you are unhappy, you want to communicate your unhappiness. If you are freaked out, you want to create your freak out. If you are lovey-dovey, you want to communicate that. Actually, all you're doing is communicating your mood. You are not communicating yourself. It is simple to communicate yourself, just say, "I love you, but I am angry. I am not in a position to tell you why at this time, but I'll talk to you later." At least in this way, you protect your personality, and you don't communicate your anger. The result of this kind of communication is that the other person will always trust you.

Communication is personality. "C" is "P." Communication is not mood. Everybody has been taught to talk ineffectively. Whenever you talk, communicate. Learn this—this is all you have to practice and understand. When you communicate, you communicate your personality. If you are an honest person, communicate that honesty. If you are a spiritual person, communicate your success. But never communicate through the channel of mood. Mood is never good. Even good mood is no good. This is because when you are in a good mood you will say things that in a neutral mood you would not mean, and it will come back to you. This doesn't mean that you should not talk when you are in a good mood, but don't talk through the mood.

When people invite you over, they ask you to have a drink. They give you wine or some alcohol. Have you ever considered why people are willing to spend $10 or $20 on you as soon as you walk through their door? They want to get you a little loose. If you are a little loose, you will loosen your foundation. That will create a certain mood. Your mood is one aspect of your life that can be your own worst enemy. If your mood comes first, you can never be happy. You will never enjoy life.

Mood is no good. Mood is no good at all. Even good mood is no good at all. It will overextend you. Convey neither good nor bad mood. Convey yourself, your personality; when personality is communicated, it becomes Self. Self is divinity, positivity, creativity, success, and influence. Influence comes to you when you communicate, "I am myself. You are yourself. I want myself to know yourself and yourself to know myself." I don't care about your damn mood! Understand this once and for all. I don't want your mood to be the friend of my mood. Moods are moods, they are not friends. "I love you (because I'm in a good mood)." Who are you? Who are we dealing with? Who is dealing with whom? Actually, nobody is dealing with anybody, because there's no relationship. There's no mutual trust.

Life is a mutual trust. Success comes when you create a real relationship of mutual trust. Success is equal to mutual trust. Mutual trust has nothing to do with mood. Just let the mood go. Say it: Mooooooood. Again: Moooooooooood. Say it enough that you will remember it. Understand that as you say it, you are becoming lighter. You need to lighten up your mood because it has a very heavy effect on your personality. It makes you crazy. Moodiness is crazy. Anyone, whether he is a millionaire or a pauper, who deals with life through mood is guaranteed to be unhappy.

Somebody once wrote me a letter. It was so heavy that the post office had to bind it. The envelope tore and the whole thing broke from the weight. When I got it, I couldn't believe that I was going to have to read it. I called the person. I said, "I got your letter. It looks like a ream of paper. What is wrong with you?"
He said, "Nothing, nothing. Everything is fine. It doesn't matter whether or not you read the letter. Don't worry about it."
I said, "Then why did you send me such a huge letter?"
He said, "I was in the mood for writing."
Somebody was in the mood to write and I ended up with a ten pound letter!

You are a human being. You have a personality. You have a Self. Personality and Self—you are a personality and a Self. The Self is always for you and you are for your Self. If your mood comes in-between you and your Self, you are gone. It is no good. When mood comes between you and your Self, it ruins your relationship—your working relationship, your friendship, your chances of happiness and your chances of success.

The consequences of mood are even greater than you imagine. This is because although mood is temporary, the damage of mood is permanent. One damage, two damages, five damages, twenty damages, until finally the self becomes totally sore, bleeding, and sick.

You are all wise, you are all intelligent, you are all intuitive; there is no dearth of that. If somebody tells me I am making you wise, I know the person is moody. How do you get a person out of a mood? First, don't speak loudly and harshly. Your personality is beautiful so you should speak beautifully. Be careful of your tone. A harsh tone has the effect of a machine gun at your ear: fire! fire! fire! rat-a-tat-tat! Never, ever speak like that. Second, never say what you need to say right away. Introduce yourself. "May I have your attention?" "Would you please give me a minute?" You need to break your approach into three parts: Speak moderately, neither too loud nor too low; introduce yourself; then say what you have to say. Say it to communicate, not to gain an effect or a specific outcome.

The biggest communication blunder that you make is communicating for effect. This comes from your moodiness. When you open communication that way, the other person communicates to reject. You communicate to affect; the other person communicates to reject. That's why life is such a hassle for you. No matter how weak the other person is, when you communicate to gain an effect, he feels that you are looking for a certain response, he thinks you want something from him. When this happens, he becomes defensive and rejects you. The right of self-defense is ingrained in every individual, so speak moderately and then, if you want to win, speak suggestively: I could say, "Would you please listen to me? If all of us can understand our own abilities and pool them together, we can have a good day tomorrow." Or, I can say, "Hey, you bunch of idiots, let's pool our strength and get going." It's the same thing. It is absolutely the same thing. But if I am direct, three people are going to say, "Sir, what you say is right, but we have our own plans for tomorrow."

Nobody is a freak, but we freak everybody out when we are direct. The reaction is not to what we say, but how we say it. Be suggestive; speak suggestively.

"I think we can be successful."
"How?"
"It's really not difficult at all."
"Well, what do you want to say?"
"Not anything much."
"Well, what is it?"
"Ah, I have a very wonderful, perfect idea of success. It just came to me."
"What the hell are you talking about?"
"I'm not talking about hell or heaven. I'm talking about success right here on Earth."
"Talk!"
"Well, I'm not sure you will like my ideas."
"Try it!"
"Well, wait a minute, it's not . . ."
"Just tell me. I'll do it!"
"Well, no. No, just understand that . . . Aren't we friends?"
"Yeah. Come on!"
"Do you think you can understand?"
"Hey, man, come out with it!"
"No. We'll go for a walk tomorrow, and then we'll talk it out."

You can appreciate what is being done. One person is trying to establish a contact of the Self. When you talk for effect, this is the sound you make: "Yap, yap, yap, yap, yap." This yapping sound upsets the balance in the middle ear. It sounds as if a duck is quacking in your ear. Then the brain sends the signal, "Get rid of that duck." The Chinese cook it. The Indians boil it. The British steam it. Duck is duck. It doesn't matter how wonderful you are, you are a human being and not a duck. I'm giving you practical, positive, suggestive advice. If you hurt my middle ear, do you think I will give you kisses in return? If you want to be successful, take my advice: Use a moderate tone of voice, introduce yourself, speak suggestively.

Something else you will need is confidence. I am always right, but still I ask you, "Am I right?" Sometimes I say I am wrong. It is wrong for me to say "I am wrong", because I am always right, but still I say it. It gives nothing to me, but it gives you confidence. Confidence is a secret of success. Not my confidence, your confidence. My self-confidence doesn't mean a thing to me. It is your confidence in me that is important. In any situation, it is not your self-confidence that is important; it is the other person's confidence in you and your confidence in him. That's what is important.

Be suggestive and polite. "Would you please be kind enough to bring me a glass of water?" I have even heard a teacher say, "Would you feel honored to bring me . . . ?" You feel honored. The teacher doesn't say, "I feel honored." This is because the teacher is a directive person.

My teacher said, "Hey, Bhajan, would you like to have the honor of grooming my two horses?"
Grooming one horse is four hours work, so this honor will be eight hours, and it's a sweaty job. I say, "Wonderful, sir, it would be a great privilege."
"Oh, and by the way, Bhajan, two miles from my place,

I have a friend who has two donkeys. Would you mind bringing them along? It will be a great privilege for you."

"Yes, sir." What else can you say? You can't say anything else. There's nothing left to say.

I groomed the horses. Then went to the other village and got the donkeys. He didn't say to ride them. I walked them. On that day I learned that even if I walk with donkeys, it affords some companionship.

Learn companionship. Communication should create companionship. "C" is equal to "C." Communication creates companionship. In life never try to control. Whatever you will control, you will pay the toll. Whatever you will win, you will lose the self. Create companionship and create companionship with communication. Purposefully in your life believe and learn that life is a communicative companionship.

Learn companionship. Communication creates companionship. In life never try to control. Whatever you will control, you will pay the toll.

Kriya to Communicate and Create Companionship
September 10, 1983

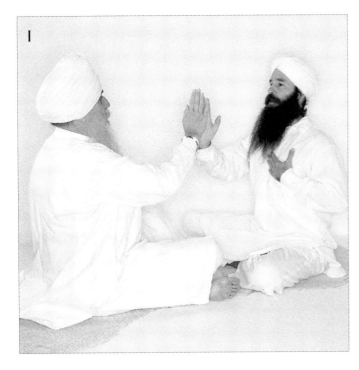

Posture: Get into pairs and sit in Easy Pose.

Part I

Mudra: Put your left hand over your Heart Center. Put your right hand out, palm to palm, with your partner. As you speak, touch hands with your partner. Whenever you speak, as the lips move, the hands must create the same effect. Let the movement of your hands reflect the movement of your lips and the movement of your conversation. Say good things. Communicate and create companionship. Practice, practice for the experience.

Part II

Now sit in Easy Pose and Repeat after the Teacher.

"I shall never transport my mood."
"I shall never transport my mood."
"I shall never transport my mood."
"My mood is not me."
"My mood is not me."
"My mood is not me."
"I shall never transport my mood."
"My mood is not me."
"My feelings are my feelings."
"I will deal with my feelings myself."
"I will transport myself to deal with other selves."
"I will not transport my feelings to deal with other feelings"
"I need harmony"
"Not clash."
"I shall not be rash and transport my mood."
"Mood is no good."
"Mood is mood."
"Mood is no good."
"Mood is mood."
"I am bright and beautiful."
"I am bright and beautiful."
"I am bright and beautiful."

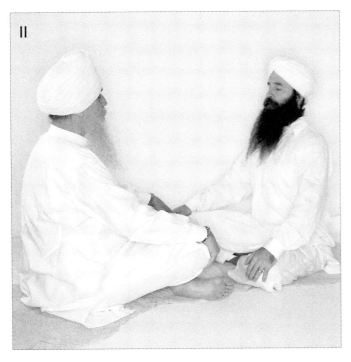

To end: Now assess yourself. Go inside and assess your gains, feel it, and understand your ability to communicate.

Comments: From the minute you start talking there needs to be a range—improvement, dis-improvement, satisfaction, dissatisfaction—in your communication style. This exercise is meant to benefit your communication style.

Time: 35 Minutes

Part III

Posture: Sit in Easy Pose, as though you were a great yogi, who has sat for 200 years at the top of the mountain through snow, through rain, and through time—and never budged an inch.

Mudra: Not specified.

Mantra: This mantra is a special sound. It is a lesson in the creation of sounds that can melt the hearts of people.

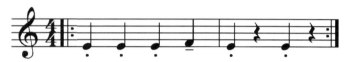

Har   Har   Har   Re   Har (pause) Har

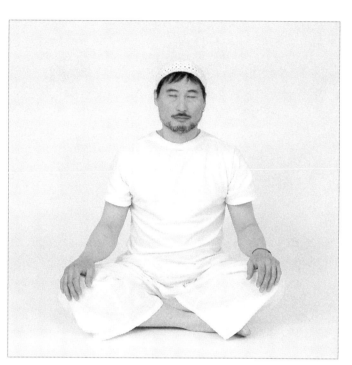

Use only the tip of the tongue. Speak evenly, with a slight emphasis on Re. (Re is chanted a half-step note higher than Har.) Feel that when you speak, you are communicating directly, face to face with Almighty God. When you utter these words, it's a communication with the Infinite, Most Beautiful Thing, which is called God. Whatever your image is of God, communicate with that. It may not mean anything to anyone else; but it means all to you.

To End: Inhale deeply and hold for 30-45 seconds. Any part of your body you feel is weak, take your inhaled breath to that area and reenergize it. Let it go. Relax.

Time: 11 Minutes

Beloved God, Merciful Creator, Lover of all Humanity, Giver of the Breath of Life, Creator of Consciousness, may Thy mercy guide us to our own self-fulfillment. May everybody be beautiful and bountiful. May we grow in peace and joy. Give us pleasantness in life and make us bright and beautiful to keep the flow of life from here to Infinity. Sat Nam.

■ ■ ■

Health Is **Flexibility**

This is called health: when you can take the maximum and your body makes it the minimum.

I need to tell you that your concept of health is incorrect. Health is flexibility. Health is not muscle, not macho, not size. I am 54 years old and I have more flexibility than any one of you. Health is flexibility and you should be prepared to take the worst. This is called health: when you can take the maximum and your body makes it the minimum. You can't avoid impact. You must remember that. Impact is when something hits you. Impact can be made by a person, a bacteria or a virus. There's no difference, the impact is there. You have to deal with it.

People are more difficult to deal with than a virus. Bacteria is all right, you can take penicillin; it will save you temporarily and your body can heal. But for people, we have found no penicillin yet. However, there is a remedy you can use to deal with people. Guru Nanak provided it. He said, "Name of the God." The scriptures said *sadhana, aradhana,* and *prabhupathi.* You are thinking that I am pushing myself to make you great, to make you something, but that's not true. I am not interested in people. I am not interested in students—and I don't love a neurotic.

When you are neurotic, you are your own enemy and you have lost track of the godliness, the divinity within you. When I think of Guru Ram Das, I say, "His Divine Majesty Guru Ram Das." That's how I look at it, that's how I feel it, and that's how I understand it. I feel that every human being, in consciousness, is a Divine Majesty. You have to recuperate yourself to be with me.

When people communicate with you emotionally, and you become emotional because of their emotionality, it is as though you are in the ocean and you can't swim—you drown. Each emotion drowns you and each time you have to rescue yourself.

A very wonderful thing happened in Europe. Somebody said to me, "I don't know what to do. What should I do?" I said, "I don't know what you should do. First, you must tell me what is happening."
"I can't say it. I just can't say it."
I said, "Have you taped it sometime so that I can listen to it?"
"You know it all. You know everything."
Now what am I going to do with this kind of person. I said, "All right. I know it all. She is divorcing you."
"She isn't divorcing me, but I can't live with her. I can't, I can't."
Then I did something very intelligent. I brought out a mirror, and asked him to continue talking. When he began to talk, I held the mirror in front of him and said, "Look at yourself. Look at your behavior. How can any woman live with you? You think she is impossible, what do you think you are? Look in the mirror. See how you are talking to me and how I am catching you."

Your power, your penetrating power, your personality, your majesty lies in what you say and how you say it. However, by the way you speak, the way you communicate who you are, you commit another blunder. Communication can give you a lot of flexibility. You can interpret and you can change the ideas, you can apologize, you can analyze, etc. because a discussion is a discussion. But you must be more careful when you write. Sometimes you write very neurotically. Written words are very heavy. If I make a statement issued by my pen, under my seal—that's it!

Credit: The Sadhana of **Maya**

When it was finally established by law, in the Western culture, several hundred years ago, that one man could not be subject to the will of another, royalty may have been overthrown, but the invisible lords evolved. The invisible lords in the United States are the big corporations.

You may have thought it was the bankers, but bankers are bankers. Bankers are the ditch of this country and once you get in the ditch, you can't get out. We have been made to live in a credit society. The shackles of credit are around our necks. When I came here, I was immediately advised to get a loan so that I could establish credit. I said "To hell with it. I don't need a loan. I don't need credit." But, "You can't buy a house, you can't buy this, you can't buy that if you don't have credit. You have to have credit."

Credit is the sadhana of maya. From today forward and for 30 years, you are tied to a pole. Every one of you go through this sadhana of maya. Systemically, to be honest with you, man is not made to have credit in maya. Yes he is supposed to have maya and yes, he is supposed to have credit—his own credit, credit of the Self. Now the battle is between the credit of the Self and the credit of money.

Your behavior is very emotional. This is dangerous, because only the emotional person can be exploited. The intuitive person can never be exploited. The whole Western society, the whole woman in society, the man in society is made to be exploited.

You are an intelligent and beautiful people. I had a great deal of trouble in India. I was a misfit there. The people there are hypocrites. They say one thing and do something different. They say, "Sweet this and sugar that. . . " but underneath it is, "I can't deal with this." Here, all I have to do is provoke you and you will come out immediately. In two minutes you are out. Your mind can be brought out in one second. You are wonderful people, a vomiting caste—it's called Elephant Kriya. You take in water and throw it out just the way the elephant does. All I have to do is put a hand on your shoulder, you feel it, and I can read everything that is going on. There's no smiling face with a knife underneath. You're good. I also like your attitude about time—you worship time. Everything about you is wonderful. I have no complaint. That's why I am sticking around. Otherwise as neurotic as you are, it would be impossible to deal with you.

I understand that you have been shackled. One time in France I saw a 15th century torture chamber. It was unbelievable to see all the instruments of torture. One particular machine operated this way: A weight was put around a person from his shoulders and each day another weight was attached. In this way, the vertebrae were broken as the spine was stretched millimeter by millimeter. When I saw it, I said to myself, "This is America!" That is how you are mentally pressured in this country, each day, one millimeter more neurotic than the next. Each day you become one millimeter more neurotic so that by the time you are 50, you are super-neurotic, and by the time you are 75 you are neurosis itself.

Let us consider one typical example of this: A person lives in a 13-bedroom home with 5 acres of landscaped grounds. He retires. He leaves the whole thing and goes to live in a retirement home. Only a person who is totally insane would do such a thing. You Americans have money, you have environments, you have earned all your lives, you live well, your children are grown and gone, you want to enjoy the peace of your whole life, and the moment you retire, you move to Miami where you sit in an aluminum chair on the beach with the other neurotics.

I don't think anybody in this country should be sick, including me. Everything is available to us. But we have been pressurized. We have been so pressured mentally that our minds are overstretched. Perhaps you have learned to control your mental and physical body. Let us get into your system and break up the neurotic deposits. We are going to do some very special exercises. They are therapeutic exercises. They are done to take away stress and strain and to restore mental equilibrium. They are called mirror exercises because they are always done in front of a mirror, or in the presence of a supervisor.

Chitra Kriya: **Mirror Exercises**
September 10, 1983

1. Sit very classically in Easy Pose. Bring your hands up in front of your eyes with your palms facing each other. Your hands are rigid and your thumbs are in alignment with the other fingers. Your hands are about 8 inches away from your eyes. Imagine that your hands are knife blades and position them so that they could cut your eyes exactly in half.

There is a specific movement to this kriya. When you do it, it must be so precise that the optical nerve takes a message to the brain that the eye has been cut in two. The cut must be clear and perfect if you want to stay young and avoid becoming old and dumb.

The movement is a pattern of exact angles that has four parts:
a. Begin with your hands in the starting position—8 inches in front of the eyes
b. Bring the hands directly in toward the eyes
c. Return the hands to their starting position
d. Turn the palms to the front and move them 8 inches left and right

Repeat the pattern: one, two, three, four. You are moving on very straight lines. You are making the turn at a 90° angle; this angle must be very precise and sharp. The first position acts as your balance. From there, you make all the other movements of the pattern. The movement is very tight. When it comes back, it must come to the center of the eyes, not a millimeter of the body's muscles should change. The brain must form this pattern. You are directing the secretion of the brain to form the blue pattern. The muscles must obey. Each time the distance should be equal. You expand as you contract; you come back as you go. **5 Minutes**

Comments: These mirror exercises are called Chitra Kriyas, the most sacred secret of India. They can change the entire chemistry of the brain. The beauty here is in making the kriya accurate. It's an electronic shock treatment. You are manipulating your electromagnetic field. You are using your nervous system to make a pattern in the brain. The pattern is making a movement and the movement is, in turn, making a pattern. It is very correlative. I won't promise you it will make you fly, but I can tell you that all your neuroses will fly, if you just go through this pattern

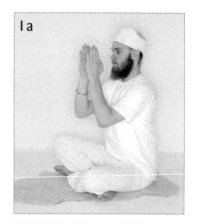
1a

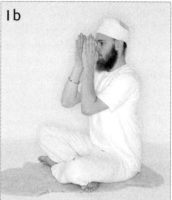
1b

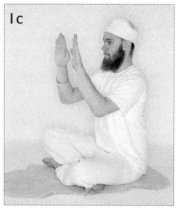
1c

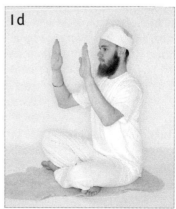
1d

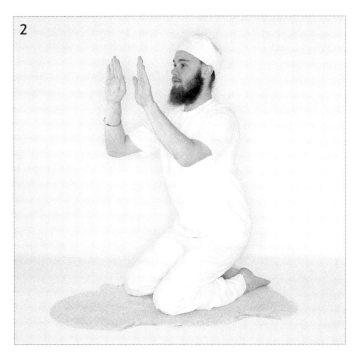

2. Sit on your heels. Continue the same pattern as in Exercise 1, with one addition: As you bring your hands to position (d), raise yourself up off your buttocks 6 inches. When your hands return to the starting position, you return to the sitting posture. **8 Minutes**

Comments: Do not misunderstand. Six inches is 6 inches, if 6 inches means 3 feet to you, you will blow up the whole universe. You must use your legs to do this kriya. The thighs will be very powerfully affected. Your legs and your hands move together; it is a rhythm. If you cannot do it, you are condemned as unserviceable. It means that you cannot kiss and cling at the same time; you are partially impotent. Coordinate! You are working on your brain, not your muscles. Make the kriya as exact as a gun shot. Measure it as precisely as a carpenter's measure. If one millimeter is wrong, the whole thing is going to be wrong.

As you exercise, your breath will regulate itself. It will give you a special Breath of Fire. The Breath of Fire will change the blood chemistry and the lungs will receive the maximum oxygen. Endeavor to complete the whole thing in one breath. Shoot the breath out as the hands come in towards the eyes. If you cannot complete the exercise with the breath synchronized, just continue to let the breath regulate itself.

I want you to go back in age ten years. I want you to feel very, very potent. Do it for your own sake, not for your neighbor's sake and not for my sake. No matter what it takes, you must coordinate. Totally time it and coordinate. Make the breath like a shot. You need that powerful breath because you may begin to experience stomach cramps. Also you will find that your calves are not accustomed to holding this posture for such a long period.

You have this mental block. You think that physical exercise is only for muscle building. This is an exercise of the brain. It has nothing to do with your muscles; they are only being used to create a chemistry. The muscles and the movements work together to create a biochemical action in the brain. I am teaching you these exercises so that you can teach them to your children and you can all be healthy, long-lived, and perfect.

This is a top-notch oriental secret. There is nothing like it in America. Kill your pain and get your scene together. You don't need acupuncture to kill pain. Relax and mentally assess yourself.

3. Lie down on your back. Put your feet together, sole to sole. Your hands are at the sides of your buttocks, cupping them slightly. Keeping your knees bent and the soles of your feet together, raise your feet 18 inches and stretch to the left at a 60-degree angle. Bring them back to the starting position and then stretch them out to the right. Continue left and right with Breath of Fire. You are moving your total pelvic area. Try to maintain the contact between the soles of your feet. **4 Minutes**

Comments: Mentally relax and take the tiredness out. This exercise will work on your creative organs in the brain. This part of the brain is responsible for things that come to you for which you cannot take credit, but you boast about.

4. In the same posture, stretch the legs forward and then back in and over your head, keeping the soles of the feet together. Move the legs straight in and over—not up—keeping the knees wide spread. Continue with a heavy Breath of Fire. **4 Minutes**

Comments: If this pattern is done for a long time as a practice, you will not grow old. It doesn't matter what the other physical conditions are. The second and third vertebrae shrink as you grow old. This causes a lot of pain and havoc. Avoid it with this exercise. That shrinking of the vertebrae is called osteoporosis. I love medical science. It always has a name for everything. You may not get cured but the doctors can let you know what your illness is called.

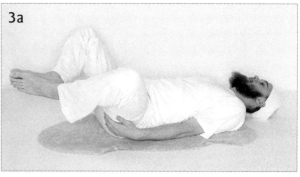

3a

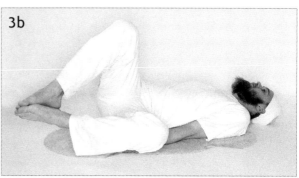

3b

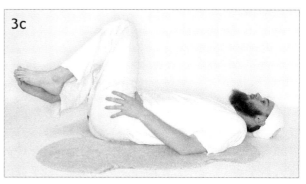

3c

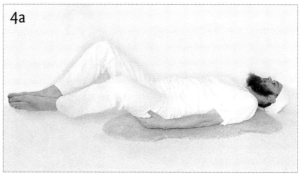

4a

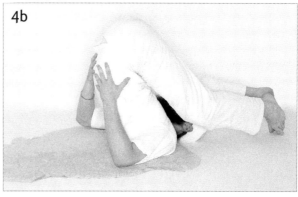

4b

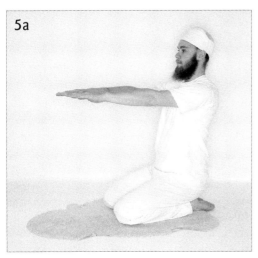
5a

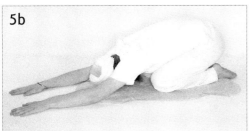
5b

5. Sit on your heels. Put your arms straight out in front of you. Bow forward and touch your forehead to the ground. Bow and rise to the rhythm of *Jaap Sahib*. Bow and rise to the sutras. The hands and forehead must touch the ground. On *namo* or *namastang* you touch the ground, then rise. Do this accurately.

Keep your hands straight. It will work wonders and give the lower back a good stretch. The prayer begins with an invocation to the gods and goddesses, then begin with the first sutra and stay steady. **31 Minutes**

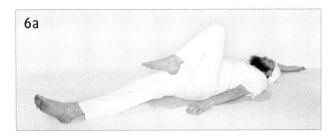
6a

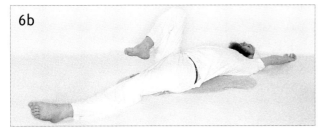
6b

6. Immediately lie down on your back and begin the cross-crawl. Work diagonally and alternately. Bring the right arm over your head as you bring the left knee into the chest. As you release them, raise the left arm and the right leg. This will equalize the energy perfectly. This is where you will gain profit for all your hard work. Don't cheat. Keep up. After **1 Minute** begin singing a patriotic song and keep singing. **4 Minutes**

7. Sit in Easy Pose. Bring your hands up and push as though you were pushing something away from you. Bring the hands back in and push again. Push hard. Push away all negativity, all sickness, all wrong. Really push. You will become young and beautiful. **2 Minutes**

Note: These are called mirror exercises because they are always done in front of a mirror, or in the presence of a supervisor.

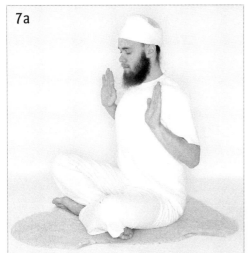
7a

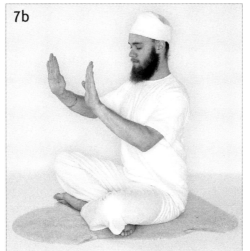
7b

Who Are You Subject To?

There are only three permissible subjections of the self. They are subjection to higher consciousness, subjection to intuition, and subjection to God. Any other subjection is not permissible.

Since I arrived in the United States, I have done two things out of frustration: One is teaching Tantric Yoga. I had decided that I would never teach it because it's very painful personally. Once the Mahan Tantric starts teaching anywhere, he must project the diagonal tantric energy and it is a costly business. It dries up your marrow and cracks your bones.

The other is Naad Yoga. Unfortunately, my experience here is that this is the only country where the employee thinks the employer is a fool: A person who works for you, whether he loves you or not, can insult you for nothing. There is no reason and there is no recourse. We have to develop a society where our communication can be heard so musically by another person that we can have a relationship of harmony and peace. This is what this Naad Yoga is about.

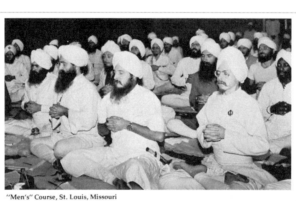
"Men's" Course, St. Louis, Missouri

The idea is to make you understand that your life is your virtue. These days, I am trying to teach so that you will understand. I have said that you are not to transfer mood. Some of you men should understand, you have fallen apart for a woman. Your marriage fails and you fail with it. That is not a true response. A woman can be your partner, she can be your love, she can be your life, she can be your anything, but she's not you. You have to understand. Anything you subject yourself to will take away your freedom and give you slavery. Then you are not a man, you are a donkey.

The question in life is simple: Who rides whom? Who you offend and who you support is not the problem. The question is whether a woman, some children, a girlfriend, a project or any temptation is powerful enough that you have to subject yourself to it. There are only three permissible subjections of the self. They are subjection to higher consciousness, subjection to intuition, and subjection to God. Any other subjection is not permissible.

You will meet a lot of women. Sixty percent of them will love you, conquer you, and make a slave out of you. Of that 60%, 40% will love you, conquer you, make a slave out of you—and then dump you. This tendency comes from their history with their fathers. Sometime during their childhood, their fathers were abnormally rude to them. Any woman whose father has been rude with her will pretend to be loving and perfect. That's the way she gets to you. This type woman gets to your guts. When she gets in there, she closes it and twists it. Whenever a woman wants to get into you, your bad days are ahead. Never let anything get to you and don't you get to anything. Life is co-existent and mutual. Anybody who breaks the co-existence is a snake. A cobra is going to bite you sooner or later, no matter how colorful it is. I know as a fact, as a counselor, as your spiritual father, as your spiritual teacher, as your friend, as your servant, as one who sees you that you are all in that danger.

There is one man who totally freaked out. His wife took away his children. He's married to another woman now. He can produce another four, and run after those children. It's crazy. When these children become 18, 19, or 20, they are going to say, "Papa, where are you?" When he says, "I'm here," they are going to spit on him. They are by their own right who they are. There is no qualification in life. Live in mutual coexistence and understand one thing: There is never a time when you should not be compassionate, tolerant and forgiving, and there is never a time when you should be angry and revengeful.

On many occasions, people have insulted me to my face. Sometimes we sit together family style. I open myself up; I don't pretend to be such a holy man that no one can talk to me. I allow people to play the game. I enjoy it because when somebody speaks insultingly and neurotically to me, I think, "Oh, God, thank you, Dhan Guru Ram Das. Almighty God, thank You that it is not me. Thank God, I don't have a trace of it." It is very fulfilling.

I want you to understand what I went through when I came to America. There were many women who brought me gifts. They were rich women and they ran after me like I didn't exist. They put money and sex before me.

One day I was sitting and talking to one of them. I said, "I would like to ask you a question."
She said, "What?"

I said, "Are you a hooker?"

"Huh? How can you ask that?"

"I don't know what it means to you but I am asking you in simple English because I speak English-English not American English."

She said, "What do you mean by `hooker':

I said. "You know. It is the person who takes the reel and puts the bait on the hook to catch the fish. That person is called a 'hooker'."

She said, "Well, in this country that person is called a 'prostitute'."

"No, you are not a prostitute. Prostitutes are very honorable. I have all respect for prostitutes. They sell themselves. They charge you money and they give something in return. It's a business. They sell their bodies; you give your money. It's very unfairly fair. But these hookers, God knows where they are going to get you that way. Then they are going to put you in a bag. How are you going to be treated? You can't predict anything. When I said, 'hooker,' that's exactly what I meant."

She asked me, "Do you know how many millions of dollars I want to give to you?"

I said, "I definitely know that I am a man in a very, very shallow pond, but I am not willing to take your bait."

Never bite the bait. If you do not know what the bait is, you are a bum. The greatest consciousness, divinity, morality, power, and strength of a man is knowing the bait. You are crazy. You think as a man you have the power to bite! You are right. You can bite, but you will not have the power to release the bite. How should one read a book? Read the lines and in between the lines. Find the bait and let it sink. Your life will be so happy, so well-admitted, so good that you will start falling in love with you. You fall in love with everybody but you have never, ever fallen in love with yourself.

Take an oath. Raise your right hand. "I shall speak truth, nothing but truth, so help me God." Now, those of you who have fallen in love with yourselves raise your hands. Start loving yourself. God gave you the gift of life; fall in love with it, go crazy for it, value it, feel it, have it, understand it. Don't blunder it. You can meditate years and years and years. What will it give you? What is divinity? What is God? Nothing! Absolutely nothing. There is no God, no divinity, and no religion. There is nothing if you cannot fall in love with yourself. You are just on the surface, you are shaky; your problem is that you love somebody else. Do you want to be like God? It's not difficult. Love yourself.

■ ■ ■

The Invincible Man **Exercises**
September 10, 1983

1. Find a partner. Sit in Easy Sitting Pose opposite each other. Look at one another straight in the eyes and repeat this mantra, "I love myself. I forgive you." As you say, "I love myself," bring your hands to Prayer Pose at the heart. As you say, "I forgive you," bring your hands palm-to-palm with your partner. Continue the movement with each repetition of the mantra. Experience what it does. Look like a man. **4 Minutes**

2. Still seated, looking into your partner's eyes, continue the movement with the mantra, "Peace". With each repetition of "Peace," move from Prayer Pose to palm-to-palm. **2-½ Minutes**

3. Come sitting on your heels facing your partner. Now come up on your knees. Bring your hands together in Prayer Pose and say, "Love." Come palm-to-palm with your partner and say, "Peace." This exercise is very important because you are relating to your sciatica. **2-½ Minutes**

4. Continue standing on you knees facing your partner, looking eye-to-eye. Stretch your arms out to each side, palms down. Move the arms up and down (about 12 inches) to a count of four. On five, clap hands with your partner and alternately chant *Peace!* or *Love!* Move the arms 1-2-3-4-Peace! (clap); 1-2-3-4-Love! (clap). Continue for **9-½ Minutes**

5. Camel Pose. Standing on the knees, press the pelvis forward and lift the heart as you reach back for your heels. Allow the head to drop back. Chant "I will never bite the bait." This is the only way you will remember it. There is no other way. **3 Minutes**

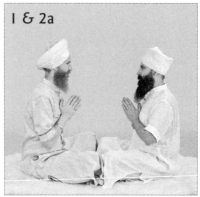
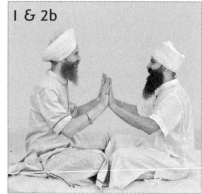
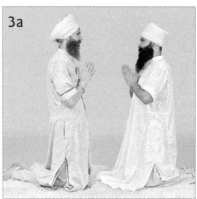
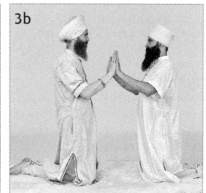
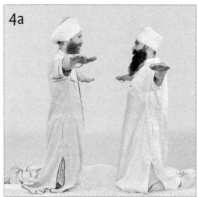
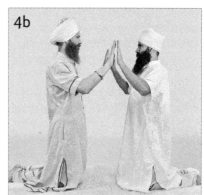
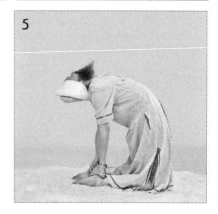

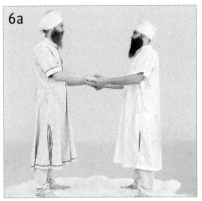
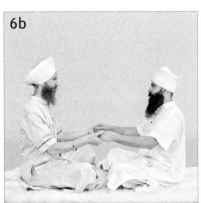

6. Come standing up and take your partner's hands. Slowly sit down and repeat, "Let us sit in peace." Slowly rise and say, "Let us rise in consciousness." **4 Minutes**

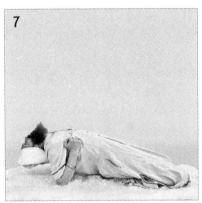

7. Sit on your heels and bend back, putting your weight on your elbows. Bring your hands into fists near the shoulders. Your head will automatically fall back. Keep this posture as you sing the entire *Ardas Bhaee* mantra. The energy will adjust itself. You will see how this burnout is going to work out. Sing with it. Hold the posture and keep the pressure. It will make changes in you. It may feel a little painful now, but it will bring fantastic strength. It is very healing, very good. Make a fist of your hands. This will break the crystallization in the muscle and the nerves. It will break obstacles in the energy flow. **5 Minutes**

8. Sit in Easy Sitting Pose. Make fists with your hands and bring them in front of the shoulders. Repeat "I am, I am." Chant loudly and powerfully as you move. Let the God hear you! **8 Minutes**

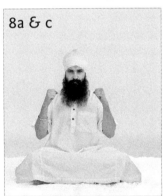
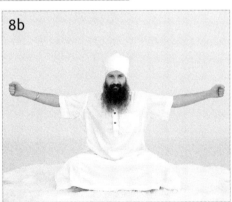

a. "I" the hands are at the shoulders
b. "Am" the arms extend out to the sides—straight.
c. "I" the hands are at the shoulders
d. "Am" the arms extend straight up

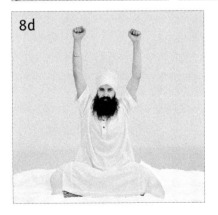

9. Sit facing your partner, eye to eye. Bring your hands into fists in front of your face—about eye level. Repeat "I am, I am." Communicate your pure "I am" to each other. As you talk, your hands should move to explain your expression. Fists tight. Talk with lips and fists. Lips and fists should indicate the language.
9 Minutes

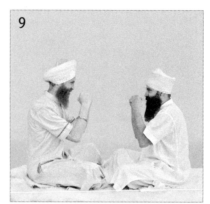

10. Sit facing your partner, eye to eye. Bring your hands up. Spread your fingers open and move the arms stiffly, forward and back. Try to part the wind. Do it fast, powerfully, and strongly. The hands must move the heavens, the earth and the stars. No bend. Powerfully and steadily. The whole body will move if you do it right. Make the whole body a unit. You must move the whole body, not just the hands. **10 Minutes**

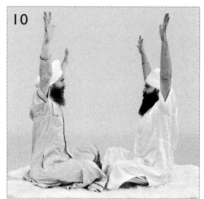

To end: Inhale and hold the breath for 30 seconds. Mentally vibrate the mantra God and me, me and God are one. Repeat. Relax.

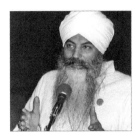

Man to **Man** 9
The Blocks Men Can't Talk About

Circa 1984

There are blocks that men can't talk about. These blocks are keeping you from achieving your potential as men. If we are not willing to talk about something, how can we get rid of it?

■ Growing **Up**

■ Living the You Within **You**

Growing Up

You cannot tolerate the fact that sometimes in order to have one thing, you must give up another.

There are blocks that men can't talk about. These blocks are keeping you from achieving your potential as men. I am going to bring them to your attention. I am not asking you to learn. I am not even asking you to listen. I am asking you to participate with me.

It is very essential that you understand the fundamental principle of life: my life is my life, it cannot be anybody else's life; your life is your life. That is the way it is. A life is personal; but you don't want to accept that principle. Either you want to take over somebody's life and control it, or you want your life to be controlled by somebody, because this is what you learned as a child from your parents. They controlled your life and you felt very secure and innocent under their control. That feeling of innocence and security that you got in the first three years became part of you. It is so deeply settled in you that you have carried it with you throughout your entire life, knowingly or unknowingly. From that experience you developed a block, the first block against being you, being yourself. When you are not yourself, then either you want to control somebody's life or you want your life to be controlled by somebody. Understand, though, that you are innocent in this game.

I am trying to bring out these blocks, which you have to understand are yours. They may be partially yours or they may be totally yours, but have no misunderstanding that you are the exception. Only those who have developed themselves to live consciously can live without blocks and none of us can live totally consciously all the time. We have not been trained to do so. Instead we have learned to be emotional. Emotional behavior and outbursts are very satisfying, and it is very, very difficult to replace them. We have been getting satisfaction from them since our childhood. Because of this we have but one intention in this human life: to continue to experience that emotional satisfaction.

We remember those times when we learned to crawl and when we walked for the first time. When we learned these skills, somebody gave us a hand, somebody gave us applause, somebody gave us a kiss, somebody gave us a hug. Somebody gave us cake, somebody gave us toffee, somebody gave us something to eat. Somebody told us, "You are the most beautiful. You are the most marvelous. You are extremely wonderful. You are my total tomorrow. I love you. I adore you. You are everything to me. You are my whole life." Whether or not you believe me, you want to hear that all the time. You are always waiting to hear it, you are always hoping to hear it, and you are always looking forward to hearing it. That is the truth. That is what you want.

You may be 5' 8" inches tall and weigh 180 pounds, but you still want somebody to put his hands under your armpits, lift you up and say, "Hi, beautiful baby." When you weighed 8 pounds that was possible, but 180? It is not possible. The problem is that you want that even now. You want somebody to hold your hand, somebody to grab you and squeeze you and mean a lot to you. This is your approach to life; this is how you started and you have never changed. You are not properly trained to change and you don't expect any change; therefore, that need, that desire, that want remains. Because you are unable to fulfill it, you try to fulfill it indirectly.

Now when you try to fulfill something indirectly that you have experienced directly you become neurotic. You become a manipulator. You wangle your way through your feelings; basically you are not very honest to your own feelings. Because you have become aware, you are conscious that what you want cannot happen. Nobody will squeeze you and squeeze you and squeeze you—nobody wants to do that. You want your wife to do it but that poor girl cannot do it. If she does it and you squeeze her, squeeze her a lot, then she gets pregnant. For nine months she is out of commission. Then there is a baby and she is out of commission for another two years. You are mad at yourself for squeezing her. That is how we get mad at life.

You have to learn to talk to yourself before you talk to somebody else—you have never learned to talk to yourself. You have not been trained to talk to yourself and you do not understand the value of self-communication. Because you do not have this experience of yourself and you refuse to talk, the block remains. You refuse to talk and life pushes on; but practically, it is no life at all.

On the other hand, we want to extend ourselves, we want to have children. We want to write our names on stones. We try to carve our names in the bark of the tree. We want to do all those things that are a part of our growth and a part of our life, but we do not want to be at all subjective or objective. We start catering to our egos because we understand that we are ego. We have a definition of a grown-up. As grown-ups we recognize that we are grown-ups. We want to be grown-ups, but there is a very powerful hook behind us, which is hanging us up midway: we want to get kissed, get hugged, get loved, get appreciated, get recognized and make sure that somebody gives this to us. This is how something that started very innocently, very normally, very naturally, has today become our biggest block and, the fact is, you don't want to talk about it.

You know about all these people who want to join nude clubs and want to walk nude on the beaches. All these people who want to show their private organs. If you look at their history, you will find that they come from families where they have been told to dress properly, behave properly, live properly. They hear that "proper, proper, proper," and when they become adults, when they become conscious, they don't want to wear anything. Not that they don't understand the morality of the issue, or understand good and bad; they are not into good and bad; there is a block, a powerful block. Nudity is the sign of a very big block. These people don't like organization. In fact they don't like God, they don't like marriage, they don't like family, and they don't like commitment. They don't like anything because they want to be one, singular, nude person. Wearing clothes, wearing churidar[1], does not mean you are not nude. Real nudity is an attitude. It is an attitude against commitment. You do not want to be committed at all. You do not want any discipline at all. You do not want any sadhana at all. You do not want to be, at all.

So the fundamental question is, to be or not to be. That is the fundamental question. This duality over commitment means that part of you and part of your life is there, but not there; and because you cannot talk about it, there is no psychology or psychiatry that can be of any help to you. Your solution is to create a drama. You get depressed, you get mad, you get angry, you get violent, you go berserk and you behave in bizarre ways. Eventually you go to a psychoanalyst or, if you are worse than that, you go to a psychiatrist. At worst, you go to a mental hospital. But do you talk? No. You don't talk. You will never talk.

You have to learn to talk to yourself before you talk to somebody else—you have never learned to talk to yourself. You have not been trained to talk to yourself and you do not understand the value of self-communication. Because you do not have this experience of yourself and you refuse to talk, the block remains. You refuse to talk and life pushes on; but practically, it is no life at all.

---

[1] Churidar are long cotton pants worn traditionally by Northern Indians, especially Punjabi Sikhs. Usually they are worn beneath a long kurta, which comes to the knees.

When I see you love me, when I see you adore me, when I see you want me, when I see you communicate with me, when I see you call me, when I see you want advice from me, when I see you yell and scream at me, when I see you become mad and abusive with me, when I see you in your many facets, I hope you will talk to me. But you don't. I know that you are blocked. I know you can talk, but you do not know that you can talk. Now, for example, I know you are intelligent. I know that. You don't have to sell me on that. I don't have to buy it. If you are intelligent, why do you make mistakes? If you are intelligent, why do you become a failure? If you are intelligent, why do you become depressed? If you are intelligent, why don't you succeed? If you are intelligent, why don't you create abundant richness around you? There is a reason for it. It is a very simple reason. Your creative nature has intelligence but you do not know how to access it. You don't know where it is, when to call it, when to talk to it or when to deal with it. It is very easy for you to deal with your emotions, with your feelings, with your environments. These three things you know how to do very well. You use your intelligence to deal with your emotions, with your feelings, and with your environments. You also use your intelligence with your problems and with your pressures. But you have never dealt with your intelligence as it is.

You have never established a relationship between you and your intelligence—not at all. You don't even let your intelligence come in. You don't do it because once the intelligence comes in, you can't be irrational, you can't get angry, you can't have commotions and you can't be emotional. You are afraid to give up your emotional satisfaction, so brick by brick, you have blocked your intelligence totally out of your life. Something that was supposed to guide you, help you, relate to you, promote you, project you, sell you, give you confidence in your personality has been, forever and ever, totally blocked out by you. You cannot tolerate the fact that sometimes in order to have one thing, you must give up another. You want the intelligence and the emotions, but it can't happen. When you are intelligent, you are not emotional; when you are emotional, you are not intelligent. It is as simple as that.

When you were a child and you wanted something, you became emotional. If that didn't get it for you, you became commotional. If that didn't work, then you became totally traumatic. You used trauma and drama and you became neurotic—then you got it. When you have had that experience, it follows that you don't use it. After all, in those days you didn't use your intelligence at all. You didn't reason to get what you wanted. You didn't argue for it. You didn't talk with your parents about it. You admitted nothing, but you got what you wanted. Now that experience has blocked any relationship between you and your intelligence. Now, whether you are 28, 38, or 48, you do the same thing. You traumatize yourself and you want exactly what you want.

When you were a little kid, your parents gave it to you out of mercy, out of devotion, and out of emotional love, but now you are dealing with Mother Nature and Father God. Mother Nature neither forgives nor forgets. Father God is inside not outside, so you are totally blocked. You cannot get anything from the outside and you do not want to touch the inside. The outside cannot give you anything. It cannot even give you your own sexual satisfaction. You can get an erection, but you cannot get sexual satisfaction. You cannot get sexual fulfillment. As a man you get nothing when you refuse to relate within. The greatest difficulty of this whole game is that you know it—that is the worst of all! You know that at the age of 42, traumatizing and becoming a psychopath, being abusive and using truck driver language, not doing your sadhana, screwing your wife, cheating your children, and conning everyone around you won't help. You know all that. You know what is good for you and what is not good for you. If you know what is good for you, then you know how to get what is good for you. But you don't want to get it, you want it to be given to you. You understand the difference?

Wishing and **Wanting**

If you want to get something you will get it. This is a law of nature. If you really want to get something, you really will get it. This is a universal law. This cannot be changed. What you sincerely need according to your magnetic field and psyche and energy shall be provided. I wanted to live in an adobe house. I never knew there were any adobe houses in America. I have never seen any adobe houses in Los Angeles. I am a villager. I came from a land where I had a beautiful adobe house, and I always wanted an adobe house in the United States. I got an adobe house, although I had to go to New Mexico to get it. What you really want shall come, but you have to really want it. Unfortunately you don't want, you wish. There is a difference between want and wish. You understand that? You wish for things and you want somebody to give them to you. You don't want anything. As a child you could only wish, and you always knew that whatever you wished for, the fairy godmother would provide it. You remember that stick with a star dangling on the top of it, and the crown and the big wings? It never leaves you; it never has and it never will.

There is a beautiful story from the orient. Somebody once pleased God. God said, "What do you want?"

If you want to get something you will get it. This is a law of nature. If you really want to get something, you really will get it. This is a universal law. This cannot be changed. What you sincerely need according to your magnetic field and psyche and energy shall be provided.

He said, "My Lord, I want to be able to close my eyes, make a wish for something and have it happen immediately."
"So be it."
One day he was just sitting and day dreaming. He closed his eyes and he said, "How great it would be, if I had all the diamonds of the world around my neck." In a few minutes he was dead because all those diamonds broke his neck. The neck couldn't take the load of tons and tons of diamonds. If all your wishes came true, you would never see the next sun.

There is a difference between want and wish. What has happened to you is that your wishing continues while wanting is blocked. There is want in men like us: We want to be successful, we want to be givers, we want to be lovers, we want to be respectable, we want to be recognized, we want to be somebody. Each of these is a want. It cannot be fulfilled by a wish. What you want, you have to get. What you wish has to be provided. The difference is that wishes are for fairy tales and wants are for men. Men want and they get it. Children wish and it is provided. You tell me you are grown up, then you were three feet tall and now you are six feet tall. I agree, you look grown up, but are you? There are tremendous blocks and you cannot talk about them. You are not willing to talk about them and you don't want to talk about them.

Religion plays a part in your behavior, too. Thousands of years ago religion took God from the universal prevailing energy, made It huge and infinite, and told man to search for It. Before that, religion was very practical. God was in a blade of grass, in the trees, in the stones. God was in everything. God was everything, everywhere, all around and that was too much. God was worshipped in different forms, shapes and situations and that wasn't tolerable. God has had to become a huge monster, a big thing out there somewhere and man is supposed to search for It, making God everything and us nothing. That is why one third of the world does not believe in God. It is a godless society, but that doesn't make any difference to God. It makes a tremendous difference to us, though. The purpose of religion is to teach us to relate to Infinity, to never ending life. If it does the job, the fear of death is taken away.

Instead you have a tremendous block—fear of death. Do you want to talk about it? There is a fear of death all the time. But are you really afraid of death? No. Do you want to talk about that either? These blocks are with us. They are a very subtle but solid part of us. That is why even those who are successful are unhappy. If all your resources and your sources are not flowing for you, you cannot be happy. If you aren't unhappy, still you will be handicapped. We are not unhappy, but we are handicapped. We are handicapped because we have blocks we cannot break through. If you really want to look at it, we have a very serious problem. This problem makes us absolutely sleepy. We actually go into a kind of drowsiness.

I say, "Hey."
You answer, "Yes Sir."
"How are you doing?"
"Fine."
"What is going on?"
"I don't know."
"What are you doing?"
"Everything. Oh no, nothing. Oh no, I don't know. I am doing something."
"Where were you yesterday?"
"Somewhere."
"Where are you going tomorrow?"
"Nowhere."
"Who are you?"
"You tell me."

And this is the bottom line, a very realistic bottom line. We have sexual experiences, we have social experiences. We have personal experiences. We have experiences we cannot talk about. We cannot even share. When we were children and we were growing up, a lot of things went wrong for us. This took away our trust. Now do we say, "I love you. I trust you. I believe in you. I am yours"? No, only a part of us says it. The major part says, "No, no, no. Don't trust this man. If he drops you what are you going to do? Don't love him. Don't love her."

Another block is a direct result of our block against forming a relationship, as a man, with our own intelligence. Our intelligence is our female aspect. We are married to intelligence and the purpose of this marriage is to produce consciousness. Consciousness is our sweet baby, our future, our tomorrow, our everything. The Id and the ego are married to intelligence to produce consciousness, but because you cannot relate to intelligence, you cannot produce consciousness. The energy is there. You have to do something with it, so you masturbate with your intellectuality. It is just like imagining your neighbor's wife and masturbating. There is no practical difference in the two. You ejaculate, you experience. You do all of that. There is a woman in your imagination and your thoughts but you cannot produce a baby. You do not want to relate to intelligence because you are attached to your emotions; you are attached to your emotions because you don't want to relate to your intelligence. I want to tell you why you do not relate to your intelligence. This is the reason: when you are intelligent, you are responsible and, worst of all, when you are intelligent, you are accountable. You do not want to answer to anybody; and when you are emotional, you are not accountable.

You know, it is very funny. Once I went to a national club in New Delhi where I saw a huge party going on. Everybody looked very fine. Beautiful people, super intelligent people, everyone came. They were respectable and very sociable. There was one man who was very well respected. He had never drunk before, but that day he went to the bar and said, "I need a drink."
The bartender said, "What kind of drink?"
He said, "Put in scotch and one whole beer."
The bartender looked at him and said, "What did you say, sir?"
He said, "Double the scotch and put one beer in it."

The bartender had never heard that order before but he put two shots of scotch into a glass of beer and handed it over. The man was not a drinker, but he slurped it down and ordered another one. The bartender gave him a second drink and said, "Something funny is going to happen." After he had the fourth drink, he started dancing, totally dancing. First he removed his coat, then he removed his tie, then he removed his shirt, then he removed his undershirt, and the moment he was going to remove his pants I had to get up. I just put my hand around his neck and I took him aside.

What you want, you have to get. What you wish has to be provided. The difference is that wishes are for fairy tales and wants are for men.

I said, "Look, you are not drunk. You are pretending and if you remove your pants here, you will lose all respect. Do you want to be respected or do you want to drop your pants? Tell me in my ear."
He said, "I am frustrated."
"What are you frustrated about?"
"Everybody thinks I am a very wise and perfect man but I am not."
I said, "I know it."
"What should I do?"
"Don't let anybody know about it."
"Why not? I am sick of it."
I said, "I agree with that. You are very sick. Nobody puts a double scotch and a beer together to begin with. Where did you learn that?"
"I went to a party. Somebody there drank a mixed drink and he did all this and nobody told him anything. They took him to the hospital."
But I said, "Nobody is going to take you to the hospital. You know what they are going to do?"
"What?"
"They are going to put a blanket around you, tie you up, put you in the back of the car, drive you home, and ask for a doctor. And do you know what will happen?"
"What?"
I said, "Nobody will trust you."

"Oh, no, no. I don't want that."
"Then behave."
He said, "Okay, okay. What should I do?"
I said, "I will pick up your clothes. Come with me. Go to the bathroom. Fix yourself up. Come out and say thank you to everybody. Explain that you just went into ecstasy and then walk away."
He said, "What does that mean?"
I said, "Say that you had an experience and went into ecstasy, that you do not know what happened to you. If anybody is offended or feels bad about it, give him your apologies. Then bow like this and walk away."
He said, "Yes, I think I have to do it."

He did exactly that, walked away and went home. I dropped him off. I came back to my house. I was lying down and thinking, "My God, what happened? Good man, very good man. Very rich man, very respectable man, absolutely social." Then I cracked up. "Ha, ha, ha, ha, ha," I said, "Oh, good, good, good." I went to the telephone and called him.

I said, "Hi, how are you? Are you sleeping?"
He said, "No, I was laughing."
I said, "I was laughing too. Why are you laughing?"
"I was just laughing. What happened to me?"
"Nothing. You got burnt out."
"You are right."
I said, "I can understand. I get burnt out too."
He said, "What do you do when you get burnt out?"
"You really want to know?"
"Yes."
I said, "When I get burnt out, I don't feel I am me. I don't feel it is me, but you feel it is you."
He said, "What do you feel?"
I said, "I feel I have no peer group, I have nobody to talk to except to myself, and I feel myself is nothing but a gift to experience myself. Therefore I respect the gift."
He said, "Where did you learn such things?"
"From my teacher."
"Who is your teacher?"
I said, "What do you want to do with him?"
"I want to find him. God, give me something. Give me a break! You know what I was going to do?"
I said, "You were going to take off your pants and you were going to dance naked. Isn't that true?"
"That is true."
I said, "You wanted social insult."
"That is true."
"You wanted people to spit at you."
He said, "That is absolutely true. I wanted to destroy myself."
I said, "Who told you to build yourself? Who built you?"
"Me."
I said, "You are wrong. You didn't build yourself. Your intelligence built you. Now you are becoming emotional and you are becoming the enemy of your own intelligence. Think about it and call me back."
He didn't call the next day, but he was at my door. He was so grateful.

When the internal block of ego communicates with emotion, it doesn't matter how wise or how great you are, you become self-destructive; and whenever your ego and your intelligence come together, you shall become successful. It doesn't matter who you are. Your ego is like the "common" wire of a toggle switch; your emotions and your intelligence are the two opposite poles. It is just a matter of blocking the current to one pole and allowing it flow to the other.

There is a difference between the intellect and intelligence. When the pros and cons relating to you are identified by you, it is the work of intelligence. When the pros and cons are identified by your emotional self, it is the work of the intellect. Your emotional self is only part of you. The total self of self, which is you, is the totality of you. We talk about intellectual and intelligent people. When we say somebody is very intellectual, we are saying that he is only two-thirds of a man. On the other hand, when we say that so-and-so is very intelligent, we are talking about the whole sum of the person. That is a very simple expression to which you and I can relate through this.

When the internal block of ego communicates with emotion, it doesn't matter how wise or how great you are, you become self-destructive; and whenever your ego and your intelligence come together, you shall become successful.

In our own understanding, in our own lives, we have a block. Though we are still children of God, we are also children of our egos. When we are children of our egos, we are afraid to even talk about our blocks. If we are not willing to talk about something, how can we get rid of it? There is a tendency in us to blame others for our faults. It is a very powerful block. It has ruined us many, many times in our life. As children we always expected to be mothered—always. When we grow up, we still want to be mothered. When things don't come through, we blame somebody. We blame somebody else because we are never ourselves. To be very honest with you, we do not want to be ourselves at all. We always want to be somebody else, to copy somebody else, to feel for somebody else, to think about somebody else, to compare ourselves with somebody else. We judge ourselves and our neighbors by whether we are rich or poor, who is beautiful and who is not. Think about it. Take a practical look at all that and ask yourself a very honest and sincere question: Who, then, are you as you?

It is a simple thing. If you are comparing all the time, my neighbor has a swimming pool, my neighbor has a Mercedes car, my neighbor has a garden—fine. You should have a swimming pool. You should have a Mercedes car. You should have a garden. But then your neighbor's wife is bitchy and that you don't want. His children are neurotic—that you don't want either. If you are getting everything from your neighbor, then get the whole thing! No. You don't do it. You want this from this neighbor, that from that neighbor. You spread yourself so thin that you never find out who you are.

Once there was a man who always felt very cold. His sister came to him and said, "Brother, you always sleep with your knees drawn up to your chest."
He said, "The night is very cold."
She said, "Okay," and she brought a big down quilt and gave it to him.
The next night he stretched his legs out. He was warm. He was happy. Six months later when she came by, she found him very happy. She said, "How are you sleeping?"
He said, "Perfect."
Six months later she came out and she found him again sleeping with his knees to his chest. She said, "What is happening now?"
He said, "I don't sleep under the quilt anymore."
She said, "Why not?"
He said, "My neighbors all sleep under cashmere blankets."
She said, "They are fat. They are slobs. They don't feel the cold at all. You are a beautiful, skinny person. Why are you doing this?"
"I don't know," he said.

That is our status about ourselves. Our answer is, "I don't know." I lived in India for 40 years. In all that time I never heard one person answer, "I don't know." Never. I have been here 15 years and I have heard nothing but "I don't know." We say that as Americans we are very educated, we are very beautiful. India is a third world country, third world economy. It is a mosquito country, if you know what I mean. But still, they know—and here we have the consciousness of, "I don't know," we have no sense of Self.

Typical **Blocks**

Americans have some fanatic fantasies. To understand this you have to understand how the country works and how the nation works. You have all come from different ethnic groups; and basically, you all came to escape persecution. You ran away from persecution of one sort or another, economic, social, religious, whatever it was. You made a conscious revolt against some persecution. You left your home, you left your country, you left your nationality and you moved in groups. It is called ethnic migration. You have ethnically migrated here, but that conscious revolt has never left you. It is with you even today, and the result of that ethnic revolt is demonstrated here:

Yogi Bhajan on The Story of **Japan**

Do you know the story of Japan? MacArthur was the Commander-in-Chief of the Eastern command. He came to Washington and talked to the President. He said, "We have occupied Japan. They are a very beautiful people and I do not want them to go Communist. I want to feed them well and uplift them." The President said, "You are mad, MacArthur. Get out of here." So MacArthur proceeded in his own way. He started producing everything that his occupied Japan needed under military command. In three years he had industrialized the whole of Japan. There is no ordinance for a factory making chocolates. Chocolate is not part of a certain gun. You can't fire with it. Yet he produced everything that the country's economy would need through his military command. He put Japan on its feet.

The Japanese people have one less block than we have. MacArthur totally Americanized them. But there was one thing he could not take away from them. It is called love. The Japanese can love without question. Their love is not conditional. That is why Japan can produce better and cheaper than we can. Their unions do not go on strike, instead their unions unite to produce more. There is a different motivation, a totally different motivation. The Japanese have unions. We have unions. Our unions are to bargain. Their unions are to make a profit, to produce and to make people rich. Our unions are a power game between labor and management. Their unions are the glue for labor and management.

They are people, we are people, but the Japanese have a tradition of loyalty that spans thousands of years. They see disloyalty as a super-death. When a Japanese man is told that he has been disloyal to his conscious cause, he is expected to kill himself. It is called, "harikari." They take their own blades and put them through their own diaphragms; because for them, betraying their conscious vow is absolute disloyalty. But Americans see it as their right.

"What are you doing?"
"I don't know."
"Why don't you know?"
"I don't know."
"Do you want to know?"
"No, I don't want to know."

This is a basic ethnic revolt against authority. We are a nation of nations but we are very anti-authority. We love God, but God is the highest authority, God is the ultimate authority, God is the Infinite. We do not want to relate to the Infinite because we will be accountable to the Infinite, and we don't want to be accountable so we become emotional.

To solve our dilemma, we spend $70 an hour for psychoanalysis, $120 an hour for a psychiatrist and $20 dollars an hour for massage. We go out to restaurant A, to restaurant B. You will find a whole world of restaurants in America because we are unable to decide what we want to eat. We are unable to decide what we want to wear. We are unable to decide who we want to marry. We are unable to decide what to do with our children. We do not even know what to do with pigeons. Test it out. Stop an American on the street tomorrow:

Say, "Thank you, hello, how are you."
He will say, "Hi, how are you?"
"I am glad to meet you."
He will say, "I am glad to meet you. Thank you very much."

Give a pigeon to him and tell him, "This is for you," and just watch what he will do and what his reaction will be. Write it down, study it and understand it. Americans can handle landing on the moon, but they don't know how to handle a gift of a pigeon. We have a block toward getting anything.

We have a block toward committing to anything. We are not committed to our children. We are not committed to our marriages. We are not committed to our homes. We are not committed to our families. We are not committed to our souls. We are not committed to our spirits. We are not committed to our surroundings. We are not committed to our neighborhoods. We are not committed to our country. We are not committed to anything. We have only one commitment. We are committed to everything—which means nothing.

We have a block against committing. When we say we are committed we feel that we are being dropped into a snake pit. For us there is no difference between a commitment and a snake pit. Someone says, "Are you committed?" and you say, "Yes." Then you feel it—that snake pit is what you feel. When somebody tells you to deal with character, you can't relate. You know what character means to you? It means doing nothing. It means being pious. Nor can you relate to being told, "Be noble." There is no worse abuse for an American than to tell him, "Be noble." He remembers the noblemen of England, the barons, the dukes, the lords. The American thinks of himself as a guerilla. This is because we won our country with guerilla warfare. We hid and we fired on the British soldiers as they came forward, line by line, in rank and file. We kept on firing and finished them off. We even got them on the run. We learned to be guerillas and now it sits in us as a façade.

If we are not willing to talk about something, how can we get rid of it?

You were not born in the 18th Century but the 18th Century is living in you. You love to be guerillas playing hide and seek. You even play hide and seek with love. You don't say, "Come, I love you." You can't say that. No, you say, "Hello, how are you? I think I met you somewhere. What are you doing? What are you doing this evening? Is it free?" You do it all in a roundabout way. You don't say, "Hello, I am so-and-so. You are so-and-so. I love you. I would like to take you out tonight. We can talk and see how we get on." You can't do it. There is no way. It is beyond your level of commitment. Once you say, "Hi, I love you. I want to take you out and talk to you," you feel that because you have made a commitment, it is a snake pit. But still you don't want to talk about it. Right?

Once I was speaking with a husband and wife. A girl came by and said, "Hi, Yogi Bhajan how are you?"
I said, "Oh good, thank you, How are you?"
She said, "I am fine. I am this and that."
We talked for a few minutes. She split. Then we split and I asked this boy, "Who was that?"
"Oh, no, no Sir, she was our yoga student at one time."
And he said this in such a way that it created a curiosity in me.
I said, "I think you know her." I was just a little direct.
He said, "Yeah, yeah, she used to be my yoga student, too."
I looked at his wife and she said, "Sir, he used to live with her."

You have learned this from your history. It is your character to hide and fire. You don't want to face the fire. You want to bite the bullet but you do not want to face the bullet. That is why you have pain in life and much less courage.

On your currency you wrote, "In God We Trust." You had to write that because you have a tremendous block against authority. It doesn't matter if somebody gives you a lot of good advice. For you, good advice is a chain around your neck. For you, good advice and a collar are no different. Imagine a dog. Imagine a huge, thick, unbreakable steel collar around his neck. Imagine hooks on that collar. There are 20, 30, maybe 40 hooks, and every hook has a chain. Imagine that. Then imagine the 20 or 30 chains being held by 20 or 30 people who are pulling the dog. That's what good advice means to you and you relate to it just like that dog, "Grrrrrrrrrrr. Arrrrrrrrrrr." If your wife says, "My husband, listen to me," you will say, "Arrrrrrrr. Why do I have to listen to you? What do you want?" If your spiritual teacher says, "My dear son, please." You will say, "What? What?" Goodness and kindness means impotency to you. It has taken me 15 years to understand what words mean to you.

God blessed me to read the aura and so I read it. One day a man came to me. He is very active, fit and all that, plus he has three children. Beautiful. I love him very much. He is a good student.
I said, "Please sit down."
He said, "No, sir, can I sit at your feet."
I said, "No." (He always comes and touches my feet.) I realized that he must know that if he sits within nine feet of me, I may not be able to read his aura, so, I said, "No, sit on that sofa."
He said, "No, no, no. By your feet, I like to touch your feet."
I said, "You are very beautiful. I understand, but just sit there." After all, what could he do? He had to sit down right there where he was, but now he was cautious. Then I could see his aura and I said, "You are very noble." I didn't say, "Are you noble or are you not?" I didn't put him on the offensive. I said, "You are very noble." I watched. I read the aura well. He became more and more gray, and then I said, "You are very kind. You are very sweet." I waited a moment and I said, "You are very darling." He became a girl. He was not a man anymore. I cracked up. I said to myself, "Look, there is nothing more to do with this guy. If he wants to fight with me, I only need to say, 'You are very sweet,' and he is going to go limp."

Your language is very aggressive and undiplomatic. To cover this undiplomatic language and your fear of commitment, you have become a first-name nation. "Hi Bob, hi Harry, hi Kee, hi Pee, hi You, hi Shit, hi Pit, hi Lit." God knows what you say to anybody. It doesn't mean a thing. What is her name? Katherine da-do-du. Who is she? Kathy. "Kathy, Mathy, Pathy, Othey, Ethy." "Me Kathy, me Robin, me Till, me Pill, me Shill, me Chill." "Hi. Hi." Nothing means anything to you. You deny the identity of others to find your identity. Others deny your identity to find their identity. You have a non-identity existence. This is because you are immigrants. You were immigrants, but you have become immigrants now and forever. You have created a tremendous block. You don't want to talk. You don't want to know. You don't want to discuss it at all.

You know if somebody dies in India we say, "hi, hi, hi." It means something bad has happened. But here this is our hello. We can't even say, "Hello." We say, "Hi." We have made our communication so shallow, so hollow, so superficial and so ruthless because we have a block against commitment. We want to have character and when it comes to character, we want to talk about it; but when it comes to commitment, we have nothing to say. We want to have a home but we don't have a foundation. We want to live the story of that man who built a house in a tree. Robinson Crusoe. You have been to Disneyland? There is no Disneyland without that house. That house is our history. I have seen a lot of homes built in trees, tree houses. We want to build a house in a tree—like birds—so we can fly away when we want to. And we do it in the name of our children. Papa builds it for the children but Papa plays in that tree house more than his children. Papa wants to be a bird. He wants to have a new nest every year—a new nest, a new mate, new eggs, hatch them and fly away. The net result is broken homes, divorced parents, half homes, half parents, half mother, half father, all that. One, two, three, four, five: meet my first wife, meet my other wife, and meet another wife.

You can be what you want to be, but you can't be what you wish to be. The time has come. We want to be, we should be, and we have to be—men.

One day I was introduced to four wives in a row and I was talking to the fifth wife. I looked around and then I stepped to the side and said, "Was that person joking?"
The husband said, "No, no. I have been divorced four times. They all came together."
I said, "Any of them married?"
He said, "No, no, I take care of them. I divorced them."
I said, "I want to know one thing."
"What?"
I said, "You have four wives, ex-wives. They don't see anybody, they don't date anybody?"
He said, "No, no, no. They don't. I take care of them."
I said, "Take care of them? Then why did you divorce them?"
He said, "That is a mystery."
His fifth wife said, "I think I am going to be with them soon."
I said, "What are you saying?"
She said, "I think this is what is going to happen to me, too."

The same cycle: every wife got divorced after the second child—every single one. Plus each one got more after her divorce than when she was his wife. When she was his wife, she was not given anything, but now she is given everything. Everything is being taken care of. Same cycle. Same orbit. Same four seasons. At its nucleus is the number one block—no commitment.

When you are married you don't pay any attention to your wife, you don't pay any attention to your children, you don't pay attention to your environment. When you are divorced, at eight o'clock every Sunday, the door bell rings. "Why have you come?" "To take my children on an outing." All day Sunday you babysit. You give up Sunday, which is practically the only free day for you. Even God rested that day, but you don't. When that wife and child were with you, what were you doing on Sunday? Watching football. Why is this? Why does this happen? Because we have blocks and we don't want to talk.

There is one story I want to tell you. A young man went to a golf club. He was hired as a caddy for $10 an hour. He was thinking and planning, "Oh yeah! Ten dollars an hour . . . $80 dollars a day. God, cash! Twenty dollars tax, $60 dollars down. Far out, man. I have been unemployed for such a long time. This is wonderful." He was doing that while fixing a golf club. He finished it. He was very happy. He came into the office where he overheard two gentlemen talking.
One said, "John, you played well today."
John said, "Yeah, but you ran off the course just a few minutes before I was finished and you didn't come back for half an hour."
The first man said, "Oh no. Don't worry. I will take you to dinner to compensate for it. Because really, I have to celebrate."
John said, "What do you have to celebrate?"
He said, "A phone call came, then I made a few other calls and I worked it all out. It is perfect. It is all done now. I think the moment I get back to the office to pick up my briefcase, the fax will confirm it."
John said, "Confirm what?"
He said, "I have been working on something and now we have an agreement and it is all done."
John said, "Well, how much have you made?"
He said, "Eighty million dollars, not more. I expected a little more but . . ."
John said, "Damn you. In half an hour you made eighty million dollars?"
He said, "I am a little sad. I expected a hundred million dollars, but you know. I was in a hurry, so I just decided to take it."

The caddy was thinking about 80 bucks while the other guy was thinking of 80 million. Both were human, both were on the golf course, and both were walking on the same trail. You can be what you want to be, but you can't be what you wish to be. The time has come. We want to be, we should be, and we have to be–men.

Living the You within **You**

You must touch the you within you. You must do your own psychoanalysis. You must come out with truthful answers and by virtue of that you shall know yourself, and once you know who you are . . . you can't go wrong.

Please try to understand one thing—and understand it once and for all. There are two ways to get the garbage out of you: one is the way we have decided to do it and the other is to go to a psychoanalyst and get the psychoanalysis done. The first is a pressure system: you are put into a mold, you cooperate, you run through it and you come out clean. With other systems you go daily, talk slowly, understand things, get more emotional, get commotional, relate to somebody, and when you are 65 you will find out what you should have done when you were 18.

This is my approach: Everybody has a subconscious, a permanent memory. It has the power to connect the conscious and the supreme conscious. There is no way their connection cannot be made if we break the block that separates them. We put you through this process so that you can reach something, so you can be happy—and I will have less trouble. My motivation is very clear and honest. If you have less trouble, I will have more freedom. If you have more trouble, I will have less freedom. I want my freedom, and I can only get it if you have less trouble. I want you to understand that it is not for money that I come here and teach a course. Neither is it to know what you are privately and what you are personally. I already know you privately and personally more than you even know yourself. I understand the patterns; the patterns are known; the patterns are no problem. It is you who has the problem. You don't want to break the pattern because that is the only thing you can hold onto. That is the biggest block! However, I have the very beautiful understanding that you have come here because you want to be here and you want to break through.

I never told you that you would have to write a long paper, but there was no other way to make you touch your own reality! [Editor's Note: Yogi Bhajan is referring to a questionnaire he had them fill out on the first day of the course.] Professionally speaking, it is very bad economics. If I make you touch your own reality, make you get out of your neuroses, then you will feel good and I am out of business. Actually, what I should do is to make you more of a mess, create more complications, make you more miserable, and squeeze a lot of money out of you. I could start selling malas (prayer beads) and other things, saying, "Put this on your wrist and you will be better for 10 days. Put this on your neck. You will be better for 20." I can't do that. It is not my style.

I believe every human being, by his own right and by his own virtue, is complete. I don't ask you to agree with it. I believe we are in the image of God. We are human beings and God created us. God is perfect so we could not be imperfect. Then where did we go wrong? Somewhere it has to be looked into. When we look into it, we find that our style is wrong and so are our patterns and our subconscious. Whenever the subconscious and the emotions get their scene together, we become beasts, monsters. Neither our rationale nor our reason works. Neither does logic, style, truth, nor lies. Nothing works. But if ever the consciousness and the subconscious touch the conscious mind, then the only thing working will be the divinity of God and the supreme conscious. The question is how to do it? One way is that I talk and you listen. I have done that for 15 years. I am getting a little bit tired of it.

"Well, I told you last Friday. Why did you do it again?"
"I don't know. I was not myself."
"Why didn't you call me?"
"Don't you understand Sir, I was not myself."
"Why didn't you call me immediately?"
"I was not myself."
"When did you become yourself?"
"Two hours ago."
"When did you do it."
"Three weeks ago."

Between three weeks ago and two hours ago there is a long time. That has to be solved, and I cannot solve it. It has to be solved by you and within you. To solve it by you and within you, I have to do something to let you touch your own self. . . . You must touch the you within you. You must do your own psychoanalysis. You must come out with truthful answers and by virtue of that you shall know yourself, and once you know who you are, then I have no problem. I am free and you can't do wrong.

The Story of **Joga Singh**

Do you know that story of Guru Gobind Singh and Joga Singh, the Sikh who left his wedding ceremony? Guru Gobind Singh was very majestic—both regal and spiritual. Joga Singh was a great disciple of Guru Gobind Singh. One day he came to the Guru and said, "Satguru, I have just received a letter from my parents. They have arranged my marriage and have asked me to come before you to receive your blessing." Guru Gobind Singh replied, "Well, there is a lot of work to be done here, but if your parents have arranged your marriage, then you should honor their wishes. Go on home. I'll calculate when you should return and then I'll send for you." "Yes, sir. I'll return as soon as I hear from you," said Joga Singh. Guru Gobind Singh replied, "So be it."

Joga Singh made ready at once and set off for his parents' village. It was about a two day journey. Later, Guru Gobind Singh summoned one of his Sikhs and handed him a letter, saying, "Go to Joga Singh's village. When Joga Singh has nearly completed the wedding ceremony, give him this letter." So the Sikh rode off. He arrived in time to participate in Joga Singh's wedding. He brought marvelous gifts from the Guru. Joga Singh was happy. Everything was fantastic.

In a Sikh wedding, the couple walks in a circle around the Siri Guru Granth Sahib, the sacred scriptures, four times, after which they are considered to be married. When Joga Singh had completed three and a half rounds, the messenger stepped forward and handed him the letter: "Message from Guru Gobind Singh."

Joga Singh stopped. He opened the letter. It said, "The moment you read this letter, stop what you are doing and proceed to me at once. Guru Gobind Singh." Joga Singh had just 20 steps more to go to complete the wedding. Without taking another step, he left the hall and began to prepare himself for his long ride back to the Guru's court. He told his wife, "The Guru has acknowledged our wedding, so everything is in order. Now I must go." "Yes, my lord," she replied.

Joga Singh figured he would ride for a day, then he would rest his horse and then ride again. He set out at full speed. On the way, he began to think. What a great Sikh of the Guru I am. I didn't even complete the last 20 steps. I am very good. Perfect! See what a wonderful job I have done. When he reached the midway point, he stopped in a town. Now, he thought, I can rest for the night, and start out early tomorrow. No problem. Let me take a look around the town. As he was looking around, he saw a house with a prostitute sitting outside. She winked at him. Joga Singh looked around. Is anyone looking at me? Then he remembered, I am Joga Singh, so he went away. Nonetheless, he marked the spot in his memory.

He wandered around the town some more. Then, in the evening, he returned to the spot again. He was fascinated. He was still aware that he was Joga Singh, he who could leave his own wedding to obey the Guru's orders, but his ego began to speak to him very passionately.

"Well, I have not yet seen what a woman is. She is available. I have money. Let me experiment. I was planning to rest tonight anyway, so I would still be carrying out the Guru's orders." Then his mind and his ego began to join hands together, faith started deteriorating, pride started going backward. When your pride becomes gay, you have nothing to say. (Don't misunderstand, when I use the word "gay," I mean happy.) Happy pride is your worst enemy. So, at about one o'clock in the morning he returned to the prostitute's house.

Just remember: there is X amount of energy in you and you are its master. You can use it the way you want and direct it in the way you want it to go.

In front of the house, he met a hunchbacked old man. "What are you looking for?" the man asked.
"I thought that one of my friends lived around here."
"No friend lives here. This is a bazaar of prostitutes. You appear to be a Sikh. Sikhs don't come to this bazaar. Go, go, go away!"
"Okay, okay, okay," he said. "I'm in the wrong bazaar."

Joga Singh went away. But passion is very powerful. I am just trying to let you know. At four o'clock, he came back again. This time, he found a very stalwart, strong man standing in front of the prostitute's door.

"You must be totally mistaken," the man said. "Sikhs don't come here. You look like a very saintly person. What are you doing? Looking for a prostitute tonight?"
"No, no, no. I was looking for a friend. I must be in the wrong bazaar. No, really . . ."
"Go! Go!" the man said. "It's time for meditation. Do your sadhana. Read your banis. You can see your friend in the morning."
"Okay. Thank you."
"Don't forget to take a cold bath."

So Joga Singh went to the river, took a cold bath, sat down and meditated, then read his banis. He reflected on what he had done and he didn't like it. Then he fed his horse, groomed him, and rode off.

When he reached the Guru's court, he told the sevadar, "I want to see the Guru."
The sevadar replied, "I don't know what happened today.

The Guru didn't get up."
"What? The Guru didn't do his sadhana? You must be kidding."
"No, look at the water pot. When the Guru gets up, he empties the pot to take his bath. But the pot is still full."
"But it's seven o'clock." Joga Singh couldn't believe it.
"I know and you know that it's seven o'clock, but the Guru didn't get up."
"But I have a letter that says, "'See me at once.'"
"Well, 'at once' means at once. Do you want to go in and sleep with him? He is sleeping. If you want to go in, go ahead. I'm not stopping you."
"No, no, no. I'll wait."
At eleven o'clock, the Guru was not yet awake.
"Is he all right?" Joga Singh asked.
"Yeah, he's all right. I hear him snoring. He is really deeply asleep."
After an hour, the sevadar went inside to check on the Guru.
"Joga Singh has come?" the Guru asked.
"Yes, master, he is here."
"Bring him in."
Joga Singh came in. The Guru said, "Joga Singh, you have come. Very good."
"Yes, sir, but you were sleeping."
"Yeah, yeah. I was awake the whole night. I was doing something. Just give me a foot massage."
Joga Singh was very happy. He began massaging the Guru's feet.
"Joga Singh," the Guru asked, "how was the marriage?"
"Lord, I don't know. I was 20 steps away when your letter came. I had to ride away."
"Yeah, yeah, you are a good Gursikh. You didn't complete those 20 steps. I know your personal control. Very good. You applied your special, personal control—along with my love, it all worked together."
The Guru continued. "You rode well. How was your journey?"
"Fantastic."
"Tell me step by step. How many hours did you ride? Where did you stop?"
"Lord, I was very tired. I rode 12 hours, and then I stopped. Then I came to that town, and . . ."
"Yeah, yeah, yeah. You went to the town. You were very much under control, right?"
"Uh, yeah…"
"What did you do in that town? Did you sleep?"
"No."
"You were running around, going to the wrong bazaar, right?"
"My Guru, you know everything."
"No, no, continue to massage my feet. The frost bit them last night. I was there."
"Were you that man who chased me away?"
"You think I only know how to stop you from completing your wedding ceremony? Don't you think it is also my responsibility to prevent you from going to a prostitute? You must think that I missed my cold bath this morning."
"Yes, that is what your sevadar told me."
"When you were taking your bath in that small, cold river, didn't you notice some person taking a bath a little bit upstream?"
"Yes, there was some person."
"The water that touched his body touched your body and the real Joga Singh came back."

The word "jogi" has two meanings. One is a yogi, one who does yoga, who is united. The other is one who is absolutely dependable. The Guru said, "Joga Singh, you are now Gurujoga Singh. From today onward, you are only for the Guru." Joga Singh didn't falter after that. He lived a very rich spiritual life. We are still talking about it today.

The idea is not to have people who are weak. The idea is for people to be strong and to let them control their weaknesses. When you want to stop water from flowing in one direction, you put up a dike to stop the flow and then open up a channel for it to flow in another direction. Human energy works in exactly the same way. You stop it from flowing to the negative or destructive side and you will have an equal amount of energy to flow in a positive direction. Just remember: there is X amount of energy in you and you are its master. You can use it the way you want and direct it in the way you want it go.

We've Come a Long **Way**

My idea is that you have come a long way in 15 years. We started from scratch. We all started poor. We have come from a class of people—twenty million Americans—who revolted. It was a silent revolt. We made a choice between consciousness and America. We OD'd on drugs. We died. We were killed. We were clubbed. We were put in jail. We were held on various charges. Even in Nixon's time, there was a scheme to pick up all the kids who looked like hippies and put them in detention camps like we did the Japanese [during WWII]. But out of all this, a new America grew. Out of the Woodstock Nation a very solid, conscious nation grew. This nation must have no blocks and all the flow that is the real flower child, blossoming with fragrance, with the delicacy of youth, attractive—not freaked out, boozed out, drugged out, cocained out.

At a rock festival, a young man, 24 years old, stood before me. "My name is Jeffrey. I am Jeffrey. Jeffrey is my name. You understand Jeffrey? Have you seen Jeffrey? My name is Jeffrey. How many Jeffrey's have you seen? You must have seen a lot of Jeffrey's. Nobody is like me. I am the only Jeffrey. Why do you look at me? You don't like Jeffrey?" I watched him standing there for 45 minutes. I saw a youth destroying himself; I felt the pain. One day, they brought to my tent a most beautiful young woman, totally naked. We put a blanket over her. When they brought her from the OD tent, all she could say was, "Oooooooooooo, whooooooooooo, mmmmmmmmmm." She continued this way all day and all night. Later, when we found out who her mother and father were, we freaked out. How could this happen to her?

Why are we failures? Why do we love depression so much? Why can't we put things together? Why don't we have the answers for so many things? Why do we continue to push our way when we know that so many times before we have destroyed so much by doing so? Why do we not take an expert's opinion? Why do we not play our parts in the education, knowledge and experience of our children? Why do we not want to relax and be good to ourselves and to others? Why do we not want peace, harmony, blessings and blissfulness? It is a big question—why?

This generation you belong to is going through a very heavy period. You have a nuclear war hanging over you. You have a television set that does not give you one piece of good news. It starts out: On the corner of Fairfax and Sixth there was a murder. Then it tells you about a bank robbery. Then it tells you about some other case going on. A train was derailed. A bus got in an accident. An airplane fell apart. God bless you, you are the only ones who can take it.

Master & Student **Dialogue**

Today we have to play a game, and it's a good one. I need someone to come forward. He may not have a block, but at least he should act like a person who has a block. I will give you a practical demonstration of what it is, how to break through it, and what it does for you through your own sensitivity.

Volunteers, please. Feel naked. Some people think, I don't want to sign my name on my questionnaire, Yogiji might read it. I read you anyway. There are six important areas I left out of the questionnaire because I thought, if I put those questions in, everyone will feel like he is being hung.

[Editor's Note: Various men came forward and explained their blocks and how they manifested them in their personal lives. Due to technical difficulties in recording their statements, we present them here in abbreviated form.]

Yogi Bhajan: This man is a qualified psychiatrist. Don't misunderstand. It is a fact that 80% of all people choose their professions to cure their own injuries. That is why you get burnt out. I am not kidding. You get burnt out because you choose your profession under the compulsion of the subconscious environment. I didn't choose to be a spiritual man under the pressure of the subconscious environment. I chose that consciously. My decision to become a customs' officer was subconscious. You have to live, therefore you have to work. You have to live to work and you have to earn. As a customs' officer I was very honest. But I don't credit my honesty to being honest by nature—not at all. You don't understand the temptations I used to go through. You can't even imagine. Neither was I honest because I was a coward, afraid to exploit opportunities because of dishonesty. Everybody else was doing it right and left, so there was no problem. I didn't do it because I couldn't do it. I couldn't do it because I never wanted to do it. I never wanted to do it because it was not my cup of tea. I was honest because I was very consciously spiritual. So what I wanted to tell you is that you can be totally in the wrong profession for the wrong reasons, or totally in the right profession for the right reasons—and you may not even know what the reasons are.

Student: *My block is that I do not trust anybody. This block has to do with my upbringing.*

Yogi Bhajan: Now, you trust. Can you believe that something in your subconscious takes away your trust? It is a very simple thing: Trust is not only trust in yourself. Trust includes trust in your intelligence, trust in your caliber, trust in your environments, trust in your psyche, trust in your penetration, trust in your intercourse, trust in the reproductive [power] of your intercourse, and overall trust in your total creativity. This is called the "assembly line" of trust. Next comes time. You trust your past; you pick up the best. You trust your present to make it best. You trust your future to create the best. All this forms a triangle. And finally, you go inward and totally trust yourself. Then the outside world totally trusts you. The most difficult thing is when the outside world trusts you, because then you have to give and take nothing. The most vital thing in human life is when somebody trusts you and you cannot consciously, subconsciously or unconsciously break that trust. Then you are real.

Student: *The block that I choose to deal with today is learning to want wealth. Most of the time, my thoughts are like stray beams of light filtering through a room. But when there is an emergency, when I am under pressure, or when I really want something, then my thoughts become like a laser beam. And I realize that I usually use only one or two percent of my capacity, and I become angry with myself and very disappointed. Why am I just spinning my wheels through life? I really feel the pain of years and years of thinking in rays in my head instead of acting in reality. Yesterday you said, "Children wish and men want. Children wait and men get." That is where I'm stuck. I know that I want to want. I know that I want to get. I'm very tired of saying this and wishing for that, fantasizing about it and not putting it into action.*

Yogi Bhajan: It is a very simple statement that you have made. You have reached "Level A." Level A is where you want to want. You want to have it. You want badly for it to happen to you, you believe it should; otherwise you will be frustrated, angry and mad. But, basically, if you want to want, and if you create calmness around you, it will come to you 10 times. Want to want. Want it badly. Then, to receive it, just be calm. That wanting plus total calmness gets everything.

Student: The block that I feel is a fear of intimacy. I was raised in a family that did not express itself physically, in fact, it rarely expressed itself at all. My father was almost always away making his millions. My mother was very upset about where he was making his millions and who he was making it with.

Most of my childhood memories are from age five onward. All my friends were girls. That is who I played with. I have a very distinct memory of trading peppermint kisses and seeing how they tasted in each other's mouths. When I was in the second grade, I used to show off by doing handstands and getting praise from the girls. Then we played a chasing game where, if I caught any girl, I would lift her skirt. The girls would scream with delight. Then, of course, one girl didn't like it. She told the teacher, and then the principal called my father, and my father was called away from his millions to deal with my embarrassment. Without much talking, he forbade me to have any relationships with girls or women again in my life. When my sister heard that, she said, "Does that mean me too, Daddy?" My father just left the room and I was left alone. My mother said, "Don't worry about it. He doesn't mean what he said."

About three months later, my parents got a divorce. I probably felt at the time that my father just didn't want to be around me anymore. And so, from that time on, I don't feel that I had any kind of intimate relationship with anyone, especially with women.

Yogi Bhajan: Intimacy, to him, is like climbing into a snake pit. Intimacy, to him, is not intimacy as you understand it. It is supremacy of somebody over him. It is love without trust. Love without trust is like a river without water. You can name it, you can feel it, you can draw it, but you can't drink out of it. Just trust—not because you want to or you don't want to. Just trust and suffer, rather than not trust and suffer.

Be straight and to the point. The greatest secret of life is, touch your own self. You know the phone company's slogan, "Reach out and touch someone?" I say, "Touch yourself and you will be picked up."

Student: My specific block has to do with a regular practice of sadhana in particular and being able to establish an ongoing discipline in general. I would like to be able to say I am going to do something and do it, and continue to do it over time. I can't think of a lot of historical background to explain why I have this problem. My experience of not getting up in the morning is kind of like a little boy pouting, a brat. "I don't have to and I'm not going to, so there." Of course, I am the only one who's losing. It is really frustrating. In my work I am supposed to help people who have problems, and yet I have this very specific thing that I want to accomplish and I can't do it, even when I focus on it and work on it and try lots of different approaches.

Yogi Bhajan: Do you like an unclean home?

Student: No

Yogi Bhajan: Then why do you like an unclean mind?

Student: I don't.

Yogi Bhajan: Then clean it every morning. That's all there is to it. I don't like my unclean mind. I know I have to face a day; and I know a lot of people are going to have to call on me. I have to inspire a lot of people. There is nothing in it for me, and yet there is a lot in it for me, because people trust me. If you trust me and I do not keep your trust, I am betraying myself. I know that I cannot afford to betray myself; therefore, I want to keep myself clean. I want to do my job, and I know that if I do one wrong job, they are going to hang me, sue me, they are going to say, "You said this!" I don't want to hear that.

So sometimes I get up at 2:30 instead of 3:30 and I meditate. I don't care. I have become so habitual in doing it that I don't go flat at all. One day, somebody gave me a Tab cola and I didn't drink it for a while. I let it bubble and then it became flat. Then, when I started to drink it, someone picked it up and said, "It's flat." I said, "What does that mean?"

"When it goes flat, you don't drink it."

Well, when I go flat, nobody touches me. So I have to be bubbly all the time. I learned from Tab. If Tab can become a teacher, I think we can learn from everything. You have to be bubbly. Something must come out of you. Just remain bubbly and clean your mind every morning. You will never be bad. You have gone through the worst. I want to congratulate you. A person of normal caliber would have gone flat. I intentionally didn't help you. I prayed for you, that is true, but I didn't come out and directly help you.

Student: I owe a lot of people money.

Yogi Bhajan: It is very simple. When circumstances go

bad, just understand that circumstances have gone bad. Don't go bad with them. It is very simple.

Student: *But the thing that bothers me is that I don't feel worthy of grace.*

Yogi Bhajan: You believe that you are not worthy of grace, but your Creator doesn't believe in it. The day you will not be worthy of grace, He will switch you off. So long as the switch is on, everybody is worthy of grace.

You know, in Canada I was hungry all the time, extremely hungry. I wouldn't eat anything because I was afraid there would be some meat in it. Then they showed me their donuts and I said, "Wait a minute, this is nothing but pure sugar. I'm on a diet." I couldn't eat the salad because it gave me gas; I didn't want to bloat up and look pregnant. So what to eat? I began to think that it was not for me to eat at all. Then one day a girl brought a big chapati with vegetables on it. I said, "What is that?" She said, "Pizza." I said "Pazza?" By the time I learned to pronounce it, the whole thing was in my stomach. I ate it so fast and so furiously that it took me two days to get it out of my stomach. That was the last time I ate fast. It is very simple. Don't eat after 4:00 p.m. I am not asking whether you can or you can't. I am just offering a simple solution. After four, thou shalt not eat.

Student: *Sir, are you telling me my feeling of spiritual betrayal . . .*

Yogi Bhajan: I am not talking of spiritual betrayal, spiritual gain and the whole thing. Just try one thing at a time: After 4:00 p.m., stop eating. The body will automatically take care of itself. There is no way out. You must understand that there was a time in the world when there were no doctors, physicians, surgeons or anything. What did men do then? Thou shalt not eat after four o'clock. The moment the sun rays fall at an angle which is below the projective angle, you don't eat. The body is bound by virtue of the sunlight, which is the meditating, affectionate supplier of prana, to concentrate and rebuild the pranic molecules to heal themselves. By healing, I don't mean physical; to heal means mental, spiritual, past, present and future.

Yogi Bhajan: (To another student) You are a nagging husband to your friends.

Student: *To my friends, not as a husband.*

Yogi Bhajan: It is the same thing. You are married, you are not gay. You are married to a woman, but you don't nag her, you nag your friends. In other words, you are married to your friends and not to your wife. Nagging is only allowed in marriage—that is it. And it is only allowed in that marriage where you are sure the woman is very divine.

Student: *The block that I am working on is fear of failure. The primary motivating force in my life has always been fear. I have always had a lot of pressure placed on me by my family to be a star. I had all these opportunities.*

Yogi Bhajan: A star in the sky or in Hollywood?

Student: *An achiever, a super-achiever.*

Yogi Bhajan: You mean like Michael Jackson who doesn't get one night of sleep?

Student: *I don't know if they thought of me as Michael Jackson, but ....*

Yogi Bhajan: Have you ever understood that all that we earn or possess or have title to is going to be left here in the end?

Student: *I sort of understand that. Yes.*

Yogi Bhajan: What do you mean you sort of understand that?

Student: *I understand, but it doesn't keep me from wanting to do it.*

Yogi Bhajan: So you want it badly. Really? Then be calm about it. Sit down and show this entire brotherhood how calmly you can sit. Put your body in a straight line. Don't blink your eyes. Calm down. You want it badly, right? Then want badly to be calm. Want badly and be calm about it. Feel good? Thank you.

The underlying idea of all these men's courses I am teaching is extremely personal and very selfish. It has been grinded into me that the time has come to do my best, by any means, to clean you out so that you can stand out and feel who you really are, and not stand out like a donkey with a load of blocks on his back. Otherwise, people will see that your tracks are very deep and your hooves are very fine, but your "upper story" will be empty. You'll be called empty headed. Most people are empty headed. They go down the pathway making the same mistakes again and again.

Be straight and to the point. The greatest secret of life is, touch your own self. You know the phone company's slogan, "Reach out and touch someone?" I say, "Touch yourself and you will be picked up."

Student: *I believe my biggest block is that I don't believe in myself. I think this feeling developed in my mind when I was very young, ages four through six. My father was very dissatisfied with his own lack of success, so he had a tendency to say I wasn't good enough. I wasn't doing it right. I couldn't make the grade. I always had to try harder and harder. Somehow he just instilled in me the general feeling that I wasn't going to make it. No matter what I did, it wasn't going to work out.*

Yogi Bhajan: It did work out for the best, thanks to your father. It was thanks to your father that you chose me as your father. Thanks to me as father, you chose Guru Gobind Singh as father. Thanks to your misfortune, you got a beautiful fortune. What are you grumbling about? You got the best thing, thanks to a bad father. Sometimes it works out well. It just takes time. You have nothing to grumble about. Ten dollar fine for grumbling! He promised me he would never grumble. He forgot. In the future, he won't forget.

(Student hands over $10.) Now take this $10 and buy sweets, distribute them to the entire ashram, and tell them why you are doing it. Tell them the story and give them each a sweet. That is how the word gets spread.

Student: *My real interest is not to be controlled by the sexual drive. I really want to transform and transmute that energy.*
Yogi Bhajan: How old are you?
Student: *Twenty-four.*
Yogi Bhajan: How can you control it?
Student: *Kundalini Yoga class.*
Yogi Bhajan: Well, Kundalini Yoga class will not give you control but it will give you proportionate use. Controlling sexual energy is inviting insanity. I don't advise you to control it at all. I want you to have it and use it appropriately. Use it honestly.
Student: *Is there a way to do that while living in your lower chakras?*
Yogi Bhajan: You don't have to live in a lower chakra, but the lower chakras are very necessary. If early in the morning at about six o'clock you don't go into the second chakra and your sexual organ does not come up, you will be bored the whole day—it doesn't matter how good you are. It is called "morning glory", did you know that? If that little thing between your legs does not become stiff at the rising of the sun, your whole day will be unsatisfying no matter what you do. I'm not advising anything. I'm just telling you a simple fact. If your little thing does not stand up by the rising of the sun, at the point where the sun starts giving its rays, it is called "getting off the disc." You may be a king or a beggar, but the day is out. The One who made you made you perfect, just channel it right. It doesn't matter that it didn't work out well with some woman.

Student: *Well, at the time….*
Yogi Bhajan: No, it is not the time. You are just creating a block. Because your sexual experiences did not work out right, you are creating within yourself a strong and powerful hatred against the sexual relationship—don't do that. Take a cold shower. I'll tell you the best thing to do when you feel horny. Go into the ocean, stand up to your chest line in the water, let the waves hit you, and just jump and play with the waves. The wave is a female and you are the male. Do it for 40 days. You will have total sexual control of your body, your semen and the movement of your testicles. You can move your testicles as you want to. Try it.

Student: *Have you done this?*
Yogi Bhajan: It is a secret that I don't want to share, but this is written in the book I am reading to you.
Student: *So what is the benefit of transmuting the sexual energy to the higher centers?*
Yogi Bhajan: Each chakra has its own supply line. You transmute nothing, but sometimes some chakras are weak enough and they start overflowing. If the city of Los Angeles starts to overflow, the whole town will be a gutter.
Student: *So Kundalini Yoga is not advisable when you are horny?*
Yogi Bhajan: Kundalini Yoga is advisable to build all your chakras. Kundalini Yoga is for those who want to be the majesties on the Earth as humble human beings. Kundalini Yoga opens all chakras, balances all chakras and makes the flow between the consciousness and the chakras very, very together. Sexual energy is the sixth sense. But don't think that it is just energy toward sexual intercourse—that is just one part. It is also mental energy, mental intercourse. It is also the psyche, the power of the soul. It is also creativity. It is also related to the future. It is also related to your Self, your balance. And it is also related to your wanting to be great.
Student: *If you do Kundalini Yoga will it take care of the Self?*
Yogi Bhajan: Kundalini Yoga will take care of you whether you like it or not. It took care of me, why not you?
Student: *No preconceived notions about what it should do or what it shouldn't do?*
Yogi Bhajan: Preconceived notions about Kundalini Yoga are the most dangerous ideas. Then you are blocking yourself from receiving everything you have gone into it for. Just do it and enjoy it, and do it more and enjoy it more. It will keep bringing you to the level where you become nothing but Mr. Joy, Mr. Happy.
Student: *Without using sexual energy?*
Yogi Bhajan: My God, don't use anything. Neither use nor get used. You must learn at the age of 24, your visit to Earth is to enjoy the Earth. The moral of it is that you must not step on anybody's toe. The grace of it is, don't hurt anyone at all.

> *Neither use nor get used. You must learn at the age of 24, your visit to Earth is to enjoy the Earth. The moral of it is that you must not step on anybody's toe. The grace of it is, don't hurt anyone at all. The majesty of it is, give—and take nothing. But when you give, you have to take; so let it be God that you take.*

The majesty of it is, give—and take nothing. But when you give, you have to take; so let it be God that you take.

Student: *I have fear. It is not fear of something. It is just fear.*

Yogi Bhajan: Fear is one. What is fear?

Student: *I don't know.*

Yogi Bhajan: If you do not know what fear is then what are you afraid of?

Student: *I don't know.*

Yogi Bhajan: You don't have fear. You just talk about fear because that gives you sympathy. When you were young, did you ever tell a girlfriend that you were afraid and she kissed you? Are you really afraid? You came all the way to America and America eats people alive. It doesn't even steam them first. In the world, we steam vegetables to eat. In America, they don't steam people, they just eat them raw. They eat people raw and you are still alive and well, and yet you say you are afraid. Are you really afraid? Are you consciously afraid?

Student: *No, not consciously.*

Yogi Bhajan: Subconsciously?

Student: *I think so.*

Yogi Bhajan: Why do you think so? You are not made to think. No human being is made to think. Only animals think of the environmental dangers and act emotionally. Humans are not supposed to think; we rationally compute. We didn't know the word "compute" so we substituted the word "think." No human being can think. We were not meant to. That is not our structure. We rationally compute between good and bad. Compute. Compute now. Are you afraid or are you not afraid?

Student: *I am not afraid now.*

Yogi Bhajan: You are not afraid?

Student: *Yes and no.*

Yogi Bhajan: Oh, my God! Next.

Student: *I can't talk easily with anybody. When I see all these people, I can't talk at all.*

Yogi Bhajan: You are a scout. A scout speaks the truth. It doesn't matter who's listening. You don't care. You are strong. You have courage. You are an honest man. Speak.

Student: *I find again and again that I can't succeed with things.*

Yogi Bhajan: You can. You are an honorable scout. You succeeded as a scout.

Student: *I knew I could succeed. It was simple at that time.*

Yogi Bhajan: That is not true.

Student: *I succeeded because . . .*

Yogi Bhajan: You didn't succeed because of this or that. You are lying. Tell me why you succeeded.

Student: *I don't even know that I succeeded.*

Yogi Bhajan: I saw that paper. You are certified as an Eagle Scout. You succeeded. Why? Because you wanted to. So, what are you telling me now? Do you want to succeed or don't you?

Student: *I want success but I don't know if I want to succeed.*

Yogi Bhajan: Son, if you want to have success and you want to experience success, you have to succeed. You are all right. You could do it then, you can do it now, and you can do it forever. You are on oath: "I am a rover on oath. I shall serve and shall hurt none." You remember that. "I shall hurt none." You take an oath, you live by it and you die by it. You are very successful, by the way. Do you know that? Tell everybody.

Student: *I succeeded.*

Yogi Bhajan: No, you are successful.

Student: *I am successful.*

Yogi Bhajan: And I want to remind you of something. You are on oath to be successful. You are on oath to put your life at stake and rescue others. Is that not true? I am on the same oath. We know no failure. And we shall never fail. Never forget it! A scout is a scout from the day he takes his oath to the day he dies and faces God. God can change because he is all powerful. A scout never changes because he is a scout. I am a rover. I am your senior. I will not let you see yourself cry again. You shall succeed. You shall never fail. You remember the last line of the "*Song of the Khalsa?*" If the Khalsa falls there shall be no world at all. Do you understand that? When a rover fails, God trembles. When a scout fails, God commits suicide. That is the loss.

Student: *One of my major problems is trusting, having faith.*

Yogi Bhajan: You see how clever I am? I removed all questions about trust from both examination papers. Did you see the word trust anywhere? I don't want to get out of this business. We'll deal with trust next time. Am I very commercial now? Go ahead. This is a very trusting and trustworthy man. Watch what he says. See how he is going to juggle the words. He is a fantastic speaker, a perfect actor.

Student: *Many times in the past, I trusted people and made commitments and found myself ending up all alone.*

Yogi Bhajan: They left you on the road. That is what they'll do if you let them. If trust means to you that you shall not be betrayed then you are pretty naive. Trust has nothing to do with it. If I want to trust someone, I will keep him awake. If you marry someone and never wake her in the middle of the night, you will never have children.

The idea of trusting someone is to see that things are

done the way you want them done. Things must come through the way they are supposed to. All of that is trust. Trust means riding a horse. The saddle is tied, your feet are set, the reins are good, things are under control. You are in trust. Beyond this, trust doesn't mean a thing. Trust everybody and ride everybody. Don't trust what you cannot ride. A bucking horse is good for a rodeo but not for a long journey. Trust what deserves to be trusted. Don't trust what you desire to trust.

That is what trust means. I definitely intend to teach you how to trust. I don't trust myself. I don't trust my neighbor. I don't trust my above. I don't trust my below. Trust is a very simple environment. Whatever you can control and use to your best advantage, you can trust. Whatever you cannot control or use to your advantage, trust not at all. Here's a story for you:

A man was sleeping very deeply, he started snoring.
His son said, "Papa, there is a thief in the house."
The father said, "Idiot, stop talking and start snoring."
"Okay, Papa." So he started snoring, too.
When the thief passed between the father and son, both jumped up at the same time and knocked the thief flat on the ground.
As they tied him up, they both laughed. The father said, "Why are you laughing?"
The son answered, "Father, I was just being kind and merciful. When I spoke to you, I was just hoping that this idiot would run away. He didn't. I knew that you never snore. I knew that you had set a trap. You understood that he would never trust you, but he would trust your snoring. That's why he is on the floor and we are standing on top of him."

Well, we have had a good time and a bad time, good news and bad news. We want to be very practical, very realistic, and we want to take all the garbage out. You know what I mean? We would like to do it as fast as we can because we belong to a healthy, happy society. We may not belong to a holy society, but as far as I'm concerned, whosoever has nine holes is very holy. Let us put ourselves on the scale now and see how we weigh in relation to our blocks. I understand you are very scared to write; but I should tell you that it is the most practical, honorable method to get in touch with your own reality and help your own self. Self-help is the best.

Sat Nam.

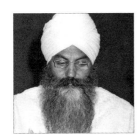

Man to **Man** 10

Being a Man

Circa 1985

The greatest tragedy that mankind was given to understand or believe was that you have to find God. You can never, ever find God. You are God—part of God. And the whole God is with you, behind you and within you.

■ Realize the Reality of Being a **Man**

■ Realizing **Success**

Realize the Reality of Being a **Man**

As a man, you have to learn this most fundamental fact: you have to carry yourself.

Today I sit among you as a man and I understand that if I share with you something that can in my eyes make you a man, I shall carry the day. Otherwise, neither my tomorrow nor yours will be good. What we are heading toward is a very unpeaceful, untranquil and dramatic situation. I am not against therapy, but life cannot become therapy. I don't believe that my life should be based on any therapy, no matter what I have paid for it. When therapy is needed I am willing to go for it. If medicine is needed I am willing to go for it. But to admit to myself that I am sick forever, I am a basket case forever, I need therapy forever, or to go through therapy just as a social thing, to let people know that I have somebody to talk to. I am willing to admit that I am not perfect, but I am not willing to admit that I am sick for all time, for all purposes, yet some of you are willingly declaring this. You are trying to tell everybody in the world that it is all right to be sick for a while but you are declaring to the world that it's all right to be sick all the time. That is not acceptable.

I am willing to agree that you didn't get parental care. I am willing to agree you didn't get parental security, I am willing to agree your wife is bitchy, I am willing to agree your neighbors are no good. I am willing to agree to anything you want me to agree to; but I am not willing to agree that all these pressures are responsible for you not being you—that I am not willing to agree to. So we are going to have a battle today, because I cannot accept that God didn't make you in His own image. *And* I do not want to accept that God could make you better than you are. I am convinced that each one of you is best in your own right. If we got messed up or goofed up, that can be handled. But the classic question here is a simple confrontation between you and you, as a Self, which you are very scared to do.

The main problem we face in life is "I don't want to confront myself. I don't want to know myself. I want somebody to tell me what is wrong with me, and somebody to tell me what the solution is, and even then I don't want to do it, and then there has to be parapsychology, there has to be psychology, there has to be psychiatry, there has to be counseling, there has to be environmental pressures or this spiritual thing."

But that is another thing. What is spiritual? And what is not spiritual? You don't want to listen to anybody you don't have to; you don't want to talk to anybody you don't have to; you don't want to be with anybody you don't have to; you want your pants and a tent, please wear it, but just carry it. Wear the pants, be the man, be the macho man, be the biggest man, but just remember, you have to carry whatever you are gracefully. As a man, you have to learn this most fundamental fact: you have to carry yourself.

You are a man, all right? Whether you have a long sexual organ or a small sexual organ, whether you are phobic or you are a maniac, whether your muscles are good or not, whether you ejaculate fast or not, whether you are dumb or silly, or whether you know your own self-condemnation or not, I am not looking into it. What I am trying to explain to you is that these things are not things at all. For every man, what I am going to share with you is how to understand that you are a man. You cannot become female. You may try, I mean to say, medically, it is possible. I am not saying it is not possible, I am not challenging the theory. I mean to say, you want to be a female, it is fine; you want to be a male, it is fine. You want to condemn yourself or you don't want to condemn yourself, that's fine, too. But God, don't you understand one thing? Now you've got it—that pound of meat hanging between your legs–what you do with it is your problem, not mine.

But that does not decide the life entirely, that's just one of the chakras. It's called the Second Chakra. You have a situation, bad and good; that's the First Chakra. You have fear and anxiety and the power to be; that's the Third Chakra. You have compassion and you want to give, or you are afraid to give, that's the Fourth Chakra. You want to speak, or you cannot speak, that's the Fifth Chakra. You want to be conscious, but you are not conscious, that is the Sixth Chakra. You want to know and you don't know, that is the Seventh Chakra. Finally, you want to be or not to be, that's the Eighth Chakra.

So every chakra has a polarity and each chakra makes you what you are; but the fact is, you are a human being and you have to carry yourself gracefully. It is not enough to be a man. You are not only to be a man but also to deliver yourself in the style of a man. It is the delivery of you, in a manly style, which is more important than your being a man, or you being phobic, you being neurotic, you being muscular, you being skinny, you being nervous, you being macho, or you being any and all of those qualities. Sand is red, green, yellow, pink or white; but sand is still sand. What you want to do with it, how you want to deliver it, which truck will carry it and which building will be built out of it, that's a different story. It is not enough to be a man that God made. Right?

Let us accept our elementary identity. That we are men is established, though you have some doubt about it, right? You even doubt that you are a man—that we will handle later. Let us read this. *[Editor's Note: Yogi Bhajan has one of his secretaries, a woman, come and read a summary from the men's questionnaires, completed earlier in the course.]*

Student: *Men seem to define themselves . . . this is based on the papers? (Students laugh)*

Yogi Bhajan: Go ahead.

Student: *Men seem to define themselves by how big or small their sex organ is; whether a woman wants him sexually or whether they want a woman; how successful they are in work; and whether they are accepted in the social group. Using this criterion, most men are left feeling very insecure and doubting themselves. No one identifies their Self through the experience of their soul. They live in such pain, holding on to the Western definitions of the masculine or manliness.*

The following are a few examples of men's thinking regarding their identity: little boys touching each other's genitals resulting in guilt or questioning whether they are homosexual; the social pecking order around me dictated subservience, abuse and humiliation; almost impossible for me to do anything but conform to peer pressure; I want to be great and don't feel like I am; I look at Playboy magazine and masturbate; I had sex three times a day; throughout most of my life people have told me I am no good.

Other issues were mother phobias. For example, I developed temper tantrums, became afraid of leaving my mother at home, but wasn't comfortable with her either; difficult time controlling ejaculation; rape-type sexual fantasies; scared to make it with a girl, mother's way to keep me by her side. Or, father phobias, for example, father was very emotional, dishonest and unreliable, used to yell and scream, wake me up in the middle of the night; I became afraid of men and afraid of fighting; father never beat me, but threatened with it a lot; my father was teaching me to tie my shoes and my father became very angry because I didn't get it.

Fear of success: My strong perseverance and determination was directed at my self-destruction; I lacked power to stay with a project or process, I am afraid to be the whole and powerful being I could be; I seem to do things that make me look bad; could not stick to something and do my best with it; I hate wealthy people but want to be wealthy, if I become wealthy will I hate myself?
(Students laugh)

Fear of failure: Great potential, average performance; afraid to demonstrate skills in group situations.

Yogi Bhajan: The ideal situation would have been for you to be honest; but the next best thing I could do was ignore what you were telling me in order to find out what you are. Many of you replied very honestly, many of you replied as best you could; reality was sorely lacking as I went through those papers, but I saw honesty and dishonesty, and I saw cheating and I saw clarity. The basic idea is not to feel that I agree with your feelings. I mean to say, it's a combat situation where you are challenging me, saying, this is my problem and I am telling you yes, these are your problems, thank you, add some more. But still, we can be successful.

Today we are going to discuss the key to success as a man. Let us turn to Mother Nature. Male is considered the Sun and female is considered the Earth. So what has happened? As males, we have visited the Earth. Our faculty and frequency of our psyche, totally, directly and indirectly, our positive and negative thought forms are practically running around a hub called female—that's what the female is. Female means the hub of the male. If you really look deep down into your successes and your failures, you will find that they ultimately boil down to your love, your anger, your feeling, your projection, and your betrayal of the female, because you are a byproduct of a female. You are born of a woman. Sun is born of Earth. In this life, you have forgotten that you are the Sun; you have forgotten your principles. Sun's only capacity is to be a light—heat, warmth and light.

Whenever you, as a male, try to succeed through any other caliber, any other capacity than being the light of day, you shall fail; because then you will be acting against your basic principle. Elementary principles you cannot cross. Whatever the situation is, you have to be warm, you have to be lively, and you have to be bright. There is no other choice. There is no other choice left for you—you must be what you are.

You are afraid of woman; you have mother phobia. You always wanted to be with your mother. But you have been made to leave, you are no longer happy with her, you can name 300 things that have been bothering you: Your mother was neurotic, she was angry with you all the time, you were scared. Now you are an adult and you have a woman and you want to be able to deal with her; but not the way your mother deals with you. Now, question is, your wife, your woman, your girlfriend is *not* your mother. Don't mix oil and water—it can't happen.

The fundamental position of failure is when you take your mother syndromes into your experience with your wife because she's available; she's the closest woman to you. It will end up a failure, because you cannot mix water and oil. It doesn't matter how much you churn it, when you leave it, water will be water, oil will be oil. Your wife cannot become your mother and your mother cannot become your wife. Reality is that you must acknowledge you are a

Meditation to Realize the Reality of а **Man**
September 21, 1985

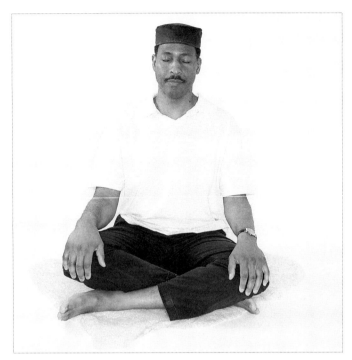

Part I

Posture: Sit in a meditative posture

Eyes: Closed

Mudra: None specified

Mantra: *I am a man, I am good.*

1. Repeat the mantra aloud three times and then meditate in silence on this thought:
I am a man, I am good.

As you meditate on the mantra, listen to the visualization: "Cross the physical level and go into Infinity on one word, one line: I am a man, I am good, I am a man, I am good, I am a man, I am good, I am a man, I am good. Create self-hypnosis. Tranquilize, go into your depth, repeat it, repeat it, repeat it, and totally go into the self-hypnotic state—every human has that right. Use just this one line: I am a man, I am good. Check your feeling, how honest are you about it? Work it out. Sit down and concentrate. Hypnotize yourself in this. Hypnotize. Go to sleep on this thought: *I am a man, I am good.*

"This is a priceless moment when you can assert yourself and bring yourself into a self-hypnotic state. Go into your deep self. Touch your soul. Touch your own Sun, your own light, your own soul. Don't let your mind create a game of you. Go into your depth. Your strength is in your life, your life is in your soul, and your power lies in your radiant body, the tenth body where your presence should work. When you present yourself before somebody, they say, Wow! The whole world should see light around you. Concentrate deeply on the self-hypnotic principle and bring your light out and repeat this mantra until you feel that stability: *I am a man, I am good*.
(**6 Minutes**)

"Begin to create a circle of light around you. Create a powerful circle of light around you. Go to sleep with the strength of this thought that you are a bright shining light. You are a man, you are a man, you are good, and you are surrounded by light. Heal yourself of any dark spot. You have to concentrate on your good, how good you are. Therefore, recite this again and again: *I am a man, I am good, I am light.*" (**3 Minutes**)

2. Stand and repeat the mantra together: *I am a man, I am good, I am light.* Repeat it several times until you experience it. In a class situation, have individual volunteers stand up and repeat the mantra and then explain what it means to them. What does it mean to be a man, to be good, to be the light? For individual meditation, state it just for yourself. Speak loudly, from your Navel Point. Declare yourself a man.

3. In the seated posture, touch the tip of the tongue with your upper palate. **Do not let them separate.** Repeat the mantra: *I am a man, I am good. I am light.* **3 Minutes**

Comments: If you keep the upper palate and the tongue together, whatever you speak you will hear. It will penetrate like a lance, right through you. You won't forget it.

To End: Inhale and relax. Take care of your face, your hands, relax your body. Feel good.

Part II

Mantra: *I am born to succeed, success is my elementary right.*

1. Repeat aloud, say it loud and clear.

2. Now put the tongue on the upper palate and speak it.

3. Speak normally: I am born to succeed, success is my elementary right. **Repeat 3X**

4. Now put the tongue on the upper palate, fix it there and say it: I am born to succeed, success is my elementary right. **Repeat 3X**

Note: Notice the difference between the two voices. Do you understand the difference of normal speaking and speaking with the tongue on the upper palate? That speaking goes right into the brain, the other doesn't. When you touch the tongue and pressurize the hypothalamus through the meridian point and the upper palate and you create this sound, you become that sound. You become that being.

Comments: Tell your children. Each man is born to succeed. Your success does not lie in how good you are in bed, your success does not lie in how rich or poor you are, your success does not lie in how much money you have or don't have, your success does not lie in how educated or uneducated you are. Your success lies in how jubilant, radiant and self-confident you are. Success is your birthright. Not to succeed is your creative habit, to succeed is your elementary desire and confirmed gift. Every man is born to succeed. Otherwise, it is an insult to God. You don't have to have prayer, you don't have to have religion, you don't need anything. Your elementary birthright is success. As a man you must succeed. You are born in the image of the Infinite, in the image of God. And there are ten trillion Gods in you. Every cell of you is a part of God. It's pranic Shakti. Therefore you cannot fail. You fail because you forget that success is your elementary right. Success is not your secondary right, success is your elementary right.

man—and even that is not enough. That's not enough. To acknowledge you are a man is not enough. First, you must acknowledge that you are a man and it is good.

Success is your elementary right. Failure is your secondary right. See the difference? It gives you a knot in your stomach to say it. If you just feel, just feel it—there is a lot of energy if you just feel it—success is my elementary right. Repeat it.

Students: *Success is my elementary right.*

Yogi Bhajan: Now you can't play the ego, because if you understand that success is your elementary right and failure is your secondary right, then you will not accept failure. That's where the ego will be helpful. Your own ego, which is otherwise a disaster will be totally helpful in this case. Understand that the will of God, the will of reality, is that each man succeed—each man is born to succeed. Did your mother tell you that?

Students: No.

Yogi Bhajan: Did your father tell you that?

Student: No.

Yogi Bhajan: Did your school tell you that?

Students: No.

Yogi Bhajan: I even didn't tell you that. I have to tell you today, because before today you were not ready to listen. But don't take it away from your children. Tell them. Each man is born to succeed. Say it loud and clear to yourself. I am born to succeed, success is my elementary right, I'll repeat.

Students: *I am born to succeed, success is my elementary right.*

Don't worry about how you feel about it; it goes right in. When you touch the tongue and apply pressure to the hypothalamus through the meridian point in the upper palate, and you create this sound, you become that sound. You become that being.

These secret yoga kriyas have been taught heart to heart, generation to generation, master to student, for centuries. I have brought you to a point where I want to give you my going-away gift. With the few years I have left, I want to give you these secret kriyas. Because you have stuck with me all these years, I want to also do my job. I want you to elevate yourself with a confirmed attitude: Success is your right; it's your primary right, it's your elementary right. It's not your secondary right.

Life is your primary right, so is success. There is no flaw in God. God is everywhere, but you can't see It, you can't

There is no flaw in God.

recognize It, because you do not have those eyes. There is bacteria in the water, but you have to have a special lens to see it. God is everywhere, but you have to see It within you, within you—with you. You have to become a lens to understand and see the dance of ten trillion cells, which is you. As those ten trillion cells can dance in absolute, successful, total rhythm, absolutely flawless, so you are the most successful manifestation of God. You are the most successful manifestation of God. The greatest tragedy that mankind was given to understand or believe was that you have to find God. You can never, ever find God. You are God—part of God. And the whole God is with you, behind you and within you. Stop searching for God and start searching to prove that God is your elementary right. Prove that the right to be successful is your elementary right.

Work is not for anything but to prove success. The whole system that is you is geared toward one point: Work to prove success. Not prove to anybody else; but to prove to you. Therefore, work is an experience of self-success. Whenever you work with the attitude or with understanding that work is an experience of self-success, you shall be successful. It is your elementary right. It is God. There is no other God. There is but one God and that is success through the experience of your work. Your work, your experience and your success is a manifestation of you and, within you, of God. It should be your primary achievement, because it's your primary right.

When you choose other things that is where you mess up, because you are manufactured. Your faculty, your quality, is to succeed. You don't have to worry about being successful. You don't have to hassle to be successful. You just have to flow with the energy of life, just being alive is successful. Just live and once you live, let others live. You will create such goodwill, everything will come to you. Live, let live. Live, let live. Every life, all energy will be with you because you are a living energy.

There was nothing, there is nothing, and there shall be nothing but you. If you succeed in recognizing you—in anything—it will become you.

Don't kill. That's why in the Bible, one of those Ten Commandments say, thou shall not kill. Once you kill, you can kill yourself, because there is nothing outside of you but you. All is you. All is the same. There is but one God. There was nothing, there is nothing, and there shall be nothing but you. If you succeed in recognizing you—in anything—it will become you. If you can see in your hands, all hands, then all hands will become you.

The greatest power of a man is when he stands before another man and he becomes that man. He becomes double, triple, quadruple, ten, twenty, hundred, thousand, million. Merge, merge, merge, merge and flow. A drop of

On Being a Man

We are starting an offensive; we want to cover all our neurosis and cleanse them out so they are no longer your problem. We want to make you capable of demonstrating your own strength.

Directions: Stand up; keep your eyes closed, speak as loudly as you can. Talk about the phenomenon 'I am a man, I am good, I am light,' as if you are addressing the entire universe without fear, without reservations, and without anything else.

Guru Terath Singh: *I am a man, I am good, I am a light. I am a man, I am good, I am a light. I am a man, I am good, I am a light.*
Yogi Bhajan: *Explain.*

Guru Terath Singh: *I am a man, God is in me and the light of God glows through me.*
Yogi Bhajan: *Keep on talking.*

Guru Terath Singh: *When I act in that flow from God, I am good. When I act in that flow, I am a light. When I act in that flow, I am a man.*
Yogi Bhajan: *Guru Bachan, stand up. Speak.*

Guru Bachan: *I am a man, I am good and I am the light. I am a man, I am good and I am the light.*
Yogi Bhajan: *Explain.*

Guru Bachan: *I am a man because God has made me a man. I am good because God only makes good and I am a light because God only makes from Himself that which contains the light.*
Yogi Bhajan: *John, stand up.*

John: *I am a man...*
Yogi Bhajan: *Loud, the whole world has to hear you.*

John: *I am a man and I work on myself all the time bringing out ... generating love and compassion, goodness to mankind ... to all the human beings throughout the world, bringing peace and happiness to the world, world in myself and world around me ... my associates. My whole life is to generate love and compassion, kindness, ... friendship, well-being amongst all to bring ... and peace to the man, which ... love and compassion as well because I am the light and I set the way. ..... It's your way ... which is not wrong, ... to generate compassion in the way, ... all the way. Without compassion, without love, without Divinity everything is ... with it the world will be saved, it takes each one of those each individual ... to generate this love and compassion ....*
Yogi Bhajan: *The other John*

John: *I am a man, I am good, I am a light. I am a man, I am good, I am a light. I am a man, my role is to uplift and to trust my brothers ... establish the trust with others and to trust others. I must have faith in God and to live with God ...*
Yogi Bhajan: *Guru Charan (Long Beach)*

Guru Charan: *I am a man. I am a man, I am God, I am good, I am the light. My light travels to the ... streets of the universe, and light opens the path before me and light touches and uplifts others, gives them hope, my light is warm, my light is everlasting, it has no beginning and no end, that light is infinite, that light is life, that light is love, that path is the destiny of the love, and destiny of service. I am a man, and I serve that light, I am that light, and I share that light. That light expands the understanding, expands, that light becomes brighter as I become a man.*
Yogi Bhajan: *Vikram*

Vikram: *I am a man because God has made me a man. I am good because I am from God and God is good. I am the light because I am the Sun. I project with the light of God, this God has given me to project, to lead, to warm, to comfort, to nurture, to teach, to help, and to give support to all around me. I am a man because I have to lead. I have to lead because that is the path. The light is given to me by my Guru. In the path of truth, as the truth is to walk as a man, the commitment and the courage to lead the way to give and share, to help, to serve. My service comes from humility, my humility comes from my strength, my strength comes from my life, my life comes from my goodness, my goodness comes from God, because I am a man.*
Yogi Bhajan: *Sat Peter*

Sat Peter: *I am a man, I am good, I am light. I am a man because I have been given a choice by freewill to choose the path projecting light, love. It's the grace of God that has given me that choice and the vision to see the power of my own soul, the power to uplift, the power to change the environments around me and the power to appreciate the light of God in every soul, the power to shine without shadows, without fear.*

rain, and another drop of rain, and another drop of rain, drop of rain, drop of rain, drop of rain, then a brook of rain, brook of rain, then a little river, river of rain, big river of rain, rain, rain, rain, ocean of rain. It's all rain, from the ocean, clouds of rain. Rain, drops of rain. River of rain, ocean of rain, it's all rain. That is the system. Drop by drop. Merge with the merge. With the drop, merge; drop, merge; drop, merge. Become a brook. Become a river, become an ocean. Same drops become clouds; same drops become rain; same drops merge, become rain. Become brook, become river, become ocean.

All is you. All is the same. There is but one God. There was nothing, there is nothing, and there shall be nothing but you.

Meditation to Turn Yourself into **Water**
September 21, 1985

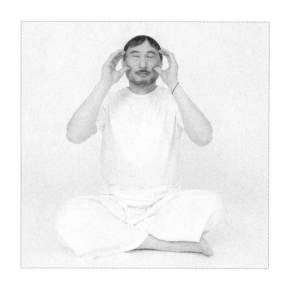

Posture: Sit in a comfortable meditative posture.

Mudra: Push the thumbs into the base of the cheek bones. Push in and up.

Eyes: Close the eyes and roll them up to the Brow Point.

Mantra: I am all, all is me.
Put the tongue on the upper palate, just behind the teeth. Keep the tongue on the upper palate as you repeat the mantra: I am all, all is me. **1 Minute**

Maintain the posture, keeping your tongue on the upper palate and pressing the cheek bones with your thumbs. Meditate. Become a pouch of water; dissolve your muscles and your bones. Your skin is nothing but a pouch of water. Pull your meridians up, concentrate, let the hypothalamus work.

Continue applying pressure and think these thoughts: "Because God cannot come to Earth and shake hands with you, God gave you a chance to make you as you. Good and bad, others may think. You are the best. If God could have produced better than you, He would have. . . . It's Almighty God, He produced you, accept it—and accept it now."

Consciously talk to yourself. Turn yourself into the *tattva* of H_2O, water, agua—that will take away the neurosis. It is a simple therapy, costs nothing. Plug into the central nervous system and just turn yourself into water. Concentrate in this position, let the energy flow. Let it rinse from you the deficiencies and defects that you create because of other people and their thoughts about you. **8 Minutes**

To End: Now inhale deeply, hold the breath and feel good. 15-30 seconds. Exhale and relax. "God has kissed you on the cheeks, right?" Shake out your hands. Relax.

Comments: Give yourself a chance. Try to understand, in a conscious way, that you can totally eliminate all your neurosis—now. Every other therapy will take about six months to six years and thousands of dollars, and still you may end up nuts. But you yourself can do it this minute. Because you have stimulated the central channel and forced that energy through the hypothalamus; you have activated both the Ida and the Pingala; all you have to do is just understand that you are you. It is a "do-it-yourself" kit. If it is true that you are born in the image of God, if it's true—first believe. It's a belief system. Then you are born to succeed. You are not succeeding because you don't understand that you are born to succeed, it's your elementary right.

This therapy has been known to mankind for thousands and thousands and thousands of years. People used to heal themselves. Water keeps all levels equal, so neurosis and wisdom will come into equilibrium.

Just understand: there is no God but one God. The only right man has, his primary right, is to be born and to be successful. Failure is your secondary thing. To be neurotic and unwise is your third. To be emotional—be a yo-yo—is your fourth. Concentrate on your first and then the opportunities will come to you. Where there is a light, all comes there.

The third project that I am going to take on with you today is fear—fear. What is fear? Oh! Give me a break! Come on, you all know English. What is a fear?

Student: Lack of trust in God.

Yogi Bhajan: Lack of trust in God. That's too philosophical. What is a fear?

Student: Lack of trust in self.

Yogi Bhajan: Lack of trust in your Self, still, what is a fear? It's an instinct to protect yourself. Fear is a natural instinct for self-protection against something that you are not sure of. It's automatic. Somebody says, "Boo!" and you blink your eyes; you close your eyes, automatically. The fear of being hurt will make your eyes immediately close, on their own. You can pick up that fear syndrome within the aura, 18 feet both sides. Fear is nothing but a self-protecting device. So if you know, if you understand, that there is nothing to protect, you will not have fear.

What are you protecting against? You are protecting against bad people. Actually, there are no bad people; every person has bad and good within him. If you know how to take the good out of the person and leave the bad with the person, you are the best. What are you afraid of? You are afraid of bad company, right? What is bad company? There is no such thing as bad and good. It's either half and half or 40:60 or 70:30; it's a proportion. Everything is a proportion. It's a ratio in proportion.

What do you have to do with the bees? Take the honey and get away. Yes. If you entangle with the bees you will meet your end. If you are not dead, you come out swollen, at least. You know what I am saying? You want the honey, get the honey, then get away. This is the fear: if I am going to get the honey, I am going to get caught. So what then? Then *earn* the honey. Don't steal it. What did man do? He created a way for himself to get the honey. He created a fire, built up a lot of smoke and when that big cloud of smoke went into the beehive, the bees fled away, giving man a chance to get the honey. That is what you do; you build up a line of activity; you build up a smoke screen. You build up an identity around you, a diplomacy around you, to cover your fear. This entire build up is to cover your weaknesses.

There is no such thing as bad and good. It's either half and half or 40:60 or 70:30; it's a proportion. Everything is a proportion.

You cover yourself against your own weaknesses. Never try to cover against your own weaknesses, just try to know your weaknesses and get rid of them. They say, "Drop them in the desert. They will die of thirst." Then you can walk straight. Whenever you know your weakness . . . Repeat it.

Students: Whenever you know your weakness...

Yogi Bhajan: Do not cover it.

Students: *Do not cover it.*

Yogi Bhajan: Get rid of it.

Students: *Get rid of it.*

Yogi Bhajan: How does it sound?

Students: Good.

Yogi Bhajan: It's very good.

The time, the money, the energy you waste to cover your weakness, is going to kill you. Listen, you may put a dead man at the bottom of the sea, but he is going to come up. Weakness is weakness, it will come up. Drop it. Whenever there is gangrene, what do they do? They cut it off. Habitual weakness is gangrene. Either cut it or it will kill you. Is that understood? Thou shall not kill; so cut it. There is no choice. Cut it. Cut—you know? You can learn it from Hollywood. When things go wrong, they say, "Cut." They do it, why can't you do it? *(Students laugh)* Call it yourself—"Cut." If there is a fight between a husband and wife, call "Cut." She says, "What is it?" You say, "That's it. No more movie." Cut.

We are not going to work on this subject anymore. That's it. Cut. Call "Cut." Make it a primary practice in your life that when there is trouble and you find yourself getting in too deep, rather than putting your head in the sand and suffocating and dying, just call cut—no more. Don't continue the drama, because each drama will become trauma. Each trauma will cost you your life, part of your life. For each trauma you pay through your life. You have nothing—except life. You turn your life into labor and your labor turns into money and money buys other services and goods to keep the life, to keep you alive. Is that true or not? So you have nothing but Life, so you had better butter it in the right way.

Never try to cover against your own weaknesses, just try to know your weaknesses and get rid of them. They say, "Drop them in the desert. They will die of thirst."

Who gave you life? God. God gave you life. You have nothing but life and you have to turn that life into labor, precious, expert, productive labor that will give you the medium, money. Money is the medium of goods and services. Money is what money does. It's an exchange store, money is nothing but an exchange store. Therefore, don't ever use money as a tool. If I am telephoning someone and somebody is listening, the exchange starts interfering, will anybody use that line? Money is an exchange, a store. God has given you life; you have nothing but life. You turn that life into labor; labor is bought and sold at a price, that's called money. Therefore in your entire life, never use money as a means to control.

But you want control. Don't you? You all want control. You cannot use money as a control, you cannot use life as a control, then how will you find control? Elevate. The only way to control things in life is to make others successful. Elevate. Don't control people to make them subordinate. Control people to elevate them; in gratitude, they will be good to you. Never ever try to control anybody. When you control somebody, even the leash on your dog, you are tied in with the dog. You can't let the leash go; you can't let the dog go; you can't let yourself go. Have you seen somebody hustling with his own dog? Dog wants to run, he doesn't want to run. He pulls on the leash, the dog pulls him. He falls down and breaks his butt. The dog runs away. Afterward, the dog comes home without a leash. He has lost the leash. Never be a leash and never put a leash around anybody, never collar anyone.

When I became a student in Kundalini Yoga, the first lesson I learned was "you are not initiated." I had to repeat that, "I am not initiated, I am not initiated" for one week. This was my mantra, "I am not initiated." Can you believe how idiotic I must have looked? I am not initiated, I am not initiated, I am not initiated—seven days. I couldn't even ask a question about why I was being asked to repeat this. And if, after seven days, I had gone to my teacher and he had asked "why are you not initiated?" and I had only replied, "I am not initiated," then I would have had to repeat it seven more days until I found the answer. As long as I didn't discover the answer, I would have to keep on initiating myself, "I am not initiated." But God was kind to me, merciful, after seven days when I went for an audience with my master and he told me, "You are not initiated." I said, "Sir, I have initiated myself, being not initiated." *(Students laugh)*

That was the answer—the correct answer; because if you cannot initiate yourself, nobody can initiate you. You have to initiate yourself, being not initiated. It means you have become fearless. You are ready for the teachings—and that was the key—that was the puzzle that each student had to solve. So you sit seven days, "I am not initiated," but if you are not initiated, then what the hell are you doing there. What do you want? There were a million questions running through my mind, a million. We went through it, I asked, I discussed, but I kept saying, "I am not initiated, I am not initiated…" I felt like such an idiot. *(Students laugh)*

I kept repeating and asking myself, "I am not initiated. What the hell I am doing here? I am not initiated. What's going on around me? I am not initiated. Why I am sitting and saying it? I am not initiated—looks idiotic to me." I had to keep on saying it and keep on questioning it and then, finally, the answer came to me: "I am not initiated, I am initiating myself. I am living myself. I am successful myself. I don't need public opinion." Nanak says, *'En janta ke paas kuch nahi.'* These people are just like you. They just pretend to be experts to take away your money. They are all after your money because money comes from labor and labor comes from life; they are all after your life. Nobody wants you. When you are dead, they box you up and put you in the ground. Don't you understand? Only a few visit your graveyard, on special Sundays, and then only to look good. Nobody does it for you. All these hugs and kisses, has anybody taken the coffin out and gone in and kissed and hugged you? How many of you have done it, huh?

This is all about life. Life is given to you as a gift and life has also been given as a gift of success; so have no fear of being successful. Fear is an instinct to protect your life. Not to protect you from being successful, you mix it up. Fear is an instinct to protect your life. If somebody pokes a finger in your eyes, your eyelid will close. Fear is an instinct to protect life, but it's not an instinct to protect you from success. You use it to protect you from success, because you use fear for anything. But it has no other purpose but for life. And life can always be turned into labor. Don't be afraid of labor: this job I am not qualified for, that job I am not qualified for, and this job doesn't make me feel qualified. You make excuses because you are afraid of labor.

You have the right to charge a price for your labor and you have the right to exchange through labor, others' labors, goods and services. But you have no right to be afraid of labor—or success.

Palate and Tongue Kriya

September 21, 1985

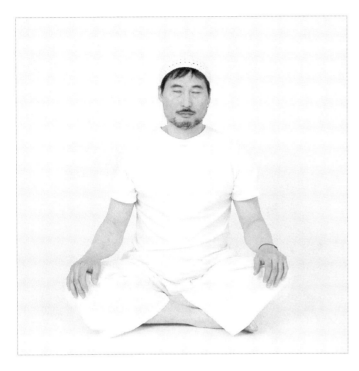

Part I

Posture: Sit upright in a meditative posture. Place your tongue on your upper palate. Don't let the tongue separate from the palate as you repeat these affirmations:
I am, I am. (3X)
I have no fear. (3X)
I have labor. (2x)
I have life. (1X)
I have profit. (1X)
Life. (1x)
Wife. (1x)

Comments: "See how difficult 'wife' is? Say life, it is convenient, say wife, it is difficult. I am not kidding, because in life you carry yourself, in wife you carry two. It becomes a double-weight sound. These words are not manufactured just because somebody spoke them, they have a certain basic meaning."

Part II

Posture: Keeping the tongue pressed into the upper palate continue with these affirmations:
With my light. (1x)
I shall carry my wife. (1x)
With my light. (1x)
I shall carry my wife (1x)
And children, too. (1x)

Comments: At this point, most of you will be laughing. "As you expand the family you will find it more and more difficult; it is true. I just wanted you to experience it."

There is one phrase, in English, called crystal clear. Have you heard of that? What do you mean by crystal clear? Guru Charan, stand up and explain to this audience your notion of crystal clear. Now listen to him very carefully.

Guru Charan: Crystal clear is when you tune-in to yourself; in tuning-in, the God exists within you. You are everything and in that clarity, you realize *Cherdhi Kala*. Maha mantra—keep up! When you experience that clarity, when you experience that 'keep up!', you have faith, you have trust, you have Divinity. You experience crystal clear.

Yogi Bhajan: Great, Sada Sat stand up.

Sada Sat: Crystal clear is without a flaw. Crystal, total clarity, like a pure white crystal, pure white light...

Yogi Bhajan: Green crystal is not a crystal?
(Students laugh)

Yogi Bhajan: No it's all right. Good, good, sit down. Now ask me.

Students: What's crystal clear?

Yogi Bhajan: That which is clear, like crystal.
(Students laugh)

Yogi Bhajan: That's the difference between me and you. You like to explain things and woman hates it when a man explains anything to her other than what it is. That's why you have such sick relationships. Women don't like you doing that. You have a sex problem, your wife is divorcing you, she calls you a shit, you say to her, 'you are an idiot, you are a bitch,' she is calling you 'a dog,' and all this fighting is only because of one thing: you like to explain to a woman the meaning of things that don't mean anything other than simply what it is. Never, ever explain to a woman anything more than what it exactly means in the dictionary, then you will have no trouble. Call "Cut!" Call it quits.

Any man who has a crystal clear consciousness will see that a woman is a lunar subject, and if he doesn't realize it, he will have her around his neck for the rest of his life, and you can't handle it. Whenever a woman talks to you, remember, and you can quote me on this: "Whenever a woman talks to you, she wants to multiply with your moon. The moment you allow her to talk to your moon, to multiply or entangle with your moon, you will become a lunatic." I am giving you a million dollar tip without even charging for it. If a woman says, "Darling, it is a fine day," she is involving you. Involve yourself first! You involve her. If you don't involve yourself in a communication with a woman you are a failure.

Just remember: Never be cut and dry with a woman. She is the lunar principle. She needs you when she talks to you; she needs you when she is with you; she needs you. Good or bad, I won't discuss today. But I will discuss this simple communication principle. She says, "It is a fine day." You reply, "Oh yes, it is." It is small, it is confirming, it is "oh, yes" communication, it is involvement. It is called buttering the soul of the mate. No commitment, no involvement, no cost, nothing.

At the same time, if you learn to say it in a way that can rebuke a woman, you can hurt her more than any rebuke you may want to give to her. She says, "It is a fine day." And you say "good enough" and you are found out, you don't have a chance. No chance. You may buy her a billion dollars worth of presents, you can do anything you want, but when you reply with curt language and then you are actually found out? You think she isn't going to wrap you up as a present? If she doesn't, she is not a woman; there is something wrong with her.

North Pole Combination: The Psyche of the Battered **Woman**

Yesterday I was counseling a battered woman. What is a battered woman? A battered woman is one who has been beaten up by circumstances; she's beaten up, gets angry and gets release. Okay? That's what it is. She has only one desire: to provoke you to the point of insanity so that you become physical. When you beat her up and you're angry and yell and scream, she loves it. Then you beat her up and beat yourself up, some men also break the walls, break the windows, the whole thing. Sixty to $600 worth of loss, plus you beat her up. After that you both get released, you may even have intercourse and go to a movie and all that; but that release ... Yeah, yeah, a lot of you do it, I know that. It's called North Pole combination; North Pole combination or North Pole connection.

North Pole combination means that you heat up, you boil over, you beat up, you create that chaotic situation and then you both trump, relax and make love, become real; and that release is greater than 100 sexual ejaculations. It is needed; it's so good for the nervous system. And that's what the battered woman does; she creates opposition, she creates that chaos. She nails you down, she pins you up, she provokes you, she does everything she can. It is so systematic. She nags you to death. You don't know what to do with it. You can't handle it, most men can't handle it. They want peace. They leave the house. The moment the dialogue starts they leave the house, they shut off the telephone, they do so many precautions. There is no precaution for it. Stay crystal clear.

Yoga Therapy Exercise for **Anger**

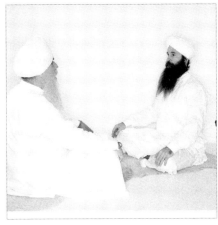

Step One: Agreement

Therapist to Client: You have agreed to this as a volunteer and you are willing to go through it.
Client to Therapist: Yes.

Step Two: Exercise

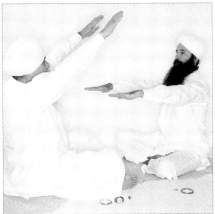

Client: Stretch your arms forward from the shoulder, fingers straight and palms facing the floor. Hold the arms as steadily as you can. Look into the therapist's eyes. Concentrate and be as angry as you can. Try to hold on to your anger.

Therapist: Look into the client's eyes. Begin by striking the back of the hands firmly. Clear your energy between each strike by gently shaking the hands. As you continue striking, the force gradually becomes lighter and lighter, moving toward a light tapping. Ask the client to inhale deeply and hold the breath. Continue tapping and then have the client exhale as you each relax.

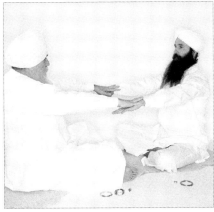

Commentary (from the Student): The first few strikes really intensify the anger, concentrating it, taking it from a diffused, undifferentiated anger toward a more compact, very tight feeling, clarifying the anger. The effect is almost stroboscopic, a flashing, as the force is applied to the hand. The first section is very intense as the feeling becomes concentrated and it starts to differentiate the experience, affecting the nervous system much like a jeweler or gem cutter fastening a stone. The right and left side begin to orient and then, after it's been concentrated, this differential begins to vibrate that anger and starts shaking different parts of it until it just crumbles, allowing it to release from a 'feeling state' and become an 'intellectual' experience that you can drop. There also seems to be a stimulation of the vagus nerve.

Yogi Bhajan: You are not angry now?
Student: Right.

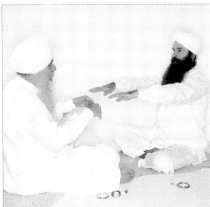 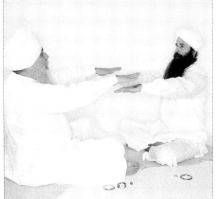 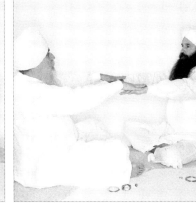

Never ever blame a woman, she is just a reflection. That's the lunar principle. That's the greatest problem you all are suffering with; you are suffering with the problem of partnership. She is suffering with the problem of reflection. Can you see through her? Can she see you through herself? Yes. If she cannot see you through herself, you don't exist. You think by money, by sexual relationship, by feeling her, kissing her, hugging her, giving her this, taking her that, you are going to continue? Forget it—won't work. Never has worked, nor will work, nor can work. Every woman desires to see a man through herself.

Let her pass crystal clear. Crystal will not burn out, it will not be scratched, it will not be roughed up. There is no problem. As a man, be crystal clear with the female you deal with, anytime, all the time, in all circumstances—personal and impersonal. If she is a neurotic help her. If she is a psychotic, help her. If she is in love, help her. If she hates you, help her. If she abuses you, help her. If she loves you, help her. Crystal clear.

You have only one role for a woman—you are a solid help. She will never trust you. She will never love you, she will never be with you. She doesn't need you. She can masturbate. She can have as many men as she wants. She can lie to you, she can make a fool of you. She can do anything she wants. But you are born out of her, she knows you. She knows you by instinct. So why play games? A woman needs in a man only one thing. You think she needs money? You are crazy. You think she needs your body? You are a fool. She needs your wisdom? Shut up. She needs your games? Forget it. She knows everything. All she needs is one thing and one thing only—you are there, always and ever—and this must be in her crystal clear. Got it? Now you understand crystal clear?

We are basically angry people. We create war, we believe in war, we believe in killing. We are angry at people whom we love. Because we use love as a hook, we want them to be under our control. We get angry when they don't listen to our line of action and we create little wars in which we win or we lose—that's the situation. Sometimes we lose, sometimes we win, but basically we are warmongers. We are warriors. We are social warriors. We keep our little world in a constant state of social turmoil, cultural wars, and we create them among those whom we love the most.

Actually, the purpose of love is to give—not to take. Don't love someone if you have to take something. Take it by right, by fight. But if you have to give, then love. Love and giving go together. Love and control do not go together. We are angry because we have been betrayed, we are angry because we have failed, we are angry because somebody pulled the rug out from under our feet, we are angry because we were deceived, we were cheated, and on and on. You can say a hundred things. But actually, if you want to look at it, you are angry because you couldn't be wise.

Wise men are never angry men. If you ever want to be wise, never be angry; that's all it takes. If you ever want to just satisfy yourself, or consider yourself to be wise, if that is ever the intention—ever—it won't happen by reading books or by following a religion or a philosophy or the greatest teacher. None of these will make you wise. You shall only be wise when you shall not be angry. Not to be angry is called being wise. Is that understood?

Suppose you are afraid and you feel the danger. The fear and the danger make you react. Insecurity and anger have to blend in order to become revengeful; they bring you vengeance and vengeance is your small scale war between you and whatever is around you. Do you understand that? But if you utter just one word—unfold. Let it unfold. Let it unfold. The secret of your success is to let it unfold. Don't use anger, don't use insecurity, don't use danger, don't use any stimulant. These are all stimulants. Vengeance is the most powerful stimulant for the human being, but it won't make you successful and you want to be successful. The key to being successful is to let it?

If you do not want the effect, don't cause the cause.

Students: Unfold.

Yogi Bhajan: Let it unfold. Let it?

Students: Unfold.

Yogi Bhajan: Let it create the environments with your patience; it will pay a lot of dividends.

Never love a woman who you do not want to unfold. Never marry a woman who you do not want to unfold, neither be with a woman who you cannot stand to see unfold herself. Let every woman unfold, because no nectar can be picked to make honey, the sweetness of life, if the flower does not unfold. Every flower has to unfold in order to give you sweetness of life. Every person is a flower, only let it unfold. Your power is in making it unfold. When the sun shines, flowers?

Students: Unfold.

Yogi Bhajan: When the sun shines?

Students: Flowers unfold.

Yogi Bhajan: And when the sun is gone, then? They close. So you can only pick the nectar when the flower is unfolded.

A closed woman shall give you nothing in your life but weight, which you have to carry, or even drag. It will make you sweat and miserable. That is where you buy misery in your life. You deal with unfolded creatures. You are the sun, you are the light. Shine and everything shall unfold. Let it unfold. The entire mystery shall unfold before you.

There are ten trillion Gods dancing in you called cells. Each human is a living psyche of the total Infinity and beyond. Holding you back is your being small, your anger, your opaqueness. Your shutters are shutting you up. Your blinds are blinding you. Let it unfold. What can happen to you? Who has ever lived? You don't want to die now, but do you want to die later? The only way to not die and to live forever—can anybody tell me? There is one way, the only way—my way—let it unfold. You will live forever.

Elevate everybody to such fulfillment that they will be left with no option but to unfold. Those who will drop, they will rot, they will stink. Bit by bit it will happen, it's just like a big huge tree. Some things do not ripen; they fall, they rot, they go away. That is the action of fate. But those who belong to destiny, they shall unfold, they shall ripen, they shall come to fulfillment. When somebody pulls a number on me, I am very happy inside and outside I pretend concern. That stimulates prayer, doesn't it? Isn't this how we work in 3HO?

Every year before Summer Solstice something goes wrong. Heavy clouds come. Everybody starts chanting, meditating, then we go to Summer Solstice, we meditate; the whole summer we meditate. Then comes the fall and we come back and we say, well, we are good and well.

The greatest thing in a human is that which is within you, which leads you to prayer. Prayer is a very humbling experience. But it's the greatest power. What is a prayer? You think it's a great thing or a small thing. It's the greatest thing, because prayer is when you tune yourself into your "real or imaginative higher Self, Infinite Self." What's a God? Bigger than you? More powerful than you? Aha! That's not true. God is within you; ten trillion Gods are within you. All that prayer does is put them together. It makes you fold your hands to unfold your strength.

Whenever you tune-in, in your strength, to Infinity and you do it in a crystal clear manner, you understand that you are part of that Divinity. You manifest you again—and that is success. Prayer is not a ritual, nor is it a right, nor is it a reality. It's an experience of folding yourself within yourself. Prayer is when you fold yourself within you and unfold your energy. It's a complete action. Prayer is a complete action. You fold within and unfold your energy. You are complete.

Prayer is not a ritual, nor is it a right, nor is it a reality. It's an experience of folding yourself within yourself. Prayer is when you fold yourself within you and unfold your energy. It's a complete action. Prayer is a complete action. You fold within and unfold your energy. You are complete.

Fear is there to protect you. Don't fear success, don't fear unfolding, don't fear cutting what is going to kill you.

If somebody thinks I am a devil, that person is meditating on devil. He is seeing in me the devil in himself or herself, through her eyes, through her thoughts, through his eyes, through his thoughts, the devil is projecting. If somebody sees me as a God, then God is projecting. I am, I am. It will never change. What you are unfolding at any given time, at any given space, is called karma. It is called cause; and for every cause, you shall reap the effect. If you do not want the effect, don't cause the cause. "So shall you sow, so shall you reap."

Then what should you sow? "Early to bed, early to rise, makes a man healthy, wealthy and wise." You don't have to go to the East, to Japan, to learn it. I mean, it's right with us here. "So shall you sow so shall you reap." If you won't listen to me, you will weep. Just understand that. Cause has an effect, equal and opposite—Newton's Third Law of Force. Or, call it theory of karma, doesn't matter what you want to call it. The question is, what you shall sow so that you can reap. You have to reap; you have to sow. Is that clear? It's clear like crystal? You have to sow and you have to reap; you are a man. You have to turn your life into labor and the fruit of your labor should be excellent. How can that happen? "Early to bed, early to rise, makes a man…"

Students: Healthy, wealthy, and wise.

Yogi Bhajan: What else do you want? If you are healthy, wealthy and wise, what is the problem then? Is there any problem? Isn't it simple?

Just remember, by early evening rest and by early morning wake up. Keep your life force in a very exalted space. The most difficult thing for a human is when the sun is down and its rays start projecting at 60° then 40°, then 20°, then at zero, then you call it sunset. In the morning, at dawn, sun is 20°, 40°, 60°, that way, until it reaches 90°, then it start sliding the other way. Just see that your energy goes that way, see that it matches the natural rhythms of the Sun. Men who are not especially careful about themselves, who are not well trained, who keep late hours, are acting against nature.

Be a compass, just point toward north. Be one pointed—always point toward north. What is north? It means nothing. Have you gone to the North Pole? It's nothing, all snow.

There is nothing. I flew over it once. The captain said, "we are going over the exact North Pole right now," everybody went to the window. You wouldn't believe what a rush it was, everybody trying to see. And you know? There was nothing but a lot of snow down there. *(Students laugh)* And if you are ever there, you will freeze to death. There is nothing, just nothing.

It's a short trip to this Earth, averaging 65 to 85 years, maximum a hundred, you got to go. Just understand that it is just a hotel, a big hotel where you live and you pay. You pay the rent. When you become a parent, that's what it is. Pay the rent—and living costs. What do you pay for living on the Earth? Pranas—the life, the pranic breath. You turn the pranic breath into labor and you pay the rent. Whenever you go, they close you like a book, put you in a closet (they call it a 'coffin') and dig a piece of land and stick you in. Isn't that your library? Earth. Then they say 'dust to dust,' soul to the rest.

There are two ways your soul can go: either to rest or to rust, whichever you want. You can cause the cause to cycle and cycle and cycle and cycle or you can cause the cause to end and end and end, forever. Why can't you cause the cause to end? Because you do not let it unfold, not only others but even in yourself. So unfold yourself. Here is a kriya for it.

Sleep Tips: Where to Lay Your **Head**

As a male, never sleep north-south. You are totally blending your energy with the axle and the axle is zero. The axle has no movement.

People of wisdom know that when a person is ready to die, they put him north and south, so that he can die easily. So the soul can leave. You need the soul, you need the energy. Sleep west or east, east or west, doesn't matter, whichever suits you. Everybody can afford a $5 compass, right? So you can always know where north is. You should always know where north is.

Kriya to Free Yourself from **Karma**
September 21, 1985

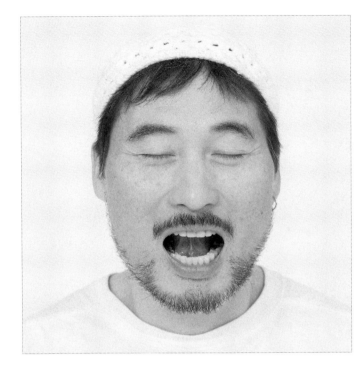

Posture: Sit straight in a meditative posture. Turn your tongue backward as much as you can, touch the soft palate of the mouth and don't release the tongue. Keep the tongue in contact with the soft palate as you chant in a monotone.

Comments: Keep your jaw as relaxed as possible. These two channels of Ida and Pingala (Yogi Bhajan touches the left and right posterior sides of his head, behind the ears) cross to the sahasrara and start activating. They will become very hot.

Chant: Har Har Gobind

Time: 2 Minutes in class. Practice until you perfect the posture, keeping the tongue on the soft palate.

Comments: Turn the tongue in, turn it really well, and hold it there. The scriptures say it's a very special kriya; they call it very secret and blah-blah-blah. They say the yogi pulls his tongue, cuts it out and turns it in, fixes it up, if you read the yoga mudra and yoga kriyas, my God! There are so many pages about it, it is nothing. It's a hatha thing, physical. But in Kundalini Yoga it's so simple. Turn the tongue in, there is a very soft place there, it is called the zero meridian. You just stick it there, back in the upper palate and if you just keep on doing it, after a while, you will find there is a little hole, then you stick the tongue in that hole. The great secret mudra—it takes 22 years for the Hatha Yogi to do it; well, we did it anyway.

"There are two ways your soul can go: either to rest or to rust, whichever you want. You can cause the cause to cycle and cycle and cycle and cycle or you can cause the cause to end and end and end forever. Why can you not cause the cause to end? Because you do not let it unfold, so unfold yourself. Here is a kriya for it."

– *Yogi Bhajan*

Student: What's the effect of this kriya?

Yogi Bhajan: Find it. You can find the weather but you can't find the effect? Cause the cause, you will find the effect. There is never a reason to cause a cause and not find the effect. You know what we were doing? What did we say we were doing? Unfold. We were unfolding our Self to our Self. First introduction between the two friends, the self and the Self; it was a meeting of the ways between two friends, the given self and the creative self. We are unfolding the mystery. These two selves react to each other and create a lot of problems and who wants problems? We want peace. There are two ways to go: you want peace or you want problems. You want problems? Have them, as many as you want. You want peace? There is only one thing—let it unfold. Isn't that simple?

I have just fallen in love with you. You have given us a paper today and we will return it tomorrow. This is a lot of work, but we want to put together your personality profile and your projection, along with your possibility. We will write you a letter, and send you a bill also. (Students' laugh) And pay the previous one! It takes long hours of typing and reading . . . those who have bad handwriting, we are going to charge you more. It takes a big magnifying glass to read your handwriting. I don't know what you write. It takes a lot of time. So make it easy for us, so that we can read your paper at least. Answer it very honestly. Then we will identify the profile and keep that letter on file. In case of difficulty, write us, if you want something sometime. We will write you back what to do. Do it or not, it's your problem, not ours.

Tomorrow we are going to talk about the path from unfolding to fulfillment. You know, we really want to do a job. God knows how many days I have more to live. Situation doesn't seem to be very healthy. So the idea is, whatever time we have out of this mess that has been created, we can't waste it on all this nonsense. The only way that we can make sense of it is to play a positive role, let it unfold and let the mysteries appear. Not very mysterious. We leave you fulfilled and strong and that's the purpose: to make you men. You are men by birth. I want you to be men by your right. That's the difference. That's the total difference. Thank you very much.

May the long time sun shine upon you, all love surround you and the pure light within you, guide your way on.

May thy grace bless us, may thy grace unfold among us, may thy grace give us the clear, crystal way of life. May the word of the Guru exalt us and may we share with all. May giving become our habit and our habitat. May we all excel in thy glory, in thy name, Sat Nam.

■ ■ ■

Realizing **Success**

Understand that the will of God, the will of reality, is that each man succeed—each man is born to succeed. Success is your elementary right.

Let me sum up yesterday in a few lines. You as you have a gift of the pranic value or pranic life. You turn that pranic value and pranic life into labor and through labor you trade for cash, and by cashing in your labor, you have services and the material things to keep your life going. But the problem is, if you do not see the pranic value in everything you have, if you do not see that it is part of your pranic life, then you basically lose the concept of happiness. The majority of people do.

As a child you grow up, and in that growth you accommodate yourself with anger, because you feel frustrated, you are not taken care of, things never happen, you were never taught, you were never told. As your passion grows, you do not find an outlet, the outlet, and you begin to feel very clogged up. Your life is not channeled spiritually, even though you are a spirit.

Your sole purpose on this Earth is that you are a soul. Ten trillion cells of you dance with the power of that one soul and you are not successful. Sometimes you hate success because when you become successful, then you have to have responsibility, and responsibility means commitment, commitment means be on time, be on time means everything has to be all perfect, all perfect means a lot of hassle, a lot of hassle means a lot of work, a lot of work means, "Who the hell cares for it? Why should I do it to begin with?" So that's it, right? Plus, when you are successful, when you are great, you are this and that, there is no sympathy. *(Students laugh)* Oh, yeah.

When emotions and feelings take over priority in work you are doomed. Totally. You have no place. You have gone and done. Tons of money and millions of friends and extreme power in your position, and still you shall be the most unhappy and upside down human being. If ever, if by chance your emotions and feelings can interfere with your work priority, you are doomed. That's how important work is.

Kirth; kirth takey dey. Jaha dana, taha khana, kirth takey dey.

Where you have to eat, only there shall you eat. You can't eat anywhere else. Time and space shall decide for you. How much you make the opportunity your own, for you, that's your intelligence.

The Principle of Eleven **Feet**

When you put the key in the car say,

Aad Guray Nameh
Jugaad Guray Nameh
Sat Guray Nameh
Siri Guru Dev-ay Nameh

"Wahe Guru Ji Ka Khalsa, Wahe Guru Ji Ki Fateh."

All that is just to give you a few seconds in space and time to be late, because time you cannot change but you can be a little late—11 feet away. It's called the principle of 11-feet distance. If a person can be delayed in such a way, so that in space and time, they have 11 feet, the accident or incident can be avoided. But it cannot be avoided more than four times. You must remember that. So there are four chances to be delayed by 11 feet.

So basically the power in you to succeed is there. You are not born to fail. But you do fail and then the question today arises, why? Because you don't let yourself unfold. Your secrets, your secrecy, your game, your chess, me, here, there, this, that, I, they, them, it is all so scattered, nobody trusts you. Listen, here is the secret of success. OPI–OPM: other people's intelligence and other people's money. If you want your money and your intelligence, then you should do one thing. Dig a hole—four feet by four feet—and sit in it. Or buy your own coffin, make a hole, break your own neck and walk in it, you don't need to change clothes, you won't have to worry, and you will be beautiful. Then forget it. Then you're dealing in the 'dump' market, not the junk market. Then we don't have to talk.

The purpose of the soul is to feel success and experience it and be satisfied. That's the price it paid for separation from God.

Success is yours in gravity, in reality, and in personality. Success is. Remember: either you shall be successful or you were born to be miserable. There are no two ways about it. That's how powerful success is ingrained in you. You are not afraid to succeed, you just don't want to succeed because you have never enjoyed what success is. Remember: there is no substitute for success and to succeed there is only one thing to do. When there are emotions and feelings in the way, jump over. Just remember, emotions and feelings are yours, but performance is also yours—and performance has to be perfect. Don't let your emotions and your feelings and your fears and your needs detour your performance. Let it not be diluted or polluted. Your life is meant to succeed. The power of success is such that, if not in this lifetime, somewhere else, some other time, somewhere you must succeed. The purpose of the soul is to feel success and experience it and be satisfied. That's the price it paid for separation from God.

Success is very vital to you. But I know you have lot of garbage, which stops you from being successful. For a few minutes, we are going to go into a trance. We are going to explore right through the subconscious mind into the realm of success. We are going to tap in; we are going to drill a well through our neuroses, through our weaknesses and through all our subconscious garbage. We are going to go all the way—deep—to fill our well, our self, with success, because success is not from the outside.

Success shall never come to you from outside. There is no such thing as success outside. There is no such thing as opportunity. We made it up. There is no such thing as luck. It's all in our imagination. There is one thing: we are born to succeed. And it doesn't matter what we do, we can't stop it. Whenever we have tried to stop it, we become miserable, more and more miserable. Why can we not fail? Because God never fails. How can a soul fail? Then why isn't everybody successful? There is water always there in the ground, why isn't there a fountain everywhere? We have to drill the pump. It is not that you are not making an effort, it is not that you are not trying to make an effort, it is not that that's not your whole motivation, it is not that that's not your meditation, it is not that that's what you want the most.

If you are a yogi sit like a yogi, if you are a bhogi sit like a bhogi, if you are a dogi sit like a dogi.

There are three things that everybody wants: love, success and good health. Everybody wants it. You can charm everybody just by saying, I'll make you the healthiest. He will be just like a puppy dog behind you. 'Oh! I love you.' In spite of the fact that you have a history of killing people in the name of love, still people will follow you. So don't misunderstand that these things don't have power. But success is a virtue which is ingrained in you and it has to be tapped.

If you are a yogi sit like a yogi, if you are a bhogi sit like a bhogi, if you are a dogi sit like a dogi.

Kriya to Unfold Your Virtues
September 22, 1985

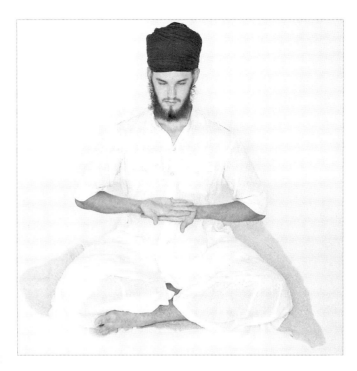

Posture & Mudra: Sit straight. Chin in, chest out. Bring your hands in front of the chest, right hand on top of the left, palms up and flat, with the thumbs pointing forward. Forearms are parallel and the hands are between the Heart Center and the diaphragm.

Eyes: Closed

1. Breathe powerfully. Breathe in as deeply as you can and exhale powerfully. Give yourself a chance. **1-3 Minutes**

2. Maintain the mudra and relax the breath, just breathe normally and meditate. Listen to the visualization as you maintain the posture steadily, like a stone:

"Start sinking in you. Sinking in you. I am the soul, I am the light and I am the success. Just concentrate, meditate and go through a self-hypnotic stage. I am the soul, I am the light, I am the success. I am the soul, I am the light, I am the success. You have to go into self-hypnosis, nobody can hypnotize you better than your own self. I am the soul, I am the light, I am the success. Penetrate deeply in you. Whatever thoughts are crossing you, penetrate through them. Drill through it. Hold your posture, hold your body like Earth. Take the mind and penetrate, tap into soul: I am the soul, I am the light, I am the success. Unfold your strength of reality, your power of Infinity, your mission to accomplish, to succeed. You are the perfect projection of success. That's why success is the one, you are the two, and achievement is the three. Within those three selves penetrate, concentrate, deep, and deeper.

"I am the soul. Go to sleep on it. Sleep, nap it. Nap it: I am the soul, I am the light, I am the success. Nap it, go nap on it. Take a nap on these three words. You hear nothing but success; you know nothing but success. You feel nothing but success. You are nothing but success. You are nothing but success. Delightful success, success forever. You. Success. You. Success. Success. You. Forever, everlasting. Honest, truthful, straightforward, direct, you are success. You were, you are, you shall be nothing but success. You are succeeding in napping. In your whole being, in your whole being feel the "Full-Fill-Meant" of success. Success is in you, coming to you, fulfilling you. Succeed, succeed, succeed! Excel! Obey, serve, love, excel! Obey, serve, love, excel! Excel to succeed, succeed to be success. Be success. Beyond you, within you, behind you, all is nothing but success. Obey, serve, love, excel! Take a nap on it, successful nap. Drill in, deepest, to reach it." **8 Minutes**.

3. Put the tip of the tongue on the upper palate. Keeping the tongue in place, chant in a monotone: **Be Success**. **1 Minute**

4. Keeping the tongue on the upper palate, chant in a monotone: **I am Successful. 30 seconds**

5. Hypnotize yourself and meditate silently on "I am successful." Whatever comes in the way, the anger, the question, the doubt, the duality, reality, non-reality, forget it, pass through it. Hypnotize yourself with these words: "Know me, I am successful; feel me, I am successful; look at me, I am successful; desire me, I am successful. Success is my essence, success is my being, success is my Self." **1 Minute.**

6. Now imagine calling out into the distance and commanding to a very distant place, far, far away, declaring that you are successful. You hear nothing but success, you see nothing but success, you feel nothing but success. You say nothing but success. When you talk, talk success. When you feel, feel success. When you act, act success. Be, be success. All is to be successful. Transform these ten trillion cells into a dance of success. Transmute the infinite power of you to be successful. Your word, which you speak, must bring you success. Whatever you see and observe must help you to succeed. Your purpose and your motive must be to succeed. Honesty is to succeed. Truth is to succeed. Self is to succeed. **4 Minutes.**

To end: Relax. Shake your hands and shake your bodies. **30 seconds**.

In our day to day life, whether we like it or not, there are challenges. The main challenge for any of us is: Is there something that can shake us from our self? You see New Mexico had a tornado? Mexico had an earthquake? But what is an earthquake, something came, shook the ground and the big buildings and everything tumbled. Exactly you are hit by the same energy all the time. It's my opinion, my counseling, my telling you, my reading you the newspaper, the radio, the television, your wife, your friend, your children, your neighborhood, your congregation, call it anything. Between me and you, there is one very important thing, can you tell me what that is?

Between two people one thing is very important. I am telling you the secret, the key to success. Between me and you there is the unknown. You and I make it known through communication, through feelings, through desires, through circumstances, call it anything. Two people can only create the known. But there is always a third power, which is the unknown. If the unknown is considered sacred, success is there. If the unknown is forgotten or not considered sacred, failure shall be there. That is the deciding line. If between me and you the unknown is sacred, we can't fail. Anything you do, anything you say, anything you feel, for God's sake, don't take away the sacredness of it. Whenever you do, you shall fail and you shall suffer. The consequences will be so heavy that you will not be in a position to handle it. But if between you A, and between you B, you respect the sacredness, then you will succeed. Everything will manifest.

If the unknown is considered sacred, success is there.

Lack of sacredness is nothing but a disaster. It is defeat. Between you and you, there is sacredness. Between you and me, there is sacredness. Between you and in this room, there is a sacredness. Anything that takes away the sacredness from you, let that thing go, period. You are born to be sacred and you are born to be successful. You want to know why you are not successful? Because you forgot that you are sacred. You always question, "Why am I poor, why am I failing, why aren't things happening? Why? Why? Why?" You have a hundred questions, but there is only one answer. You forgot you are sacred.

You forgot that you received the sacred trust of the pranic breath. You forgot that the body was given to you as a gift, a sacred gift. You were sent to Earth on a sacred mission. You were provided all the environments. You were born, you were in a very, very cozy pouch. After you were born, you had beautiful milk; you can't buy it, can you? Even if you try, you can't. You have a priceless nurse, later on you may hate her or like her, I am not into it. But at that moment, when you were innocent, she was a divine nurse, and there was a father, no matter how much of an S.O.B. he was, at that time he was the representative of the Divine and you called him pitha, papa, whatever. You had that.

Kriya to Realize **Success**
September 22, 1985

Posture: Now sit and transform yourself into your Navel Point.

Eyes: Closed

To Begin: Inhale Deeply, Exhale Deeply. (3X)

1. Chant: I am, I am from the Navel Point. Transcend your feelings. Hypnotize yourself with the sound. **1 Minute**

2. Sit at the navel and from the navel see your entire life. Listen to the affirmation read by the teacher:

"Sit in your navel and see your entire outside world, day by day, minute by minute. Hypnotically sit with your navel; the moment you hypnotically sit with your navel you can see all sitting there, because that's the source of pure energy where you could live without breath. You can connect and coordinate with the entire universe.

You are a gift of the divine; your visit here is a gift of the divine. Concentrate deeply and excel. See from your navel all your deceit, your weakness, your treachery, your lies, and laugh at it.

Because you can sit in the navel, you can be as secure as God is. Experience security—that you don't have to cheat. You cheat because you are insecure, you lie because you are insecure, you deceive because you are insecure, everything wrong and rotten you do because you are insecure. Navel is the security. Sit deep in your navel and look at your world around you and laugh at it. You don't have to lie, you don't have to use diplomacy, you don't have to crisscross yourself, you don't have to cheat, you don't have to sin, you don't have to be wrong, you are to succeed. Being straight, direct and honest. Sit in your navel and succeed. Sit in your navel and succeed. Succeed!" **4 Minutes**

3. Open the eyes and roll them up toward the Third Eye Point between the eyebrows and the root of the nose and declare to yourself that you are successful. Silently meditate: I am successful, I am successful, I am successful. **2 Minutes**

Comments: Because you have seen the success in the navel, you don't have to hide, you don't have to lie, you have to declare: I am man, I am good, I am successful, I am man, I am good, I am successful.

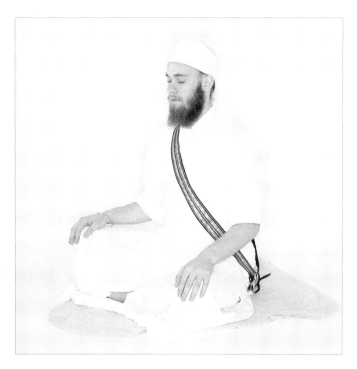

4. Repeat very loudly from the Navel Point—Cannon it out: Man, good, successful, man, good, successful… **1 ½ Minutes**

Comments: Cannon it so powerfully, within five to seven repetitions, your tongue should start getting dry. That's how effective it should be. Cannon it means fire it like a cannon.

To End: Meditate. Hear what you have said. Hear it in your bones, feel it in your bones, be it in your bones. Relax and move your shoulders, your hands, shake it out.

We have a basic creative caliber. It is not only a basic creative caliber, but also basic human criteria to create the environments, and be so bountiful and so beautiful, that we can profit. God knew. We may forget, but God knew that every pranic life has to be transformed into energy and services and must have the criteria of desire—to want more, need more—and these must be paid for. This way our livelihood is taken care of.

We went to collect roots, fruits, and wood to live. Then we started going out and hunting. We never wanted to go collect roots and fruits and wood every day, every week. So we started hunting, killing other beings, breaking harmony and in this way, we began creating our own domain. When we started hunting, we were hunted, too. Tribes would come, take over the other tribe, run away with their children and their women and kill all the men. Or, men who could be subdued were shackled and turned into slaves. So we started manufacturing inferior humans out of ourselves.

That was the game then; but today, in the modern world, we are creating inferior children. We are unhappy, we rock our marriage, we come from broken homes, broken hearts. We have neurosis to deal with, we have a life full of duality and then we have children who do not know what is tomorrow, what is today, what was yesterday. "Who is my father?" "Who is my mother?" "Why is my father doing this?" "Why is my mother doing this?" "Why are my neighbors like this?" We have created a generation of questions and no answer. No answers, no insight. We belong to the era of the most selfish, self-centered, angry, unsocial hypocrites. That's what we are. Our smiles are not real, our talk is not real, our relationships are not real, our commitment is not real. We are just passing the time.

We want to know who we are. But even when we are told who we are, "you are the light of God," the tragedy is, we say, "What do you mean by light of God? What is light? What is God?" You have duality about every reality. You have a question about everything, because you have a potential fear. You are haunted by fear all the time. You never believe and you cannot be made to believe that God created you in His perfect image and God is in love with you. You don't believe in love, in God. How can anybody else believe you are in love with them? If the glass is empty, what can it give?

To cover yourself, you play a lot of games, you say a lot of things. You have become wrappers. You know that wrapper game? Give somebody a big present, unwrap it, unwrap it, unwrap it, unwrap it, unwrap it, after an hour and a half you will find a little rubber rat at the bottom. Have you played that game? It used to be very common in the 60s. Send somebody the biggest gift, so big it would come in a cart, you know, in the back of the truck—that big. So you open up the first box, then you come out with another and you open that, you come out with another and on and on and on. Ultimately you will find some scummy little rat, twenty cents worth, wrapped up at the bottom.

Somebody was listening to a conversation, he was going on, wrapping the words and you go on unwrapping, and he goes on rapping, ultimately, at some point, you say, "What do you want to say? What is it?" Because you are scared, you can't say, "I am through, I am done, I don't want it, I can't do it." You don't want to take the responsibility and you feel that by spinning the lies, and gaining time, and twisting things, and manipulating the situation, you will get away. But you don't recognize one thing, you are nothing. All you have is your reputation. You have to learn one fundamental thing: all your cleverness and all your wrapping and all your talking and all your gaining time and all your scheming and thinking and playing games, your saying and not saying, your undertow and over-tow, within the lines and over the lines, and right on and not on, and all that, it's just bad communication. There is no need to talk. If your presence cannot work, you cannot work. If your presence?

Students: Cannot work.

Yogi Bhajan: You cannot work. If your presence cannot move, you cannot move. If your soul doesn't shine, you are a dead person. With all this manipulation, which you can do because you have the most fertile brain, you can work and talk and cheat and play and tie the knot and do the whole thing; you have to do it.

You know, one evening I told somebody in confidence, I said, "Hey, you have some time?"
He said, "Yes sir. What I can do?"
I said, "Take me to a bar, a single's bar."
He said, "Sir!"
I said, "This 'sir' is a very difficult person sometimes. Take me to some single's bar, if you know any here."

So we went to a single's bar. To begin with, the entry was horrible. We arranged to sit on one side; there was so much noise, so much talking, and nothing meant anything. They were all drinking, all talking, talking and drinking and drinking and talking, but there was no juice in it. Why? Because evenings are very painful, evenings belong to honest people. Evenings belong to strong people. Evenings belong to people who are pure and self-possessed. Otherwise it's very difficult to pass an evening. Evening belongs to those who have gained their strength in the early morning.

You store energy in the morning just to pass an evening. Your destruction is by night; your prosperity is from the morning. Every fault you have ever committed, every mistake you have ever made, you've done it from 4 pm to 12 am, watch it sometime, circulate yourself, put it on your own computer, check it out. It's very difficult to make a man commit a mistake at 11 o'clock in the morning if he is not dumb. If he had a good night's sleep and he woke up as a normal person. You meet the guy at 11 am and ask him to commit a mistake, forget it. But if you get somebody at 11 pm, you can twist him around like a yo-yo because there's nothing there.

So to be prosperous, which you want, you have to balance your energy. You have to gain it in the morning and you have to lose it in the evening, not to the extent that you lose your case. There is one thing that you all need—and it's called freshness. When somebody talks to you and somebody is with you, you should meet and feel fresh. If you talk to somebody, yes, yes, what do you want to say? "Oh! You want to talk to me about God?"

The guy will say, "Hell with you, I don't want to talk about God; you give me a God? I don't want it from you." Why this reaction? Because there is no freshness about you; it is called the vibrant self. We want to test it out.

Kriya to Awaken the Vibrant Self

September 22, 1985

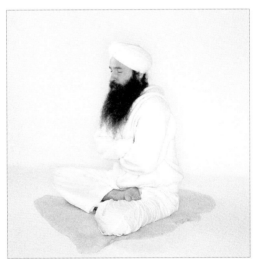

Posture: Sit in Easy Pose or other cross-legged posture.

Mudra: Cross your arms across your chest and lock your hands under your lower ribs.

Eyes: Closed.

Movement: Jump like a fish. Jerk your whole body, keeping your hands locked onto your opposite ribs. **1 Minute**

Rest and **Repeat** the exercise for **3 Minutes**.

Comments: It is just spinal energy you are going to create, that's it. Come on, do it! If this exercise were easy everybody would do it. It's pretty difficult. But jump up, give yourself a chance.

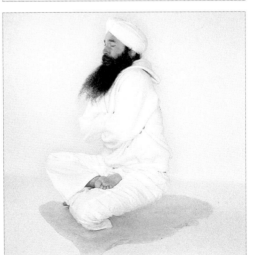

Do it during the day sometime or at night or in the morning. It reduces chances of insanity. It is very powerful. But just remember: there is a rib here, it's called seventh rib, put your hands on both sides, lock it and then do it. When the hands are locked on the lower rib it means there is no space for you to stimulate your own insanity. Your problem in life is that your main movement in life and the majority of your movement and purpose in life is your own insanity. It is called purposeless pursuit. It's an emotional non-reality. It's a commotional release. And it's a total waste of time—a total waste of the most beautiful life.

Sometimes people go back and forth to the same place to look for something that never existed. It was just a thought. It's called pursuit of non-reality. You know how much it is in you? Eighty percent.

"Aah! I saw that girl."
"Where?"
"Oh on 7th or 8th Street."
"When?"
"Oh, just a while ago; let's go."
Idiot, it costs gas, it costs time and she may not be there. But no, you are stuck on the idea to go. And now that guy is going to lie.
"Hey, there she is."
"But let's go anyway."

Eighty percent of you pursue imagination and then you pay bills, you burn gas, you have wear and tear, you have laundry and you have clothes to fold and iron, you have to eat, and on and on. Eighty percent of you pursue dreams— 80%. And then you complain that you are poor? How can you be rich? Who can make you rich? Every pursuit has an expense and every expense should be exactly two percent of your gross income. There should be a minimum of 30% profit. It's simple, damn economics. Otherwise don't move; don't do anything.

"I love you." What for? Take her to dinner, take her to this, take her to that. For what? So you can sleep with her once? Spending $280? That's one week's worth of work.
I asked somebody, "You went to a movie?"
He said, "Yes sir."
I said, "What did you learn?"
"It was good."
I said, "What? What was good?"

If I am going to spend five bucks, I want to see what's what. I want to see something. If you go to a movie and you don't come out with $15 worth of an experience, don't go to the movies. You have to get three times your actual expense; and if you get popcorn and a soft drink or cold drink or nachos, whatever, then it should be five times. I am not kidding. I am telling you, don't change clothes on the day you cannot earn $50. Because it takes $5 to change clothes, $1 to take a bath, and you must earn $30 that day. Otherwise you have wasted precious city water. You have no right to switch on the light if you cannot make $100. Don't make a phone call that is not essential, otherwise you have to fly and go and talk to that person, that's when I talk. When I feel the situation has arisen that I have to fly, take a plane and go and talk to that guy, I will pick up a phone. Every expense where your actual money is spent, 15% must produce 250% gross. It's simple damn economics. Your emotions, your dreams, and your desires included. Don't follow shadows, you are the sun, you are the light, and you are the success. Wasting pranic energy on non-productive, non-profitable ventures is a treachery to God. It's a betrayal of the gift of the pranic values, which is life. You betray life, you won't be happy.

Multiply doesn't mean produce babies. Multiply means to produce profit from your time and your space. Every breath you consume, inhale and exhale, should produce ten bucks. You are thinking what's wrong with me? You want to know what's wrong with me? You are idiots. Out of $10, you pay Uncle Sam the tax, you pay the pension fund, you pay the insurance. Just look, if you make $100, you pay $50 federal tax, $11 state tax, $9 you pay to the accountant and CPA, $10 for the insurance, $10 for the wages of your staff, you are only left with $10 per every $100. So when you give somebody ten bucks you have paid him a hundred dollars. It took a lot of pranic breath to create that hundred dollars; it took a lot of pranic breath to get $10 for you. And you go and take a neurotic, idiot girl who has no values, who doesn't understand what the hell she is doing, and you waste a dinner on her? You must be blind and crazy. Whosoever doesn't produce, doesn't get paid. And if you pay them, you are nuts. It's a simple law of life.

If you give, then don't call it a business. Give because you want to. Give and then forget it. Give as much as you can, because God gave you a gift, then don't do business. Don't mix giving and business. Giving is good, give as much you can; give yourself. No problem, but that's not business. Business is for a profit and giving is for satisfaction—divine satisfaction. But what do you do? You mix it. You give and take and take and give and give and take. You give, and if you can't take, then you look around for when you can. You become thieves, you become cheats, you become liars, you become dishonest, you become dishonored and that is not a man. Don't learn treachery. Give—give and be graceful about it. If it's a business, it's cut and dry, straight and honest, absolutely productive and profiteering rules. Is that understood?

You want to do seva, do seva and leave $20 for having the opportunity to do seva. Nobody is going to bother you. But if somebody says, "Come and work for two hours," just tell the guy, "Okay, for $150 an hour." "Why?" "Well, don't hire me." Or, if your value is $10 an hour, take $10 an hour, whatever, but be exact. Don't waste any time in non-productive ventures.

You are wasting your life. Emotional and commotional feelings, imagination, and all that, do not bring profit. If you sit down on water and start writing scriptures, who will read it? Who will read your writings on the water? You need paper, you need a pen. Just please remember, life is nothing but a gift of pranic life from God and life can be transformed into labor and labor can be sold and bought and it will give you money, the medium of exchange, and through the media you can buy material and services to keep life going. So each life has to be sold profitably. Each labor has to be sold profitably and every venture has to be business-like, honest and straight. Any work you do must make for you between 10% and 30% profit. If the capital is 10% and you make 10% profit, you make nothing; you are going to die hungry. Because 10% is the interest and 10% is the wear and tear of you, you need 20% on top of the 10% in order to live—that's 30%. So everything you do must give you at least 30%.

If I am willing to go to dinner with somebody, the person will spend money on the dinner right? Number one—that's 10%. Then the person should give me enough company that I should be totally recuperated within my work load and I should feel fresh and young, that's another 10%. And the final 10% I should feel that it was really worthwhile. That is my 30%, that's what going to dinner is worth. Otherwise if I start going to every dinner, I will be dead in six months. Because I'll eat like a pig and I will become a pig; and I am already pretty fat.

But I am just explaining to you that for going, for making small talk, for being with somebody, just find out if it's profitable, spiritually, mentally, physically for you. Otherwise don't move. Shallow talk, pep talk, table talk, this, that, is a pure waste of precious time.

Somebody once asked me, "I cannot think, I cannot plan, I cannot talk, I am not successful, I don't know how, nobody taught me. You came in such and such town, I met you, I happened to be there, I made you my teacher, now tell me! I want to be successful." Now can you believe this dialogue? But there it was, a lot of pain, a cry for help.
I said, "What do you do best?"
He said, "I can sleep. That's all I can do."
I said, "Then all right, sleep."
"What will happen?"
I said, "I don't know. But whatever you can do best, just do that. Be at your best."

He slept and he had a dream. Watch this: he had a dream that he had a grandfather who is very sick and is dying and he is remembering him and he should go wherever he is. He first took two to three days to find where his father is. He never knew what a father is, or where he was. But somehow he found it out. Then he found from his father where his grandfather is. He said, "I don't know where that old man is. He must be dead; he used to live in such and such…" Somewhere remote. So then he asked his friend, "You want to go on a trip and hitchhike?" He said, "Yeah."

Well, he is pretty rich now. His grandfather met him, felt him, called the justice of the peace, wrote down the whole thing in his name. Told him he is my grandson and he is going to inherit everything. On the third day he died, leaving him a chunk of money and land you can't even buy today. So, even if you only know how to sleep, sleep good. That will serve you. Don't do things halfway.

When you motivate things emotionally and try to make a business out of them, you have already failed. When you motivate things because of your ego and you want a business out of it, you have already lost. This is not a business course, I am not going to teach you all that. That I'll teach in the business course. Now, today, I am teaching you as a man, as a successful man. You are born to succeed. God wanted it that way. Then why do you fail? You fail because your motivation is wrong. You love and you fail, love can fail? Never. Love can never fail. How can love fail? Love is giving, not taking; you take, you don't love. You fail. Love is the name of giving. Not giving as charity but offering. Giving voluntarily, to feel honored, that's love. Love is not taking. If in love you take, you shall fail, because then life shall turn into a poison. *Peta* they call it.

Bait pranan ki ahuti deit, prem ke sagar mein aisa tartayiye, sada sukh jeevan, subhaydaan, hoye sang, apne sang, apan navariye.

"…in the game of love make yourself and make the whole self an offering, in this there is no limit, no thinking, no feeling and no defeat."

But in business, as a man, you must have 30% profit and 20% margin. You know, you go to a wholesale factory, they don't even bother. They jump the price 100%. You come to a retailer, he will try to jump it 100% and then, when he cannot make it, "sale," some kind of sale.

What kind of sale is that? There is no sale, it's just to make you feel that you are gaining something. The one who wants to make a profit from you is telling you that you are profiting from him. You know what this gimmick is, this sale? He couldn't reach your pocket in a straight manner, so he reached it in an indirect manner. He is telling you "I am reducing the price 50% for you," because you are his cousin's uncle's brother-in-law. That's not true. He is really telling you, "I am sorry I couldn't make an idiot of you. Come in, though I couldn't get you totally, half is enough, come in, there is a sale." When there is a boarded up sign, "going out of business", you go in the shop and look at their faces—they are sitting shiva. Oh!! We have to sell it, the bank is tight on us; they make every excuse to get sympathy through apathy. But the fact is that the price was originally up 200%. Only an emotional creep will sell at no profit.

When you sell yourself at no profit who are you? You are a man and you sell yourself at no profit? Who are you? You, the man, the majesty of God, the highest incarnation, the most successful, the most wonderful brain, pure and simple, light and delightful, and you sell yourself for bloody small, creepy emotions and feelings. You sell yourself all for your neurosis and your emotions and commotions. What do you bring home? Your psychotic, neurotic self. Then what? You will hate yourself and everybody will hate you in return.

So you are a confirmed, hate-filled, angry, absolutely... now I am not going to say that word, I remember I am a holy man, so my apologies, you can fill in the blanks. That's not even God, that's not even man. Man must excel. There is a one quality of a man—you must be in command.

Kriya to Develop the Art of Selling Your Self
September 22, 1985

Posture: Sit in a comfortable cross-legged posture.

Mudra: Cross your arms across your chest and place your hands on your opposite shoulders.

Eyes: Closed

To begin: Inhale deeply and exhale deeply (3-5X)

Listen to the Affirmation:

"Sell yourself at absolute profit. Sell yourself, value yourself, profit yourself. Price yourself and sell yourself; come on make the self-sale. You shall make the profit. Sell yourself, price yourself, value yourself, present yourself, wrap yourself, negotiate about yourself, and sell it for a profit. Profit! God doesn't send the profit, you are the profit! Sell it for the profit.

Price it, value it, negotiate. Bring profit home. Shine up, brighten up. Value, value, value. Qualify the values. Qualify, qualify the values. You are real! Qualify. Value. Price each value, plus it, total it, add profit to it, negotiate, sell yourself. You sell other things, but one who cannot sell himself can't sell anything.

Develop the art of self-sale. If you do your own PR, the whole world will do your PR. If you sell yourself, you can sell the whole world, you are God! If you can sell God, you can sell everything because everything is God, understand? It is a simple science. If you can sell God,

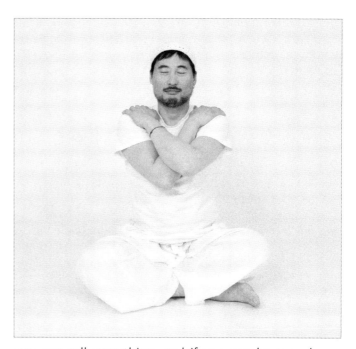

you can sell everything, and if you can be sacred, you can sell everything anyway. Because if sacredness gives somebody junk, it is called blessing. When somebody gives somebody something it is called a thing. Things are questioned. Blessings are never questioned, gifts are never priced. Selling is a gift. Value yourself. Add your values, price yourselves, add profit. Negotiate and sell. You are priceless anyway, you sell your pricelessness.

5 Minutes

To end: Inhale and relax. Shake up your hands.

The United States is a beautiful country, very beautiful. It is a democracy, it's a beautiful country, it's the "home of the free and the brave", and whatever. There are so many adjectives. We agree that the United States is great country, and the USSR is a great country and that Luxembourg is a great country. It's not the area, it's not the people, it's not the geography, it's not the politics, it's not the economics, but you Americans should not forget one thing: We discovered America as trappers. It is in our genes to lay traps and then catch life and sell the hide. Don't forget that.

We are bird lovers and animal lovers out of necessity, because we are neurotics. We don't have any constant, consistent love and togetherness in the family, therefore we have to raise dogs and cats to counterbalance our inefficiency and deficiency in our human love relationships. In our sincerity of communication, in relationship and in our power to be human, we are defective, third grade, rejected human beings, unloved, and in terrible pain, constant pain—constant pain.

We hurt ourselves socially, we hurt ourselves economically, we hurt our self in every aspect. Not that we want to be hurt, that's not our problem. We do not know where to find satisfaction for our ego. By sleeping with 300 men or 600 women, or doing big deals and small deals, or isolating, going somewhere where nobody can touch us, or living in the middle of New York, we don't know. We will never know. Because somebody has failed, somebody has not given us the basic elementary values, who we are and how we can be who we are. If a man has money, he wants to buy everything with money. If a woman is sexy, she wants to buy everything with sex. A man with power wants to buy everything with power. It's all garbage.

There has to be someplace where one can learn to stop and evaluate one's self; give yourself the values you need to give yourself. You always start by giving other people your judgments, your values, your relationship, and all that. Sometimes I really wonder if you even know that your own evaluation is in a mess. You have not done your own homework.

I can teach Kundalini Yoga in hell and in heaven, exactly the same.

Somebody joins 3HO, somebody joins Sikh Dharma, somebody is a Hare Krishna, somebody is a born-again Christian, somebody is a Catholic, an Espanolian, a this or a that, God knows what you are, but actually, to be factual, you are nobody. Your quantity may be anything: how many people are in this religion, how many people are your students—damn the whole thing—is it the quantity or the quality? Is it the money, is it the power, or is it the sacredness? It is the space you enjoy, the time you have, or is it the wisdom? You have to decide. If somebody can shake you and somebody can crack you, then you have not yet found yourself.

You know, when I became a Sikh, I didn't become a Sikh because . . . well let me be fantastically clear, I mean, I don't make any reservations about it and a lot of these Sikhs are very mad at me for it. "Why do you say that?" they ask. Well, I say what I want to say and I say it anyway. I don't care. One day I was sitting and lying down and looking at the roof, and I said, "O God, what a funky job you have done? What have you done? I mean, what are you trying to do? You want to be appreciated and praised, couldn't you do better than making all these creepy people and then getting them into the mess, what is this way? Okay, I will get up and chant to you. But you have to do some good too, once in a while be a good God."

If somebody can shake you and somebody can crack you, then you have not yet found yourself.

I had a feeling, I said it. I am not worried about it. It's not that I am reconfirming myself that God is going to curse me. Who the hell cares whether He curses me or He appreciates me? I can teach Kundalini Yoga in hell and in heaven, exactly the same—and after you teach in America you don't need any other proving ground. If one can survive in this country for five years, one can survive everywhere.

There is a trap in every step—you lift and you place. We are trappers in talking, we are trappers in our movement, we are trappers in our relationship, we are trappers in the beginning, we are trappers now and we are trappers in the end. We want the skin, we want the hide and we want the meat. We do not know what to do with the meat, but we definitely know what to do with the hide. That is flat consciousness; we have to grow above it.

The only way you can identify yourself is to identify your Self. Evaluate yourself, assess yourself, and feel yourself, for once, for God's sake! I am a Hare Krishna, I am a Sikh, I am a Hindu, I am a Muslim, I am a Jew, I am a Christian, I am the God—you are nobody! You are fooling around. You have theories and you have projections. You place a trap and cover it with grass, make it look good. But you are not doing yourself any good, neither are you good to anybody else. Therefore you have to understand that you have to evaluate yourself. In you, the very birthright is to be sacred. You cannot be successful, you cannot give anybody anything, if you do not have that sacredness ingrained in you. It is ingrained in you to begin with and you let it go to waste, it's not fair.

Somebody once said, "How can I raise my Kundalini?"
I said, "What do you want to raise?"
He said, "Kundalini."
I said, "Why? What is the idea?"
"I understand it's a power."
I said, "What do you want to do with power? Run a grinding mill? Or a jackhammer? What do you want power for?"

If your power is not in your grace, every other power is as useless as you can name. If your consciousness does not clearly help you to be compassionate, you have not even learned to be as worthy as an animal, which is your own pet. If you do not understand that it's your birthright to be happy and successful, you have not evaluated yourself.

Whenever you value yourself, you will find one fundamental thing: it is your birthright to be happy and it is your birthright to be successful. Anybody who complains and says, "I am not successful and I am not happy," he is treacherous to God. He is unsacred, unholy and a crazy person. If an American says, "I deny all the fundamental rights," then what is America? It's better to be Russia.

The difference in this country and any other country is that it has a Bill of Rights. We trapped ourselves so well that we gave ourselves a Bill of Rights. We knew we were not going to be real. We were going to change, we were going to fluctuate, so that's what we did. We knew that "absolute power corrupts absolutely," so we divided power into legislature, into judiciary and into executive, we separated it. We knew we were trappers. Everybody couldn't be Abraham Lincoln. And we knew that the people's will shall decide the fate of this country, but we wanted to give the people a channel.

Also we are immigrants and we knew we had to succeed. So we recognized two things: we have to evaluate our self and we have to succeed. We have to succeed to be happy and we have to be happy because we are succeeding. So basically we are in good shape. But individually, we do not evaluate our self all the time. Because as children we were unloved, uncared for, there was a little coldness, that has made us a little shallow, it's given us a little pain, and we have developed the habit of complaining.

When I came the first time to America, my experience was very harsh. Somebody said to me, "Who are you?" I mean in the whole world, you won't find one person who can ask that except in the United States. Then I realized that this country is 200 years old, it has no culture and I have never forgotten that. What are you doing? Where are you going? This is the only country where people say "I am starving." They will never say "I am hungry, I need to eat," or "I feel like having some little tidbit or something." No, "I am starving. I am freezing." I always say, "Why not say 'I am dying' and be dead?" I mean, who wants you? Can you believe how sick your children become when they hear those words from you? How insecure they become, how insane they become, how perverted they become? Have you ever thought about that dreadful word you use, what effect you cause? I want to show you, just a little bit, by experience. Sit down.

If your power is not in your grace, every other power is as useless as you can name.

Meditation to Move through the **Ethers**
September 22, 1985

Posture: Sit down in a meditative posture and close your eyes.

1. Listen to the Guided Visualization: "Go in trance, it is all cool, it's all vast, it's all blue. It is the infinite, it is the infinite, the infinite. Transmute yourself into the first layer of blue ether. Blue ether, the vastness, the blue, the lively, the life, the first state of impact of a soul. Transmute, transmute and intertwine yourself into the second blue ether, the self-realized, self-purifying, self-vastness of Infinity. In the sacredness of that, swim, feel, fly, be loose, get lost. Nap it. Repeat it, repeat it mentally. The vastness, the beauty, the Infinity of the blue ether.

Transmigrate into all facets of it, enrich yourself like a light, blue light of the gas-burning furnace. Heat! Transport yourself beyond that. Beyond that! Beyond that! Feel starving and hungry. Feel starving and hungry, feel the skeleton, the feebleness, no strength. Hungrier and hungrier and hungrier. Starving and starving and starving and starving and starving! Freezing and freezing and freezing and freezing and freezing!

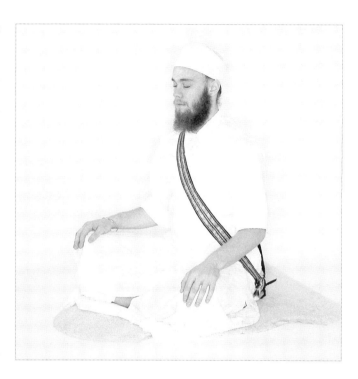

Return, return to the third ether. Warm and cozy, radiant and innocent like a child. Beautiful, beautiful, soft, beautiful, radiant, content, contained, satisfying, content, contained, satisfying, successful. Bright, full of light. Bright, full of light. Bright, full of light. Feel it, experience it. Move, move into the joy of it. Move. Let your anger go. Let happiness return. Let hatred go, let love return. Let defeat go, let success return, you are now living love." **5 Minutes**

2. Very sweetly sing, in a monotone: **I am living love**. **3 ½ Minutes**

Comments: Hypnotize yourself. Let heavens and angels hear it.

3. Go deeply within yourself and Sing: **I am man, I am good, I am living, I am love**. **1 Minute**

Comments: Go deeper and deeper into a deep hypnosis of you. Touch your goodness, touch your manliness, touch your love, touch your living faculty. Give yourself all the good values.

4. Inhale and meditate in silence. Count your virtues as you listen to the visualization:

"In the vastness of the sky spread your wings. In the vastness of the sky spread your wings and let yourself fly the flight of victory. Over all, above all, with strength and merits, with success and love, celestial being, born in the will of God with the light of God, with the life of the breath—pure, simple, honest, celestial being. Light and vast. Powerful and pure. Excellent and excellence. Excellence be your virtue. Excellent be yourself."

To End: Inhale deep and hold it. 30 seconds. Feel that you are filled with excellence, light, beauty, power, strength. Exhale and relax.

May the long time sun shine upon you, all love surround you and the pure light within you, guide your way on. Feel good, feel good, don't try to be too holy. It's all right. Everybody who supervises the nine holes with the tenth hole of consciousness is holier than anything else.

Well, God willing, we will meet again, we will teach again and be again.

■ ■ ■

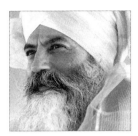

Man to **Man** 11
The Qualities of a Successful Man

Circa 1986

Nothing in the world can destroy you. Nothing in the world can build you. It is only the art of communication.

- Communicating **Successfully**
- Claim Your **Virtues**
- Communicate **Prosperity**

Communicating **Successfully**

Woman is not worried about the fact that you are saying something. She is not worried about what you are talking about. She just measures the heat, the life, the love, the force in you.

I would like you to understand something. I am going to do my best to make you understand, because I am very sick and tired. With all the intelligence and the commitment, we still have broken homes and divorces, and we are poor and some of us cannot pay our bills, and some are still angry. The problem as I see it is that we are professionally doing all that; we are professionally weak. It is not that we have been made to be weak. That's not true. I don't agree with that.

In this course I am discussing with you the basic faculties, which you innocently ignore, or don't take care of, or let build up in your personality through a very slow process, like gangrene. It kills your psyche and it forces you, as a man. You must understand that there is a difference between a man and a woman. Let us deal with that basically: A woman is conceptive. She can conceive. She can deliver. She can bear. It is inward world. She's a person. She is human. I am not discussing that part today. But in a man's life, she is the axle. She can bring you a lot of grief and influence a lot of your decisions in life. So much so, that she can damage you permanently. On the other hand, this woman, this axle of the male psyche, can give you growth, can give you strength.

Two things woman cannot do: She cannot sprout the seed and she cannot ripen the seed, remember this. To think that she can is your own foolishness, because the moon cannot sprout the seed. It is the sun's energy that will sprout it and it is the sun's energy that will ripen it. Now if we understand that, if we know that, and then we don't want to use that in our life, we are the craziest people in the world. There is a part in your life that woman can play and there is a part in your life that woman cannot play, and you don't want to accept that. That's why in our whole life, we live in conflict, and it is that conflict, which takes away the power of prosperity from us.

It is very shocking when you say. "Oh! I love her very much." Sometimes, the way you say "I love her very much," it looks like an insane person is talking. It doesn't make any sense. It has no logical sense. It is a consolidated, concentrated, emotional expression. A man should never have an emotional expression—write it down. It is the greatest folly to be a man and to talk in a consolidated, concentrated, emotional way. What happens when you do that? If you think you are great Romeos, which I doubt you all are, but I presume you are, because you feel you are very great Romeos. You believe you have to give an impression of a very consolidated, concentrated, high degree, hi-tech emotional response. Now, I am asking you, what will happen? You shall always live as a divorced idiot, lonely, and you will always be abused one way or the other. Because the moment you give an emotional, concentrated response to a woman, she will measure your temperature. She doesn't care what you are saying. All she cares about is the temperature. How much heat is in it? And after that, she knows she wants more. There is nothing to want. You are already a paper bag, used toilet paper. Do you want to do this to yourself? I am asking a question.

Woman is not worried about the fact that you are saying something. She is not worried about what you are talking about. She just measures the heat, the life, the love, the force in a male. Woman is not interested in how you look. Sometimes you see a weird man married to a very pretty girl and you ask, "Who is this?" She replies, "This is my husband." You look into the features and the facts, those false and right things yourself. Now, woman is governed by the heat of the Sun. Moon is governed by the Sun. What is in the heavens is on the Earth. The same principles apply. I am not telling you something I've made up, or pulled from a book yesterday, or God spoke to me at midnight and I am telling you now. No, I am just talking to you about certain basic realities—fundamental realities.

A female, what is a female? Business is female. Profession is female. All deployment of personalities is female. All employment of your wisdom is male. You walk through your life in deployment and employment; and they are off balance. You cannot just be you. If you presume in your mind, in a certain, distant image of you, that you have any value, it's not true; because in that image of yourself, you have only the value of a statue. Are you a statue? So it is the heat in you, by your feminine expansion and sustenance, that is the criteria and measurement of your value as you. Remember two things: expansion and sustenance. It is by your profession, by your family and by your influence; those three things are female. And those three things do not know whether you have a business degree in administration or you have a science degree in engineering. That is your own you.

Success is not by your caliber. Success is by the deployment of your caliber and the continuity in it. In the middle of the night, in the month of January, suppose your heater blows up. Let us put it that way, okay? What will happen? By 3 am you will start shivering; by 4 am it will be unbearable;

and by 5 am you will have to leave because that one cozy room will be freezing, am I right? That's what happens to your life. The coziness, the heat, the strength, the value of life, which is in you—you don't have to borrow it, you don't have to get it from somebody, it is you—that is female. But it is in how you deploy it, how you employ it, and how you bring it to balance that is male. If male is not a male . . . look, these are little rhymes we used to use.

> When male is not a male
> and he doesn't have a nail
> then he is a snail.

These three little lines—when we put these three lines before you and you look at them, you will find out what I am saying.

Now—immediately your mind has gone toward your sexual gland when I said the word nail. I can understand; but here that nail means the rhythmic axle and snail means snail. Snail cannot walk straight like an arrow; it goes like this, in a zigzag. It is a vibratory content. You walk two ways: One is rhythmic and one is straight. So your power to grow is *Pratyahar* and *Pranayam*—call it contraction, call it expansion, and together call it deployment of diplomacy: Where to say what? How to say it? How good you look? How bad you look? How do you want to look? It's diplomacy and that is what you call vibration, but even with all the diplomacy there is a strength, a fundamental strength, which is *you*. When *you* become diplomacy, the game is lost.

That is the greatest problem that you all have now, because first you say, let me have a career, let me have something, let me have another thin wafer. "Let me have" is a state of mind in which you push yourself to the hilt; it can be a very aggressive, moderately aggressive, or politely aggressive state. There comes a real stage of life, when you have a career, when you have a life, when you have your deployment and employment, when you are in balance or you're not, but at least you know where it lies, and *then* you goof. That is what I am going to handle today. Life has no place for mistakes. To err is not human. Normally we say, "To err is human." You understand? It is a consolatory statement. To err is not human. Only you err, when you do not deploy yourself in the basic strength and the outside deployment—inside strength, the axle, and the outside deployment must balance.

Don't you think that you are one person, a person based on the totality of your outer world? Any crack in the outer world can bring a flood into your life. The problem that all men of all walks of life have is that they don't care for their outside world; they care for themselves. I care for myself and when I care for myself, then I care about what I want and what I don't want. I will be a failure. You can't do that because what you want is just part of the whole thing that you are: You are a householder, you are a leader, you are a business executive or a laborer, you are a husband, you are a male chauvinist, you are a male macho, you are a meek, humble human. You can make as many categories as you want and then list them from A to Z, all the way to the bottom, and you will find out that all that you have put together relates to you, one way or the other. Sometimes in the morning you can't get up because there is nothing to get up for. Why? Because you do not analyze your life by categories and by steps. At night you cannot sleep because there is nothing to sleep with. You object and say you sleep with your wife, but that is not at all sufficient, my friend. You only sleep at night with your satisfaction and you get up in the morning with your spirit. You get up with your soul and you sleep with your achievement. You don't sleep with a female; it's a very wrong diagnosis.

You only sleep at night with your satisfaction and you get up in the morning with your spirit. You get up with your soul and you sleep with your achievement.

During the day, when you meet anybody, you do not meet anyone you know or don't know. You don't know if a person is a friend or an enemy. You do not have anything to do with whether a person is good or bad. Then why do you meet? And what do you meet with? You meet with an opportunity—taking it or missing it—that's your day. Are you shocked? You are. You don't meet with anyone. You meet everybody either to cash in on or lose an opportunity. If you don't have that strength, that grit, that power in you, start crawling—don't walk. It shames the human race. You crawl, nobody will mind. It doesn't take much, two pads on the knees and two pads on the hands, and then crawl. If you want to crawl in your life, it's your option. It is not anybody's affair; it is your choice. It is neither compassionate, nor is it a kindness, nor is it a great, generous, human divine work.

You cannot cash in on the opportunity if you do not have the spirit behind it—and you cannot have the spirit if you get up in the morning with a body and then a cup of coffee and then a vodka mixed with gin and orange juice. I have seen people. I know a man, he gets up in the morning, puts a glass of orange juice, and then one or two or three eggs in it, then he puts a cup of vodka in it, cup of gin in it, and then sometimes just for color, he adds some red wine.

I said, "Crazy! What are you doing this for?"
He said, "If I don't do this, by 11 o'clock, I will just go to sleep."
I said, "Have you used sometime hypnosis?"
He said, "No, what's that for?"
I said, "Just get up in the morning and stretch your legs and put your hands over the headboard like this sometime—try

that. Stretch your legs and put your hands straight, make a straight line and just say to yourself: let me be with my spirit, let me be with my spirit, let the sun shine in me, let me be with my spirit. In just about one minute, you won't be in a position to lie down straight. You will just get up like a straight arrow. You will be up on your feet."

Also, watch out if you are sleeping north and south. The worst thing a male can do to himself is sleep north and south. Your axle and the axle of the Earth will meet together and you will be a dead man in the morning. Female can tolerate north-south for 70 hours, male cannot even tolerate it 3 hours. The moment your energy and the energy of the axis, north and south, of the earth meets together, you become a blotting paper, soaked with the entire universal negativity. Still, man has not learned.

You know it is very funny, the Aryan used to be very strong. They conquered the world and they traveled the world. They were even worshiped, considered men of God; but they used to do Surya Kriya every morning, those exercises with the Sun, certain postures, certain powerful prayers, certain powerful thoughts, which in our language we call sadhana. What is sadhana? A bunch of exercises? No. Bunch of mantras? No. Bunch of people getting together? No. That's not true. Sadhana is nothing but a tendency, a tendency to get up in your own spirit.

Sadhana is nothing but a tendency, a tendency to get up in your own spirit.

What do you get up with? With work? For work? You get up for sex? You get up to make a telephone call? Whenever you get up for something other than your own spirit, you have ruined the day. That day you will be poor. There is nothing you can do about it. I can't help you and you can't help it, because you have set the clock. If you are so naive that you can't get up with your own spirit in the morning, then what will you remember? It is a fundamental question. Where is your strength? In your body? No. When you are dead, the body will be there. Nobody wants to keep it, unless you have said that it should be sold for $1200 to a hospital. Your strength is in your spirit and I just don't want you to underestimate what I am saying.

Whenever you get up for something other than your own spirit, you have ruined the day.

Kriya for Infinite Strength and **Communication**
September 21, 1986

Posture: Sit straight.

Mudra: Lift and spread your arms; the elbows are lifted with the hands slightly higher. Bend the elbow at 90° and bring the palms to face each other. Touch the pinky finger to the thumb. Touch and release, touch and release, move quickly.
3 Minutes

Comments: I just want you to be practical. Concentrate and see how much clarity it brings to you. Don't believe my words. I want you to know. I am not asking you to buy a machine or invest in a computer. I am trying to explain to you what your body can produce for yourself—how much infinite strength you have. How cheap it is to get rid of the confusion in your own self. That's what I am trying to explain. You don't have to telephone me when you are confused, all you have to do is this thing, by yourself. It takes exactly three minutes.

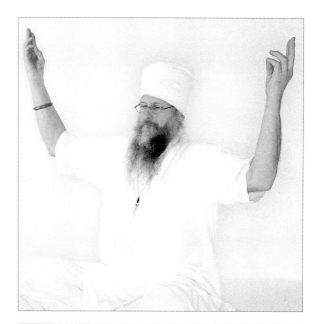

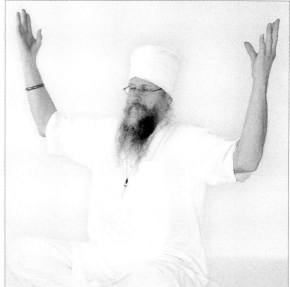

Business is not just going somewhere or everywhere to try to make a fool of ourself. Business is also female, which reorganizes and regenerates your own self, your being, your *bij* or seed. It is also business to be very strong, to not show your weakness, to be great when you are confronting someone or facing something. Being afraid is not a man.

Within your body there is an inflow of power of the Mercury, which is represented by your pinky and your Id, which is represented by your thumb. When they both connect and disconnect, for about three minutes, the brain has no other option but to manufacture a total clarity of your heaven, of your hell and your Earth—high, low and neutral—that's the law. Don't feel bad about it. Your strength is in your projection, not in you. Here's a simple example: suppose one of you has a bow and an arrow and someone else is bringing a cobra in his hand and is going to strike you with it and put you to death. All right? When you see the death coming, where is your strength? Your strength is in your body. Now, your strength is in your body whatever it is, big or small, but what's more, your strength is in how you stretch the bow and shoot the arrow to stop the incoming enemy.

Now you all know that fighting is a mess and nobody knows whether you will win or lose, but if you have common sense, your projection can stop the negativity before it touches you. It is very natural for a bird to make a nest. You have the home. Home—you have a home. In Punjabi, 'ego' is called *homey*. So home is nothing but a *homey*, an ego where you confine your physical material. That's why you have doors. That's why you have fences. That's why fencing is the law of life; you fence yourself. Sometimes we are very stupid. We make just a little fence, just four feet; cats can jump over it, dogs can jump over it, anybody can walk over it just by stretching. I mean, there is absolutely no keeping things out. I don't understand it.

Real fencing is called seven layers of fencing. First fence is your identity. Write it down. These are the secrets of success and it will work for you. First fence is your identity. Examine yourself; is your identity well respected, well established and well understood? Mostly your identity is not well understood by the world you belong to and that's where the problem is.

Second fence: your purpose to achieve is well contained; you should receive consciously. Do not ever take another person for granted. Never, that's the biggest mistake a male can do—and they all do it. I am not saying that it's the biggest mistake a male can do and you don't do it. You do it in spite of my telling you! In spite of your knowing it, in spite of your writing it down! Someone even wrote it on the back of glass through which he could see, and still he did that. We are very short-tempered individuals. Just meet the world with reception, receive the world.

Third is your first impression, the first word you utter, first statement you make, first communication you establish. It should be short and balanced. In this way, life is a great pleasure to have a few moments with you. You have already said you are short on time. You have already said you are meeting. You have already said that it is a great pleasure. It means you want to achieve everything quick.

Fourth is a very vital situation called inquiry. Inquire everything first. Fifth is judge it for you and without you. Sixth is, if you are lucky and you have a consultant, consult. Seventh is act.

7 Layers of **Fencing**

1. *Identity–Be well respected, well established and well understood.*

2. *Receive the World Consciously–Don't ever take anyone for granted!*

3. *First Impression–Your first communication should be short and balanced.*

4. *Inquiry–Ask, research, know everything you can about the situation.*

5. *Judge it–For you and without you.*

6. *Consult–If you have a consultant, seek their advice.*

7. *Act–Take action.*

Now tell me honestly, in your everyday walk of life, do you go by this procedure? In your walk of life, you have to train yourself in this whole thing; it should be your attitude. You know what these seven things are called? It is called male attitude.

Whether you are gay or you are straight or you are a pervert or you are macho or you are normal or you are heterosexual or monosexual, God knows what you are? You think you are brown, yellow, skinny, black, it doesn't matter. This is a male attitude. Okay. Now you remember those seven things? If you just remember some of them—that's not enough. Repeat them until you can recite them from memory. That's how you are going to be.

Dialogue **Exercises**

Watch. Just see—this is a most academic person. They both are very academic. It is not as if we are talking to just anyone from off the street. Both are college graduates, let us put it that way. You will see the most fascinating thing right now; you will see it happening. I am showing you the practical side of it right now. Ask him question.

Question: *Are you a Sikh?*
Reply: Yes, I am Sikh.
Yogi Bhajan: Have you gone through the seven steps? You didn't know I can read the aura. Now watch when he questions you. You just thought for a moment what should I say and then you said it. No, don't do that. He is asking you a question, it could be any question. You go through the seven steps as quickly as you can and then reply to him. Communicate now. It is a simple debate of the subject. How do you know? In my destiny? When you ask the first question and you use the term, 'Sir', it means you have already subjected yourself. Question is gone. Sir means sir. Sir just means sir. Reply is, "yes, sir." Then you have no grounds. Come on.

Indeed, as a man of practical wisdom and action, I practice those seven rules and when you practice these seven rules, life becomes humorous. Your communication improves, your effectiveness becomes spontaneous, and that is the one secret step of success; but you look around and try to find answers, you look confused and go through the jumbo jet of your own conflicts, you are already lost.

All right change subjects, any subject, and you have the right to start the dialogue. You can ask any question you want. It's a very rare opportunity and a good day. All right you say "Sir" and sit.

Student: *Sir, are you a man or not?*
Yogi Bhajan: My God! That is what God made me. You can't see? You have bad eyesight? I thought you had good eyesight. Then, correct. That's how I made me, too. A real man. Are you real? You are? So how can you see me and even ask the question, Am I a man or not? Where is the doubt? Oh, but this was the simplest; it was very simple to doubt my gender. Fantastic, please don't spread it around that you have a doubt about you, even now, keep it a secret.

Do you understand on the simplest question that we have communicated about—what laughter came out, what life came out, what joy came out—have you understood? It will always come up, exactly like this, if you practice this procedure in timelessness. Make it a habit.

Student: *Should we tell our partners, our wives, about what we're learning?*
Yogi Bhajan: This is a men's course. Have you come to Ladies' Camp to talk about the woman? This is a men's course. Do you find any woman here? Are we crazy to talk about our self and give our secrets away to our opposite sex? Impossible. Later, they can find out if they want it.

Let us dialogue because communication is what a male is. Male minus impact and interlock of communication is nothing but a virtual mockery. Not only do you have to have an impact, but also you have to interlock the other person. You have to bring the other thing to zero. Have you no shooting experience? What do you do? You bring focus on that point and then you fire. First is the interlock and second is the impact; and the procedure is this. Go ahead.

Student: *What is a teacher?*
Yogi Bhajan: Teacher is what teaches.

Student: *What does a teacher teach?*
Yogi Bhajan: What do you want to learn?

Student: *I want to learn what a teacher is?*
Yogi Bhajan: What you want to learn, the urge of you to learn, is what a teacher is.

Student: *But what makes me a teacher?*
Yogi Bhajan: You are a teacher by your very existence, by your urge to learn, your urge to grow. Your urge to expand makes you seek a teacher. How do I seek it is your question; why you are stopping it I can read. How to seek—that's what you actually want now. I know.

Seeking is within your own strength within your own soul. You shall get what you seek. The reality of seeking is the identity of your existence. If you seek wrong things you will have wrong things. If you seek right things you will always have right things. When you seek a higher Self, then you shall seek a teacher. Seeking a teacher is not a reality of normal life. Seeking a teacher is seeking the reality of your higher Self.

Student: *But I see myself slipping away . . .*
Yogi Bhajan: Slip away? If you don't want to seek your higher Self, then slip away. There is always a start and a stop. Anybody who wants to start his higher Self will start seeking, and as they seek, sometimes they just stop. When

If you seek wrong things you will have wrong things. If you seek right things you will always have right things. When you seek a higher Self, then you shall seek a teacher.

they stop things will slip away. Because the law of life is that destiny and faith run in parallel—that's a parallel force. Blessing through grace is a perpendicular force. Power and projections and pleasure, happiness, is a diagonal force. When these three forces start acting in centrifugal and centripetal dynamic, the entire universe is manufactured. So is the business and so the blessing and so the boys and the girls and the homes and the towns and the cities, the rain, the water, the mountains, the plants, the forests, the birds, the underworld, the fishes—the whole life—are a projection of those two dynamic fields, run by the three-dimensional force, and in that is a human criteria to seek a higher Self.

As long as there is an urge to seek a higher Self, you shall, with your teacher. The moment you have urged yourself to be perfect, you shall become a teacher. And because only God is perfect, they will keep on seeking. Those who stop, they don't stop in the power of the time and space, they hang themselves as ghosts. So, there is no stopping. Nobody stops. It is just like a divorce. You divorce your wife but then you pick up your child on weekends and child custody and child support and then the real game starts. If you see how much time you spend on being married and how much time you spend being divorced, you will be shocked how intense being divorced is over being married. So basically, if you look at the time you have to spend being divorced, if you had spent that much time being married, your marriage would never have had to face a divorce—it is true. Try it. When you are married, you forget you are married until the divorce hits you. Then you start—and the problem with the divorce is, you can't forget anything. You can't stop the child support, you can't stop picking up your children. I mean, really, how many of you, being married, take your children to the park every Sunday by yourself? Give me a break.

How many of you give $150 to $300 extra to your wife, saying, "Honey, this is for the child and you." Come on, name me. How many of you have developed a reserve so that when you are extremely hurt, totally angry and you want to blow up like a cannon, you don't have to talk the way you talk to your divorced wife. Have you ever talked to your own like that? No, because you do not communicate with this law of seven. You do not process things quick. You do not go through it quick. You have not developed it as a mental habit. You have not let it become a mental tendency.

If you do not read behind the words and between the lines and all that, you will be sold for pennies. You have to go through the internal process. You can't help it. I am going to deal with this practical thing we have just started, establishing communication, between two boys. Okay. Ask him a question on career and thoroughly examine him.

Student: *What is a successful career?*

Reply: What did you say? Successful career is one in which I can pay my bills plus I can pay my neighbor's bills plus I can pay bills that I don't want to pay.

Yogi Bhajan: Successful career is when I can pay my bills, pay my neighbor's bills and pay my bills, which I don't want to pay, and still there is a little surplus. Successful man is where his environments, his deployment, money, profession, whatever, it is always there to give extra support than needed. This is what he said? You said that? Well, how did it get complicated? Do you think that anything, which is complicated, can be successful? So how did it get complicated?

Student: *I'm just following it to the best of my knowledge.*

Yogi Bhajan: Follow what? I asked you to follow those seven rules. Did you follow them? It is not to the best of your knowledge. It is just your knowledge; it became your knowledge—that is your knowledge now. There is a grape in the mouth or a grape in the stomach. Grape in the mouth is not food. Grape in the stomach is the food. Knowing the wisdom and not applying it, not applying it in timelessness, is a waste of knowledge—and it is a super waste of life. Let every man know that the faculty to live as a man is to process life in the space of timelessness. When any man processes the life in time, he will just live in pain.

How many Virgos are here? Okay, doctor Virgo. Correct, that's a good match. They are very critical, self-critical Virgos, and normally they are obsessed with the details in any situation. If they are lucky, then they get out of this. Okay. Doctor you have the right to bombard him, question after question, and he has to reply as fast as he can.

Students: *What about your future?*

Yogi Bhajan: Wait a minute—that's a non-Virgo answer. I have no problem that you said that, and when he asked that question, question was correct. The answer was, I want to avoid having a problem in the future. You are guarding your future. You don't have to go into an intellectual wrap. Instead, you have to go inside and see that you are confronting a future—that's where you missed the fifth point. Whenever you answer without the fifth step, the internal examination and guarding, from there on, your answer will never have an impact. He will ride on you like you are dust and he is a chariot and you don't want that, correct? You will start feeling depressed and after a long fight with depression, you will become confused, and after a long confusion, you will say, "My God, there is no God," and the moment you start going into those kinds of thoughts, you will be using your life force six times more than you normally use in proportion.

If you go through this kind of coincidence once a week, you need seven days to recuperate—which means all you have is four days a month. The entire month is out and you can't afford it. It is called mental fatigue, like fatigued iron, you will become brittle. The people who are brittle in attitude, they are brittle with their life. Those who are brittle and fatigued in their life are those who do not assess their communication; they don't use proper communication techniques. Nothing in the world can destroy you. Nothing in the world can build you. It is only the art of communication.

Art of communication can take away your entire strength and dump you. Or, it can give you your entire strength and place you in the heavens. Between heaven and hell hangs one thing called word, what you speak. You are what you speak. So answer immediately with that rule because proportionate depression will make you proportionately aggressive; and when you are depressed you are not acting. When you are proportionately, equally aggressive, you shall act—and that will be madness. You will act madly and you will think you are bringing your own wisdom. Not possible. So when you talk and act and fight and walk in life, just have two principles: casual and schedule. Go by the seven principles and look very casual, very normal, calm, unimposing. Go on doctor, he is yours.

Student: *How are your finances?*

Yogi Bhajan: Too long. The pause is too long. You can look like you're thinking, you can look imposing, you can look calculating—but not too long. When you take too long, then you are confused, you do not know, and you are lost before even uttering a word. Answer him quickly. Repeat the question.

Student: *How are your finances?*

Yogi Bhajan: By the way he has no money problem. They are well off.

Student: *How is your wife?*

Yogi Bhajan: He is discussing your blonde; be careful what you say about her.

Oh, by the way, this is one gentleman you should learn from. The way he behaved and treated and progressed toward his wife, he deserves many, many thanks. His life is now well-balanced, happy and the way he made it happen is real charisma; it is a real art. Why I am giving him credit now is because he was in a situation, which is called super impossible, and now it is so tamed, so well-balanced and so beautiful that he deserves great congratulations as a man—and he did it single-handedly. That's what I appreciate in him.

Subject is sex.
Student: *Do do you like sex?*
Reply: Yes.

Nothing in the world can destroy you. Nothing in the world can build you. It is only the art of communication.

Student: *Why?*
Reply: Because

Student: *How do you like sex best?*
Reply: The way it should be done.

Yogi Bhajan: All right let us save the opportunity for someone worthy. He is too humorous.

The debate is about, "I shall rule."
Student: *Am I asking the question?*
Yogi Bhajan: Yeah, you are the winner or he is the winner. Who rules who? Between two men there is a conflict. You are ruling him or he is ruling you.

Student: *What is your problem?*
Reply: There is no problem.
Student: *I feel that you have a problem with me.*
Reply: That would be *your* problem.
Yogi Bhajan: In a short time . . . He is very expert on a long communication in a short time.

Now pitch in against each other and try to attack the integrity of each other. It will be quarrelsome, and don't use foul words please. He shall attack your integrity, you shall attack his integrity in a defensive manner, but no foul language will be used. You are both highly educated. I think you can do this performance.

[Students go through exercise.]

No, no, you are not intense enough. We have to find somebody who can fight really loud. The character you are representing is intense attacking but not using any filthy or ugly language. He is educated. He doesn't need instructions, but I think between two well-balanced, educated people, a communication can happen in a state of anger, which the audience will benefit from understanding. You will communicate in a very, it is called Aries communication, head-to-head manner. You know what it produces? That kind of impact we need—interlock. He will be interlocking you on that issue. What subject do you think will be enough to provoke you?

Student: *It's hard for me to be provoked.*

Yogi Bhajan: Yeah it is difficult to provoke you, that's your problem. Don't look to me, provoke him. Your job is to provoke him. He is a very unprovokable personality and your job is, within the realms of etiquette, to provoke him. That's all.

[Students go through exercise.]

Okay, okay, thank you, it was beautiful. It was very good. I am trying to give you what a common man, under confined environments, will want to establish a communication with. [To a student] Give them a lecture on why they should not eat carrots.

Student: *Everyone, it's best if you do not eat carrots. In fact, in order to maintain improper liver function, please don't eat carrots. Also, each year there is arthritis, rheumatism and possibility of constipation by not eating carrots. Because the carrot doesn't make the skin clear, if you have a skin problem, too, stay away from carrots. If there is any possibility that your hair is going gray or if your hair is falling out, you also want to avoid eating carrots because carrots help the scalp and you want to keep your hair from growing better later in life. Does anybody have a question so far?*
(Students laugh)

Yogi Bhajan: Thank you sit down. A subject, which was impossible not to admire, even among all the people of faculty here, why we should not eat carrots, because of the way he prescribed it will let you know that it's not what you know, it is what you deliver and how you deliver through your words. Knowledge is not enough. You did not understand his joke? He was breaking rules and pretending not to be provoked. He was telling you not to eat carrots; but instead, I feel the impact of that is an interlock that all you want is to go right now and eat a carrot each. You understand?

So you must understand where lies the success and where lies the strength in life. Success lies in saying it with a smile. Success lies in interlocking the word with a smile. Each word you speak, interlock it and deliver it with a smile.

Life is no different whether you dramatize it or you traumatize it. If you dramatize your life you will not have impact. By dramatizing you can interlock. But as you have seen, you must have seen a drama in your life, when you see a drama you always hear—oh well, this is it! But there is something behind it; somebody is acting; it is not real. In a drama you feel that reality is being communicated to you, but you don't have to take it or you don't have to experience it. In trauma you don't feel anything except anger toward it. So what is the best secret of life: communicate exactly as you. That is the second phase we would like to practice. Just say "as you."

More Dialogue **Exercises**

One: *Speak very angrily, almost near abusive language, but without jeopardizing your image as being nice and kind. Choose anyone you feel comfortable with.*

Two: *Choose two people who have great art and intellectual sense, who are uncomfortable using aggressive language. The discussion is about impact and it's an aggressive communication, using the question: Is life art or misery?*

Three: *This is a straight negative fight. There is no rhythm or any place for any positive baiting. Baiting is considered positive. Be negative without baiting.*

Ask yourself a simple inner question, I am real? When you say that, when you will speak this, also concentrate, synchronize and feel it. Before you finish this sentence, synchronize, I am real. I am real. Each of you will say it and each one of you will synchronize to feel it in timelessness, in sharpness, in reality.

Kriya: Communicate as **You**
September 21, 1986

Posture: Sit in a meditative posture.

1. Repeat loudly: I am real, I am real . . . **30 seconds** to **1 Minute**

Comments: When you say that line, I am real, concentrate, synchronize, and feel it. Before you finish the sentence, synchronize I am real. I am real. Each of you will say it and each one of you will synchronize to feel it in timelessness, in sharpness, in reality. Say it loud in your real voice, in that communication that is your real communication, in that projection that is your real projection. Synchronize timelessness to experience it.

2. As you repeat the line, I am real, mentally vibrate the mantra:

Aad Sach Jugaad Sach Hay Bhee Sach Nanak Hosee Bhee Sach

"In the beginning I was real, through the time I was real, now I am real, and Nanak, real I shall be." 30 Seconds

3. Repeat: I was, I shall be, I am real. 1 Minute

4. Repeat: I was, I shall be, I am, I am. 1 ½ Minutes

5. Now sing the line, I was, I shall be, I am, I am, as if you were an Italian Opera singer. See what it does to you. **1 Minute**

Comments: Do you understand the difference? One is affirmative, the other is very positive, futuristic, musical. When you talk to somebody in a musical, futuristic situation, you create chaos because musical communication has to be rhythmic and futuristic communication has to be very exact; and sometimes you can't deliver that. If you don't have the capacity to deliver in that way, you create confusion; so it is always better to be very low-key, mono, affirmative. It won't make you feel bad and it will get you everything you need—and that's all life is about.

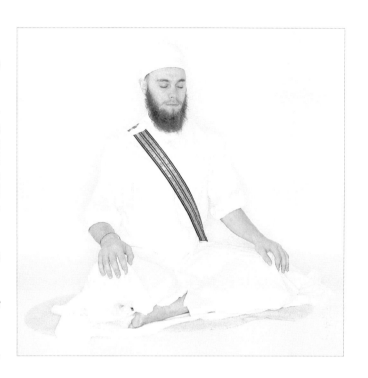

Claim Your **Virtues**

Four or five flowers to have in your life are tranquility, trust, faith, integrity and divinity.

The Lesson of the **Sword**

This is what I want to teach today. This is a very finely made sword. The cut is here and here, on the opposite side. So strength in the opposite is a parallel strength, they call it. Until the parallel strength is built, there is nothing strong. That's the law. You think strength has to be the same, both ways. It's wrong. It is never right. That's where you goof up in your life, you can't cut negativity strongly. The lesson of the sword is to cut negativity and make a path. Lesson of the sword is not to fight. It was a symbol of honor. It was a symbol of knighthood. It was a symbol of initiation. And this is an African spear, you will find the chieftains, how much family power they have, is listed on it. So the sword and the spear are symbols, the symbolic carriers of your strength.

Lingam **Kriya**

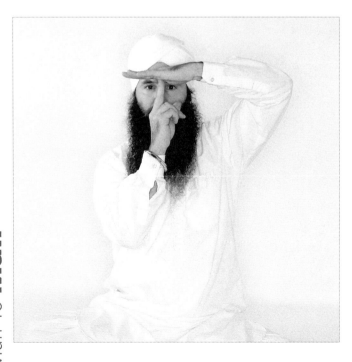

Posture: Easy Sitting Pose

Mudra: Bring the left hand up above the brow line, palm down. Take the middle finger (Saturn) of your right hand and make a T with your left hand, placing it in the center of the palm of the left hand, aligning the right middle finger with the bridge of the nose. The right middle finger should be very straight. Curl the remaining fingers of the right hand (right palm is facing toward your left). The tip of the nose and the root or base of the middle finger should be on the same level.

Eyes: Stare straight ahead through the middle finger.

Mantra: I was, I shall be, I am, I am, Har Haray Haree

Comments: Take a bath. Then prepare for meditation, sit in a comfortable seated posture, and practice for 62 Minutes, from 11:30pm to 12:32am. It is called transit-lock time—from evening to morning.

Yesterday we talked in detail about what are called symbolic situations and gave you something to go do as homework, so that you can understand where the strength is and how to build up the strength so that you can call on it anytime. Was that clear? How many of you did the sadhana last night? There were so many in the ashram I could hear it. Did you feel the strength or did you not feel the strength?

Too much energizing with it is not very advisable, but energizing with it anytime, as a male, whenever you want is okay. It will give you the potential of opening like the bud. You know what that means? The life of a male is like a bud. If doesn't open, it doesn't let the fragrance get out. You don't rule by the strength of your muscles or the game of your mind or even the power of your soul—that's for you to live. It has nothing to do with anybody. Your greatest virtue is how your fragrance travels and how it affects other people. In other words, man has his own smell, without it he is a living hell. It is a simple thing. Man has his . . .?

Students: *. . . own smell.*

Yogi Bhajan: Without that, life is a living hell. That's what word is. So basically what you are trying to understand within yourself is that you have your own smell. Don't substitute it and don't alter it.

I was counseling somebody this morning, and while counseling I said, "Is it true you had intercourse with somebody for a short while just out of passion." Answer was yes. So I said, "You know what it did to you?" The answer was yes; then his question came, "How much time will it take me to recover?" I said, "Next life time." Three days of physical, commotional intercourse brought to this person 15 years of aging and dullness, which he does not know how to get rid of. So actually, because of your odor, you can be blinded by passion. Your smell, your fragrance does not qualify the relationship. You are calling on nothing but the long painful self.

Kaam Kaaya Ko Gall Hei

It means "passionate living destroys the physical body." It is not that you are not intelligent, it is not that you cannot be successful, it is not that, as a male, you are not productive, it is not that you have to go out and study the whole world and universe and come out to be somebody, it is not true. Actually your passion blinds you and your fashion destroys you, because in passion you make up a fashion, and in that fashion you build up your style, and in that style you fly. You move like your fragrance. The net result is that you endure nothing. You become self-critical. You become a self-depressed person. You cannot share with anybody—and that pain is enough to kill you. You have two worlds to live in: One is the world of your head. The other is the world of your heart. I am asking you: if you cannot put your head and your heart together, what can you put together?

There is no camouflage in my mind. I am not willing to misunderstand you or your pain. For example, let's just take this one example:

A man's wife says, "My dear, do you expect to eat at home or are we going out?"
His reaction is "Maybe at home, maybe we will go out."
She says, "Are you sure?"
"Don't be my mother; I am sick of it. I told you."
"Okay, fine, you have told me; but what exactly do you want? Are you going to eat at home or are we going to go out?"
"I am going to eat at home, home, right here."
So she gets up, she cooks, and everything is fine. He puts on the heater, fine.
Then he asks, "What time is it?"
"It is nine o' clock."
"All right, let's go out and have a bite and then go to a movie."

Now this woman doesn't have the spear that I am holding, which she wants to put through your heart. She has spent two hours cooking the whole damn meal and now you are saying "I am going out and then I am going to entertain myself." You understand what this does to another person? It is not that you do it to your wife; I am just using that example. This is also what you do in your business. Exactly. Your pattern of behavior with your wife and your pattern of behavior in your business and your pattern of behavior with your success is the same pattern because it is all female. You cannot deal with your domestic government; you cannot deal with your administrative government; you cannot deal with your totality, governing your whole universe, because you have to understand that you have to deploy yourself and employ the means to secure your deployment, so that it won't tear everything apart. You must employ means; you must use your fragrance.

This is a building. You see it? You see the whole thing. It's based on four walls but if we extend it beyond this, we may need pillars. There must be weight-bearing walls. Have you heard of the concept weight-bearing walls? That is a criteria; it is a character in life. It has to have commitment. That commitment must come from your communication. Your strength is not in your muscles or your brain or your this or your that. The fragrance, which I am referring to that of a flower, is from your words: what you say and how you say it; when you say it and why you say it. One slip of the tongue—one—I am not talking of two. One slip of the tongue can bring you from the top to the bottom. And one use of the tongue can take you from the bottom to the top. Power of the word is unseen like the power of God, but it has mileage in it. You want to ask me to prove it. You will ask me tomorrow. The bird flew from the air. Where? Show us. They don't leave any sign but everybody knows they fly. But when you say "I want to see whether the bird flew through the air or not," people will think you are crazy. Everybody knows that birds fly through the air and leave no sign. Exactly in this way, the universality of God and universality of fragrance is exactly yours. It can never, ever be anyone else's.

You can change your culture. You can change your attitude. You can change your country. You can change your way of dressing, eating, living, you can even change your way of sex, commotion, emotion, everything, but one thing you can't change—your fragrance. For that there are only two things to do: either it is there or it is not. You have to decide today one thing: are you in command or are you not? Now the problem with you is that you want to be in command but you don't want to do all that needs to be done, which a commander must do. That's your problem. That's your duality. You want to be in command. But you do not want to do the homework.

I have seen a very beautiful father; he is very loving to me. I love him. One day I was at his house and his child came and started created a big drama. He couldn't handle it. He was just fighting back, yelling and screaming, and calling his wife's name. The child was taken away. "Don't you know the Siri Singh Sahib has come?" I thought to myself, my God.

I pulled him aside, "Hey, come here."
"What sir?"
I said, "Deal with that kid and calm the whole thing down. I want to know that you are in command. Otherwise, I am leaving in ten minutes. I will give you ten minutes."
In ten minutes the kid was nice, the home was calm, and everything was normal. This is how you act under fear. Threat. Then I cracked up.
"Ha ha," I said.
He said, "What?"
I said, "Why didn't you handle it to begin with?"
And you know what he said? He said, "I was irresponsible."

"I was irresponsible"; now I am asking all of you from here to there, can you honestly tell me that most of the time you are irresponsible without any reason or cause, but you want a responsible life? You want a responsible life and you deal with it irresponsibly. You want to grab an opportunity, you want to have success, and then sometimes you talk and you don't even know what you are saying. This is normal. I don't understand it. I will think about. I can promise you straight. You know what you are doing to yourself? You are just doing to yourself . . . how do you say it? You are doing yourself in. No male has the right to be doubtful in communication. Your doubtful communication is the only enemy for which you will pay in blood. Now we are not discussing right or wrong, believe me. I am just discussing the truth. You cannot talk in your life the way you talk. You cannot dramatize in your life the way you dramatize. You have to be exact. Repeat after me: exact, authentic.

That's your problem. That's your duality. You want to be in command. But you do not want to do the homework.

Students: Exact. Authentic.

Yogi Bhajan: And on the spot a leader, now repeat it again.

Students: Exact. Authentic. And on the spot, a leader.

Yogi Bhajan: Say it again.

Students: Exact. Authentic. And on the spot, a leader.

When you go home from here, check it out. All your misfortunes are because you disobeyed these three laws: Exact. Authentic. And on the spot, a leader. Just work it out deeply in you and you will find it so. Just remember, when a man is a yo-yo that's what he gets. You can play that. You can play your insecurities with your self. You cannot play your insecurities with the world around you. Do you understand the difference? You can play your insecurity with yourself. You can discuss them, deal with them, and find out where your strength is and what you are going to do. When you plan your life, you need to know your insecurities. But you cannot deploy them in the world around you. When you walk out of the door, you are dressed up. You don't walk naked. But in the bathroom, you don't take a shower with your suit on. You understand the difference? Am I correct in description? How many of you have ever taken a shower in a three-piece suit and a tie on? Can anybody raise their hand? Is there any insane person here? And how many of you have walked totally bare naked with a tie around your neck and gone out into the street to do shopping? Now, those two things you can do but you wouldn't. But mentally, when you communicate, that's exactly what you do. You talk bare naked with somebody where absolute diplomacy is required; and you get uptight and square in situations, that is totally combative, analytically covering yourself, when something has to be very free, casual, and frank.

Now tell me how can life be cozy at all? I am just asking a question. That mental stress and that physical exploitation of the pranic energy, that confusion and that duality doesn't let you live to your full potential—and that's why you become a victim of vulturing. Vultures come and say: "I will make the best out of you. I will do wonderful things to you. I will do that to you." They paint such a Garden of Eden and then they steal the few flowers you have collected with a lot of hard work. Four or five flowers to have in your life are tranquility, trust, faith, integrity and divinity. Say it again: Four or five flowers to have in your life are tranquility, trust, faith, integrity and divinity.

When you are divine and you have divinity you are not

divided. Some people do not understand what divinity means. Divinity means you are not divided. Tranquility means you can take it—doesn't matter what. What is next? You know what trust is? Trust is the total thrust in you. You know? Have you seen some cars, when you try to go uphill, they can't go. They say, "put-put-put." These cars cannot be trusted; don't you say that? "I can't trust my car to go uphill." Is that understood? That's what it is. Trust in yourself. Now ask me the question. What do we have to trust in our self? That's a very fundamental question. Trust in yourself—trust that you are very divine and let everything be judged by that touchstone. I am not open for discussion.

If you want it, I have the answer for your neuroses. I am willing to work with you because I just want to tell you: If you want to drop neuroses, you can drop them just by dropping them. By discussing it, you can drop it. You have a fear of alienation, which you are unable to overcome. I am not saying you are the only one. There are a lot of people who have this fear. Fear of being alien. Fear of not being successful. Fear of their own guilt. Fear that they will offend the world around them. Fear that their relatives will leave them. Fear that they will not have enough money and support for their old age. Fear that their enemies are going to get them. Fear of the darkness. Count how many I said. You are a mathematician. You were not listening? How many fears have I listed? Count. Did somebody write them off? Is not what I am teaching you timeless? You should be sharp and quick to grab things that are readily available and useful. Each male has fears and one of them is very prominent. If that fear is not encountered then love cannot flow from you.

Four or five flowers to have in your life are tranquility, trust, faith, integrity and divinity.

Dialogue **Exercises**

There are two mikes. I need volunteers: One person will stand up and spontaneously speak. I am afraid of _____ and the other person will totally destroy that fear. That is what I want to happen. Get on those two mikes please. Quick. Each one will say their most prominent fear. And the other one immediately attacks it and proves it wrong— I want you to prove it is wrong.

Student: *I am afraid of success.*
Reply: Then succeed.

Student: *I am afraid of closeness.*
Reply: Then come closer to yourself.

Student: *I am afraid of death.*
Reply: Then live life to the fullest.

Student: *I am afraid of failure.*
Reply: Don't fail, succeed.
Yogi Bhajan: Continue—there are so many fears you know? You read it from the book. You see and say.

Student: *I am afraid.*
Reply: Then simply be yourself and rise to the occasion.

Student: *I am afraid to succeed.*
Reply: Just simply succeed.
Yogi Bhajan: How?

Student: *You have the ability.*
Yogi Bhajan: Where?

Student: *In your mind, in your heart.*
Yogi Bhajan: What is my mind? How do you know about it?

Student: *By working.*
Yogi Bhajan: What work? Birds don't work; animals don't work; worms don't work; human has to work? What you are talking about?

Student: *That's nonsense, you can succeed.*
Yogi Bhajan: You can say it is nonsense. There is nothing to succeed at; it's not worthwhile; life is just a pile of shit.

Student: *That's not true.*
Yogi Bhajan: That's very true. I know, I realize, I feel it, it is understandable.

Student: *I don't believe it.*

Yogi Bhajan: You can't believe because you don't know what belief is. Spell it.

Student: *B-E-L-I-E-F.*

Yogi Bhajan: See, you are just equal to a kindergarten child; you started spelling it. That's why you don't know what you are talking about. Where is the belief? In your head, in your heart, in your toes?

Student: *My heart.*

Yogi Bhajan: How many times have you listened to your heart? How many times have you listened to the cry of the heart of the whole wilderness of people? How many times have you gone out and listened to the prayer, the heartfelt prayer of those who are ugly, who are unseen? How many times have you gone into the park to see the bums and hear their prayer? What made them to be? How many times have you walked out of our secured world to the insecure world and seen how much pain is there and how much have you done to relieve it? How many miles have you gone on your own to play for those who couldn't walk? How many times have you washed your hands for those who do not wash? How many times have you not eaten for those who are hungry? How many of you have done anything, risked yourself for any reason, which is real, which is of the unknown?

Student: *Not enough.*

Yogi Bhajan: Don't agree with me. Be yourself. My vastness doesn't mean your defeat. It is a father's death when he sees his son being defeated under pressure. My vastness is useful to combat it and you will become equally vast. If an airplane, hundreds of pounds, can take the weight of the wings and carry it through the air to that height? Exactly you can go to the highest. It is through combat with the opposite that you combine to excel to the highest. That's why the time has come when they will kill me, because now I am a source of threat. I came in this country to create teachers and now they know it. They don't want it, because a teacher of consciousness can live and let many live. Consciousness and intelligence are two ways to combat the fear. There is no other way. When you are no longer afraid, you will have no vengeance; and only then can you enjoy the tranquility and the peace.

Yogi Bhajan: Why did you agree with me?

Student: *I don't know.*

Yogi Bhajan: Why don't you know? What is it that you don't know? Because everything that is attacking you has its own death in it. Remember that! Anything that brings death to you, also carries its own death. Just turn it around. God couldn't create one thing. You know what God could not create? God cannot create one thing—square or triangle–God has to create everything round, complete, because It is the perfect one. If somebody who is created by God brings death to you and you just turn it around, he shall die in itself.

Paapi Ke Marne Ko Paap Maha Bali Hei

"To kill a sinner, his own sin, is the extreme power."

What do you want to know? You want to know whether your heart is made of plastic or of rubber? What do you want to know?

Student: *Right now, nothing.*

Yogi Bhajan: There is nothing to know because everything is hanging in the knowledge. Even not to have knowledge is a square from which you can go to all four sides of the town. You feel weak?

Student: *No.*

Yogi Bhajan: Every week?

Student: *I don't understand.*

Yogi Bhajan: I know you don't understand, but you are standing up. Why do you use negative words? To get out of the proposition? "I don't know." "I don't understand." God gave you the brain, the best computer. To build this computer and the most modern chip 100 years from now would require an 80 mile by 80 mile square, and 10 mile high building to store it in—and you are carrying it in your skull. Why you don't understand it? Why are you waiting to answer my question?

Student: *I do understand it.*

Yogi Bhajan: You do. How?

Student: *I was just insecure.*

Yogi Bhajan: Again insecure is a negative word.

Student: *I understand what you said.*

Yogi Bhajan: You didn't care?

Student: *I didn't care.*

Yogi Bhajan: Have you understood or not?

Student: *I am glad I understood.*

Yogi Bhajan: Why you are not happy about it?

Student: *I am happy about it.*

Yogi Bhajan: Well, what is the basic of your life? What is the foundation of your life? One word—I need the answer. I don't need a lecture. Give me one word. What is the foundation of your life?

Student: My soul.
Yogi Bhajan: Not true.

Student: God.
Student: Not true.
Yogi Bhajan: What is the foundation of your life?

Student: Happiness.
Yogi Bhajan: Nonsense.

Student: Sadhana.
Yogi Bhajan: Forget it. Too gross. Sadhana is a perfect, selfish act to qualify oneself in strength to match up with the world. It has nothing to do with anything around. It is an act, which we do for ourself, because we want to survive and live, excel and become powerful. It is our power grasping trick; it has nothing to do with your base. What is the foundation of your life?

Student: Creativity.
Yogi Bhajan: You are drowned in hell or heaven, I don't care. What creativity? God is Creator and now you are in competition with that guy?

Student: The God gave me creativity.
Yogi Bhajan: Well, that's a long philosophy. What is the foundation of your life?

Student: I am, I am.
Yogi Bhajan: Too much of a bible. You want to know?

Student: Yes.
Yogi Bhajan: A little smile. True. If I am wrong drag me out of this place. The entire foundation of this whole male human life is one little smile. Not a big one, little. That's all it takes. There is no more powerful winning chip within you as a male than a small smile, like a small salad. What you call it? You know. Dinner salad—just a small smile. That's the foundation of this whole male syndrome.

You lose when you become tense. You are responsible for your own loss. You are neurotically defeating yourself all the time. Smile and let the whole world smile at you. Now it is a negative thing. You don't want people to smile at you. You don't and you are losing something very precious. You are losing something very precious. In the kingdom of God, plus and minus creates neutral. Attention creates grace. If you smile with people and people smile with you, at you, after you, behind you, over you, under you, that's all you are. That's your strength. Is that understood? So when you communicate, do not, for God's sake, communicate one word with which you cannot smile.

All right, both of you now talk to each other and just understand, you are not going to say one word in which you both can smile.

Student: You are married?
Student: Watch.
Student: How are your insecurities?
Student: What insecurities?
Student: Good.
Student: How is yours?
Student: I am fine.
Student: Great to hear.

Yogi Bhajan: Any person who wants be successful in life and has no degree, no art, no nothing, all he has to do is talk with a smile and not say those things with which he cannot smile. Success will be yours forever. Those who call themselves Sikhs must understand: there is something very common between the Sikhs and the Christians, which nobody even understood when the Christians were real Christians, not Roman Christians, when they were being persecuted by Romans. They stood being persecuted with a beautiful smile on their face. And in Rome, that coliseum stands today as a symbol of that. All holy places in Sikh Dharma are standing as a symbol of that smile on the face of a Sikh when he was facing and combating death.

Whether you are a Christian, you are a Hindu, you are a Muslim, you are a Jew or you are none, or you are other, whatever you want to call it, I am not discussing your religion; I am discussing your faith. Faith only means when you can combat the life. How serious can it be with a little smile on your face? You must remember, the higher you go in life, the higher shall be the penalties, higher shall be the dangers, higher shall be the confrontation, and higher shall be the schemes to destroy you. It is normal. Can you face life with a smile or not? That is the purpose of this living. Today the entire world doesn't understand you at all, but I have heard one comment: "God, to whom these angels belong?" They don't care what nonsense neurosis you are carrying inside—nobody cares.

Once, by mistake, provoking some lady, she said, "Who are these people? Beautiful, I love them. How can they keep their clothes so white? How they can be so shining and radiant?"

I said, "My lady, they are very ordinary people."
She said, "God, you don't have to tell me that. They are not ordinary people. In this world of today they are living above the trend, above tradition, above everything which America stands for. What is above the man?"
I said, "Tell me."
She said, "The crown. They are the crown of our civilization"

Sadhana is a perfect, selfish act to qualify oneself in strength to match up with the world.

I just wanted to share that with you. So God knows when you stand before a mirror and you look at yourself what you call yourself, but I am telling you what people say about you. At first sight, when they look at you, they see you are special. You are someone. If a person doesn't appear to be someone, he has no right to invite opportunities. When you are someone and you invite opportunities, immediately, those who want to destroy your opportunity shall appear. War is on; and those who do not know how, in the middle of the war, to be peaceful, they are the ones who are wrong. That's why in the old time, the law used to be that the armies would front each other. They used to have their breakfast, brunch, whatever. Take up their arms, fight the whole day, and when the sun went down, they used to lay their arms to rest, heal their wounds, recuperate to fight the next day.

Many of us fight our sleep. We do not know how to sleep. We do not know how to rest. Rest and work have equal forum and need equal attention. You know the problem with you? Oh, Mr. Unsuccessfuls, let me tell you what your problem is. All of you who are unsuccessful are those who say we will rest tomorrow. We will rest later. You know that syndrome? In the middle of the rest, when you are just enjoying it, he will say, I will do it tomorrow, let me work now. The highest priority of work is to rest. That's why you don't rest when your wife is all right, your children are okay, your family is okay, your home is all right. You are in a peaceful tranquility, but you don't rest with it. You bring more garbage into it. You pick up somebody's garbage pan on the street and bring it and put it in the living room. You start the war.

You are successful in business. You experience tranquility. You are peaceful and then you get somebody's nuisance in it, in partnership. You blow up yourself and blow up somebody else. You look at somebody and look at his smile, and look at his success, and look at his beauty, and look at his wonderful things, but you do not investigate. Then after you talk to the guy, he says, "My God, I am suffering from cancer. I have an ulcer in my stomach. I have had six operations on my intestines; they are cut down by six feet. I have three brain tumors and my one eye is totally false and I do not hear from my left ear and my right hand works half way and three fingers in my left arm are also numb." And you are competing with that guy? You understand what I am saying? Do you hear me?

Not to value your value is the biggest fraud a male can play on himself. The biggest nonsense in a male's world is not to value his values. You are always willing to barter and sell yourself out for a momentary passion, momentary kiss, momentary high, momentary telephone call. Once, you know, Narad said to Lord Krishna, "Wait a minute, these 1800 women dance around you. They never stop. What is the secret?" Lord Krishna replied, "Because I play my flute in the center." My dear men, you can't be off center. You have no center. When a man goes off center there is no place of holding yourself. You may say, "just for a moment" or "It was only that hour. It was that minute. It was that situation." No my son. There is no error. There is no place for error in life and love.

How many times have you committed errors and still you are surviving. Aren't you a miracle people? Combine your intelligence and your consciousness with purity— and purity means don't add nonsense to your life. Don't support those who cannot support themselves. Support them and teach them how to support themselves. "Don't give somebody a fish to eat. Teach them to fish and they will eat forever."

Don't give somebody grain and then enjoy his or her being dependant on you. Teach them how to grow the grain so they can prepare a breakfast for you to honor it. Tell all those you know and tell all those you don't know how to be great. Make your enemies great so that you can have a good fight. Now you are saying, "That's not true." But the law of being great is to have great enemies. No plane can ever take off without the opposite wind. If you think you can change the law of the universe then you are not a part of the universe. Two things my sons: Never let kindness and compassion slip from you. These are the two legs on which a male stands—not the muscle, not the money, not the technology—compassion and kindness. Be kind to your enemies and be compassionate to those who are out to get you. This is the highest state of mind in which a male can always be shielded.

Two things my sons: Never let kindness and compassion slip from you. These are the two legs on which a male stands—not the muscle, not the money, not the technology —compassion and kindness.

You know how protected you are if you are compassionate? The entire universe has to change environments to protect you because Mother Nature cannot let two things be destroyed, kindness and compassion; and God the Father is beyond Mother Nature, so you can't reach it. Never be rude to those who have been mostly rude to you. That's what Guru Gobind Singh said. When everything fails, your hand going to the sword is not so very bad, because what is the sword. Sword is anointment—knighthood. You cannot be a knight until you have knelt and been touched on the shoulder by the sword. Isn't that true?

The greatest thing, which is a defect in your life, is when you have to do something and you don't do it. You've got to do it. You've got to do it and you are the only one whom time has chosen to do it. Compassion should not make you compromise. Fight life compassionately, kindly. Be casual on your schedule. No tension. The only thing that the enemy will defraud himself of is his own strength, when he cannot or she cannot figure out where you stop and where you start. But if you are calm, quiet, peaceful, kind, keep going. You shall be kept going. You don't have to ask anybody to give you an injection for strength. You ask yourself. Where is my strength? Your strength is in tolerating the attack of the opposite, taking it on the shield of your grace and then counter attacking so that it may not happen again. Don't go for the sword of the enemy, go for the arm. Swords don't fight, arms do. Just learn. When your life, your family, your children are very tranquil, peaceful, growing, at that moment, you will find something will try to walk in the center of it to create a ruckus. Believe me or not, that's exactly when it will happen.

When you are on the way to your prime success, when everything is calm and cool, then comes the hailstorm. You can deal with it commotionally, emotionally, justify yourself with angles, ifs and buts. Or, you can say this is not my cup. I shall not compromise. Nobody can blackmail me. Nobody can steal away my smile. I am not going to hide anything. I am not going to be a rat running into holes.

Kriya to Claim Your **Virtues**
September 21, 1986

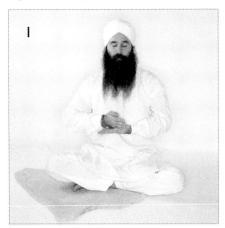

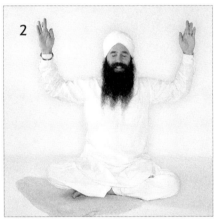

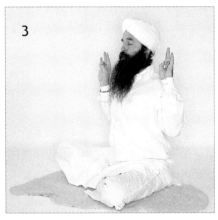

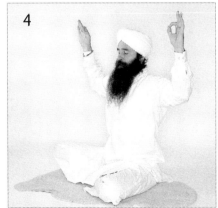

Posture: Easy Sitting Pose

1. Bring your left hand palm up in front of the navel. Place the pinky side of your right hand, the edge of the hand, and cross it over the palm of the left hand, as if you were chopping it, and rest it there.

Chant: I am a virtue. I am virtuous. I am, I am. **1 ½ Minutes**

2. Cross the Jupiter and Saturn fingers and bring the arms up so that the elbows are at a 90° angle and the mudra is about a foot away from each side of the head. The palms are facing front.

Chant: Meeeeeeeeeeeeeee.
Thouuuuuuuuuuuuuuuu….
Weeeeeeeeeeeeeeeeeeeeeee….
Iiiiiiiiiiiiiiiiiiiiiiiiiiiii….

Continue repeating the sequence, Me, Thou, We, I.
3 Minutes

3. Sit straight—macho. Chin in and chest out. **Buddhi Mudra:** The Sun (ring) finger is caught by the thumb, make sure the thumb covers the nail of the Sun finger. The other three fingers are straight. Allow the elbows to relax down and have the palms facing forward.

Chant: Har Hari
When you say *Har*, use the tip of the tongue and chant in a deep voice.
When you say *Hari*, use the tip of the tongue, but use a female voice, a high falsetto. **3 Minutes**.

4. Gyan Mudra in the hands, thumb and Jupiter (forefinger) together; bring the arms up so that the elbows are at a 90° angle and the mudra is about a foot away from each side of the head. The palms are facing front.

Chant silently: Har Har Deva
Pump the navel four times as you mentally chant the mantra. Keep the posture and don't let any muscle move. **2 Minutes** in silence.

Then play *Walking Up the Mountain* by Guru Das Singh and Krisha Kaur as you continue meditating silently and pumping the navel: *Har Har Deva*. **8 Minutes** (10 Minutes total)

Comments: It is not to do anything. It is just to let the knowledge come to you. It is the posture to bring unseen knowledge. You can go to the library and read the books, but this is bringing the libraries to you. *Har Har Deva* at the Navel Point in absolute silence. Nothing should move in the body except the Navel Point.

5. Play with the energy between your hands. Hands are in front of the body, palms facing each other, just play with the energy. Feel the ball of energy and play it. Your hands have to move powerfully, forcefully to control it—as much strength as you bring into the hands that much shall you increase your sensitivity. **2 Minutes**

6. Make your arms into a bow. The left hand is pulling the arrow back: the thumb and the forefinger are pinched together, the other three fingers make a fist. The left elbow is pulling back behind you and the hand is at the left shoulder.

The right hand is stretched forward and to the right, at an angle. The thumb and forefinger make a "C" shape, with the three remaining fingers curled into a fist. Stretch the arms away from each other. Stretch across the chest. Your torso may naturally twist as you stretch across the chest and create the angle.

Breath of Fire. Heaviest Breath of Fire you have ever done. **3 Minutes**

7. Interlace your fingers above the crown of your head; your thumbs are relaxed and separated gently. Round your mouth and breath heavily in and out through the mouth. **2 Minutes**

To End: Inhale deep, hold the breath and maintain the posture—go through your fears from your childhood—day one up to today—and get rid of them. In one breath you have to get rid of all your fears in timelessness. Exhale. Repeat twice more.

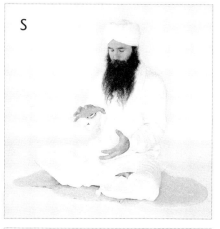

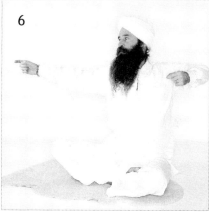

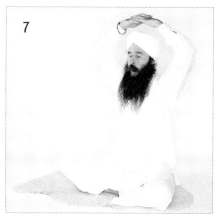

Communicate **Prosperity**

Give people the bounty the God has given you.

There are a lot of opportunities in the world. One is you can dig trenches to lay the wire and you can be paid $5 an hour or you can bill on one final invoice for $60,000 and you might never put in more than half an hour of work. Do you know what I am saying? Go for the opportunity. Go for the scales. Go for the strength of it. Go and time will go with you. It is a very simple world. You have one unique thing—that you look unique, you look special. The price of looking special is a heavy price but if you want to deliver special, positive, maturity to anybody, you must understand this simple law of life. Give everybody 10% success, he will give you 4% percent. Simple law: *hei*. Don't deal negatively with situations.

If a person is rotten, negative, that's why he wants you. People want you because they have a hope that you can give them something better, you can put their line back on the track, you can help them, you can make them rich, you can make them feel hopeful. Do that. Heal people mentally. That's the job of spirituality; otherwise you are not spiritual. You are a phony, you are a demagogue, you are a hypocrite, whatever you want to be called. Heal people mentally and far more in return, they will be grateful to you.

If somebody says I am drowning, I am sinking, I am bad, I feel terrible. Tell them that after every storm there is beautiful sunshine and the air looks clearer. Give people the bounty the God has given you. Just remember: Give people the bounty the God has given you and that will make you the most beautiful person on the Earth. If you give people the bountiful God, God will make you beautiful. That's the bargain.

Therefore, never utter, never speak, never say anything negative. Is that understood? Just remember, when you are listening to negativity, you have the right to listen and you must listen. As the person grows more negative, gets on the scale of 1 to 10 and their negative is 8, 10, 10+. Your job is not to examine the truth, whether the person is negative or very negative or truthfully negative or not; that's not your job. Your job is to turn around and sometimes, with ease, say, "What did you say?"

This morning I had a big fight. The person convinced me that they were angry. "I didn't come through, I this, that…", the whole anger was laid out flat. You know what my reply was, "All right, that's your anger, that's your feeling and that's your decision, is that true?" The person said, "Yes."

I said, "That's not real. Reality is that you are trying to be angry, you are trying to be not realistic. The reality is that in your calculation you have goofed and you can't find anybody to blame now and blaming is not a realistic attitude. It is a common attitude. People do blame. People do accuse. People do allege. People do a lot of things but question is not what people do, but what you do and how you meet it?

Question is what your strength is? What your grit is, not what people are doing to you. People will always do things, weird, negative things. They will always be jealous. They always lie but lies do not live very long. They will try to bring you down. Their anger can reach a capacity, an animosity and vengeance, such that if their situation is interlocked in vengeance and anger, interlocked in life, you don't have anything to go for. But don't do away with it; instead, as it is being presented to you, just laugh it away. Somebody said to somebody, "Hey, you shit, son of a bitch, you rascal, you idiot, oh, you cursed devil." Now can you believe all this was said in one breath? But just see what his reply was. You know what he said to her? "Oh man, that's a wonderful script," and he walked away. I couldn't believe it. I couldn't believe it, in my whole life I had never seen something like this. The man had been accused, abused and faced and he said, "Oh man, that's a wonderful script." Doesn't fit me and he walked away. He didn't bother to say why are you abusing me? Why are you accusing me? What wrong have I done? What is this? What is that? Not a word! He said, "Oh man, oh man, it is a wonderful script" and he walked away smiling. That's called endurance.

You know when I used to be a uniformed officer in the academy, Mr. Webber who was my training officer, he said to me, "Put the uniform on and come in, very good uniform, very well pressed, totally hard and done well." So I appeared, "Yes, sir."

He said, "That's good" and to my surprise he started abusing me left and right. I didn't know what to do. It was a new experience. I stood like a solid rock. In the end he said, "Did you hear me?"
And my reply was, "No, sir."
He said, "Why not?"

> *Just remember: Give people the bounty that God has given you and that will make you the most beautiful person on the Earth. If you give people the bountiful God, God will make you beautiful.*

I said, "I didn't."

"Why not?"

I said, "I don't want to waste my mind and time. That's why, sir."

He looked at me and laughed, then we sat down, we had a cup of tea and I said, "Why did you want to abuse me like that? Why did you caution me? You know, anybody can be angry and react."

He said, "Whatever comes to you, it is not you, it is the uniform, it is the star. If that cannot protect you and you can get provoked, you are not an officer. So write it in your book. If anybody can provoke you and anybody can make you react, you are not you, then you are just a slave of anybody. That's real slavery."

Real slavery is when you can be provoked and you react or compromise your values. That's the real slavery. You can lose a case but you cannot lose the grace. You can lose this Earth but you cannot lose the heaven. Losing is as graceful as winning is and mind you, in losing and winning, it is the deployment of your energy. Sometimes it is better to retreat, sometimes it is better to advance; but you must know what the weather is. Some of you feel that being macho all the time is the only way of life. No, my dears, macho and meek live in you.

Use it when you want it, but don't intermix it. Don't be "macho-ly" meek or meekly macho. You know what I am saying? There is a situation called compact. You know what compact means in English. In terms of law, compact and impact are interlocked. You must use both the inductive and the deductive method. Deduce and induce the judgment. Don't be hasty about it. What you have to do is bring their solidity in. You must understand the secret of strength is in your word—not in how much impact it has but in how much trust it can produce. If your statement, your word, cannot have the impact of trust, you are wasting your time.

Dialogue **Exercises**

Come to the mike. Sell him on going to Las Vegas to see a show.

Student: *I got a great thing for us to do tonight. Let's go to Las Vegas and see a show.*

Reply: You got what?

Student: *Let's go to Las Vegas tonight and see a show.*

Reply: What's the show?

Student: *What kind of show? Let's just go see it.*

Reply: First you tell me the show?

Student: *Famous movie stars!*

Yogi Bhajan: You lost. You've taken too much time to describe the show, you didn't do your homework. When he says what is the show, you say, dancing girls, charming situations, lots of partying, great food, wonderful room. No charge. You should come with that naturally. It is the impact. When you say "what is the show" then you look like a "what" is the show. You lost the show. Just understand. Give a gap only where a gap is necessary; otherwise the gap is nothing but eroding your capacity of impact. Start again.

Student: *Let's go to the show tonight in Las Vegas.*

Reply: What's the show?

Student: *Oh dancing girls, dancing elephants, dancing horses, dancing geese, dancing birds, all free, all the food we want, all the drink we want, all the yogi tea you want.*

Reply: Let's save the time. Watch a dance here.

Student: *Oh it is not the same thing. There is a band there. The Beatles are playing; they are all together, Elvis Presley is there. Buddy Holly is there. Mick Jaggar is going to be there, Jim Morrison is going to be there.*

Reply: And?

Student: *And that girl who sings that song you like is going to be there.*

Reply: What's the song?

Student: *Come on let's go.*

Reply: You want to hear ball and chain?

Student: *Come on let's go.*

Reply: Why?

Student: *Tonight only, one night only. You are never going to have another opportunity in your whole life to see these people all together in one place. I got two free airline tickets round trip. I got a room at the Imperial Hotel. Top floor. Let's go.*

Reply: You haven't sold me.

Student: *What are you going to do?*

Yogi Bhajan: Wait a minute, wait minute, you sit down. Now, match. You sell him Las Vegas show and you sell him the other town, Reno.

> *Real slavery is when you can be provoked and you react or compromise your values. That's the real slavery.*

Student: Hey let's go to Las Vegas tonight.
Reply: I am ready.

Student: But after we go to Las Vegas, we also have to go up to Reno. Have you seen Lake Tahoe? Have you seen how beautiful the silver is on top of the mountain of snow?
Reply: Once you've seen the Golden Temple who wants to see silver?

Student: Oh the Golden Temple, of course we will go there third.
Reply: I agree I will go to Las Vegas.

Student: I want to go to Las Vegas but also there are some very far out things to see going up to Reno and since I have a ticket, we can get a round trip—and they have offered us Reno for no additional charge. I think we can also take one day and go up to Reno and Lake Tahoe.
Reply: I can't go to Reno; I have a party I'm supposed to go to.

Student: I will drive don't worry about it. You don't have to worry about it. I will take care of the expenses—all expenses paid. I will take care of it. I know it is like a story book. Everyone thinks I am everywhere else. Reno is great. We will enjoy it. Let's just go.
Student: I can't go. I can't go to any to city that begins with an R.
(Students' laughter)

Student: Well, if you come to Las Vegas, you know they call it the City of Enchantment, so it doesn't begin with an R so you don't have to worry about it. Besides being precious work, it is going to be a great time. We will spend our day and a half in Vegas. We can go up to Reno. We have our rooms covered. Our airfare is included. I know a great Italian restaurant called Leonardo's. There is a Golden Temple restaurant up there that's also very good that used to be owned by our Sikhs here, I say it will be fantastic. From there we can just fly back to San Francisco.
Yogi Bhajan: And it doesn't start with R. It is the City of Reno, it starts with C.

Student: Okay, let's go to Las Vegas. We will do that.
Yogi Bhajan: You are losing.
Reply: We can go to Las Vegas and do that thing and then after we go to Las Vegas, then we can decide where to go. Let's not make any hasty decision now.

Student: What hasty decision? Why make a decision. You will come as my guest. You don't have to decide anything. There is no decision. What is there to decide? You are not paying a dime extra. We'll go to Reno. It's very beautiful.
Reply: We are going to Las Vegas right?

Student: We go to Vegas then we go to Reno. No problem. Compromise situation.
Reply: We are going to Vegas, right?

Student: Oh yes, we are going to Vegas. I want to go to Vegas.
Reply: Okay, let's go.

Student: Great? All right, I got tickets for two to Reno. What's that? I mean we are going to buy the tickets to Vegas. It's no additional money to also buy it to Reno. So what do we lose? Why do we want to have an additional cost deciding later. It is decided we go to Vegas together, then we go to Reno together.
Reply: I tell you that?

Student: I know wait, wait, wait a minute. I know this one place there that you have never seen, but you have to come to see it; but if I tell you beforehand it's going to lose the impact. You are going to love it.
Reply: I will tell you what.

Student: You are going to love it. You'll love the food; I know you like pizza. I know what you really like and I know the food that is available in Reno.
Yogi Bhajan: Okay sit down. Very good, thank you. Thank you. Next scenario: You sell an apartment. He sells a house. Go ahead.

Student: How would you like to make the best investment of your life?
Reply: I am interested.

Student: I have got a beautiful house at upper Ram Das Puri.
Reply: Yeah?
Student: Yeah.

Reply: Well, you know, I just found an apartment and the price of that apartment is going for, in that same area, probably right where your house is, $1200 a month.

Student: I could sell you a house for a $1000 a month.
Reply: Well, that sounds like a pretty good deal.

Student: I can put a Jacuzzi in it. It will have a view of the valley of the Khalsa. You won't have to travel far to solstice, and I have to close on this house by next week. You have to decide right now if you want to buy.

Reply: Well, I am not really interested in living at Ram Das Puri because I have got a lot to do in Los Angeles. I really need to be connected there; but there is a permanent Ram Das Puri where you are living, it is a very, very good deal and now you are talking about a Jacuzzi. Well, I can't put a Jacuzzi in the apartment but they have a set of Jacuzzis downstairs and all the amenities that you can imagine.

Student: This house comes with a plane and private pilot, who lives up in Ram Das Puri. His name is Ek Ong Kar Singh. He will be able to fly you to Los Angeles, or wherever you need, to deal with business and come back and forth, instead of back and forth to LA.

Reply: You are trying to sell me a house or give me a house? How come a plane service? Something sounds fishy about this deal.

Student: There are a few amenities involved. Yeah.

Reply: I see. Well it sounds like a very good deal for somebody.

Student: Don't you agree that the house is a better investment than an apartment?

Reply: Well, it all depends on what you are paying for the house and what you are paying for the apartment.

Student: You can write off your interest on your income tax every year. Your house is going to appreciate greatly in that area.

Reply: Yeah that's all true, but sometimes it doesn't always fit your needs. Now this apartment, where things usually go for $1200 a month right in the area where you are living, what do you pay now?

Student: I am paying $500 a month.

Yogi Bhajan: Now, that's too much. Okay sit down. What we are driving at from this conversation is that we live as sales people. We do not live as people. We sell our things. We sell our self and that's why the game of life is profit and loss. It's not compact and impact. Think about it. I've shown certain examples to make you understand that both knew what they are doing, both did it professionally, and gave us a lot of laughter; but neither there was an apartment nor there was a house. Neither he is going to Las Vegas nor he is going to Reno. What I am trying to draw to your attention is that basically man is a man and sales are sales. Sell commodities but not your manhood. That's the total difference, Don't sell another man his integrity, his peace of mind or his grace. Commodities are meant to be sold but don't sell your soul, don't sell your mind, and don't sell your body. If you are very successful in selling these three things, just remember you will be left with nothing. And you cannot live with nothing. Self-impeachment is not a way of life; it is a curse of life, so please remember.

You know how the biggest store may just put the word sale on it. You know what you feel? Things have gone cheap. You know what I am saying? Commodities, it is all right. You have already priced them to sell—jacked them up. They bring the price. The pricing is your game but when it comes to the Self, Self is never for sale. Just remember this. Write it down in your heart. My Self is not for my sale and now we will do the closing kriya.

Suli **Chadana**

Suli is when a big, one-inch thick, iron nail is put through the First Chakra and goes to the skull by your own weight. That death is called "Suli Chadana" and they performed the Suli to Christ. Christ bhee suli chadya, put it on a suli, but instead of putting the nail through, they tied the person to the cross and hang him so that his own water, his own belly kills him.

They thought that when people were put on that nail they would take a lot of opium and then the person with opium won't feel the pain he will go through. It's a slow death; and they die in about three days. They expected people to bribe the executor and give him a lot of opium, hoping he will give the man to die a big dose, even to die by the opium, that's how much opium was given. But the death was supposed to be cylindrical. A person has to go through that ring by his own weight, otherwise it can be a very painful death and the whole village has to visit. I mean this was just a fear of association, if you do something and you are condemned, this is what will happen to you. So nobody dared to do it. However, this was and suli means needle, so instead of going through that whole drama you may just be pricked by the tip of a needle and you may bleed.

Drib Drishti Kriya to Show You the Future
September 22, 1986

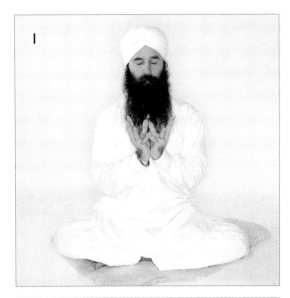

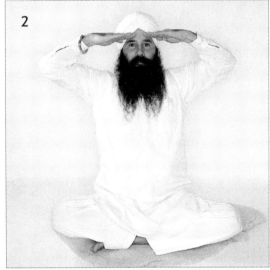

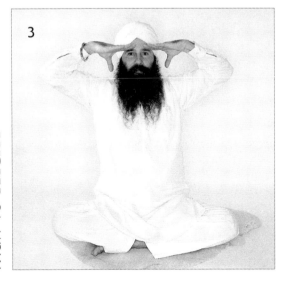

1. **Mudra:** Lotus Mudra at the Heart Center. Bring the heels of the hands together with the tips of the thumbs and the tips of the pinky fingers touching, the other fingers are spread evenly.

   Eyes: Closed, looking down toward the center of the mudra behind closed eyes.

   Mantra: I am, I am, myself is not for sale.
   Chant in a monotone for **1 Minute**

2. **Mudra:** Bring your hands just above the eyebrows, palms down, as if you were shading your eyes. Thumbs and fingers are straight and together; the fingers point toward each other and remain about an inch apart. The hands don't touch the face.

   Eyes: Look straight ahead

   Mantra: Har Hare Hari
   Chant very methodically, not too fast. **2 Minutes**

3. **Mudra:** Keep your hands above the eyebrows, but allow the thumbs to drop down.

   Eyes: Look straight ahead

   Mantra: Har Hare Hari Wahe Guru

   Chant aloud: Har Haray Haree and then press the Navel in toward the spine. Then chant silently Wah Hay Guroo. Then release the navel and begin the sequence again. These two mantras should be done in 4-beats each; they should balance each other.
   Do not exceed **31 Minutes**.

   Comment: This secret kriya will remove your fear of the future. You know what the future is? This kriya allows you to start seeing the future; it brings you the future today. If this kriya becomes perfect, your future will always be known to you. In fact, if you do this kriya, the future will not only be known, but also, that part of you which is negative in the future will be eliminated, only a token shall remain. For example, you were to lose an arm in an accident. When the accident takes place, you receive only a scratch. Instead of losing an arm you may have a little cut.

Commentary on Drib Drishti **Kriya**

The whole universe can do it. Even the parrots can be taught to do it. No, I am not kidding. Pundit Ram Lal's parrot exactly used to do this kriya, more perfect than a man can sing and say. He trained him but I told him Pundit Ji, it is not complete. Because he is my *jyothishya*, what you call this, astrology teacher. I learnt from him numerology, astrology and all that stuff, so I corrected it. Just understand the impact. He told parrot one day how to time it and next day parrot could time it accurately, but he could not say Wahe Guru in silence. You could see the hiss in his sound. I mean, understand there is a difference between a man and a parrot, but that difference you have to give.

Har is translated as *Har*, *Hare* is *Hare*, mantra is mantra, it cannot be translated. *Har Hare Hari*. What are you? English these days? There are a lot of words. *Tu mera gur haai*, *haai* is an English word; it is in Sri Guru Granth. *Tu mera gur haai*, *haai*: H-I-G-H. Guru High Guru, *tu mera gur haai*, it is a totally English word; they took it from us or we took it from them. What are you going to translate, let me see? *Har* is *Har* you can't translate. *Har* is basic God. *Hare* is the expanded God, future God, future in relationship. *Hari* is the Creator God. There are three forms of it: *Parsa Parsu Parsraam, Iss Maaya Kay Teen Nam*.

You know what the future is? That's a kriya because you start seeing the future; this brings you the future today. If this kriya becomes perfect with you, the future will always be known to you. If you do this kriya, the future will not only be known to you but that part of you which is negative in the future will be eliminated, only a token shall remain. For example, a token would be, if you were to lose an arm, in an accident, you get just a scratch instead. Instead of losing an arm you may have a little cut.

No, no the hands don't touch. The thumb stretched down. They don't touch. Fingers cover one third of the eyebrow. That's how it is. That's why I told you it is a very special place and you look straight and you look at nothing. You just look. And if you perfect this kriya, things will start coming to you. *Drib Drishti* they call it—knowing all through sight. This is the most sacred kriya of the great, those who call themselves saints, yogis, naths, anything.

May the long time sun shine upon you, all love surround you and the pure light within you, guide your way on.

You are men of God, may you recognize it. You are men of the universe. May you deal with it in the light of God. You are men to be men. May you feel the pride of it, to be in grace. You are the men of success. May you accomplish it. You are the men of self, light and respect. May you understand it. You are the men of merits. May your virtues be known. You are the men of knowledge. May your compassion be known. You are men of absolute determination. May your kindness be known. May you be men whom the world, the Earth, the Universe, may be proud of. Sat Nam.

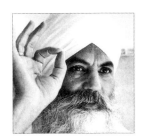

Man to **Man** 12

Excel as a Man

Circa 1987

What is a man? Man is a living experience, which can confront every temptation and still resurrect itself…It is an endless seed; it lives to seed. Its faculty, its quality, its generality, its temperament, its achievement is not mortal.

■ The Faculty of **Man**

■ Three Kriyas to Become a **Man**

The Faculty of **Man**

Do you believe yourself to be a man or don't you? That is the question. Can you be questioned by the whole world and have an answer for it? And is your answer—I am a man of Infinity.

These kriyas, which you are going to go through, are the most beautiful things I could ever have done in my life; there is no claim to them except they will cleanse the serum system in the body. It gives you—absolutely—a stress-free experience. Sometimes I wonder that my body, and what you call in English, death, or what I call, permit to go home, is slowly making me close up shop; but at the same time is opening up a new era and technology that is to teach you through the tube, television. You will go through the exercises and these meditations and, as God is your witness, you can go through it and you will be very happy. It's my belief that it doesn't matter how strong or virtuous a man may be, there comes a time in life where you will have to face a twist in yourself; and we do not have the strength to take care of our own twist. Man is a marvelous machine, a seeder, he has the capacity to implant the future of his own self; it is the seeding capacity of God. Man has never valued its virtue, he has always valued his paraphernalia and his victories and his conquering nature and his territory and his possessions, but he has never valued his principles.

What is a man? Man is a living experience, which can confront every temptation and still resurrect itself. Giving in is not a man; getting out is not a man. Man is an infinite fountain and source of that courage which has no end in itself. It is an endless seed; it lives to seed. Its faculty, its quality, its generality, its temperament, its achievement is not mortal.

I will share with you the story of a man called Nanak, who lives today as powerfully, as youthfully, as he lived then. When he lived in his body, it was to question him. Today, there is no question. Each one of you has that capacity to live, beyond question; but you can start today, now that tomorrow will not question you. In life, men are questioned, challenged, and tested. Do you believe yourself to be a man or don't you? That is the question. Can you be questioned by the whole world and have an answer for it? And is your answer—I am a man of Infinity. If you don't want to call yourself a man of God, then call yourself a man of Infinity, then your love is with Infinity and nothing else.

You inspire people to love, like a big ship takes all its cargo in its hull and carries it to its destination, but it doesn't get attached to the cargo. Taking people to their destination is the destiny of the man; it is the dignity of the man; it is the divinity of the man. Man is not what you think man is: man is an institution of grace, not reaction. When as a man you react, doesn't matter what the temptation is or how hard the button is being pressed, remember this, then you are not a man. The difference between man and animal is so little, there is such a fine line you can't believe it. If you react or provoke to react or ask to react or make to react, you are not a man. Man never reacts to environments, circumstances and pressures. Man accepts the challenge and makes his own way. I hardly believe that you understand what I am saying, because what I am saying is that people look like men, they even try to act like men, they even talk like men, and they believe and feel they are men, but the reality is they are not. Take it upon faith—that doesn't mean he is real.

The first faculty of a man is that he must not react, by all provocations of the Universe, and he must not react to any and all the temptations of the universal Self, including God. You can call me an atheist, but it will not be true; because God, through His nature, also makes man to react. Therefore, where you will be tested you never know. What you think is gold may be only glitter; every temptation has a very charming glitter to it that can make you blind, but that does not mean it's gold. Silver and platinum are very different but the only way you can tell is by weight and gravity, they look alike most of the time. Zirconium, the man-made diamond, and diamonds have all the faculty of diamonds, it's just that nature has proper laws of deflection and man cannot produce those. Otherwise, mind you, a $10 zirconium is sometimes clearer, better than a diamond; but it does not have the flaws, the reflections, that the natural diamond has. Even in hardness, a zirconium can now be proven to be just like a diamond, it is made just like a diamond. Therefore, man can be a man. Man with this man, that man, God man, president man, noble man, holy man, call it anything, I have no objection. Man is only a man when he can experience everything going on and he does not react or attract. Then what does he do? He accepts the challenge. Accepting the challenge of good and bad is the first act to be a man.

Accepting the challenge is the first act of the man and converting any adversity into prosperity is the second challenge of the man, which he accepts. Nurturing and caring is the third challenge of the man. Kindness and compassion is the fourth challenge of the man. Being noble and honorable is the fifth challenge of the man. These are the five challenges, which every man has to accept in his life whenever they come head on. Otherwise, you can call yourself a man but you are not. For that, you require

The Five Challenges of the **Man**

1. *Accepting the challenge*
2. *Converting any adversity into prosperity*
3. *Nurturing and caring*
4. *Kindness and compassion*
5. *Being noble and honorable*

character, instinct, intuition, intelligence and knowledge. I understand that poverty is a curse and richness is a way of life. What makes you rich is not what you are, what makes you rich is your richness in proportion to your intelligence and your happiness in proportion to your consciousness. You can be intelligent and be very rich, but you may be very unhappy, if you are not conscious. There is no other way around it. A lot of people feel they can goof around and then have their lives make sense. Everybody wants to take, nobody wants to give; so sometimes you take the mistake. The problem is that whatever you take you can drop; but when you take the mistake, you cannot drop it—you have to pay for it. Therefore, in every man there is no place for mistakes. You can turn yourself into anything, but there is no chance for a man to have a wrong turn. Any wrong turn will change your direction in life, any change of direction will always pollute you, make you impure, and any pollution will make you weak and no weak man enjoys the experience of being a man. Impotency in action, in challenge, in creativity, and in success are torture, a slow death, to every man. Dying is not difficult for a man, suffering is. Every man suffers by the glory of his weaknesses; every man enjoys by the glory of painless living.

You must understand, as a man, you can limit yourself or you can expand yourself. The basic strength in you is the reality of the religion. Religion is nothing but the science of reality, which gives you a practical experience to understand whether you are getting into something that doesn't belong to you. If it belongs to you, does it accept you? If it accepts you, is it with you? If it is with you, then is it within you? If it is within you, it is around you, it has taken your character and faculties to the extent that it becomes you. If that is not possible, get out of it as fast as possible, otherwise you will not have even a chance to live in peace. Without harmony, without peace, without grace, and without dignity, please don't call yourself a man. Assessment is virtuous. God gave Its own face to a man, that's why we look saintly. By age and maturity we become gray or silver, which only symbolizes our purity, our piety and our projection. It gives us the strength of character that belongs to a man by right. But there is a yo-yo in a man. He fights his own brain with the strength of his balls and he loses his balls because he has no strength—that's the bottom line of this asshole called man.

Ninety-six percent of the human race, which is man, belong to this category. Man has to draw himself from this pit, and pit against it, walk away from it, spitting at it, and try to release himself and relate to his own higher consciousness—that is called the beginning of the man. In that beginning, we need a meditative strength. To that end, I am grateful to God and Guru that I could sit down and give you these two hours, which you are going to face very soon and go through these kriyas. I hope you will remember me by the end of it and you will appreciate what, as an humble man, I have done for you. You are fortunate to have chosen to come here and spend your time; you will experience something which I wanted you to experience. I wanted to share this with you and I myself shared it before. Just understand—expansion, expansion and expansion—there are three words, which make M-A-N: There is morning, there is afternoon and there is night. That completes the word man. All three have extension, extension, extension toward excellence, excellence and excellence.

What you want to find in love is to eat your own shit. Every man does it, every man lives on his own stool. In America, stool is not understood; you think it is a little wooden chair you sit on. (Students laugh.) So I have to use the word shit because that you understand. Well, sorry for the language, I have to speak in the American English, your own roughage, which comes out of your anus. And man lives on the roughage of his consciousness. Every man answers the call of nature or creates bowel movements and faces his balls—just remember, this is a psychological phenomena and biological fact. It is the pituitary that gives you the hardness of the penis and the pleasure of the ejaculation of your semen. And it is the same pituitary that controls the sixth sense. So sex is a sixth sense; I am not wrong. Scientifically I am right; medically it is true.

But basically, just remember, your excellence does not depend on who you are, but on how much you love your excellence. Whatever else you love is minus your excellence, because excellence does not tolerate any second-rate love. Every man has to love his excellence, and, therefore, fall in love with his consciousness and subject his intelligence to that consciousness to exceed, so that he can succeed in excellence. There is no secret about it. Love for the material world and love for the Earth—as much as you do and as long as you live—is confinement. Living on the Earth and loving everything and looking toward the heavenly abode, called resurrection, is an excellent way of subtlety, in which you can radiantly shine.

It is not you and your heart that matters, it is the opening of your heart, in whose fragrance the virtues will come. You can't attract one person, but if your heart opens and the fragrance of the heart blossoms and releases, whosoever will touch it, feel it, smell it, shall be yours. It is the values and the virtues of men that matter. The dawn of life is the morning of life, rest of the life is the afternoon of life, and recuperation is the night of life. Those three words make the word man: morning, afternoon and night. There is a relationship between them as a man. If you do not equally recuperate and blossom like the morning and rest and take the taste of restfulness—mental rest, spiritual rest, physical rest—you cannot be a man.

I went to Spain; I went to that fort and I bought a cannon, unfortunately in our negotiations and deciding to buy, the clock struck one. The gentleman we were talking to took a chain and put it on a hook and stopped talking. I tried to persuade him, all right now it is done, give me the cannon, take the money; but he won't speak. I was very shocked, what happened?

So I called another guy I said, "What is the matter?"
He said, "He won't talk now; it is his siesta; he is resting. He won't—doesn't matter whether you buy it or you don't buy it. Come five o'clock he'll talk to you."

We went to test him out five minutes before five; he looked at us, smiled, but won't talk. (Students laugh.) So we waited until five o'clock and at five o'clock he pulled that little chain this way, opened the door and he said, "Thank you very much; it was very kind of you to wait so very long. I really want to sell it. I'll give you five dollars off. Please have it, it is yours."

I was shocked. After buying that cannon I gave him ten dollars. I said, "This is a tip for practicing rest. You have taught me something in practice, which I never learned from the books."

To remind me, I have put that cannon in the secretariat. Whenever I visit the secretariat, I remember the man who sold it to me, because he also sold me a thought: there is a relationship between work and pleasure, work and rest. My condition today, the reason that I cannot be with you, is because I did not rest properly. If being a yogi and having much more—a thousand times more—strength than an ordinary man, if I break the law of nature, if I can be talked into that misery, you cannot be an exception either. That's why I have personally appeared before you, to let you know that rest is as important as work is. Man, in a word, is a constituent of three things—M-A-N—morning, afternoon and night. As the brilliance, calmness and coolness of the night is the doziness and the coziness of the afternoon, and the brightness and beauty of the morning, if these six things don't touch you, you will never experience yourself as a man.

I wish I should stay longer with you; but you have to start and you have to practice what I have laid down for you and I should be leaving you so I can work through my subtle body at a distance. Sat Nam and blessings, blessings, blessings.

Three Kriyas to Become a **Man**

These kriyas, which you are going to go through, are the most beautiful things I could ever have done in my life, there is no claim to them except they will cleanse the serum system in the body. It gives you—absolutely—a stress-free experience.

Becoming **Divine**
circa 1985

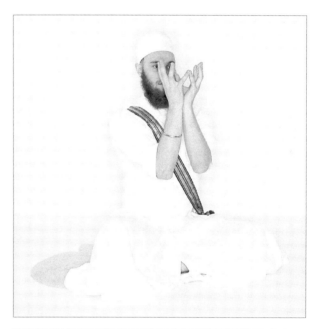

Posture: Easy Sitting Pose

Mudra: Lotus Mudra. Bring the heels of the hands together in front of the chin. Spread the fingers evenly, and bring the tips of the thumbs and the tips of the pinky fingers together.

Eyes: Fix your eyes on an *imaginary* partner, a beautiful human being of light.

Music: Humee Hum Toomi Too Wahe Guru

Chant aloud with the music.

Time: 31 Minutes

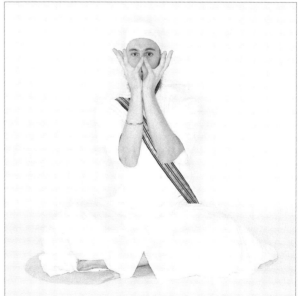

Balancing the Apana **Energy**
circa 1985

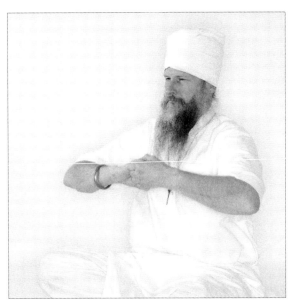

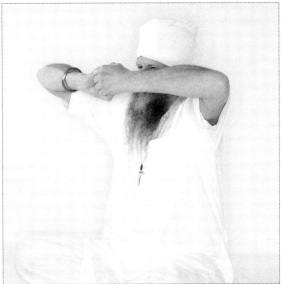

Posture: Easy Sitting Pose

Mudra: Bear Grip: Piston the arms up and down from the Heart Center to the Third Eye.

Eyes: Not specified

Breath: Not specified

Music: Sat Nam Wahe Guru (Indian Version I)

Time: **31 Minutes**

Comments: You will never fall apart as a man unless you have too little or too much apana. It makes you do things incomplete, unaccomplished, half way. This exercise will make you a man.

How to Overcome **Crisis**

Posture: Easy Sitting Pose

Mudra: Bring your thumbs to the base of your Mercury finger. Your hands are in front of your face, palms facing each other, framing each side of your face. Move your hands rapidly 6 to 8 inches out and back to the starting position. As the hands come toward each other, use force; but do not let the hands touch. It will discharge all the energy.

Eyes: Open

Breath: Not specified

Music: Sat Nam Wahe Guru (Indian Version I)

Time: 62 Minutes

Comments: One wrong after another, one mistake after another, causes a man to question himself, "Am I a man?" I am here to tell you, "You are a man."

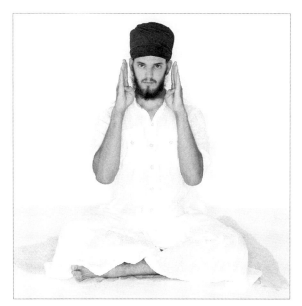

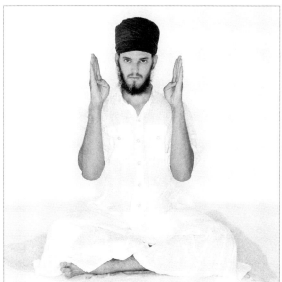

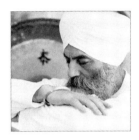

Man to **Man** 13

On Being a Spiritual Man

Circa 1997

If you can nurse, nurture, love, take care, make a person grow, and from the heart, the person says "thank you," there is no more blessing than that, there is no more prayer than that, there is no more goodwill than that.

- The Technology of Being a **Man**
- Wake Up Like a **Man**
- Life in **Balance**

The Technology of Being a **Man**

It is not the story of penis or Venus; it is the story of glandular health.

Now, imagine, you have a business [penis] there (See Figure 13.1) and you have two testicles, called balls, correct? That's how God made men? Now, these are two balls [the eyes], same size, same density, same working, same vibration as the testicles; and this nose, is exactly, from root to end, the length of the penis, carbon copy. This is the pituitary gland, which controls your sexuality. It can also have a left side and a right side, you follow what I am saying?
Students: Yes, sir.

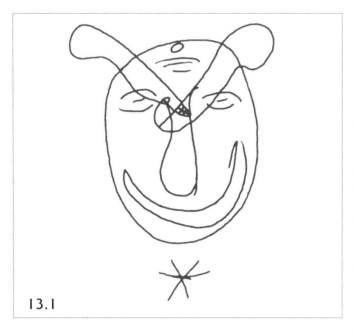

13.1

You are sexual. Normally, it is a biorhythm, a rhythm of the pituitary. There is nothing down there. When men get impotent and get bogged down and all that, medically, they feel miserable. Their misery is not whether they can perform sex or not. There are people who are 80 years old who can't perform sex, but are still very jovial, very healthy, very sparkling, and very light. The misery happens because when you are not in good sexual condition, your sixth sense sensory system is also not in good condition. The pituitary does not consolidate you. It is the master gland; it tells all the glands to secrete and to join in the blood. If you do not have healthy blood chemistry, you will be handicapped.

It is not the story of a penis or Venus; it is the story of glandular health. Glands are the guardians of your health; and it is the glandular system that makes you men. It is the secretion of the glandular system in your blood, which makes you strong men, medium men or weak men. Sometimes people ask, "Why should we get up in the morning and have a cold shower? What for?" It's a very simple thing. Don't see it as a torture and don't fall in love with it. Just understand the truth of it. First thing, you get up from the bed, you stretch yourself, is that true? Then you walk and you get under a cold shower. The cold water gives a shock to your body. The entire blood from inside comes out to the skin to protect it; and you massage and you go under the water; and you massage and go under the water; in and out you go, three or four times, and your coldness will be gone. You will feel warm later, because all your blood has come to the skin and the capillaries are all rushed opened.

Some people say, "Why can we not take a hot shower and then follow it with a cold shower?" It is because that shock value is gone. You need that shock. You need that challenge, you need that strength, so that you can face your day. One thing God has made, which is very powerful, is called a towel. You towel your body and make it red. Third thing is you should have a blanket. You put on a blanket and you get warm, as if you were in a heated cubical. When your outside is warm, then blood rushes inside and feeds all the organs, including your testicles. At that time, your testicles change size. You know, testicles are like a kind of grandfather clock pendulum, which goes up and down. Sometimes the left is down, sometimes the right is down. Their circulatory power depends on which side—left or right—is higher or lower.

You have a thing called a prostate. The prostate is a gland that for any sexual desire, it secretes. So, the urethra is oiled by that secretion before your discharge, and after you finish intercourse, you must go and urinate. This way, you will never have a prostate problem. Simple precaution. There is nothing to it.

The difference between intercourse and masturbation is that you must play the game of love with your opposite partner, and that should take enough time so that it will keep her smell in you. This way, your pituitary can come through. Otherwise, it doesn't matter what kind of sex you are having—you are just masturbating. And mind you, any sex that is of the masturbating capacity or quality, or actually masturbating, will take away the entire balance in the system as well as the gray matter. The gray matter, which is part of the brain and floats in a serum, will be unable to swim and move and change. So, what will you get out of it? Irritation—men should never feel irritated.

You have another thing that you waste your life on. When you want to have sex, you find a way to reach it. Sometimes you use anger, sometimes frustration, sometimes sympathy, sometimes empathy. You use all that psychology, all those words that you know without going to a class and without going to college. So, on the day you feel horny, you bring her flowers, you do this for her, you do that for her. The day you don't feel horny, you don't even bring her leftovers. Therefore, men are not generally trusted. Because your emotional swings are so painful for a woman, she doesn't understand who you are. When you want sex, you kiss her, hug her, you go upside down, in and out for her, hallelujah, hallelujah, all that stuff, and the next day—what? What are you saying?

Now, the trouble is that the woman has a problem. Because every woman has an apparatus to be a mother, she is 16 times more sensitive, 32 times more protective, and 64 times more territorial, so she can guard her little ones she calls family. So, if you do not give a woman the family accuracy or family behavior or family manners, it doesn't matter how rich you are, how poor you are, you are not going to have a woman, one way or the other.

You cannot buy certain things. You will not learn through this course by money or by youth or by being macho. There are solid principles of a wonderful man. Man is one who mans himself. There is just this one line. Man is one who mans himself. A man is one who 'wows' the woman: wow woman, man and woman, male and female. You are in it. Even the word, 'she' contains 'he', 'female' contains 'male' and 'woman' contains 'man,' Where are you going to go? Look at your tragedy: You are born, you have a mother at your head. She nurtures you, but she controls you, right? When you grow up, this thing starts standing up a little bit, then there is a smell that controls you. Then you go after 30, 40, 60 relationships, you get ready to settle down, then that relationship controls you. Hey! What should I do? I will get it, then you get it. Then you go out, work hard, you want children, you have a home. You are tired. You are over-anxious, over-pushing, absolutely over-tired. You have burnt your fuel very fast and then you come home.

You see, the funny part that you don't understand is that when you come home and your wife comes home, if she is working, she will still immediately cook dinner, feed the children at night and in the morning, do everything, and with all the complaints, she will do it exactly right. And then you will complain—even after having a sex! If she wakes you up in the middle of the evening and says, "hey, up, up, up." You say, "I am very tired, I have an 8am appointment the next morning."

If you have sex and you can't make up the energy in the day, you are empty. You have no reservoir and you have no fulfillment. You know what sex is? *Ojas* they call it. *Ojas—Jas* means supreme happiness, that which gives a man supreme happiness, *ojas*. If you put your finger behind your ear and rub it, and smell it, you can smell your *ojas*—and smell how ugly it smells. Smell, smell, smell, smell! Figure it out. That smell is the exact smell of your discharge. This *ojas* is not there, it is charging from here; it's evident all over the body.

So Fresh and So **Clean**

It is required of a man to clean his armpit with the coldest possible water, at least three times, if not four times. Huh? When? What? You mean in one year? (Students laugh.) Each day, each day, each day, because armpit sweat is nothing but the exhaust of the brain and cleaning it keeps the pituitary very alert during the day. Once you have experienced it, you will clean them 22 times, it's the best thing people do. I'll tell you I have seen people who are practicing this. I have so many students, they go in the bathroom in the middle of the office, right? They take very, very cold water, take off their shirt, clean themselves here and there, massage their face, and come back fresh; it is so easy. There are people, who don't have much water, you know how they smarten and freshen themselves? They take a little water, clean their mouth and brush their teeth. They use that wooden brush and they wash their hands and their face and they are fresh. Your charm as a man, not you as a man, but your charm is the freshness that you bring to yourself. Fresh, very fresh. If there is an old banana, are you going to eat it? Fresh banana is all right, not that it should be too fresh.

You need to establish play with your mate. You need a soul mate, you need a religious mate, you need so many things to mate. There is one word for every man that he must have—a playmate. Playmate is a very polite wrestling match, in which a man and woman induce their integrity, their divinity, their love, their touch, their feeling, their smell and over all, their understanding. Am I too quick? You are digesting it or it is going over you? Men are in the rhythm. You have a rhythm and then the rhythm becomes your habit; you feel comfortable. Once you have a habit, you are very uncomfortable to change the habit. Woman has no habit and no rhythm. Woman wanes and waxes, fluctuates like a moon. So, if you look at the heavens, as a man, then it is simple. Sun is warm, stationary, bright and it is steady in its body. Moon is cool, bright, shiny, but it wanes and waxes in its body. Sun wanes and waxes by degrees—60°, 90°, 60°, and finally down, and goes to the other side of the world. These are the two differences between men and women.

You should be fresh and young when you talk, when you seduce, when you pursue. I don't know what you want to call that word, but when you want it. You understand? Secondly, you should always be available, flexible, but very firm. Number three, you must have spontaneous noble manners, so that victory shall be always forever. Spontaneous, noble manners, remember, there is not one woman born who will not test you on that. Woman will test you with three things: Are you noble? Are you courageous? Are you a man of your word? You can never escape this test.

This love business: "I am falling in love with him," "I am in love" and "She is in love." It is a temporary endowment. She has youth, you are horny; it is a sexual endowment. You have an imagination of facts and features, and she has those facts and features; it is a temporary endowment. You need someone that has a catering manner, and she has a catering manner; it is a temporary endowment. You feel in your head and heart that she is yours, and she feels in her head and heart that you are a possibility. You feel, with this combination, that you are on top of the world, and she feels, with this combination, that she will put you on top of the world. She will put a stick in you, so that you will always be up, not down.

This is a very unfortunate part of women. And this is where men fail—that's where you fail. She puts you on a pedestal, you know, a woman can kiss you, hug you, sleep with you and the next morning she will say, "I am going to go see my elder aunty and I will see you in the afternoon." It turns out that her boyfriend will be there, she will have sex with him and then come back the next morning, acting very righteous and so noble, you can never find her out.

What can happen between men and women is constant bickering, constant nibbling, constant question and answer, constant doubting and shouting. It creates the environments that go from good to bad and bad to worst. Man, who wants to live a very normal, safe life, should not indulge it.

"Murkhey na ulajiye"

"Don't entangle with a foolish person or foolish situation."

If a situation is foolish, just say, well, we will consider it, we will think about it. Your macho ego is mainly the problem. You only want to think about right now. If she says something, "David, you look very weird today." You can't take it. "I am not weird, what the hell are you talking about? Where I am weird? What? Who told you I am weird? Where are you going? Whom are you meeting? Who are you comparing me with? What nonsense is this?" You get your own answer as well, "Oh, I am weird and I am lonely and I am very low and I don't know, but perhaps you, who have seen me, are not going to be mean. You will raise my consciousness and give me hugs and kisses so I can feel good."

Woman is a mother, she has a nurturing capacity. You can lay everything on her and get out of trouble. She says, "Oh, yes my darling, really I am very tired, my head is aching" and still you can end up with sex. But for you, first your body has to ache, or you pretend it is aching, you pretend you are not feeling good, so you can go to bed. If she knows you are going to go to bed straight, but she knows what you mean, that you're avoiding her, then she can put a condition on it. If you want love with no conditions, always remember, it is not big love and humor and dogma, and all that, and don't read a lot of poetry or love stories. Love is a simple attraction of the momentary, biorhythm of the body. It is nothing more than that. You may read all the books and you may see Romeo and Juliet and romance and everything, but when you are not feeling good, you are not good.

Woman has a gender problem. She wants a mate who can meet her demands of security of health, security of wealth, security of senses. A woman, who will be with you, will want to feel proud of you. She should be in awe of you, "wah" of you, she should appreciate you, she should have great reverence for you; but when you act like a woman to a woman, that's where you mess it up. Remember, woman is not a man.

Students: *Woman is not a man.*

Yogi Bhajan: And man is not a woman. Let's talk about the gay community. They are men and men, and women and women, but even there, one is male and one is female. I studied the gay community while I was in Los Angeles. I was living in the community where everybody was my neighbor and they were all very open gays, very simple. Among them, there was a male and a female, you can simply look and you can tell. Though instinct is there, the bodies were different. They enjoy life, they have been married, they have a home, they sometimes adopt children, they invite guests, they do everything that we do. Because a female in the body of a male and a male in the body of a female, correctly act, exactly the way others act; or female body, which has a male in it, they have some words for them, I think they call them "queen" and "butch"[1] and this and that. They have a whole science. They have a whole language. But what do we do? We put them down. If we are not gay, we say gays are bad. And the gay thinks you are weird. Actually, this is an imbalance of the pituitary. It's not

---

[1] These were the colloquial terms at the time; they change constantly and he always spoke in culturally relevant terms.

> *Woman will test you with three things: Are you noble? Are you courageous? Are you a man of your word? You can never escape this test.*

gay and hetero- and all that, there is no problem like that. It is the pituitary, the secretion of the pituitary gland, when it is off, the other glandular systems are off. [Editor's Note: Yogi Bhajan refers to the pituitary as the body's command center for glandular balance and function in the body. All of our behaviors and feelings, including gender expression, have a base in the glandular and nervous systems.]

All habits, where you cover yourself up—to extend or to contract—are the habits of the pituitary. What is the most effective organ? It's the liver, and when your liver is in trouble, you have no appetite for sex. Because the liver will ultimately affect the lung, lung will affect the spleen, spleen will affect the immune system, and body repair will not happen immediately, so there will be long-term stress, and finally, you will be so stressed, that you can't perform. It doesn't matter to me whether you take your underwear off and, in just two minutes, discharge or you take your underwear off and you don't come for two hours. Abnormality is abnormality. Reality of a man, which is glowing and glorious and shining and absolutely shrewd, is one who becomes a man of his own manhood. You watch yourself, as a man, and you watch under the hood, you are a man. When you have a headache, you take Tylenol or Advil, you think those things take away the pain? No, they take away your senses. Sense of pain is gone, pain is not gone. Pain is very much there.

When you fight, have you seen those people who always fight with their wife and then have sex? Why? Because they can't have sex successfully without that aggressive projection. You have seen people who go very methodically, and then once they get up, they grab it, and like a rabbit, in-out, in-out, in-out. You develop all these patterns through your pituitary command center—it's called the command center or Agya Chakra or *ajna*, Third Eye—that's what they call it.

The problem with you is, psychologically, "I want to do it, I didn't do it, I want to do it, I got it done, I have got to do it, it's not satisfactory, I couldn't respond, she couldn't . . ." You have such a mathematical, accounting department up there. What for? Two testicles and a little penis and you have got this whole stuff, this mind, working, thinking, imagining, what is the deal? When you got to go, you got to go. When you are horny, stick your horn somewhere and get it out; but not with all the paraphernalia and all the attachment and all the sensory system.

Sex is very regal—regal—when there is no attachment, when you are stress free, you are personally free, and you just love the joy of doing it. But don't forget, woman must excite. Start with a little foot massage, back rub, whatever, keep playing. Now, you don't have to learn everything from me. There are pictures everywhere: Chinese, German, French, Indian.

The tragedy, which you will face in life, and which nobody will ever tell you except me is that when the female is a virgin, her hymen is there. You know what I mean? When a man enters her, the hymen gets torn and that's why the blood comes. But it is not whether she is a virgin or not, it's about when he enters her, is he perpendicular to the hymen, which catches the penis and pulls on the inner cavity. That's why your penis has a little ring on the end. It can lock in, so that if you are circumcised and you lock in, you can come out. That's why there was a little meat to move around, to give you a margin. Whenever you go in, it catches it, and once the hymen does that and the inner organ locks it, then the rest of your life, you have a great sexual life. But if the hymen is broken wrong, we call it bucket love. You know? Put a bucket, water and sugar and everything and take a spoon and stir it. You won't have that grip and she won't have that strength, neither she can lock with you, nor you can lock her, then what shall we do? I do not know why God goofed and made it this way. He should not have. I was sitting there when God designed a man and I was watching. Maybe one day I will have to create the man and we'll do

---

Good Things for Great **Sex**

Good Hygiene: *The temperature of your testicles should be one centigrade lower than your body. The worst thing you do in the West is that you do not clean your anus. You clean it with paper and what is left there gets dried up and the entire area tightens up. How does it make you feel? That's why French men learned that they can't perform sex without keeping that area clean; they started using a bidet. Americans have started doing the same. That's also why there is the coffee enema, so that those inner membranes get tightened and disinfected. Men, in the old times, took castor oil once a week to clean this area. Keep it neat and clean so that when you are sexual, all your nerves, energy, and blood has a chance.*

Good Foods: *Sweet potatoes, water chestnuts, and one of the cheapest, but best things in the world is beet soup. Beets. You know what they call Borscht? It should be written on the wall, if you are a man, you must eat Borscht. It is a must. At night, when you have to have sex, then you must wake up for sex that morning. Don't start aiming toward it; your performance will not be one hundred percent correct. If you are not sure, not ready, the best thing is to take a big bowl of lettuce soup and you will get up the next morning maybe—and at least you don't have to face the shame of you did it, or you didn't do it.*

it differently; but God didn't design it differently. So, I am telling you what the reality is. Today, 99% of women don't care what virginity is, and men don't care either. I was asking a man a question once, I said, "You know, she has about 60 friends and boyfriends." He said, "Well, I am very lucky, she is experienced."

So, anything or everything we say, talk about or understand, you have an argument for it. Sixth sense has no reason, no argument and no contraction and no projection. Sixth sense is totally your own royal, gracious truth. If your sense, sixth sense, is not developed toward the reality, "I am a man, and I have to be a man myself, with my mannerly manners," you don't have a chance. Okay, we will stop here, you can ask questions. If there is anything I can explore or expand for you, I will be grateful.

Question and **Answer**

Student: *Do you have to wear a shawl or blanket after our cold showers?*
Yogi Bhajan: Yeah, you have to. It is called a Jewish shawl. You see Jews, when they pray, they put something on their shoulders? Because your shoulder becomes cold and then your blood and the spinal serum won't go to your brain. It is not a religious thing, it is simple science. You put a blanket around you and you sit. Enjoy it one day, see how good it is. Experiment with it. Especially in Española, where the water is pretty cold.

Student: *How do I know when I'm really meditating?*
Yogi Bhajan: Until you become totally, unbearably lofty and heavenly; I sometimes sit down and I space out so badly, I don't want to come down. That doesn't mean I stay up there, I have work to do. Meditation is not what you know of meditation: meditation is when you calm yourself down and sit peacefully, all the negative thoughts will start coming, "oh, she escaped me . . ." Every bad, negative thought, like shit, floats, and you say, "Wahe Guru, Wahe Guru." You take a higher sound, higher word, higher thought, and use it to override a low grade, negative thought. That's meditation. When people come and ask me, "Oh, I meditated, I was in ecstasy . . . ," I say, bull, liar, nothing, it will never happen. When you are meditating, you really come to a state of no-thing-ness, you don't know what is going on, you are just You. You are very beautiful when you are You. When you become You, the entire Mother Nature and the entire Universe, start dancing around you—that's You.

Student: *How soon should we urinate after intercourse?*
Yogi Bhajan: Whenever you can. Faster the better, because you have already been lubricated, so ejaculation has already taken that lubrication to use, and thereafter urination should follow. If you urinate quickly, you will not have urethra problem and it will also not allow the glands to relax and expand and become out of control.

Student: *What was that drink you recommended with castor oil?*
Yogi Bhajan: As far as I am concerned, I don't teach it, teachings are there, I just repeat them. They say, ounce of castor oil with cardamom in boiled milk. They drink it and they must have had a good experience, otherwise why should they put it in a book—and in a spiritual book. They must have had good feedback, so that's the way it is.

Look toward me, good. You are asking a question right? And you don't care for the environments? Care for the environments—as a man, it is your first faculty to care for environments, care for your position and care for your projection. Those three things are a must for a man. Before you utter a word or before you act.

Student: *Sir, is there any food that we can eat to heal our prostates?*
Yogi Bhajan: What we can eat? To heal the prostate—any food that has zinc, it is very useful. There is a medicine in India, which is very effective. In case you are in trouble, you can get the name.

Student: *Sir, could you please say something about birth control? The pill, condoms and abortion.*
Yogi Bhajan: Birth control is a very wonderful idea. It can be done many ways, one is, withdrawal, second is by moon cycle calculation, third is by using condoms, fourth is very smart on the part of woman, moment you finish, she goes and douches herself, so these are four, five, six ways, that birth can be controlled. But, there is one personal risk in everything, and you have the right to use any method you want, but it must be synchronized with your partner, and female and male must understand what their purpose is in doing it.

Some people religiously feel that we should produce as many children as God sends us, but if God promises, I will send you the children and also the food and everything else then He is gracious and you have the capacity to raise your children. These days though, it is very unfortunate: you have two people working, raising children, seeing to their education, dealing with the neighbors, going to the parties. Have you ever considered all that work and where it goes? But you can conquer all this as a man—if she just puts up a smile, fakes it—you will make it.

Student: *Sir, you said, a man is a man who mans himself, and just before you arrived, we were talking about the man's mission. If a man has a mission that takes him away from his marriage or his children* *to build his domain, how can he remain noble, spontaneous?*

Yogi Bhajan: Very, very simple, my wife knows what I am doing and my children know what I am doing and if they come in the way, I will bulldoze it.

No nonsense. Man is not afraid of losses nor is he afraid of greedy gains. You know, I have built this whole domain. When I came to America, first thing I wanted to do is put all the businesses, which I started, not in my name. Then I fought the point of paying all the ordinary business taxes, but that's why I paid that tax so the profit would not come to me, profit will go to the dharma. So, I set up a president and I set up the businesses, and I set up everything for it. Because I want my children to get what I think is right, but those who have worked with me and sweat and given their life and blood for it, must have, in the long run, the ownership. From them will grow the other people, they will have it and on and on; it's nothing personal. What price I have to pay for it, I don't give two hoots.

Mission is mission and that's a man, but my manners are very polite. I just do what is called justice. When I die, they will get their portion, other portion will go to the dharma, and those who work with me, day and night for 20 hours, for the past 25 years, shall have the ownership. Those who have shown their back and said, "screw you" and all that, they will get the news. Don't worry about it. If you are very straight, you are very straight. You should never be late to be straight. That's man's biggest fault. But if your wife says, "you have two jobs," and you say, "yes, I have two jobs just to provide all this," and then she finds out there is a girlfriend, then is the tragedy. It is not that I am not straight, but I have lawsuits and I have been put through the mill. But it doesn't matter, what can I do? It comes with the territory.

Suppose you are going to Saudi Arabia and they do not allow women. Tell your wife, this is the salary, this is the job, I am going there, I promise you nothing but that I will be your man. That's all—not more than that lesson. But if you find I am not your man, you just tell me; if I find you are not my woman, I will tell you. Relationship will never break. I went through this hell for 28 years, doesn't matter. Who cares? Die by the dozen, but don't kill your honor and don't drag down your grace and don't barter with your courage. Take a stand, take a stand! You don't have to yell and scream to take a stand, just say, "I feel this is right," or "I feel this is wrong."

Men must speak politely—that's the main thing—and speak with a lot of romance. Dance through the words, start whistling, start singing, start catering, start looking at her eyes, you know, "when I met you at the railway station, remember, we were in the general compartment." My God, even your eyes can't believe it sometimes. Then soon enough, they become bigger and bigger and bigger. Now I can see clearly what I've fallen into—wow. Woman is done. Don't fuck a woman; cook a woman with the fire of romance. Just romance her, and cook her with the fire of romance.

There is a man, a friend of mine, I asked him today, "How are you doing?" In the past six years, he has not had intercourse once, because he doesn't want to. He appreciates her and at night he talks to her so much, but after a few minutes, he is snoring. The next morning, he says, "I am sorry, I was tired, I slept. No, no tomorrow, another day will come, don't worry about it." But the fact is that he doesn't want it. It is not that she doesn't want it or he doesn't want it, but that in the past so many years, he has been unable to know that he doesn't really want it.

Never, ever, as a man, in the presence of your woman, nibble at any moment, participate in cheap jokes or try to look in wonder.

You are poor or rich, that doesn't mean anything; or you have good character or you have loose character, that doesn't matter; a woman has a sensory system to choose a mate. It's just like the whole world: strongest is best. It's a genetic thing, every woman in her caliber and psyche, shall choose. I don't do it anymore. In the old days, I can see two people then say, "go, get married, you will be fine." Psyche meets. Anything else? You can ask me your question, so you can go from here satisfied because we only have three or four days together and we must do it right.

Student: *Sir, before a baby is born, does it know that it's going to be aborted? If a baby is going to be aborted, before incarnation, do they know it is going to be aborted?*

Yogi Bhajan: The child?

Student: *Yes.*

Yogi Bhajan: That's the theory of karma. Some children come, never to be born. Some children come and give a message and leave the grief. There is one woman, 18 years ago, she was pregnant and she aborted the child; she is still lamenting and crying today. The doctor and the psychologist and psychiatrist say that if she relaxes, she may conceive again, but she is unable to relax. Children happen, that's why there is a marginal gift of 120 days. You build a house, then you move in. That's why, a child is built and after that 120 days, the soul moves in. That's why after 120 days, they don't push, they don't do anything, it is settled.

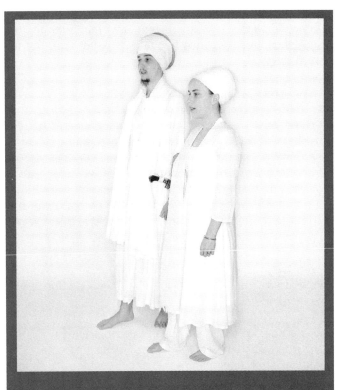

Flourishing the Soul of a Child: Charan Japa

If you walk a lot, with your woman on the left side, hands locked, and on the left you say, Sat Nam, and on the right you say, Wahe Guru; it's such a Japa, it's called Charan Japa. It is the oldest method, in which a couple brings in a very easy, most beautiful child, and their own self is improved, too. It is a very realistic science. Woman on the left, man on the right, walking this way. On the left is, Sat Nam, on the right is Wahe Guru. Step by step by step, until the child is born. Three to five mile walk is essential, necessary, needed, wanted.

Student: I am interested in your view on marriage.

Yogi Bhajan: Marriage is a carriage in which two people either live in bliss or in hell. Marriage is not an institution; marriage is a beginning of sensual, sexual, social partnership. If it is based in honor, grace and togetherness, then you will be prosperous and comfortable. If it is based on selfishness, like you have to date somebody, you lie to somebody, and you must know, every date has a pit. You must not harpoon or bait a partner, you should be very straightforward; it's good enough, because every man has a woman right there, you simply can't see it.

Marriage is the most wonderful institution. As a married woman or man, you are a householder—you pay the police, you pay the thieves—what is that which doesn't live in you? But still, you are together—that joy of being together is one of the happiest joys. Marriage is wonderful institution, very wonderful, no doubt about it. But it should be a carriage to carry you both, not to play games. Treat the wife, as a wife; the moment you start saying, why and if, you are wrong. That's enough of a signal to correct yourself. Woman doesn't have a long, war-like quality. She picks it up slowly, ever so slowly, until finally, she becomes a warrior. Man is a warrior in nature, very glowing and beautiful; there is no reason for a man to be upset.

If woman can upset you, you are in deep trouble. Because man, like the sun, has to keep his setup, doesn't matter what. That's the price you pay for marriage. When you have a girlfriend, you can go and take her to dinner and all that, all those lies you tell her and all those lies she tells you, that doesn't settle the issue. Sometimes you make mistakes, blunders, and then you go under. Marriage is a very vital issue. Marriage is a balance sheet, which everyday must be done: Where are we? What are we? Where are we going? How well are we doing? How bad are we doing?

Women will take a long time to attack you; men always take a very short time to attack. Men are very much in an attacking mood: they get angry, they get jealous, whatever you call that, and then say whatever comes out. Whereas, woman is very slowly simmering and heating up and one day, all of a sudden, you will feel that she, who is somebody you never thought of as having a tongue and a mouth, will serve you notice.

There are four or five things that a woman will feel deserves an outburst to do you in. One is when she feels you don't love her, you love somebody else. Second, you are not very careful of children; third, you threaten her home, her security; fourth, you do not care for her personally, instead of helping, you put more pressure on her by bringing friends, relatives into the whole thing, where she does not feel safe. Safety, family, children and herself, that's all. It's all covered by these things.

Student: When you were talking about playmate, did you mean . . . do you have an opinion that it is better to have a marriage or better to just have a girlfriend?

Yogi Bhajan: They say marriage is something we don't want to live without. Or marriage is something you cannot live with. It is in-between. It all depends on you, your manners and your management of yourself as a man. As a man, if you've got your environments and your manners, you will never fail. Man will never fail. A man who mans himself and who is married doesn't need anything. Once your woman knows that you are decisive, she will never provoke you. Once you know you are courageous, she will never stimulate you. Once you know how to protect your territory, she will never cross you. Woman is a reflection, like a moon, moon reflects the Sun's light; moon doesn't have its own light.

Student: What do you do in an argument with a woman?

Yogi Bhajan: Go, play football. When you are attacked by a woman, never, if you want to win, never respond. She attacks in order to get a response, right? She will say, "You son of a bitch, God, you are the ugliest man I ever married." And you say, "Thank God you are married. We will discuss that later—bye. I have something to do, some place to go. Don't worry, I am a son of a bitch, I am the ugliest man, but when I come home, be ready to hug me." What can she do? But if you respond and say, "I am not ugly, I am not this, I am not that," she will say, "Your mother is ugly, your grandfather is ugly, your neighbors are ugly." I mean, she will rub you so badly . . . what is the idea of getting rubbed? She will provoke you, provoke you, and provoke you, and then you will end up beating her up. Then she calls 911 and you end up in the cell. Woman can provoke and 911 is there to oblige.

One woman, a man never said anything, but she called and said, "Oh, I am dying, I feel giddiness, I…, my husband, my husband my address and I…, 332, 1st Lane." They recorded it and went to the address and found him at home, sleeping.

They said, "There is a fight."
He said, "Where? Where is my wife? Where is my wife?"
They said, "What do you mean? Your call came from here."
He said, "No, she is not at home, the call couldn't have come from here."

The telephone call was forwarded from somewhere else, where she called. So, they investigated the servant, asking, "Where is the wife?"
"I don't know."
"What time did she leave?"
"11 o'clock"
"Where is she now?"
"We don't know."

It was a puzzle for the police, they didn't know what to do. He said, "There is a fight with what? With my wife? Absolutely not. I came home from the office, I am tired, I am sleeping, anything else I can do for you?"
They said, "But there is a complaint."
He said, "From whom? Bring her before me, I want to see what wrong I have done."

She had forwarded the call to some friend's number and then from there, connected back and played this drama. When the police reached her, she said, "I wanted to test whether 911 comes or not."

Yogi Bhajan: They are moon, they can go anywhere, do anything. There is no end to their charisma. Manu wrote a very beautiful thing. He is a law giver like Moses. They call him, in India, Manu, that's Manu's law. He writes this thick tome, pages of paper in the scripture, praising the woman; everything is great, good and wonderful. But the last line, he writes, "Oh, woman, when your brain hemisphere falls in your butts, you do not know where your heels are." That one line, nothing else, everything else is in appreciation of the woman—inches and inches thick—but the last line is what made history.

Student: Sir, as we switch to the Aquarian Age, what are the top values or rules for a man to deliver in the Aquarian Age, as opposed to the Piscean.

Yogi Bhajan: For an Aquarius man, he has to have an experience with a woman, not understanding. He has to have merger with a woman, not communication. He has to have deep understanding with woman, and not just association of time and space. Aquarius man who does not rely on experience will falter; he will not be glorious. Piscean man is logic, reason, discussion, time and space. Aquarius man is a royal man; he is established like a king in the palace and over all the territories; he is a king, he doesn't go visit personally to make it that way. That's just the way it is. The man, like the law, must rule the domain.

Student: So will there be any special challenges to us, as men, to deliver …

Yogi Bhajan: No, it is not challenges, it is a death. It's not a challenge. Either we live above it or we die under it—we don't have a choice. Our only choice is to create our caliber, our concession to caliber and strength to caliber. We must develop a meditative mind, which is the only privilege of the Age of Aquarius man, and he should get an answer quickly. No motions, no commotions, no feeling, no this, no that, it won't work. You should be very meditatively equipped, with your mental mind as a meditative mind, and you should have an answer right before you.

Student: What characteristics should a man cultivate in relationship to his family?

Yogi Bhajan: Humor. Three things a man has to get—humor—that's number one. Experience and kindness are the others. Some men pitch their children against their wives; some wives pitch their children against the man. Some feel bad, don't say it and then, in the end, burst open. All those extremities are not righteous, they are not royal, they are not glorious, they are not desirable, and once you start missing the bus all the time, everybody can see it.

Student: Sir, you know, when I feel challenged at times, frequently, I call on Guru Ram Das or Guru Gobind Singh and I …

Yogi Bhajan: That is where you mentally stretch outside of you. There is a friend of mine, he is a gambler, professional gambler. All his life he has done nothing but gamble, I asked him, "Why do you gamble?"

I met him down there, in the Caribbean; there is an island where they invite special gamblers. So, we went there to meet somebody and he met me there, and he said, "I have come here to gamble." They paid his room expenses so he would come and gamble.

I asked him, "Is that your profession?"

He committed and admitted to me, "I don't want to gamble, but I can't stop it."

I said, "It's a very simple thing, whenever you have the urge to gamble, sit down and meditate, gamble with the lord, see who wins."

Today, he has the best meditation, he is the best man. He has money, he is rich, he has all that the world can give him. So, why do we gamble? We gamble with everything in life, because we refuse to relate to our higher Self. We have a higher Self, why should we be mediocre? Always look to your higher Self—always. There is one thing in Sikh religion, which I particularly like and that is, *Cherdhi Kala*, exalted spirit, that will give you charm, that will give you a smile, that will give you humor, and that will give you excellence. Not one woman will follow you—50 will.

Student: *In terms of us having ten bodies, sir, if we are calling on Guru Ram Das and Guru Gobind Singh, I mean, you have encouraged us to call on Guru Ram Das for assistance in various situations.*

Yogi Bhajan: That is where your subtle body will become shining and the radiant body will become a hundred thousand times stronger, then you get protection. It's a simple formula; it is not something fake or made up, or a philosophy.

Guru Ram Das is the Lord of Miracles—that's all he is. The moment you call on him, you are out of the picture, he is in. There is no escape, matter will go away. That is my very personal experience and absolutely very well tried and tested. Also, the words of Nanak are very beautiful,

"Dukh parhar, sukh ghar lai jaa-ay."

"Give your worries, pain, all misfortune to God, and take happiness home."

What is God for? What do you love Him for? What do you worship Him for? Hand it over to Him. One friend of mine, he was drinking all the time; everybody tried to cover for him, recover him, everyone by him. One day, I told him, "Why don't you go to the gurdwara and give your bottle there to the Guru."

He did it. He has never touched it since then—that was seven and a half years ago. Because, you know, to take a bottle of wine through the whole congregation, all the way to the altar, and put it there, requires courage, and he said, "Unto my lord, I give this to you, I am saved, I am honored, I am exalted."

Student: *Sir, why do we develop our humor?*
Yogi Bhajan: Okay, attack me, be nasty and attack me.

Student: *You are a very ugly guy.*
Yogi Bhajan: What did he say?

Student: *You are very ugly.*
Yogi Bhajan: What?

Student: *You are very ugly.*
Yogi Bhajan: I am? Am I ugly? Good for you, so now, you have now an ugly yogi. That's good. Enjoy him. You know karate and the martial arts?

Student: *Yeah*
Yogi Bhajan: When somebody attacks you, take that force and throw them over. Confront only where you can elevate, otherwise, never confront, bypass it. It's a simple rule in order for a man to have good sexual energy, good personality, good environments, and a good home. Confront where you have to elevate and if you can't elevate . . . you know how many people call me names? "You are a womanizer," "you are a charlatan," I don't know even those words, but it's a long list. I don't think that means anything. I think they are seeing their face in the mirror. Somebody once told me, "I have heard you are a womanizer."
I said, "I have not heard it."
"But have you heard from me?"
I said, "No, you have heard; I have not."
"Why not?"
I said, "I don't have ears for this kind of stuff."
"I have heard, you must have heard."
I said, "That's true, you have heard and I am confirming you have heard. I have not heard, that's okay."

Student: *Sir, what is the relationship between a woman's actions as a moon and a man's subconscious as the Sun.*

Yogi Bhajan: Woman's actions are to provoke you consciously and get you out subconsciously and make you unconscious. She is a very, very deep, well-grounded animal, if she comes on with her beastly animal nature, you don't have one part, one ounce that can protect you. Thank God it comes only at times; otherwise man, when a woman gets wild, even the wilderness cannot protect you. That's true. So, it is better to be very gentle, safe and play the role of kindness. Play the role of kindness, not blindness. Mostly, you are very blind to woman. You never find where she can hit you or where she can harm you. You only want to please her. When you please her and please her, then you want to police her and police her, then she gets you; be very normal.

I am going to talk about all that tomorrow. If the woman would like to just present a father image, woman can follow the father image, then she will go against father phobia and father mania, or for father phobia or father mania. There is a girl I have been talking to for three days, I asked her, "What is your problem with your boss? He is so wonderful, so well read, so gentle, so beautiful."
She said, "Yeah, he is gentle. He is like my ex-husband, who was very gentle; he was a banana."
I said, "What do you mean? What's that? He is not your husband."
"He is just like him, though, I can't like him."

Some women have seen their father flirting and sexing left and right, they will never trust you. In the middle of the sex, she will say, "I have cramps," just puts you through misery.

Student: *Sir, I just don't understand one thing you said, you said it should be written on the wall that a man should eat what?*
Yogi Bhajan: Beets.

Student: *Thank You.*
Yogi Bhajan: Beets will beat out from you the weakness in your blood. Beet greens will strengthen your digestive system.

Student: *When dating, what do you recommend? You said something about no hassle, no hassle, no fuss whatever.*
Yogi Bhajan: Dating is a blind date, a friend fixes the date, you fix the date, there is a chase date, blind date, fixed date, circumstantial date, there are so many ways of dating.

Student: *Right.*
Yogi Bhajan: Right? You have to be super gentleman. If you are a super gentleman, on any date, the other partner, if she is not admissibly correct, will leave you. Then your choice of marriage will never be wrong. But if you date for sex, or you date for a party—or any other reason than marriage—I have seen people living eight, nine years together, and all of a sudden they break, because they never understood each other. It was a marriage of living arrangements for convenience, for insecurity, whatever. That's not dating. Dating is going with somebody to lay out the analysis of our plus and minus and come out with the balance sheet.

Student: *Thank you. Sat Nam.*
Yogi Bhajan: See, what we are teaching here, 30 or 40 men, do you know what the idea is behind it? You do not have a basic definition of a man, his activities and projection, his strategy. That's why. We are trying to remedy this lack of fundamental understanding. There will be certain definitions and homework so that you will understand it and become a totally wonderful man.

Student: *Sat Nam, Sir, can sex help you get liberated? How does that work for a spiritual man? Can sex help to liberate?*
Yogi Bhajan: What?
Student: *Can sex help you get liberated?*
Yogi Bhajan: From where?
Students: *(Laugh)*
Student: *I mean, can it be a part of the spiritual practice?*
Yogi Bhajan: No, it is a part of a very powerful domain of yours. Liberation? You can be liberated out of sex by a divorce, or you can be liberated from sex by getting HIV. Sex is not a small thing, sex is a sixth sense. If you are together and your juice is together, you feel wonderful. If you are not together and your juice is not together, you will do weird things. Sex affects your behavior, your feeling, your projection, your strategy. Sex is the most dangerous thing man has got, but it is the best thing man has got.

You are born by sex, you pursue sex, and you die by sex. Now I will read you something very funny today, you all will be shocked. This is America talking, not a yogi from India. Healing diseases with body and mind, San Francisco, researchers at the University of California, San Francisco, are going beyond the physical to help patients deal with disease. They are starting to incorporate spirituality and alternative therapies along with traditional medicine, into a complete healing process. UCSF offers 8 weeks of a trans-reduction course to patients, and earlier this summer, some of the 30 HIV infected individuals attended this center. It is the first of its kind and will provide a healing retreat for the participants. For AIDS patients, Dr. Johnson Tokmato, the UCSF clinic director said that a survey has shown many patients are into alternative methods of healing, not only our patients are becoming more aware of these alternative methods but also more and more health care providers and medical institutions have recognized the benefit of some of these methods. The focus is on meditation.

But why do they have to make it so difficult? Because they are doctors?
Students: *(Laugh)*

> *Sex is the most dangerous thing man has got, but it is the best thing man has got.*

Yogi Bhajan: So, spirituality and personal empowerment, personal identity...empowerment is such a dirty word, used for all purposes. It implies that you have to be bigger than somebody. Identity is when you are smaller than the other person so that person can bend on you, depend on you, be dependant, not be dependable. This empowerment these days is getting really..., well, now there are pages and pages and pages. What good have they done? As he puts it, "our programs are not about illness or dying but rather about the quality of life, no matter what the circumstance are."

Student: You said something about the passages on the right or the left, and is there any difference?

Yogi Bhajan: It depends upon which nostril is working.

Student: And which one is more dominating all the time?

Yogi Bhajan: No, if your right nostril is working, you have to, you want to go and ejaculate immediately, if your left is working, you want to take time.

Kriya to Create a **Saint**
August 14, 1997

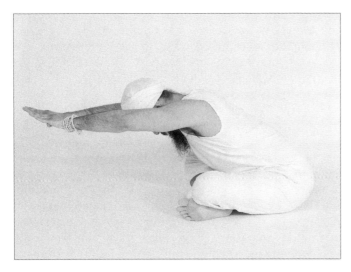

Posture: Sit in a cross-legged posture. Chin in Neck Lock. Fold forward, putting your chest on your knees. Only fold as far as you naturally can, keeping the spine as straight as possible.

Mudra: Stretch your arms straight out in front of you. Lock the left thumb into the right hand, placing it between the thumb and forefinger (Jupiter finger) of the right hand. Fingers are straight and pointing forward, arms are straight and locked. There is no bend in the elbows.

Don't let the arms drop to the floor; keep them in line with the spine, stretching forward as an extension of the torso.

Time: 62 Minutes

To End: The final 11 Minutes is done with Breath of Fire.

Comments: This is your sexual age. I want to see your sciatica stretched and opened up through this posture. To create a saint, base is a man, or base is a woman. So we are dealing with your very elemental things, defining them, explaining them, then through these kriyas, we want you to experience that.

Commentary on Kriya to Create a **Saint**

The pain you are experiencing is because the flexibility of your sciatica and sexual nerve has gone much more off than it should have. You are governed by two things: the sciatic nerve and the central nerve. Over the years you become frigid and overdo when it comes to food; you eat a lot, good dinner, good breakfast. That which tastes good when it goes through the mouth will start hanging here (the gut) and that is bad, because when it grows larger, it puts pressure on the diaphragm.

You are very incompetent sexually, this so-called 'sexual act,' insults your sexuality. You don't care for your sexual form, you don't understand that it is fundamentally correct to keep yourself in good sexual form. Once you have incorrect sexuality, even with all the grace bestowed on you, you will still be angry, frustrated. There is a word for it, what do they call them? Irritated, groggy, foolish. Actually, there is no perversion but this: when a male cannot undertake to nurture his own central nervous system and cannot afford to utilize the power of his own sensuality. You always think in the West that sex is just having intercourse, but intercourse means also my talking to you now—this is also intercourse. Intercourse means exchanging between two people. Intercourse has a lot of manners and meanings and understandings. Cohabiting means sex, but cohabiting also means living together. Get it together to be together— that is what together is. It has to be general, absolutely general. You cannot love me and hate B and love C and hate D, because the hate is the part of you that makes you an inferior man; and love is what makes you a superior man. There must come a balance. Suppose you have three people and you love two, you are minus one, and that stress you can't understand, but it contributes to your entire grace and you will be handicapped in this race called life.

You may try to go to a doctor or a psychologist or a psychiatrist or a swami, or a yogi or a teacher; but nothing will help you, because you are stupid about yourself. It's important that you be very wise about yourself. It's not what you do—it is what you think! Your thinking will come from your physical projection and your self-importance, your self-importance will increase day by day and as it increases, your nervous system, your sciatica, your central nervous system, will not hold out for you and you will start acting out. Your friends and your relatives will feel it first, then everybody will feel it and you know what they will do? When you talk to somebody in a very non-coherent way, the other man looks at it. But this doesn't have to happen. This isn't a valid way of living. The price you pay for a good life is life itself. I repeat: the price you pay for a good life is life itself—and you cannot pay with anything other than goodness.

I will tell you my experience of 28 years and I say it openly; I have said it so many times. If you want to make the best of me or some statue of me, thinking I am a great teacher and all that, fine, but take the peanuts. Take so many that that many peanut shells, that many scabs, I have got on me. You know what I am saying? If there is an intense insult, it is my glory. It is the glory which kept me alive and made me go through this:

"Dukh parhar, sukh ghar lai jaa-ay,"

"Give the pain and calamity to God and take happiness home."

All those who are my students, I have done them a favor. I put two 6' 2" gray headstones where there was no place for a grave, but I thought this is enough, stone can stand. I wrote The *Song of the Khalsa* on the back and engraved on the front, the line,

"Ketiaa dookh bukh sad maar. Eh bhee daat teree daataar."

This is the sutra on which I live. *Ketia* means many, many; *dookh* means discomforts, painful discomfort; *bukh* means hunger, painful hunger; *sad maar*, if it's multiplied a hundred thousand times, God it is your blessing, thank God that you feel me fit or make me deserving to go through it.

Those of you who do not believe in God, you do not believe in calamity, you do not believe in reality, you do not believe in any ethics or your higher morality. No, this is all there is: if God has found you, He will test you out, through a very vulgar, unsophisticated, inhuman, small situation. The funny part is, when you smile, it will disappear. Calamity has one situation: it creates a climate of terror, horror, fear; but the moment you say, "Unto God it goes, God is with me, *Ang Sang Wahe Guru*," it will practically disappear. Because if somebody comes to your home and you do not open the door, you do not welcome them, you do not feed them, they will disappear won't they? So when calamity comes, don't receive it, don't associate with it, don't feel that you can't do the same thing you would do as a man with a woman.

Student: *So, I think, in sex you should try relaxing and going to the left nostril.*

Yogi Bhajan: There are lots of things we are going to learn in four days, I shouldn't teach you everything today. I know that you are all very eager for me to show you a movie: here the mouse is going in, here the mouse coming out. But I have a very simple, gentle way of teaching, so that you can understand with a lot of grace and honor. Once God has made you a man, he has made you a successful man. The Lord Infinite cannot create damaged property. Whether you believe in God or not, somebody created you, whosoever created you, as an artist, has created perfect art in you. So there is no need to be handicapped. Now, let's meditate a little bit so that you may not get off scot-free. Let us see how manly you are.

Student: *What does this meditation do?*
Yogi Bhajan: You should tell me in the evening, rather than my telling you what it does. You can't escape the answer. You see, you have come here in a wonderful situation. Here we are, everything is at stake. This men's course is not a joke. This is about everything we have and if we can make men out of you, we will have a very powerful future and wonderful peace of mind, a wonderful legacy. Because to create a saint, base is a man, to create a saint, base is a woman. So we are dealing with your very elemental things, defining them, explaining them, then through kriyas we want you to experience that. Is that all right?

Student: *Sat Nam, how does a single man know it's appropriate to pursue a relationship with a woman that he is interested in?*
Yogi Bhajan: *"Beej mantra sarb ko gyan."* Every spermatozoa knows how to reach the egg and go eight times around. All men of all quality know, from the very sight and smell of the woman, what is what. They may not get it, but they know it. When rhino is excited, he doesn't need a horn, he is the horn. Some things excite a man, some things depress a man, some things coordinate with a man, some things are friends within man, some things are against the man, some things only cater to the ego of the man, and some things totally destroy the ego of the man. Man goes through all the facets but with all the facets if he can remain a man, he shall have no problem. Whether married, unmarried, single, multiple.

You know, royalty, they have what they call a harem. What is it? Nothing—it is just a show. They have as many women or they have as many servants—all this paraphernalia—to glorify themselves. But when a man glorifies himself, then he becomes a real man. Then all prosperity, virtues and things come to him. That's the beauty of a man.

"Tehal Mehal Thanko milae, Jahan pe hai Sant Kripal."

"If the self saintliness has blessed you and you live under that, then all the palaces and servants will be at your door, all will be yours. Then you become very radiant."

I remember this story and I always tell it. An Archbishop came from Japan, he was friendly, he wanted to have a kundalini experience. He came all the way from San Francisco, put all the presents and pearls and God knows what. I was dying and lying down in the middle of room with three quilts and two blankets on me. When I took a breath, my entire chest hurt. I had just come from India with influenza, and with this and that virus, you name it. They had given me an injection so I couldn't feel the pain and I could sleep. Before I was going into deep sleep, I was told that he had arrived and they couldn't cancel it, they couldn't call. So I asked him, "Krayapa, you have come to have a kundalini experience."

He said, "Yes, Master."
I said, "Put your hand in the quilt, take away my right hand and put it on your forehead and then go."

He did as he was told and all of a minute later, in his Japanese, he started praising the Lord and was so happy. He didn't want to leave; I was told he wanted to stay with me. I said, "Get rid of him as fast as possible. It happened, that's all he came for, we don't want him here." Then, a couple of years later, he was very loving and he said, "Master, I have got one wish in my life."
I said, "I know what wish you have: You want the biggest temple in Japan."

He said, "Yes. But I have books and I have done so many things, but it is not happening." There was, in the corner, a big spoon and in the spoon, the Adi Shakti was carved. I said, "Krayapa, why don't you pick up that spoon?" So long as this spoon of wood will be with you, you will be the richest and the temple will be complete. It is true. Today, he is so popular, he is so good, he is so wonderful, he forgot who is who; but whenever one of our students goes, he pays them very special respect and recites the story.

This energy, which you have, is priceless, but you need the proper attitude and manners to use it. It is your energy, not anybody else's. Whatever you have is all inside you, if you try to find it outside, you are just living in doubt and wasting time.

Leader, Protector, and Provider— Along with a Little **Humor**

Don't acclimate yourself, associate yourself, with anything other than humor.
"Hi sweetheart, how are you my moon?"
"Doing well."
"Are you waning and waxing?"
You can pull a woman from a mile away to two hundred million thirty-six miles, just with two seconds—simply expand her horizon.

"George, don't you think we should go eat outside tonight?" You don't want to go out, so what do you do? You take the leftover food out, heat it up, and put it on the porch that's outside; you obey. She will laugh and you will laugh. But if you say, "let's go and eat outside," then eat in a café where everything is outside. Don't go to a fancy restaurant—tug her into it—you are picking a fight. You are not manning your man; you are not straightforward;

you are just under a very negative, depressed influence which supports your fear. You are afraid and fearful and you are overdoing it. Never, ever overdo and overact with a woman. These are some faculties men have to learn. There are some responsibilities men have to learn. For example, never sneak into the bed of a woman if you have come home late and she is sleeping. Take a glass of milk, go sit down, sip it, whistle, play a song. She must get up and acknowledge you. You think, "Why should I trouble her?" because you don't have a relationship with her.

She will say, "I am sleeping and you are whistling?"
You say, "I am missing you and you are sleeping; let us both whistle."
(Students laugh.)

You have to understand. You have to interlock with a woman. Interlock socially, psychologically, systematically and personally.

There was a guy once, he came to bed late one night. He had his shoes on, the whole thing, and he went flying onto the bed, shouting, "Aaaaaa," and it broke.

His wife was in it; there was total disarray, headboards flying, and she said, "You know what you have done?"
He said, "Your Tarzan has come."
(Students laugh.)

That's it! They pulled the whole thing outside and they both slept on the floor.

Your fears are very, very, very, very, very, very annoying to the woman and your aggressiveness is very annoying to the woman. Sometimes, you must understand, there are some women who are, by nature, better women. So they will provoke you, right? You will get hot and beat up and whatever you do, it is your range. Then you both must have sex and you will have sex—in 99.9% of people this happens. Woman has a very provocative range of words. I will give you an example.

Somebody's father came to see their son and daughter-in-law. He came from the office and she gave him a bottle and a nipple and said, "Well, normally your mother is here, so it's better you suck on this to enjoy your day. I am going out to my friend's house to have a good meal."

Do you know what the net worth of that man is, who she said that to? Six hundred million dollars. She gave him practically a baby's bottle with baby formula in it and she left. Well, he called the butler, he called the maid, he said, "What is the problem?" They said, "Your parents were very hungry and they asked to eat early and we provided them some food but the mistress got mad. She was totally unaware of what was going on." You know what he did the next day, foolishly?

He took his parents to a hotel and moved himself. These are the kinds of reactions people have. I mean to say, if some good people had not intervened, it would have been a final divorce. You overcompensate with your relatives and your family and your environments and your children. That is a very, very cumbersome situation. As a man, you like it or not, you believe it or not, you can do it or not, but you are supposed to be the guardian of security and justice. That's what is expected of you.

I asked somebody, "What you do every Sunday?"
He said, "I go to synagogue."
I said, "You? I mean, you and synagogue? You are an atheist; you are not even Jewish, you were just born Jewish."
He said, "No, no, no don't say anything; it keeps my wife calm."
I said, "I know you are an atheist and you don't believe in anything, forget about this synagogue; you don't even believe in God."
He said, "I have started believing, after discussing with you for a few days, but the fact is, where is God?"
I said, "Here you go. What do you do in synagogue?"
He said, "I go and sit down and sleep. It's very calm to me, but my wife is fanatically religious."

So some things people do actively, because man is a leader, protector, provider and the most graceful institution of all, put together in a family. There is no irrelevance in it. If you understand yourself as a man, you understand what sexuality is, what the senses are and what the sixth sense is, you will totally understand that you are not going to put yourself under such a burden that you may regret it later on. After all, to become rich, rich, rich, rich, you have to think rich, rich, rich and you have to act rich, rich, rich and you have to be rich, rich, rich and you have to carry people rich, rich, rich; there are so many facets to it and you have to come through. Therefore, it is obligatory for you to understand your glory; you must be a royal, glowing person. You must be a competent person. Your answers should be short, precise.

If you want to help somebody in the kitchen, just say "may we." You understand what I am saying? "May we"—not "may I." These little things make a difference. In the conversation between you and your reality and your personality, you must understand that you are a man first, you are a man in the middle, and you are man in the end—that you cannot change. You have a pound or half a pound of meat hanging outside of you—that you cannot change. You don't have a breast, you have a chest—that you cannot change. You cannot become pregnant and you cannot menstruate—that you cannot change. You understand that?

Students: *Yes, sir.*
Yogi Bhajan: When that is there and you do not compensate for it while dealing with a woman, it makes

you a small, little man. You understand what I am hitting at? Every woman wants a big man whether that thing is big or small, doesn't matter, man should be big, big, big. You understand that? And when you do that, you cannot be big enough.

Student: *So are you saying that a woman who wants a man, a big man, wants a good partner sexually also?*

Yogi Bhajan: Sexually, sensually, it's very little stuff, it's very little stuff. What I'm saying is to always be vast. Don't waste your life. Be vast, big, excellent, excel, it's natural. No female can ever tolerate a grouchy, complaining, crying man. This is the faculty of the female, which you have adopted. No, I am not kidding. It is the faculty of the female to be complaining, to be insecure, to be grouchy, to be saying, "My hands are hurting, I mean, my legs are falling apart." It's her problem. She wants the Eiffel Tower and to rule over the whole of Paris. Women are very, very well inter-created, inter-decorated human beings. What they want is what glorifies them. If you are glorified and you are royal and you are great, they will give their life to you.

Look at Princess Diana, whatever she is, if Charles had acted as a king and a man, if he would have manned his man, he would not have seen this day. So there is an insertion of perversion, because it comes to you out of fear and fear is one process that brings insecurity, and insecurity is one process that builds a degree of impotency. If you are worried too much or you are sad too much or you corner yourself too much, then it will bring you grief and then it will give you diabetes. It will be a very different situation. If you are very angry and you are holding it in and holding it in, it will give you cancer. That's where men die fast. Relax. Never start a fight with a wife or woman—learn from this preacher today.

Anything can happen to you. It's not that it will always be right, it's not that it will always be wrong, just understand what is happening to you. If you do not have flexibility, if you are angry or full of grief and insecurity, you know what you lose? You lose your security, you lose your flexibility, you lose everything; insecurity is very essential. When you find yourself insecure, you try to be secure, you understand? You want to be secure if you are afraid; because everything has a polarity. So, you must use your common sense, your sensual sixth sense to grow out of it. But if you don't even know where her "buts" are, you are in damn trouble. See that everything that goes on between you and any person doesn't have any negative thought of your own. We will work that out right now, to get it out of your system for a few minutes and you will be fine.

Kriya: The Faculty of a **Man**
August 14, 1997

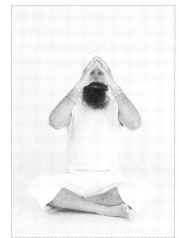

Posture: Sit in a meditative posture.

Mudra: Bring your hands up in front of your face, the tips of each finger are touching the tips of the opposite fingers; the fingers are spread apart and there is space between the palms, about 3-5 inches, the hands are slightly rounded, relaxed; that is, don't hyperextend the fingers by pressing too hard. The tips of the thumbs are just in front of the tip of the nose.

Eyes: Closed

Breath: Long Deep Breathing or One Minute Breath

Music: Tantric *Har*

Time: 18 Minutes

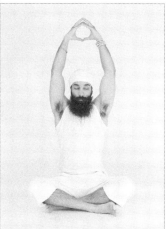

To end: Inhale deep and stretch the spine up, stretch the arms over head, maintaining the mudra. Stretch up. Exhale. Inhale and stretch from the base of the spine. Exhale. Inhale, continue stretching and twist left and right. Exhale.

Comments: One minute breath is twenty second inhale, twenty second hold, twenty second exhale and the balance of this at the frontal lobe creates a separate electro-magnetic field. It will give you a very calm, beautiful experience and take away from you the initial subconscious stress, after a while you will relax and enjoy it.

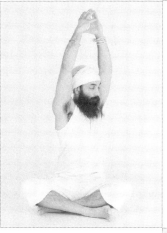

This mudra is called the "Touch of Health." It takes away disease from the body. This kriya gives you an experience of the faculty of a man. It balances the frontal lobe and gives you a separate electromagnetic field and takes away from you the initial subconscious stress, which after a while, relaxes you. It is the faculty of a man to worry, but it is the reality of a man not to worry. After 40 days of this kriya, you will be a different person.

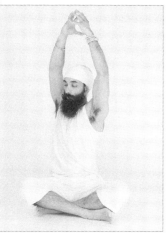

It is faculty of the man to worry, but it's the reality of the man not to worry. God made man and woman in His own image, so He knows better. You know better, but never, ever in your life say anything bad, because what you say is the sound current which makes you.

Realize that you cannot even think of not appreciating everything. Appreciate your blessing, appreciate yourself, appreciate your commitment, appreciate your surroundings, appreciate your challenges, appreciate everything. In 40 days you will be a different person, that's how powerful self-appreciation is.

Somebody broke his leg, went to the hospital, the doctors fixed it up as much as they could and the person came out not walking straight. One friend said, "Hey! This accident, it is horrible, you are limping."

He said, "Well, that's a blessing in disguise; now I have to walk carefully and slowly."

He did not take it as a negative. Never let down anybody, never let down yourself and never participate in a let down; in lieu of that you will be a royal, glorious, glowing Knight of your own championship of character, characteristic and sense of justice.

May the long time sun shine upon you, all love surround you and the pure light within you, guide your way on.

Lord God, give us the extra strength to be of any service to any and all where we could be serviceful. Give us the character and the strength to do good to all those where we can be serviceful. Give us the intelligence and wisdom to serve all those where we will be serviceful. Give us the personal strength so we can be wise and serviceful. May the long distance of this destiny on this Earth complete with a royal glow, grace and character. Give us the strength to live behind legacy that our verdict may not become fruitless, give us the strength to make a mark for which we and our generations can be proud. Sat Nam.

Wake Up Like a **Man**

How to invoke from inside and bring it out in order to serve the outside is your success as a man. This is your criteria of life.

The subject I am covering with you today is that before you can take care of yourself as a man, you have to act like a man; so you should learn to get up like a man. Your concept is to sleep at night, is that true? And in that moment of sleep, you do not know whether you are a woman or you are a man or you are dead or alive. When you are sleeping, you hope you will get up, but if you don't get up—and many don't get up—it's ok. So, everyday when you open your eyes and you feel you are alive, it is a new day.

Get Up Like a Man: Wake Up **Exercises**
August 15, 1997

1. Open your eyes into the palms of your hands.

2. Cat Stretch: Stretch left and right. Stretch thoroughly, hands, legs, toes, fingers.

3. Stretch your hands and your legs upward, try to reach 90°, if not, do what you can to bring your legs up and your hands up. "You will make a U of your body, if you are 'You' then make a U of the body."

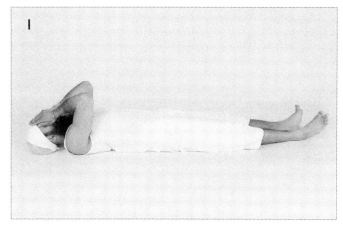

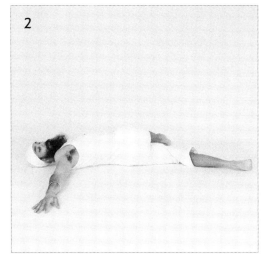

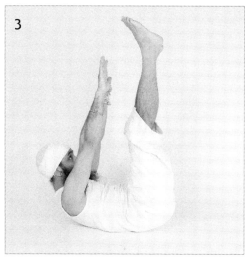

continued...

4. Cycle your legs while lying down on your back.

5. Sit up and make fists of your hands, holding your arms out as if you were picking up a large barrel. Begin to twist left and right, creating a rhythm.

6. Cobra Pose with your tongue extended out like Lion Pose. **3 Minutes**

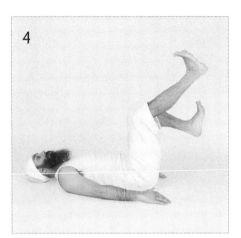

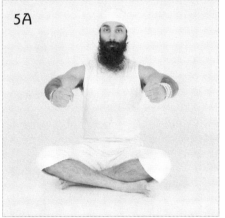
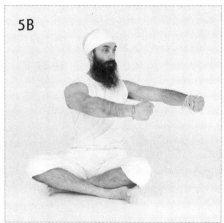
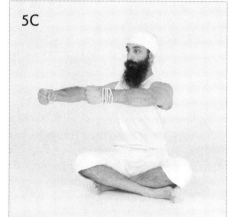

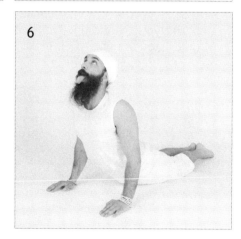

7. Cat/Cow Pose: Flex the spine and make it beautiful.

8. Baby Pose with your hands by your hips, palm up. Rest for **3 Minutes**

9. Come sitting up and pull and stretch your ears

10. Activate your ida and pingala: massage the outside of your nostrils with your forefingers, then the root of the nose with your thumbs, vigorously vibrating each side of the nose at the corner of the eye.

Comments: Everyday when you open your eyes and you feel you are alive, it is a new day. Your body must be activated by you. When you get up from bed, you will *not* get up from the bed, you will stretch your entire body like a child when it is born, he stretches himself. And wahhhhh! that first cry, that will stretch your lungs.

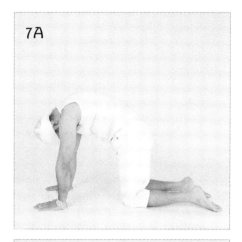
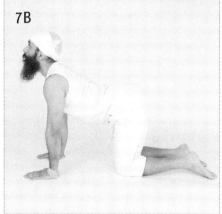
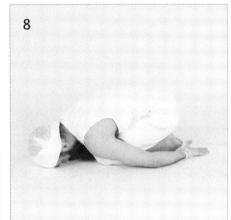
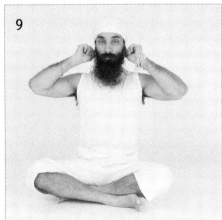
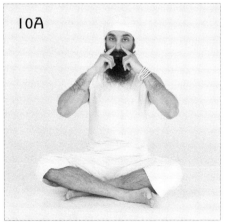
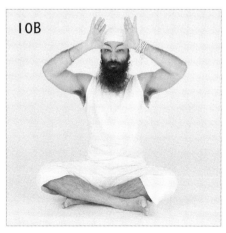

At night before going to bed, you must meditate and relax yourself completely. Brush your teeth, wash your face, your hands and armpits, your feet and your calves, otherwise you will have no sexual activity—and that sooner than you think. At night your testicle temperature should be one centigrade less than your body. So take a very cold cloth and clean and wash yourself, then keep it there for a minute or two, that's what you need to serve them, if you want them to serve you. In the morning also, please remember to do the same.

There are certain places for you as men, which need a cold cloth. If you have it, you take Narayan oil and put it on the back of your neck and then you put an ice cold towel there. You can get all the blood of life there. What happens, which people do not recognize and where you fail is that all these muscles become so tense, they restrict that flow. Some get migraine headaches, some get headaches, some get tired, some go totally berserk, all these symptoms are just from not having this flow of blood. Blood flow will be there but not totally, as it should be. The muscle is restricted and the majority of men get tension in the neck. Like that day a person came to me with a very powerful migraine headache, you know, when the migraine headache starts and it never ends? So I said, just do it. She came to me and I pressed the meridian point, she is fine. Can you understand why the person had to suffer for a week or two? Sometimes the medicine works, sometimes not. Because the problem is basic. As long as you do not stretch your body, and you are still on top of it, you should not touch the earth. So these are bed exercises.

Going to take your cold shower and doing all that, that is separate. Your body must be activated by you. The greatest mistake men make is they drive the car when it is still cold. You drive your life, to the full swing, when you are not even awake yet.

As men, you must get up as men. Then, as men, you must walk like men. Your hands and your legs must cover equal distance. Your hand and legs?

Students: *Must cover equal distance.*

Yogi Bhajan: Those who do not move their hands with their legs, ultimately have no friend called brain. That is why you become senile and you don't know why. That's why you think you are an eighteen year old, when you are not. Hands and legs?

Students: *Must cover equal distance.*

Yogi Bhajan: Walk like a man always and please, from the heel of your shoes, find out whether you are putting a balanced weight on each foot or not. Walk on your toes and not on your heels. Men who walk on their heels—in the army we trained them to walk on the heel—will be dumb. Ladies were asked not to be dumb and walked on their paws; that's why they started wearing high heels, rather than walking on their paws.

Exercise for **Clarity**
August 15, 1997

Hit the base of the hands and then the base of the fingers and the tips of the fingers (together). As the fingertips strike each other, the hands pull away from each other and the fingers fold. Makes a clapping rhythm: "poka-la-la". Don't meditate. Keep your eyes open. It will sharpen your IQ.

When you are confused or depressed, somebody has stabbed you in the back, you don't know what to do, put some beautiful, meditative music on and do it for **31 Minutes**.

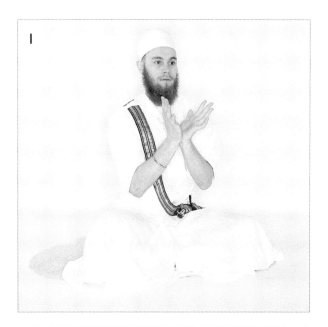

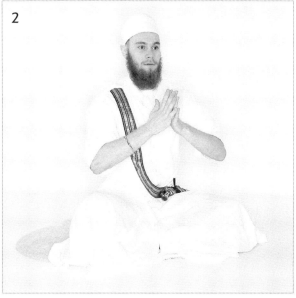

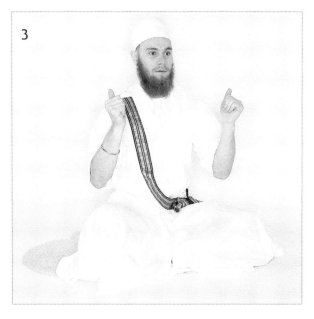

Relaxation **Exercise**

August 15, 1997

Take your left hand, put it behind your neck, and squeeze the muscles tight. Inhale deep. Hold it and press the neck forward without letting the head drop, the neck should resist the pressure of the hand. "It is a competition." Exhale. Take the right hand and do the same thing.

Repeat the cycle three times. Witness your body's recuperative powers.

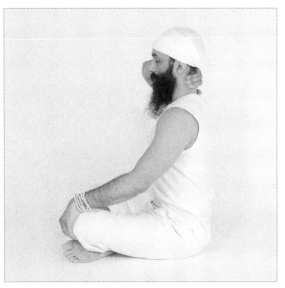
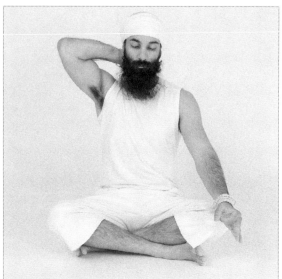

Kriya to Invoke the Internal Power of a **Man**
August 15, 1997

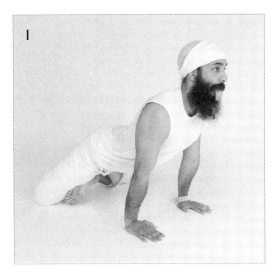
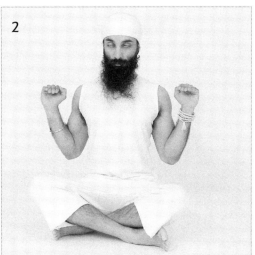

1. Lion Pose: Cross your legs in Easy Sitting Pose, Half Lotus or Lotus Pose. Put your hands on the ground in front of you. Lift your weight off your buttocks and come onto your knees, with your legs crossed. Put your weight into your hands as you drop your hips forward so that the knees, hips, and spine create one line. Extend your tongue in Lion Pose and chant with the music. Chant with your tongue extended; it will be awkward but just practice it. Music: Wahe Guru (Siri Nagar Singh) **3 Minutes**

Comments: One day your tongue can be out and you can chant the *Tresha Guru* Mantra:

Waah Yantee, Kar Yantee, Jag Dut Patee, Aadak It Whaahaa, Brahmaaday Trayshaa Guroo, It Wha-hay Guroo

It is not a Sikh Mantra. May I tell you all that? Patanjali, thousands of year ago, wrote about this mantra. This mantra belongs to God. God is what three letters, G-O-D, one who Generates, one who Organizes, and one who Destroys and Delivers, that is the faculty of God, and he has three identities. One who does this, this is their personal mantra, "Wahe Guru".

There are only six letters in the whole world that can give you mastery over the universe: Har, Hare, Hari, Wah-Hay Guru. That's it. This will bring you all the knowledge in the world and anything you want. These are sounds and the universe exists on sound. The universe is running on a sound psyche, not on any other thing. It has a sound psyche. With words you can win the world, with a word you can lose the world.

If your tongue can be out, and in this posture you can chant it, one day you will be really very grateful to me. It gives the *Vaach siddhi*, whatever you say happens. Your words penetrate into the heart rather than the head. You become a winner—and that is the faculty of a man.

2. Sit in a cross-legged posture. Chin in and chest out. Make your hands into the shape of a hooded cobra and bring them up beside your shoulders, fingertips pointing forward. The elbows are down by your ribs. Squeeze your shoulder blades together behind you, taking the elbows and hands back as far as you can. Squeeze. Close your eyes and breathe long and deep. Go into absolute silence as you listen to the mantra. Music: Wahe Guru (Siri Nagar Singh) **38 Minutes**

3. Maintain the posture. Stop the music and begin chanting aloud. **90 Seconds**

To End: Inhale deep, hold, Cannon Fire exhale. Repeat twice more and relax.

Comments: There is no power outside of you. Says Nanak,

Sab kuch Teri ander anther vey baye, bahar tuneto param pulay

"Man has all the power inside the man and what he finds outside, he just goes into a zigzag, there is nothing outside you, which you can get."

How to invoke the power within you and bring it out is your success as a man. This is your criteria of life. Some people think that we are foolish to chant mantra every day. That is not true: *man tarang*, man is *mind* and *tarang* is a wave. Mental waves becomes purified with the excretion of the sound. Then the sound conquers things for you. You don't have to do anything.

"In the beginning was a word, word was with God and word was God." John said one thing in the Bible that is true; but Nanak was very good with it, too. He said, *Asankh naav asankh thaav* . . . the whole *Japji Sahib*[1] he relates to that, explains it.

How to invoke from inside and bring it out in order to serve the outside is your success as a man. This is your criteria of life.

Mann tarang, tarang is called wave, mental waves become purified with the excretion of the sound and then the sound conquers things for you. You don't have to do anything.

---

[1] Written by Guru Nanak Dev Ji in the 15th Century, it has become the first prayer of the Sikh and is known as a universal song of the soul in praise of God and the experience of ecstasy.

Kriya to Prevent **Impotence**
August 16, 1997

1. Come into Triangle Pose. Lift your left foot and your left hand and stretch your toes. Hold.

2. Lift your right foot and your right hand and stretch your toes. Hold.

3. Lift your left hand and your right leg. Stick your tongue out and breathe through your mouth. **3 Minutes.**

4. Switch sides. Lift your right hand and your left leg. Continue breathing through your mouth. **3 Minutes.**

Comments: Sex is not what you think sex is. Stabilize yourself, stabilize. How can you stabilize yourself in bed if you cannot stabilize yourself here. As a man, if you do not stretch yourself diagonally, you will be one third impotent straight. After the age of 45, you will be ejaculating less and less and less, at the age of 54, you will want to be very passionate sexually, but you will experience a reaction and you will not enjoy it if you are not diagonally stretched.

It applies to Muslims, Jews, Christians, Hindus, Buddhists, everything. It's the story of the man. It's not a story of faith. Life is not story of a faith or trust or religion or any other b____t. Life is just a story of life itself.

The diagonal stretch (exercise 3 & 4) was originally practiced for 2 ½ hours on each side. We would help each other out of the pose, receive a massage, take some juice, relax and practice on the other side for 2 ½ hours.

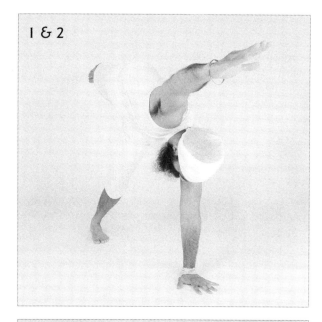

1 & 2

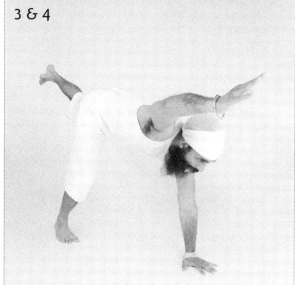

3 & 4

Commentary on Kriya to Prevent
Impotence

I know that it is easier [opposite arm and leg lifted], I used to do it. I never said it is shocking. You think I just fell out of the banana tree? *(Students laugh.)*

Yogi Bhajan: Somebody once saw a banana tree and there were so many bananas hanging there. He said, "God I have one dream."
I said, "What is it?"
"That I should have that many penises hanging."

Men have fantasies, you can't believe it. But they can't do this simple exercise, that's the problem. You are going to learn everything without even reading a book. Don't worry. Your capacity of inheritance has gone weak in your sixth sense. Some doctor was telling me that sex should not be called sex, it should be called sense. So it is—the sixth sense. Sex is not what you think sex is. How can you stabilize yourself in the bed if you can't stabilize here.

Student: *When do we switch legs?*
Yogi Bhajan: Not right now. You switch nothing. You kill yourself and totally let the central nervous system give you a diagonal push. Mouth open, tongue out, breathe. The penis has no other chance; it has to be done this way.

You have got to know what a man is. Don't watch those cartoons and their little gadgets and feel that you are men. I mean, there are woman who have nothing invested in you and you just get horny and mess around and that's how you call yourself men? You are just a little crow, nibbling at the pussy—shame on you! Come on now. Show me how much you love your penis. I want to see it right straight direct. If you, as a man, do not stretch yourself diagonally, you will be one third impotent straight. One third?

Student: *Impotent straight.*

When we practiced this kriya, we were supposed to practice two and half hours on one leg. And we did—I did.

Hair and the Technology of the
Turban

I am not selling turbans to people and nobody should take it to heart, but facts are facts. These are the facts. There is nothing I can do about it or you can do about it. We have the longest hair on our head. We have 26 parts to the skull. You understand? When the blood does not reach the gray matter in which the brain is sitting, your brain starts compensating and the psyche is affected.

Hair is pure protein. Remember, just as you need heavy water to generate atomic energy, hair provides the scalp and the brain with absolutely pure protein. If you take your hair and put it in mulch, that plant will grow better than any other. That pure protein, which should be there, isn't there because you cut your hair every week or every month, whatever. But you can save yourself once in a while, by wearing a scarf at night, like the old times. Put a scarf on at night—that you can do. Scarf should be cotton, silk or wool and it will give you a personal adjustment, a cranial adjustment, so the gray matter and the brain can sustain itself normally well.

I have long hair; we braid our hair and then we just wrap the scarf and tie it, cover yourself. The idea is to cover this part, from here to here (across the brow and behind the ears, covering the crown). Tell your wife to pull your hair, massage your head, and little by little, pull all your hair and then put a scarf on.

Somebody once said, "I am bald."
I said, "That's your bad luck. I can't change that." Then you have to do it with your hands. It is most important for a male that the cranial adjustment should be absolutely correct. Scarf will provide some help.

What is a turban? You think it's a cloth? People thought of wearing a turban because of what some God told them? No, it was known that the male's cranial adjustment shifts and he cannot perform his duties. Because his left part of the hemisphere is subjective, it is not equal. The turban is a very personal, pressed scarf; it is just a cranial adjustment by a man for himself. He crowns himself.

Scarf at night is required, it is necessary. Normally at night the scarf may go away or not, but once for few minutes, you tighten this area. It is even good for bald headed people, because this is how it is, this triangle, where the bone is porous, it gets the Sun. People think that the Sun is only there when he is up there, Sun is everywhere, all the time. A reflection of the moon is everywhere. It's the moon and Sun which play us. If you don't want to wear a scarf, then comb your hair and pull them together, the 26 parts of the scalp must be brought into one order—before getting up and before sleeping. You will have very easy day.

Don't get fanatic about it, it's just a science. I am not putting turbans on people. That's not my purpose. But a lot of people will wear it; I did it because I used to have sharp, splitting headaches. Sometimes it happens. Kundalini Yoga is not a small thing, it's a power. I used to have a very splitting pain here; but it's not because I run a boutique shop.

Woman has both hemisphere's of the brain equal—you don't. She grows breasts, you don't. There are certain fundamental differences. Men are from Mars and women are from Venus. Somebody stole those words, which I spoke 28 years ago or so, in New York, and has written a book. I have no comment, read those books, if you can't make sense of them, then come and call me. Men are from Mars, dry, arid, spirit. Mars is habitable. All seven planets have their souls transparent, totally transparent soul, clear. They don't have a body like this. They have subtle bodies and they are all there.

The planet Mars is called Lord of War and Joy, Lord of War and Joy. Planet Mars is very rough, rugged, the word is rugged; it's not sandy, it's not watery, it is rugged. The man is basically rugged. Moon is the reflector, moon is?

Students: *The reflector.*
Yogi Bhajan: So, a female, when she reflects—look at you, watch this—when female reflects, the man's ruggedness cannot catch. You bring her all the flowers, you have all the intercourse with her, screw the whole world for it, but she will not, shall not, respect you; because it's a natural law; that is the natural cohabitation; that is the natural intercourse. There is a transcontinental psyche and body language and biorhythm. You know what happened? Your mama said, "Now, you are born a man, now you've disobeyed me, now tell a lie, say I am not at home, tell this, tell that, get this grade, do this, do that." It's no fault of yours; you were four years old when you were taught this.

When I was young, we attended a special class. In our domain, a boy would go to school at five years old, before that he was basically taught with pictures and drawings. I am unfortunate that Pakistan came and I don't have any of my notes. If I had shown you, you would have flipped, every detail.

Yogi Bhajan on Alcohol and Other Intoxicants

You drink? I have no objection to drinking. Drink, it's your money. But you drink and your sensitivity is gone. You know, Newton's Third Law, action has a reaction, equal and opposite, is that true? Now when you drink, you accelerate—isn't that true? You are going to fall. But where you are going to fall? How far you are going to fall? And how often you are going to fall? That you can't control.

If you ever want to drink, some people have that urge, that compulsion. Some people are neurotic, psychotic, but just take a cup of milk with cardamom. Boiled milk, that's good for you, with cinnamon boiled in it. Cinnamon, cardamom and milk, then take a dropper and put ten drops of gin in it—that Bombay gin has 26 herbs that was made for man for healing, made from juniper berries, which has become a drink—ten drops, your kidney will start improving, your circulation will start improving, and you will start improving, but put someday eleven drops and see what happens. It's so accurate. But remember that eleven drops will act adversely and one ounce will do you in. Gin was made for kidney disease. Its dose was ten drops. Now people take a bottle and "glug-glug-glug." What is that? What's going on?

Rum was made to soothe the nerves and accelerate the circulation. Malt vinegar was made first, thick. Have you seen malt vinegar? Originally, it was thick and that was to clean out the dirt from the body.

Maple syrup is the most powerful thing on the Earth for men. Have you ever made boiled milk with cardamom and then you put maple syrup in it, stir it, and then let it cool, and put two to four scoops of ice-cream in it, and let that become a little pulpy? Drink it. See in five minutes where you go, just five minutes. You will be dissolved. Or, take this iceburg lettuce and you put the whole head in a steamer—whole head in the steamer and then take it out, cut it in half like a turkey and put gravy on it and then you eat it. You will be gone. It has a natural opium. It relieves tension in your muscles, it gives relief to your penis muscles and what is penis? It doesn't have a bone, it's just a muscle. Blood, ordered by the pituitary, goes into the penis and makes it hard and strong. The tragedy with you men is that you think the penis is hard. Penis should be at your control at 40°, but once it goes into the cavity, it should start working with the heat of the vagina. Some people can't even get it in, they just pre-ejaculate because of overexcitement. If you have a meditative mind, you can control the action of pituitary, you can control the universe. Accurate?

I am just giving you some examples. You must understand, it's not true that I have not practiced them myself. It's also not true that I don't have the experience of it and also know the benefits of it. Religion is not what you practice, religion is a personal reality, an experience. This whole philosophy, the whole thing is cheating, everybody wants your money, everybody wants you—it is a slavery. A person who is a slave to religion or religiously fanatic is already cursed; there is no solution for such person. You have never understood the totality of God, the reality of God. You will never understand, and life will go away.

The idea in this next kriya, what I am trying to do to you is teach you to speak from the *Anahat*. *Anahat* means limitless, that's what Kundalini Yoga is. It works on the *Anahat*, everything. You know, in Hatha Yoga, you practice postures; but it will take you 22 years to practice one posture—and then you can be a master of it. In Kundalini Yoga, time limit is three minutes. Only as we practice, we get 31 minutes or half an hour or 40 minutes—whatever people can adjust to—or 62 minutes is our maximum. Because this is the yoga of the householder, people with penises and pussies. Yeah, it's true! It's the yoga of a householder. It's not a yoga for those, "don't touch me, don't see me." What is that pound of meat God has given there and has created in his own image, how can He be wrong? Then you do too much or too little.

Kriya: To Be a **Man**
August 16, 1997

1. Fish Pose: Come onto your back and lock your feet behind your head. Place your elbows on the backs of the thighs and lift your hands; the elbows make a 90° angle and the hands are up and flat, facing toward your buttocks. Sing with the music: Wahe Guru. 1-3 Minutes (Done for 1 Minute in class)

Comments: If you can sing in this posture from the navel, *Wahe Guru*, you will be appreciated among the enemies, among the demons, among the most negative evil. I am not telling you something that I have just learned in the newspaper yesterday. I am telling you something that has come from centuries of practice, demonstrating the power of the man by the will of God.

2. Virasan: Sit on the left Heel, with the heel between the two 'sit bones', right at the anus. The right foot is flat and the knee is up by the chest. Hands are in Venus Lock, lifting up behind you. Chin in and chest out. Sing with the music: *Wahe Guru*. **1-3 Minutes** (Done for 1 Minute in class)

3. Come into a deep squat—feet and knees together. Wrap your arms around your knees and lock yourself into the pose. **15 Minutes**

Comments: Religion is not what you practice; religion is your personal reality, your experience. What I am trying to do to you is teach you to speak from the *Anahat*; *Anahat* means limitless—that's what Kundalini Yoga is. It works on the *Anahat*. Everything in Hatha Yoga takes you 22 years to practice, just one posture and then you can be the master of it. In Kundalini Yoga, the time limit is 3 minutes. In practice we can get 31 minutes or 40 minutes, whatever people can adjust to, or 62 minutes is our maximum, because this is the yoga of the householder—people with penises and pussies. It's not a yoga for those who say, "don't touch me, don't see me."

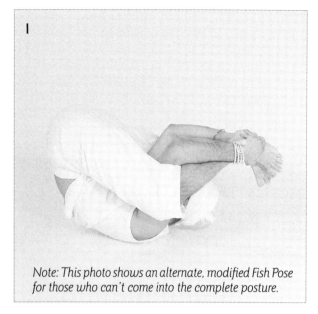

Note: This photo shows an alternate, modified Fish Pose for those who can't come into the complete posture.

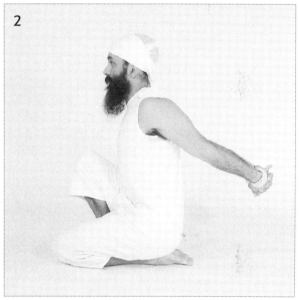

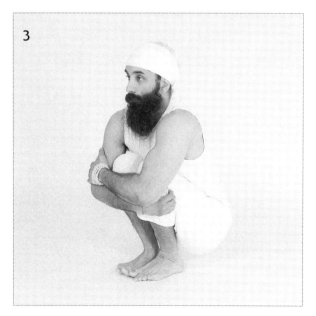

Now, technically speaking, the construction of the penis is very simple. Blood comes from down there and there are cells that hold the blood; but the command is from the pituitary, the master organ in this whole sexual thing. When you get older, what goes bad? The prostate. The prostate first lubricates the penis, lubricates the whole area and prostate lubrication must stop in the vagina of the female. Otherwise, you will never be loyal to you—you can go and do whatever you want to do. But if that prostate doesn't secrete enough in her, and her vagina doesn't sense the smell of it, and your ions don't mix with hers, nothing happens. If she doesn't do anything, look, it's very simple, whatever credit you want to give her, but the rule of the prostate is, it post dates you to infinity—that's why we play all this hugging playing game, simple. Hugging, playing, all that kissing game—what's it for? To stimulate the prostate.

Penis: *Pe* means urine and *nis* means the artery. It's normally a urine artery, but other purpose of the prostate and the penis is personal. So, it must lubricate. Now, the woman, in this whole thing, this intercourse, will be lubricating also, you know? But if that prostate drop gets into her, she becomes stimulated and contracts, then you have to pull the whole thing; there will be no water bucket sex, absolutely not. And if you get caught in her—have you seen the animals who finish this thing? Have you seen their expression? There are tears in the eyes and they say "ooooo". Seen that? That's it, I mean, don't torture a woman, that's not right. Don't torture a woman. As a man, manage yourself and treat a woman as woman. Do something, just do it, and turn around and sleep.

Fatigue **Fix**

You want to get out of fatigue in a small, smart way?

Take orange juice, put half a banana in it, blend it and put black pepper and a little black salt.

Now, this is one of the most exciting things in your life. Your working capacity, your analyzing capacity and your projective capacity of the brain, depends on the biorhythm of the testicles. Try to test it out. When you are really miserable, you can't think, you are flat out, right? Understand that? Take a cold ice cloth and put it around the testicles, watch the time and watch the time when it starts telling you, you are okay. Don't go to any doctor, don't go for any special injection, you don't have to do anything. The moment the testicle temperature becomes equal to your body, you are impotent and naïve, you are an idiot, irritated, frustrated, depressed and abusive.

Breakfast of **Champions**

What should be your breakfast as good men? Half a melon with cottage cheese and a teaspoon of black pepper. You can take with it pure yogi tea, with lemon and unheated honey or maple syrup. You shall never have a problem in your whole life.

There are things to do, there are things to know, and there is experience to be gained. This class will be of no use if you will not practice and experience yourself. Just now, I was coming here and we were discussing something very serious. At 2 o'clock I decided, okay now I will get ready and we'll go at 2:30 but I have to be fresh, I have to be young, I have to be totally in my sense, so I can pull the tapes from the heavens to speak to you free and clear, far or near, doesn't matter. I wanted to have a bath, I have a very deep tub, manmade, it's just stone. I had a Jacuzzi put in it, which puts 25 pounds of pressure per square inch. I timed it, about 10 minutes, took a bath, water was warm, I was very relaxed, and I let the water go and let the cold shower bother me. I became younger and younger and younger and brighter and brighter and brighter—except, if I had continued for a few more minutes, I would have been hornier and hornier and hornier. *(Students laugh.)*

You must know you, as a man. You must know. You must have the experience. You must. You don't enjoy any one thing, you enjoy your experience. And if you do not know your own experience, within yourself, the whole outside world is nothing for you. This hush, hush, sweep it under the rug is the most cowardly act of all of you. To say you have not learned—learn it! Learn it wherever it is available. A man who is not learning and is not learned has a most difficult life. What is your value? When you are talking bullshit morning to night and think this, think that, what the hell you are? You are born, you obey, you grow up, you earn, you die in an old home, what's all this for you? Thank God woman is now becoming an equal earner and she will also face the music.

You have to understand that you are you. Woman has four ways of liberation: she can marry a God man, she can serve a God man, she can give birth to a God man, or she can become a God man. You have only one way: become a saint and a devotee and divine. So, what are we talking about? Your right brain is powerfully projective, your left brain is powerfully supportive, subjective. It's a fight of objective and subjective. We have to call it quits until tomorrow. I have to close your session for now but I will not be as nice as I am today. I don't want you to not enjoy your afternoon because of your thighs and all that.

When a man fights, he says, "Come on!" and slaps his thighs, right? See that? Why it is? There is power in the thighs, it's called domain of the sciatica. We will discuss it tomorrow. Today is enough, you have become a kind of man. There are few books you should have as men. There is a business law book, how to set up business, how to run a business, how to be a businessman; and there are also books on these men's courses, and if you acquire them, learn them, experience them, they will be with you. There is one thing that will give you all knowledge. There is one thing that will meet all calamity head on—your experience.

May the long time sun shine upon you, all love surround you and the pure light within you, guide your way on.

May the bliss of life, balance of life and bounty of life that is with you, remember, in the image of God, there is no handicap, it's true, it's virtuous, it is powerful and the Mother Nature serves you, if you just remember, that it is all God's own thing. Even when you play your personal ego, that was given to everybody so they can recognize the God's will, which will demonstrate a painless life. May this day bring you a painless life, virtuous, and gracious and may you be in beauty, bounty and bliss. May every breath of life be with you as that of God's extension. Sat Nam.

Life in **Balance**

We have to understand who we are. Answer is very simple, am I a noble man? If you are a noble man, then you need a noble woman.

This is what I am going to conclude this course with. Your life shall face odds and evens. It's a continuous process. Sometimes it's good, sometimes it's bad. Good and bad are the two sides of the coin; therefore, if there is a good, there is a bad, too. If it's good for you, it's bad for somebody else. The entire universe is in balance, so it cannot be that everything is good for you and everything is bad for everybody else. With some people, even though they've faced the worst, they learn toughness, they learn self-empowerment; on the other hand, people who are very rich, well-cared for, they are very stupid, a little bit can bother them so much that they don't understand what to do and what not to do. A yogi is the one on whom the pair of opposites does not act, the pair of opposites do not affect him. Neither good affects him nor bad affects him, what affects him is the accomplishment.

In fact, accomplishment is for your own nobility or for somebody's nobility, that's what makes it an accomplishment, otherwise it is not an accomplishment. If you can nurse, nurture, love, take care, make a person grow, and from the heart, the person says "thank you," there is no more blessing than that, there is no more prayer than that, there is no more goodwill than that. But if your actions make a person go crazy and create fear and insecurity, anger and dirty language, then there is no better curse than that either.

So, technically speaking, we are in a world today where we have to understand who we are. Answer is very simple, am I a noble man? If you are a noble man, then you need a noble woman. Your nobility can always be challenged by a woman. Therefore, you have to have a noble woman to keep your nobilities within your own security, not in anybody else's. There is a lot of work, which you can get done, if your woman is bright, beautiful and noble, full of character and characteristics, outgoing, outstanding. If she is not, push her to be, for your sake. Help her to be, push her to be, guide her to be, encourage her to be, all this can work with a woman.

Never, ever participate in the negativity of a woman. A woman loves to talk. You see the whole newspaper—that bus got turned around, that boat got sunk—every bit of news is negative and death. So, too, woman has a very sick mind because she has a balanced mind. She is going to draw on your attention, she is going to tell you everything, which is nonsense, negative and unbecoming of a person—and not noble. Mostly women say, "you didn't do enough for me," "I didn't take enough of a rest," "I have not eaten, I am hungry, I am starving," "I don't know what I am doing." These words, which totally put you on the spot, like this, "what am I doing?" They do it because they talk too much and they have to talk too much, they have to draw attention. They are very attention hungry. If this disease, attention hungry, in a woman becomes serious, then they become flirts. If that becomes more serious, then their sexual relationship becomes ignoble.

So technically speaking, in your life, when you deal with a woman, you deal with one simple parameter: you remain noble and you inspire her to be noble in your whole conversation. I want to remind you well, with a clear heart, woman will not like it. You should know that. Woman doesn't like nobility; she likes flirt, flattery, and if you have any iota of sense of nobility in you, never flatter a woman, then she's got you by the testicles, then you are finished. Be noble with her, neither flatter her nor curse her, neither flatter her nor curse her. Just be noble with her.

Student: *Sir, we shouldn't tell that she is particularly wonderful, radiant, beautiful?*

Yogi Bhajan: That day you are horny, that day you will tell her. Every idiot knows that when a man is horny, he is very flattering. Fucking is[1]—there is no book on fucking, but everything is fucking and every language is fucking and the difference between intercourse, cohabitation and fucking is that fucking is just on the spot—that means you are fucking yourself. Actually, you are not fucking anybody because your projection, your horizon, your alma mater, your dynamics, your psyche, your reality, your geography all will change, if you do that sexual act by flattery. You get it done, flatter a woman, seduce her, bring her over, fuck her, then what? You are lost, she has a few minutes, she has few minutes of what? You are a man and you have a few minutes of what?

If you have to have intercourse with a woman, actually speaking, it is called intercourse; intercourse was never a word for sex, never. It became intercourse, just like cohabitation, those who live in a deep understanding of the self and their self becomes an amalgamation of each other, word was called cohabitation. When? What? This is how you can understand the real woman: the real woman is she who will take your pain, which is coming to you, as a priority onto herself. They are more sensitive—sixteen times more sensitive.

[1] Editor's Note: Creative use and impact of using curse words by Yogi Bhajan was calculated, artful and effective for reaching his audience. It could be shocking but was also received and perceived as being earthy and real.

You are crazy when you look at a woman and say, "you look very pretty," pretty for what? Do you look at a picture, then say, "picture, you look very pretty?" Woman is a living organism, a mammal, you deal with it. What she does for you is a totality, reality, projection, power; she makes your thoughts and their accomplishment. Woman is not just meat and bone, and sex and sensuality, woman is actually your alter ego, your sixth sense. It is very important and very few women can play that role. So, you are handicapped because your selection of a woman is handicapped. Your investment in a woman is handicapped. You are not result-oriented. You are scared and afraid in relationship, whereas, you have to be very straightforward, firm, noble. You must have a standard. As a man, you call her your better half. She is the better half, so she had better be better, as your better half. There are a lot of ways to appreciate a woman. Can somebody tell me, if you sincerely want to appreciate a woman, how you will do it? If you want to appreciate a woman, right on this spot, what you will say?

You must start with humor with a woman or she will get you. Give her a crack; she is already in there. What will you say? You may want to have a relationship with her, sex, whatever your intention is, I am not talking of intention here. I am talking about what you will say, what she will understand, and are you a man? Look at this flattery, "I thought God made me handsome, but God, He made you really good." Match it. Match the sentence. Say to any woman something like this and she will understand that you are a man, you have a standard, you have a commitment, you are divine, you are real. It may be a bogus statement, doesn't matter, but even if you fake it, you will make it. Woman is herself a very crooked and complicated creature; therefore you have to learn to be straight with her. The moment she knows that communication with you is only straight, straight, straight, you've got it all.

Never flatter a woman in the morning, "Oh, you are the prettiest thing I have seen this morning, you are so shiny" and then, in the afternoon, you say, "You bitch, God! I know you. Now, all of this, for a woman, is a totality—not reality—totality. She will never forget it. If you ever abuse a woman, she will never forget it. If you ever appreciate a woman, she will always forget it, the very next day.

Appreciation she digests in hours; depreciation is what she hates. You see, they don't tell you their age. No, ladies don't tell. They don't even tell that they are grown up. They are so unrealistic. If somebody asks me, what is your age? I say, I am 67, going to be 68. They won't, because maturity is not their way of life. Less than maturity is not your way of life. You have to be mature, saintly, confident.

There are four things a man cannot afford to do: a man cannot be cheap, he cannot be crooked, his body language has to be very firm, and he has to be direct. If he avoids these four things, one way or the other, the woman will immediately know it and she shall not trust you. What are those four things? Repeat.

Students: *A man cannot afford to be cheap, he cannot be crooked, his body language has to be very firm and he has to be direct.*

Yogi Bhajan: Now I will tell you a real-life story. A man was very, very rich, he was so rich that he bifurcated his wealth, some in Europe, some in America, some here, some there, but he never wanted to be known as a rich man. But he was very rich, he was very intelligent, and his time of marriage came and he was only 27. All these bogus Americans, you see, they have all kinds of money, they have paper money and factory money, but this man had real cash money. He was so rich that his money was earning money, can you believe that? (You are rich only when your money earns money, not when your work earns money. Then you are still poor.) He met a woman and they talked and they met and right away, straightforward, she said, "I hate these macho rich people." One, two, three—shot.

He said to himself, "Well, she doesn't like rich people." But he discussed with her, he said, "Rich men with the power of their money can . . . " Whatever she said was very correct. Romance started and finally he came to an understanding, you know what he did? He brought her a silk rose, one, and put it in water. They put that silk rose in a vase with water and he said "I am so poor that I can't even buy a rose, or a bouquet, so I decided to give you this silk rose, which is nothing, but it has one character in it, it will last longer. I tried to make it real but I want to tell you it is not, but still, it will last longer." She married him; a week later, they went to church and got married. Marriage was very private, no invitations whatsoever, and then he said, "My friend has invited us to use his jet; he's given us a honeymoon." My friend has?

Student: *Given us a honeymoon.*

Yogi Bhajan: Then on the Caribbean Island, there was a friend's boat, then in the Mediterranean there was a friend's ship, then in every town in the world, there was a friend's five bedrooms, biggest residence, and then there were another 50 servants on this honeymoon tour; they were the friend's servants. *(Students laugh.)*

Whatever he was buying was on a friend's cards, so in the four months of their honeymoon, she became accustomed to certain things, and one day she asked, "Your friend is so rich, why can't you be?" *(Students laugh.)*

"He doesn't mind, look what I have bought, what we have bought is so much and he doesn't mind," he said, "No. I am the poor polarity of my friend; he is the rich polarity of me."

She said, "If he's so connected, why couldn't you be very rich, too?"
He said, "I am."
She said, "I don't believe it."
He said, "Read the card." On all his cards, his name was written backwards, you see, but the name was real. So, then he said, "Actually, I love you very much and I wanted to marry you; but you told me you hated rich people, so I didn't want to confront you on that. First I wanted to know you and then I wanted to prove it to you and I wanted to see whether you liked me or not, my sex and my way of living and everything, and then I planned to let you know that I am the richest man on the earth."

And she said, "Where did you get this money? You are so young."
He said, "Hard work."
She said, "I never saw you working in all these four months."

He said, "Honey, you were sleeping and I was working." Today, his wife works more than him. He taught her everything and when we met, I was joking with him, I said, "Well, you have married a woman or a secretary?"
He said, "No, Secretary General."

It's a very clever way of flattering, but very real way of flattering, very heart to heart, no nonsense. That's what you have to learn: to be realistic, to deal with every woman directly, because you cannot deal with a woman directly if you are not direct.

I was taking a phone call this morning. It was the ugliest phone call I have received in my life and I was telling this lady, "Love your husband, cool down, you know."
She said, "No, suck him, f___ him, love him, this is not for a woman."
And I said, 'Who told you that?"
She said, "You."
I said, "I never said a word, I just said."
"I mean you, all men, you are teaching men's courses these days, and you are nothing for women."
She started yelling and screaming with the top of her voice.
I said, "What happened?"
She said, "My husband, he is not learning anything in that course; teach him some manners."
I said, "What went wrong?"
"Nothing."
(Students laugh.)

I said, "There must be something wrong."
She said, "Why you teach these men? They don't know; they should learn from their mother or from their wives. You are charging them and they are going to come home and discharge trouble for us."
I said, "Wow, what an assessment, correct."

What I mean to say is, when you go home and you don't discharge yourself, that is, keep your battery charged up and use it until you come to the next men's course and get better, all these exercises I have shared with you, it is better you do them there. This is our last meditation that we will do as a man.

Meditation: Tantric Yantra to Receive All Knowledge
August 17, 1997

Posture: Sit in a meditative posture. Your right hand is up with your thumb touching your Third Eye Point and the other fingers are together, pointing straight up. The fingertips of the left hand are together and touch the base of the right hand. Concentrate.

Eyes: Tip of the nose.

Breath: Breathe long, deep and slow.

Music: *Tuniya*

Mantra: Sat Nam Sat Nam Sat Nam Ji Wahe Guru Wahe Guru Wahe Guru Ji

Mentally Vibrate the mantra for 20 Minutes; then begin chanting aloud, **4 Minutes**, whisper **1 Minute**.

Time: 25 Minutes

To End: Inhale deep, concentrate on your spine, exhale. Inhale deep and pull your spine, vertebra by vertebra all the way up, hold the eyes at the tip of the nose, concentrate. Exhale. Inhale deep again, maintain the mudra and bring your shoulders up to your ears—tight! Cannon Fire Exhale and relax.

Comments: If nothing works out in your life, and you can't read all the books, you can't go to all the libraries, you can't visit every place, you can't go through every woman, there are things you can do. There is a written procedure of a picture, a tantric picture, this is the mind's tantric picture.[1] Even I meditate on it; it isn't something to take lightly. Meditate according to that procedure and God willing, you will get all the knowledge. It gives you three things: the unknown will be known, unheard you will hear, and not to happen will happen, if it is in your interest.

You know, life is square, which stops—and triangle gives you elevation, prosperity and goodness in life. But, just remember, when a square is cut diagonally, it becomes two triangles. That's why tantric energy is the most powerful energy, it is totally divine energy, it cuts through everything and that you have to understand once and for all.

Sat Nam means your identity is true. *Nam* means identity, *Nam* is a noun: name of person, place or a thing. *Sat Nam* means your identity is true, it is five sounds, S-ah, T-ah, N-ah, M-ah. These are five sounds. *Wahe Guru* is a *trikuti* mantra; it's a mantra of the *agya* command center (the Ajna Chakra) and it is in three letters, Wah-hay Guroo.

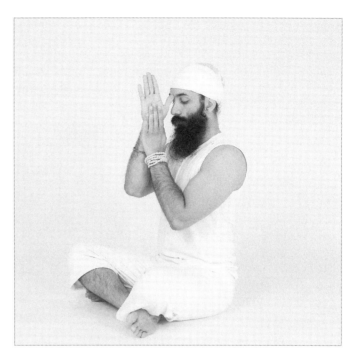

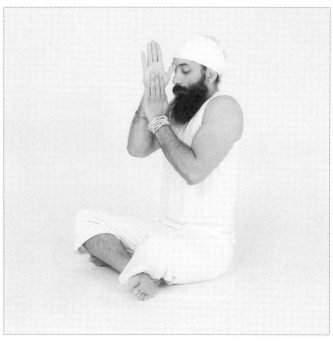

[1] Yogi Bhajan is referring to the Tratakum photo and meditation. Available from www.kriteachings.org.

For the Age of Aquarius, if you want to enter peacefully and righteously, we are preparing people for the Age of Aquarius by giving them 11 minutes each of Kirtan Kriya, Sat Kriya and Sodarshan Chakra Kriya[3]; 33 minutes in the morning, 33 minutes in the evening, it will open up the chakras and it will take care of your *tattvas* and it will give you power in your own being. Sa-Ta-Na-Ma (Kirtan Kriya) balances the *tattvas*. Sat Kriya absolutely energize the *tattvas*. Sodarshan Chakra Kriya opens up the chakras in absolute balance, so you are never going to be in trouble. Have a nice, wonderful day. Thank you very much, God bless you. Sat Nam.

■ ■ ■

---

[3] See Appendix A for these three kriyas for the Aquarian Age.

Appendix A: Additional Recommended Kriyas

- Hidden Self **Kriyas** 1 & 2
- Sat **Kriya**
- Sodarshan Chakra **Kriya**
- Kirtan **Kriya**

Hidden Self Meditations

I. Meditation on the Hidden Self
July 26, 1982

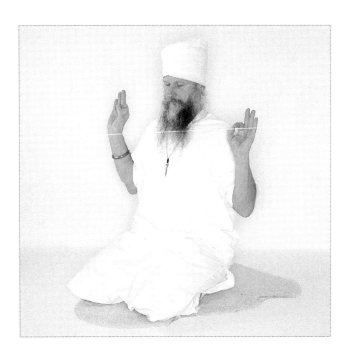

Posture: Sit in Rock Pose, on your heels.

Eyes: Look at the tip of the nose.

Mudra: Bring the hands up next to the shoulders in Gyan Mudra, other fingers are straight and the palms are facing forward, elbows are relaxed down at the sides.

Inhale deeply and exhale completely. Pump the stomach as long as you can on the exhaled breath while mentally chanting 'liar' with each pump. Inhale, exhale and continue.

Time: 11 Minutes

II. Kriya to Invoke Balance in the **Psyche**
July 31, 1982

1. Sit in Easy Pose. Put hands in Prayer Pose either with the fingers against each other as usual (single lock) or with the fingers interlaced but kept straight (double lock). The thumbs are crossed. The hands are held about midway between the heart and navel center. Keep the base of the palms together and shake the hands vigorously. The wrists are loose and the whole body should shake. Carry on for **5-7 Minutes**. It can make you sweat.

2. Stretch your arms out to the sides, parallel to the ground with the palms up. Maintain the posture through Exercise #7. Pump the navel while doing Breath of Fire. Continue **2-3 Minutes**.

3. Inhale and exhale with the mouth open, accentuating the breath in the throat for **3 Minutes**.

4. Breathe powerfully through the nostrils for **1 Minute.**

5. Concentrate on the Navel and the Third Eye Point while literally chewing on the hidden self for **3 Minutes**.

6. Inhale and hold the breath, then exhale. **3 Minutes**

7. Experience your radiance and crystal clarity. **3 Minutes**

8. Lower the arms and feel that you are Sat Nam. **1 Minute**

Comments: It is to be used to invoke psychic balance and to get out of depression. It also works on the hidden self. It promises that you will never have a bad nervous system. It is a very exhilarating meditation and very potent. Yogi Bhajan recommended that it only be used when needed and not done every day.

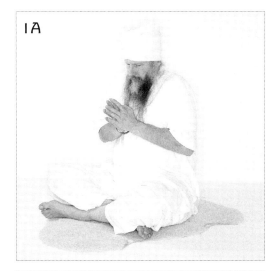

1A

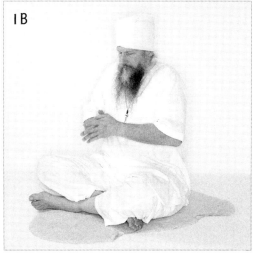

1B

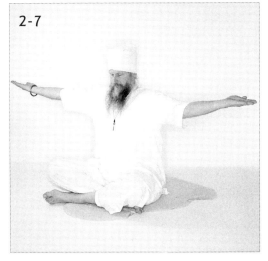

2-7

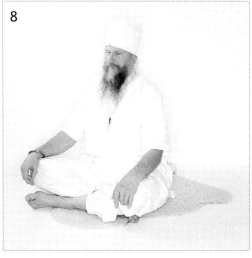

8

Sat Kriya

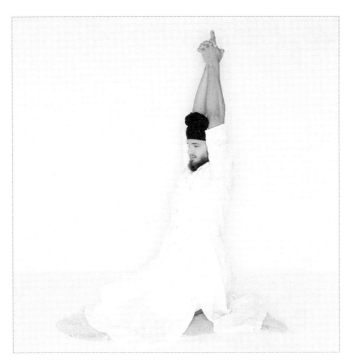

Sit on the heels and stretch the arms overhead so that the elbows hug the ears. With the palms together, interlock all the fingers except the index fingers (Jupiter) which point straight up. Begin to chant **Sat Nam** emphatically in a constant rhythm about 8 times per 10 seconds. Chant the sound **Sat** from the Navel Point and solar plexus, pulling the umbilicus all the way in toward the spine. On **Nam** relax the belly.

Continue at least **3 Minutes**, then inhale and squeeze the muscles tightly from the buttocks all the way up the back, past the shoulders. Mentally allow the energy to flow through the top of the skull. Ideally, you should **relax for twice the length of time that the kriya was practiced**.

Comments:

Sat Kriya is fundamental to Kundalini Yoga and should be practiced every day for at least 3 minutes. If you have time for nothing else, make this kriya part of your daily commitment to yourself to keep the body a clean and vital temple of God.

Notice that you emphasize pulling the Navel Point in. Don't try to apply *mulbandh*; it happens automatically if the navel is pulled. Consequently, the hips and lumbar spine do not rotate or flex. Your spine stays straight and the only motion your arms make is a slight up-and-down stretch with each **Sat Nam** as your chest lifts.

Sat Kriya's effects are numerous. It strengthens the entire sexual system and stimulates its natural flow of energy, relaxing phobias about sexuality. It allows you to control the insistent sexual impulse by redirecting the flow of sexual energy to creative activities and healing in the body. People who are severely maladjusted or who have mental problems benefit from this kriya because these disturbances are always connected with an imbalance in the energies of the lower three chakras. General physical health is improved because all of the internal organs receive a gentle, rhythmic massage from this exercise. The heart gets stronger from the rhythmic up-and-down of blood pressure you generate from the pumping motion of the navel. This exercise works directly on stimulating and channeling the kundalini energy, so it must always be practiced with the mantra *Sat Nam*. You may build the time of the kriya to 31 minutes, but remember to have a long, deep relaxation immediately afterwards. A good way to build the time up is to do the kriya for 3 minutes, then rest 2 minutes. Repeat this cycle until you have completed 15 minutes of Sat Kriya and 10 minutes of rest. Then follow this sequence with an additional 15–20 minutes of deep relaxation. Do not try to jump to 31 minutes because you feel you are strong, virile or happen to be a yoga teacher. Respect the inherent power of the technique. Let the kriya prepare the ground of your body properly to plant the seed of higher experience. It is not just an exercise, it is a kriya that works on all levels of your being—known and unknown. You might block the more subtle experiences of higher energies by pushing the physical body too hard. You could have a huge rush of energy or you may have an experience of higher consciousness, but then not be able to integrate the experience into your psyche. So prepare yourself with constancy, patience and moderation. The end result is assured.

If you have not taken drugs or have cleared your system of all their effects, you may choose to practice this kriya with the palms open, pressing flat against each other. This releases more energy than the other method. It is generally not taught this way in a public class because someone attending may have totally weakened his nerves through drug abuse.

Sodarshan Chakra **Kriya**
December 12, 1990

Posture: Sit with a straight spine.

Focus: The eyes are focused at the tip of the nose.

Meditation: Block off the right nostril with the right thumb. Inhale slowly and deeply through the left nostril. Hold the breath. Mentally chant "Wahe Guru" sixteen times, pumping the Navel Point once on "Wha", once on "Hey", and once on "Guru". (You pump the navel three times with each complete repetition of "Wahe Guru" and you chant "Wahe Guru" sixteen times. Therefore on each breath, you pump the Navel Point 48 times.) Unblock the right nostril. Use the right index finger (little finger may also be used) to block off the left nostril and exhale slowly and completely through the right nostril. Continue.

Time: 31 or 62 Minutes a day. There is no time, no place, no space, and no condition attached to this mantra.

If you are going to clean your own subconscious garbage, you must estimate and clean it as fast as you can or as slow as you want. You have to decide how much time you have to clean up your garbage pit. So, start with 31 Minutes, then after a while do it for 40 Minutes, and then for 62 Minutes. Take time to graduate in it.

If you can do this meditation for 62 Minutes to start with and develop it to the point that you can do it for 2 1/2 hours a day, it makes out of you a perfect superbeing. It purifies, takes care of the human life and makes a human perfect, saintly, successful, and qualified. This meditation also gives one the pranic power. This kriya never fails. It can give one all the inner happiness and bring one to a state of ecstasy in life.

To Finish: Inhale, hold 5-10 seconds, exhale. Then stretch and shake every part of your body for about 1 Minute so that the energy may spread.

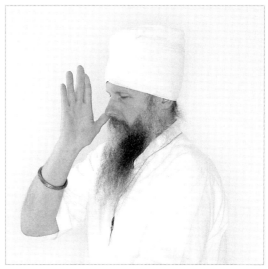

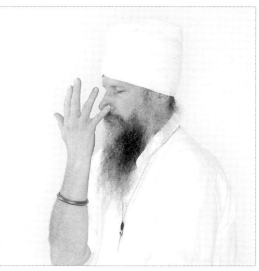

Of all the 20 types of yoga, including Kundalini Yoga, this is the highest kriya. This meditation cuts through all darkness. The name, Sodarshan Chakra Kriya, means the Kriya for Perfect Purification of the Chakras. It will give you a new start. It is the simplest kriya, but at the same time the hardest. It cuts through all barriers of the neurotic or psychotic inside nature. When a person is in a very bad state, techniques imposed from the outside will not work. The pressure has to be stimulated from within. The tragedy of life is when the subconscious releases garbage into the conscious mind. This kriya invokes the Kundalini energy to give you the necessary vitality and intuition to combat the negative effects of the unchanneled subconscious mind.

Yogi Bhajan

Kirtan Kriya

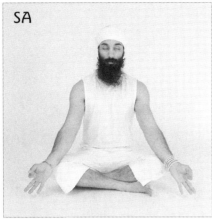

SA

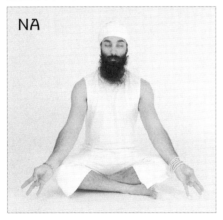

TA

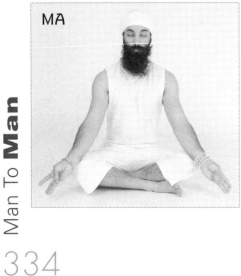

NA

MA

This kriya is one of three that Yogi Bhajan mentioned would carry us through the Aquarian Age, even if all other teachings were lost. There are four principle components to practicing Kirtan Kriya correctly: Mantra, Mudra, Voice, and Visualization.

Mantra

This kriya uses the five primal sounds, or the *Panj Shabd*— S, T, N, M, A— in the original *bij* form of the word Sat Nam:

SA — infinity, cosmos, beginning
TA — life, existence
NA — death
MA — birth

This is the cycle of creation. From the Infinite comes life and individual existence. From life comes death or change. From death comes the rebirth of consciousness. From rebirth comes the joy of the Infinite through which compassion leads back to life. Chant the 'A' as if you were pronouncing 'mom,' in the following manner:

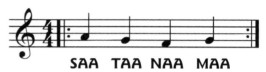

SAA TAA NAA MAA

Mudra

Each repetition of the entire mantra takes 3 to 4 seconds. The elbows are straight while chanting, and each finger touches, in turn, the tip of the thumb with a firm but gentle pressure.

Sa — the index or Jupiter finger touches the thumb;
Ta — the middle or Saturn finger and thumb;
Na — the ring or Sun finger and thumb;
Ma — the pinkie or Mercury finger and thumb; then begin again with the index finger.

Visualization

You must meditate on the primal sounds in the "L" form. This means that when you meditate you feel there is a constant inflow of cosmic energy into your solar center, or Tenth Gate (the Crown Chakra). As the energy enters the top of the head, you place **Sa**, **Ta**, **Na**, or **Ma** there.

As you chant **Sa**, for example, the "S" starts at the top of your head and the "A" moves down and out through the Brow Point, projected to Infinity. This energy flow follows the energy pathway called the golden cord—the connection between the pineal and pituitary gland. Some people may occasionally experience headaches from practicing Kirtan Kriya if they do not use this "L" form. The most common reason for this is improper circulation of prana in the solar centers.

Voice

We chant the mantra in the three languages of consciousness:

Aloud	the voice of the human	awareness of the things of the world
Whisper	the voice of the lover	experiencing the longing to belong
Silent	the voice of the divine	meditate on Infinity or mentally vibrate

To Begin the Practice

Sit straight in Easy Pose and meditate at the Brow Point.

Chant aloud for **5 Minutes**, then whisper for **5 Minutes** and then go deeply into silence, mentally vibrating the sound. Vibrate in silence for **10 Minutes**, then whisper for **5 Minutes,** then chant aloud for **5 Minutes**.

Close the meditation with a deep inhale and suspend the breath as long as comfortable—up to a Minute—relaxing it smoothly to complete **1 Minute** of absolute stillness and silence.

To end: Stretch the hands up as far as possible and spread the fingers wide. Stretch the spine and take several deep breaths. Relax.

Comments:

Each time you close a mudra by joining the thumb with a finger, your ego seals the effect of that mudra in your consciousness. The effects are as follows:

SIGN	FINGER	NAME	EFFECT
Jupiter	Index	Gyan Mudra	Knowledge
Saturn	Middle	Shuni Mudra	Wisdom, intelligence, patience
Sun	Ring	Surya Mudra	Vitality, energy of life
Mercury	Pinkie	Buddhi Mudra	Ability to communicate

Practicing this chant brings a total mental balance to the individual psyche. As you vibrate on each fingertip, you alternate your electrical polarities. The index and ring fingers are electrically negative, relative to the other fingers. This causes a balance in the electro-magnetic projection of the aura. If during the silent part of the meditation your mind wanders uncontrollably, go back to a whisper, to a loud voice, to a whisper and back into silence. Do this as often as necessary to stay alert.

Practicing this meditation is both a science and an art. It is an art in the way it molds consciousness and the refinement of sensation and insight it produces. It is a science in the tested certainty of the results it produces. Each meditation is based on the tested experience of many people, in many conditions, over many years. It is based on the structure of the psyche and the laws of action and reaction that accompany each sound, movement and posture. The meditations as kriyas code this science into specific formulas we can practice to get specific results. Because it is so effective and exact, it can also lead to problems if not done properly.

Chanting the *Panj Shabd*—the primal or nuclear form of *Sat Nam*—has profound energy within it because we are breaking the *bij* (seed or atom) of the sound, *Sat Nam*, into its primary elements. You may use this chant in any position as long as you adhere to the following requirements:

1. Keep the spine straight.
2. Focus at the Brow Point.
3. Use the "L" form of meditation.
4. Vibrate the *Panj Shabd* in all three languages—human, lover, and divine.
5. Use common sense without fanaticism.

The timing can be decreased or increased as long as you maintain the ratio of spoken, whispered, and silent chanting—always end with **1 minute** of complete stillness and silence. Yogi Bhajan said, at the Winter Solstice of 1972, that a person who wears pure white and meditates on this sound current for 2½ hours a day for one year, will know the unknown and see the unseen. Through this constant practice, the mind awakens to the infinite capacity of the soul for sacrifice, service, and creation.

Appendix B: Healing and Healthy Foods for **Men**

Food is the medicine which creates essential energy in the body and creates essential rest in the body to bring an equilibrium—that is the beauty of food—and all food was considered as human medicine to begin with, and to live with.

- A-Z Foods and Supplements for **Potency**
- Fasts, Recipes, and **Remedies**
- Rejuvenating Foods from Around the **World**
  Presented by Soram Singh Khalsa, M.D.

Editor's Note: Over the years, Yogi Bhajan provided literally hundreds of recipes, remedies, and fasts to cleanse, tonify, and purify the nervous, glandular and digestive systems. He gave specific remedies for men to strengthen and balance their sexual energy, tonify their nervous and uro-genital systems for longevity, and generally increase their vitality so that they could enjoy a happy and healthy sex life and experience the greatness of being a man. He emphasized, more than once, that we are Healthy, Happy, and Holy—in that order, Healthy comes first for a reason. The following lecture, notes, and Q&A are taken from all the various men's courses over the years. We have tried to consolidate the information so that it's accessible and user-friendly. Recipes have been compiled for your convenience. For a complete survey of Yogi Bhajan's dietary recommendations, see *Foods for Health & Healing: Remedies & Recipes.* These herbal remedies and recipes are suggestions only; we make no claims to cure. Consult your physician prior to any dramatic change in your diet or exercise regimen.

A-Z Foods and Supplements for **Potency**

It is a creative energy. Sexual energy is nothing but creative energy. Don't mix up these two energies and think one is creative and one is noncreative. Both are creative; it is all in how you use it.

Asafoetida

Sometimes you have wind in your stomach. This indicates your *apana* and *prana* are not in balance. A lot of wind can make you bulky and fat. Asafoetida can help with this problem.

Asafoetida is very good for sexual potency. It is called the 'diamond to the poor'. It is one of the best things for procuring your sexual efficiency. It gives you mental balance. Take asafoetida, sauté it in ghee and add it to your food. Potentially it is very healthy, but it does have a very powerful odor.

Asafoetida also comes in a homeopathic form; 6X or 12X can be taken twice a day to take care of wind problems. However, this form is not useful in building potency.

Bamboo Juice or Tabashir

Supports the liver. When you add tabashir to a masala, any sexual problem due to the liver will go away.

Castor Oil

It is the most strong, potent oil. About one ounce of Castor Oil in your mouth with a glass of cardamom milk; it is a miracle work, it will do a miracle. You can also use it to massage the anal sphincter and keep the tissues of the perineum healthy.

Chawan Prash

Another very good remedy for men is chawan prash. It's like a black marmalade, which comes out of the bamboo shoot. In India it was known before the time of Alexander the Great. Just spread it on a piece of toast and eat it.

Chestnut Milk

Another simple recipe that is pure sex food is water and chestnuts. Soak the chestnuts in water overnight, then blend and strain.

Cauliflower Parantha

"Don't misunderstand—I am a married man and I learned all these things by the goodness of God to share with you. So I would mix the masala with the cauliflower and put a little black pepper with it and make a stuffed chapati. I would make it with ghee and eat it. After eating I would usually sleep and God, when I would get up from the bed, I would go up to the roof and then I would look around for someone who would want to talk to me. Can you believe that?"

Cheese

Some of you are creating another problem. You're eating too much cheese. I know it tastes good, but it is also very heavy to digest. The best cheese is panir, homemade cheese. Once in a while commercial cheese is fine. Cottage cheese is okay.

Q: What about cheese made from wheat milk?
Yogi Bhajan: Oh, *nakasta*. *Nakasta* is very good. It is very good for the lower back.

Diamond Dust

Diamond dust is a reddish powder that has been used for centuries in India. It is used with certain abnormal conditions. Before age 35 it is used once in a while, and after 35 it may be taken daily for 20 - 40 days and then stop. The best times of the year are spring, fall and winter. It must not be taken in the summer.

Eggplants

Eggplants are called the 'testicles of God.' (See Recipe Italiano)

Figs

Figs can make you a sexual pig. In the book from the Women's Course, I have taught how to inject saffron in the figs and preserve them in the refrigerator, and people do enjoy it. They get beautiful results from it. But today I will tell you what else you can do with a fig. Take figs, maybe 20-25, blend them with yogurt and drink it.

Q: Does it matter if these are the dry figs or the fresh figs?

Yogi Bhajan: Absolutely fresh: One cup of yogurt to ten to fifteen figs is good. It becomes thick and can be eaten with a spoon. In the scriptures, it is said that if there is any sexual or nervous disability, this can correct it. Eat this with nothing else. It's a complete mono diet.

Try it for one week; I prefer two weeks myself. It's good. You must understand when you work hard, you need the energy. Without hard work, you can't make your life and without life you can't have hard work. So you need the energy for creative purposes.

It is a creative energy. Sexual energy is nothing but creative energy. Don't mix up these two energies and think one is creative and one is noncreative. Both are creative; it is all in how you use it.

Q: On the yogurt and fig diet how much can you eat of that a day?

Yogi Bhajan: A normal, sophisticated human, should decide the amount, the quality and quantity. Don't overtax yourself.

Ghee

When a man uses more ghee in his food than any other oil, normally he will not have any problem in his sexual life. Ghee is very compatible with the body and it does not create an over or under weight condition. It creates healthy semen and you avoid potential problems.

Gold Leaf

Gold leaf is only recommended to eat with a few things— one is papaya and the others are fig, apple and also carrot— and for longevity and good health, gold leaf with date.

Golden Milk

This is a drink made from turmeric, milk and oil. It is very good for the spine and lubricates joints, helping to break up calcium deposits.

Lotus Root

A very good food for sexual potency as well, can be eaten fresh or steamed, if you can only find dried lotus root, it makes a great tonic when cooked in soups or teas.

Mango Powder

Mango powder is a mine for sex; it triggers, or initiates balance in your sexual capacity. It won't let you down, when they want you up. Take a banana and split it down the center; put mango powder in the center of it, fill it up, about two tablespoons, and then put lemon juice on it. You are set.

Masala

This is the basic foundation of a vegetable curry dish. It is usually made of onions, garlic and ginger with various spices. This particular spice combination is recommended for men to recover their energy and potency.

Ground fennel seeds mixed with nutmeg, cinnamon, cardamom and clove. You can also include poppy seeds and oregano for a more savory, less sweet masala. When you use cardamom, any problem with the area around the spleen will go away. Poppy and oregano seed are used when the digestive tract is not digesting well and it gives you wind (gas), which can create problems sexually. They also help in cases of hernia and moderating your sexual discharge, when you are either over stuck or too stimulated. Also, use these seeds when you are nervous and you need the stimulant strength of your nerves; you can mix them in. This masala can be used to make cauliflower chapati or parantha.

Q: We have a list of things for special effects; shall we throw them all in together?

Reply: No, sir. It is better to deal with one at a time. Too much atomic energy can make a cinder out of the whole thing. So don't make a Hiroshima out of yourself.

Q: After eating the stuffed chapati, and after you sleep, what happens?

Reply: It gives you a very balanced sleep because it stimulates the entire system; it tunes up the nervous system and you get a very good sleep and after that you have a good day at work and after that you know what you do, you know what I mean? Create first what you want to use. Don't overtax your body's system. That's what I'm trying to tell everybody.

Q: Can women and children eat these kinds of foods?

Reply: I would suggest that women can and I'll suggest that a child between 12 and 15; it's a stimulant food. There's no doubt about it. It can give him a good nervous strength but it may make him more horny and the guy may go berserk. I don't think that you should stimulate children too much.

Mung Beans and Rice

Mung beans and rice is a very standard fast, it's a very cleansing fast. Mung beans and rice and yogurt is known to be the fast of the angels. It's a simple, poor man's fast—mung beans and rice with yogurt—you can live on it. You can live healthy for years and years and years and you'll never be sorry for it. I have seen a very saintly person—in summer he had mung beans and rice, he would make it at night, and early in the morning eat it with the yogurt. Then the whole day he wouldn't eat anything. But during the winter, when it was very, very cold, he would grind chilis and make the mung beans and rice very hot, and eat it with yogurt. God, you can't believe it. In the whole house where that man sat, he created a radiant light. And he did nothing else. Just from food. That was his specialty. Early in the morning, there would be a line, half a mile long. He would cook enough to feed that many. People would bring milk, mung beans and rice to him and tell him of their wishes and have them answered. They would say, "Sir, I have this sickness, or I have that sickness." It didn't matter. He gave everyone mung beans and rice and yogurt. Everybody. People were cured and that is why they call it "food of the angels." It's very simple, it's very honest, and it's very easy to digest. It has protein, it has the carbohydrates, it has all the combinations you need. I recommend when you make mung beans and rice, put a lot of vegetables in it. Make it a little tasty. Americans are rich, so you should make that food rich, too.

Q: Should we use spices?
Yogi Bhajan: Yes, you can add spices. As a mono diet, it is a very cleansing diet.

Nut Paste

There are certain foods that are a must for you. There is a potency food made of onion, ginger, garlic, saffron, pistachio nuts and almonds. (see recipes)

Peaches

Peaches do not grow on the beaches but eat them. Peaches have to teach you how to be a man. All "P" fruits (peaches, plums, papayas, pineapples, pears, and persimmons) are good for men's creativity. The best way to eat them is to blend them well with yogurt. If you are not hypoglycemic, you can put honey in it.

Q: Could you use kefir instead of yogurt?
Yogi Bhajan: At that time I did not know about kefir and I cannot change what I have been taught by my teachers. It is written yogurt, so it has to be yogurt.

Pistachios

Pistachio is another nut I recommend to you. Eat a handful of raw, unsalted and unskinned pistachio nuts daily.

Poor Man's Diamond Dust or Hot Golden Yogurt

Now we come to what you call the "poor man's diamond dust." Blend a glass of milk (16 oz.) with 10 green chiles and turmeric.

Q: Are we to use jalapeños?
Yogi Bhajan: Yes. I mean real Mexican chiles. After it is blended, boil it and make yogurt out of this mixture. Next put some turmeric in it. In the morning, eat 8-10 ounces of this yogurt. Then put some weights on your feet or you may end up flying all around the room.

Q: The turmeric gets boiled in?
Yogi Bhajan: Yes, turmeric is boiled in—a tablespoon for 16 ounces of milk will make two servings.

Q: Should the chile peppers be raw?
Yogi Bhajan: Yes, raw.

Q: Do you have to sauté the turmeric to make it digestible?
Yogi Bhajan: Turmeric is always best cooked. You can either boil or sauté it. If you boil it, boil it in water. If you sauté it, sauté it in ghee.

Potent Potatoes

By the way, don't forget potent potatoes. Some people are so funny. Some people take potent potatoes without yogurt. Potent potatoes must be eaten with yogurt to balance their energy. (see recipes)

If you want to be potent, food is the stimulant of life. Food is like gas and semen is like oil. If the oil and gas are ok and engine is working right, you'll have an easy ride.

—Yogi Bhajan

Saffron

It is written in the scriptures, "Go to the valley of God which is in the area of Kashmir and take the saffron which will keep you young and alive."

Saffron is a very beautiful God-given gift. Depending on the quality it will cost a lot, but it does cost as much as a pure gold, although it works better than gold. Your health, your sexuality, your sensuality, in the sense of a preserved energy, is your greatest decoration, and it the greatest ornament. If you want to be something, be something as a man—creative, protective and potent.

Shala-jit.

Shala means stone. Shala-jit means that which can win the stone. It is actually the milk of the stone and is black in color. It must be boiled with equal parts of black pepper in milk. Take a glass of milk (about 16 oz.) and put almost equal part of black pepper in it and let it boil and it will leave a reddish streak in it. Then drink that milk. It is great for the lower back and for sexual weaknesses. If Shala-jit is not available you may use Garlic Saffron Almond Rice with Yogurt. (See Recipes)

Ter

In India there is a thing called "ter". I ate it in Albuquerque. So if it can grow in Albuquerque, it can grow everywhere. In the back of your garden you may be able to grow it. It is a cucumber-like vegetable; it is long and edible. This vegetable is very cleansing, it is very good. It is very cooling and very beautiful for the sexual nervous area.

Turmeric

Turmeric is great for the joints. Take it in Golden Milk before bed or simply make a paste and take it as a supplement in the mornings.

Whey

A great source of protein and should be a staple in the diet.

Zucchini

For imbalances and abuse of your body, go on a raw zucchini fast—eat nothing else. When zucchini is in season from the new moon to the full moon or the full moon to the dark night eat as much raw young zucchini as you like—there's no limit.

Fasts, Recipes, and **Remedies**

Don't go on a crazy fast without preparing for it and without having the capacity to go through it. Fasts can mess up the metabolism and the body rather than being beneficial.
—Yogi Bhajan

■ ■ ■ Fasts

Banana Fast
Nine bananas daily for fifteen days from the new moon to the full moon.

Fruit Fast
One kind of fruit at each meal; three or four meals each day for one month, preferably between April 15th and May 15th.

Tomato Fast
Eat only firm, ripe tomatoes, garnished with lots of powdered, dried, mint leaves and tamari to taste; remove skins from tomatoes by scalding them briefly; start Monday morning and end Sunday at midnight.

Banyan Milk Fast
Eat banyan milk with yogurt for six days. This is especially good in the spring.

Raw Zucchini Fast
When zucchini is in season, eat nothing else, from the new moon to the full moon or the full moon to the new moon. Eat as much raw young zucchini as you like—there's no limit.

These next four diets, recommended for men, can be done whenever you like. They can be done together, one week at a time, for a full month of fasting.

Potato Peel Soup Fast
Potato Peels and vegetables (Choose any kind you like.) Take 2/3's potato peels to 1/3 any kind of vegetable you prefer. Make an ordinary soup out of this. Then eat only this for one week. This fast can be done any time of the year.

Watermelon Fast
Anytime in the year, but especially when it is summertime, you can go on a watermelon fast, but it must be done alone. Eat nothing else. A mistake commonly made is you mix melon and watermelon, but actually watermelon and melon are two different things. For one week eat as much as you want, but do not do this diet for more than seven days. You do not need to eat the seeds, if you do not wish.

Melon Fast
For one week eat melons (not watermelons). This is a very good fast for the male human being.

Seed Fast
Walnuts, almonds, pistachio nuts, and melon seeds (not watermelon seeds), in equal weight. Soak them at night and remove the skins. In the morning, before using, place them into a blender and blend them up with either skim milk or water. Strain (if you do not want to drink the fiber), add honey, and its ready to drink. If you want to drink it cold, you can add ice before you blend.

This drink can be taken one time in the morning, afternoon, late afternoon, and at night, but do not drink it more than four times a day. There is no quantity restriction of how much to drink at each meal. Only do this diet for 5 days.

■ ■ ■ The Basics

Ghee also known as Clarified Butter

Simmer sweet butter (unsalted butter) for 10 minutes over medium heat. After it has settled for a few minutes, remove all the white foam from the top. A clear yellow ghee will be left on the bottom. Pour this into a container, not allowing any white sediment at the bottom to slide in. Ghee will keep on the shelf (unrefrigerated) for several weeks and it is very low in cholesterol.

How to Make Your Own Whey

Use one-half gallon milk and the juice of two lemons. Bring the milk to a boil and then remove from heat. Add the lemon juice and let the mixture sit. Curds and whey will form. The liquid is the whey. The curds can be strained through cheesecloth to make panir.

Masala Spice Mix

- 1 Tablespoon nutmeg
- 2 Tablespoons cinnamon
- 1 Tablespoon cardamom
- 8 Tablespoons fennel seeds
- 15 Clove pods

This is the ratio. Mix and make a powder of the ingredients. You can also use poppy seeds or oregano seeds, and the juice of the bamboo, tabashir.

Chapati

Chapati flour is the best if you can get it. Otherwise, whole wheat flour with a bit of pastry flour and a pinch of salt. Add water until it holds together like an elastic, bread dough. Knead it for about 10 minutes. Then let it rest. Take a pinch of dough and roll it out into a circle and bake it on a flat iron skillet. Cook it dry on one side until bubbles form and then turn it over and finish on the second side. Stack with ghee if you're making multiple chapatis at once.

Parantha

Shallow fried whole wheat bread. Make a chapati dough and then fold a teaspoonful of set ghee into it. Also spread a little more ghee over the outside surfaces and double-fold it lengthwise. Roll it flat, approximately 5 in diameter. Heat the griddle and apply a little ghee to it. You will use a slow fire. Cook as you would a chapati. Serve immediately as it tends to lose its crispness if stored.

Mung Beans & Rice

A perfectly balanced protein dish, easy to digest, and very satisfying. Good any time of the year, but makes a particularly good winter diet.

- 4½ cups water
- ½ cup mung beans
- ½ cup basmati rice
- ¼ cup ginger root, finely minced
- 1 onion, chopped
- 3 cloves garlic, minced
- 3 cups chopped vegetables
- 2 Tablespoons (40 ml) ghee or vegetable oil
- ¾ teaspoon turmeric
- ¼ teaspoon crushed red chilies
- ¼ teaspoon ground black pepper
- ½ teaspoon ground coriander
- ½ teaspoon ground garam masala
- ½ teaspoon ground cumin
- ¼ teaspoon cardamom seeds (2 pods)
- 1 bay leaf

Rinse mung beans and rice. Add mung beans to boiling water and cook until beans begin to split. Add rice and cook another 15 minutes, stirring occasionally. Now add the vegetables. (Alternatively, one could add the vegetables along with the rice.) As the mixture cooks, it will start to thicken. Heat the ghee or vegetable oil in a frying pan. Add onions, ginger, and garlic and sauté until clear. Add spices and cook 5 more minutes, stirring constantly. Add this to the rice and beans. The final consistency should be like a thick soup. Total cooking time is about 1½ hours. Add salt or soy sauce to taste. Serve plain or with yogurt. Makes 4 servings.

■ ■ ■ Vitality Drinks

Restorative Drink: Sesame-Ginger Milk

Take this drink immediately after having intercourse. This creamy and stimulating drink is nourishing to the nervous system and the male sexual organs.

- 12 ounces of milk
- 2 Tablespoons (or 1 3 inches) of fresh ginger, peeled and finely chopped
- ¼ cup of ground sesame seeds
- 2 teaspoons of maple syrup or honey

Blend until frothy in a food processor or blender; to serve warm, add a Tablespoon of Ghee and heat gently and enjoy. A simpler version is to put a tablespoon of raw sesame oil (not toasted!) in some warm milk and enjoy.

Yogi Tea

Everybody's favorite! Good for the blood, colon, nervous system, and bones. Good for colds, flu, and physical weakness.

- 10 ounces (315 ml) water
- 2 slices fresh ginger root (optional, but excellent!)
- 3 cloves
- 4 green cardamon pods, cracked
- 4 black peppercorns
- ½ stick cinnamon
- ¼ teaspoon black tea (a teabag)
- ½ cup (125 ml) milk or equivalent
- Honey, to taste (optional)

Bring the water to a boil and add the spices. Cover and continue boiling for 10-15 minutes. Remove from heat, add black tea, and let steep for 1-2 minutes. Add honey and milk, bring to a boil, and remove from heat. Strain and serve. Makes about 4 cups. It's often easier to make a gallon at a time and store in the refrigerator (without the milk). Then it can be taken cold in the morning as a liver cleanse—and heated up with milk as you like.

Yogi Bhajan's Morning Lecithin Drink

- 8 ounces cucumber juice
- 2 tablespoons liquid chlorophyll
- 2 tablespoons protein powder
- 2 tablespoons lecithin granules or liquid lecithin

Blend and drink

Vitality and Weight Loss Drink

This drink is very good. It has helped me to survive working 20 hours a day, running from airplane to airplane, and all the nonsense that I have to go through.

- 8 ounces orange juice
- 2 Tablespoons of protein powder
- 2 Tablespoons rice bran syrup
- 2 Tablespoons chlorophyll
- 1 banana

Blend. You can live on this drink, if you take it four times a day and eat nothing else. If you are young you may drink it three times a day and you can lose weight, be healthy, and take care of yourself.

Weight Gain Drink

Make split milk (whey) and to the split milk add:
- 4 Tablespoons rice bran syrup
- 4 bananas
- 4 teaspoons solid protein powder
- 2 ounces chlorophyll

Drink this four times a day and you can become an elephant.

Q: How much milk?
Yogi Bhajan: It depends upon your capacity.

Q: Do you think taking a protein powder that has saccharin in it is a bad idea?
Yogi Bhajan: If possible avoid saccharin, but if it is required medically, go ahead.

Jaalaa Jeeraa (Cumin Tea or Cumin Water)

- 1 pound of Cumin seeds, whole.
- 1 ounce Tamarind, fresh or frozen
- Black salt, sometimes called Sulphur salt. Use only a little because of its strong odor.
- One half lemon per 10 oz water.
- Black pepper (optional)
- Peppermint leaves
- 8-10 cups of water

Place all of the ingredients into a pot. Bring water to a boil, then lower the flame and let cook at a low boil for 4-5 hours. The idea is to take the extract out of the cumin seeds. It can be drunk hot like a tea, or cold like a drink, but normally is taken cold.

Do not throw away the seed mixture after you have boiled & strained. When you are ready to make more tea, use these old ingredients and add fresh ingredients to them. This tea can be made in a large quantity ahead of time and stored in the refrigerator for up to a week.

Benefits: Jaalaa Jeeraa can be used by anybody, male or female, who has fat on their body. If you take 2-3 glasses a day, all of your fatty tissues will be dissolved, and it won't let fat deposit anywhere in your body.

This tea can also be used to improve the beauty of the skin and to maintain the youthful appearance. For this purpose, drink 2 glasses a day.

It also improves the digestive system. It has been called the 'buddy of the colon', since it cleanses all of the mucous out of this area.

The tamarind in this recipe is a good source of Vitamin C. One ounce of tamarind provides about a hundred thousand units of Vitamin C.

Golden Milk

This delicious hot drink is very good for the spine. It lubricates the joints and helps to break up calcium deposits.

- ⅛ teaspoon turmeric
- ¼ cup water
- 8 ounces milk
- 2 Tablespoons raw almond oil
- honey to taste

Boil turmeric in water for about 8 minutes until it forms a thick paste. If too much water boils away, add a little more water. Meanwhile, bring milk to a boil with the almond oil. As soon as it boils, remove from heat. Combine the two mixtures and add honey to taste. If you like, prepare a larger quantity of the turmeric paste. It will last up to 40 days if refrigerated.

Banana Nutmeg Ice Cream

- 1-2 Cups of Milk
- 3 bananas (Use 2 if they are large)
- Nutmeg. (Take 2 whole nutmegs, and grind them up fresh. Do not use powdered nutmeg from a jar.)
- 1 fresh apple
- Honey

Blend all the above ingredients together. You can drink this mixture as a hot drink, but it can also be made into ice cream.

To make "Ice Cream": Powdered cinnamon must be added to the above ingredients. Freeze and then eat.

Benefits: This recipe will keep a normal person young for a long time. Freshly ground nutmeg must be used, because non-fresh nutmeg is very intoxicating to the point that it can make you totally dizzy and you may not come out of it. The effects of the nutmeg can be quite heavy if taken straight. It will make you forget this world and the world to come after. Nutmeg, when used with banana, is a tonic. Nutmeg used without banana is just nutmeg and can even make you go crazy.

If you are a person who does not drink milk, you can substitute almond milk instead. Almond milk is very good in hot weather and can give you a lot of energy.

Nutmeg as **Medicine**

Karta Purkh Singh Khalsa
Yogaraj Ayurvedic Herbalist
for the
Kundalini Research Institute

Yogi Bhajan recommended nutmeg many times, principally as a relaxant. Nutmeg is appropriate for people who have trouble staying asleep. The sedating action of nutmeg begins after a predictable delay of 3½ to 5 hours, depending on the person, and results in a prolonged somnolence of a predictable 8 hours. For insomnia, begin with a dose of one half teaspoon of powder at 6:00 p.m. The next night, increase the dose to one teaspoon. Continue increasing incrementally. Adjust the time of administration slightly to promote proper time of initiation of effects. You should feel profoundly drowsy at bedtime. Adjust the dose for the desired depth of sleep.

Nutmeg is a valuable sedative. Because it has a delayed action, it can be taken in divided doses throughout the day. A larger dose at night will produce a latent morning anti-anxiety effect. A typical dose would be one teaspoon of powder at breakfast, lunch and bedtime. As the metabolism of nutmeg is gradual, you might experience a sustained feeling of relaxed ease throughout the day, even if the doses are irregular.

Nutmeg effectively lowers blood pressure and pulse rate. If you increase the dose too quickly, the side effect is extreme fatigue.

This herb excels in treating premature ejaculation, for which Yogi Bhajan recommended it many times. Presumably the effect is from reducing blood pressure. The most effective use is a modest daily dose that does not cause undue sedation, say one half teaspoon of powder, over a long term. Ejaculation begins to be delayed after taking nutmeg for about 30 days, and this effect continues.

A home medicine for diarrhea includes ghee, ginger powder, raw sugar and nutmeg. The addition of the ginger increases the digestive fire,

continued...

to treat the underlying poor digestion, the cause of the diarrhea.

As a digestive aid, Ayurveda considers nutmeg to be similar in action to cinnamon and clove. If necessary, any can be substituted for the other. It reduces high air tattva. A typical combination for suppressed digestive function includes dry ginger, caraway and nutmeg, taken before meals.

Nutmeg is cultivated in Southern India, but most nutmeg in the United States comes from the Caribbean. The vast majority of nutmeg in the world is cultivated and harvested for culinary use. Seek out fresh, quality whole nutmeg nuts for maximum benefit.

Whole seeds preserve the active ingredients well, but the active ingredients degrade rapidly upon grinding. Use bulk powdered seed, freshly ground. Nutmeg has a very strong taste. Capsules prepared from seeds that are freshly ground and immediately encapsulated retain the medicinal effects.

Compared to other common herbal relaxants, nutmeg is very powerful. If used in an excessively high dose while awake, the user will feel stupor and disorientation from the sedative effect, as with any other powerful relaxant. Smaller people and those with low blood pressure should start with smaller doses and proceed with caution. Also, those with a history of drug abuse or alcoholism should approach using nutmeg with caution.

Lassi

When there is a slight kidney pain either left or right, for which you have no reason, and it goes away and comes back and goes away and comes back, it means the kidneys are fatigued. For this there is nothing better than this simple lassi:

- 2 ounces of yogurt
- 10 ounces of water
- Pinch of black salt

Blend and place outside by 4pm until 8 am the next morning. Then in the morning sip it slowly, let it mix with your saliva.

You can supplement this lassi with a second drink:

- 2 ounces each:
  Pomegranate juice
  Cranberry juice
  Pear juice
  Orange juice
- 1 to 1 ½ bananas

Blended until smooth. Drink this after the lassi and you will have 'wings' all day long.

Other Great Foods for **Men**

The Best Way to Eat Brewer's Yeast

- 2 quarts milk
- 6 ounces brewer's yeast
- 2 ounces dried mint leaves
- 2 ounces cinnamon

Bring all ingredients to a boil; cool; make a homemade yogurt from the mixture. Serve it for breakfast, with honey to taste.

Potent Potatoes

This recipe has its roots in the tradition of yogic cooking. The spices help to purify the blood, stimulate digestion, and increase energy. You may decrease the amounts of pepper and cayenne to suit your taste.

- 4 large baking potatoes
- ¼ -½ cup (65-125 ml) ghee or vegetable oil
- 2-3 onions, chopped
- ¼ -½ cup (65-125 ml) ginger root, minced
- ¼ teaspoon caraway seeds
- 1-2 Tablespoons (20-40 ml) garlic, minced
- 1 teaspoon black pepper
- ¾ -1 teaspoon turmeric
- 1 teaspoon cayenne or crushed red chilies
- 8 whole cloves
- ½ teaspoon ground cardamom
- ¼ teaspoon ground cinnamon
- 2 - 4 Tablespoons (40-80 ml) soy sauce or salt to taste
- ½ pint (500 ml) cottage cheese

Optional:
- ½ pound (225 gr) cheese, grated
- 1 red or green bell pepper, diced
- ½ cup (125 ml) chopped pineapple, drained

Scrub potatoes, rub with small amount of oil and bake at 400° F (200° C), until well done. Heat ghee or oil in large skillet. Sauté onions and ginger until they begin to brown, then add garlic and spices and cook for 4-5 minutes longer. Add a little water if necessary. Add soy sauce (optional). Stir and remove from heat. Cut baked potatoes in half, lengthwise. Scoop out the insides and combine with onion mixture. Add cottage cheese. Mix well and refill potato shells, covering each with grated cheese. Broil until cheese is melted and bubbly. For a nice touch, garnish with bell pepper and pineapple. Serve with yogurt. Serves four.

Italiano

This recipe applies to men and women alike.

Make a pakora of the the eggplant: Slice an eggplant into thick slices, and dredge it in garbanzo flour. Then deep fry them for about two or three minutes.

Then take 40 pistachio nuts, 40 peeled almonds and 20 figs and blend them together until it becomes like a jam. This jam is put on the pakoras. Eat this dish with one perfectly ripe banana. The banana is essential for potassium.

Nut Paste

Steam onions, ginger and garlic in the ratio of 3:1:2 and saffron, in a ratio to the ginger of 1:8 but no more than 15 grains. Blend this with a maximum of 50 pistachios and 40 almonds and a little honey. Eat this mixture on toast. The saffron and the nuts are soaked overnight in a little milk.

Q: *Do you blend the milk with it also?*
Yogi Bhajan: Instead of water use a little bit of the milk.

Q: *Sir, what do you mean, it's a sex food?*
Yogi Bhajan: It will keep you going. It will give you substance and endurance. It gives you good nerves, good semen.

Q: *How often should this food be eaten?*
Yogi Bhajan: I recommend eating it no more than once a week. It's quite hot stuff. I recommend that you eat it on Sundays, or a day that you can play, run around, or go to the beach. Exercise so that this food is digested and is excreted in your sweat. You should have milk with this meal.

Q: *It is made with three onions?*
Yogi Bhajan: No, that is the ratio of the ingredients by weight.

Khoa

On low heat, bring milk to a boil, until it reduces and becomes thick, which is called khoa, saturated milk. Add 10-15 grains of saffron to that milk, just enough to give it a golden color. Then add crushed pistachio nuts, ¼ the weight of the milk and continue cooking. As the mixture cools, add honey, 1/8 the weight of the mixture. Spread it in a pan. It makes a kind of milk candy. It's very heavy, you can't eat it all at once. At this point you may add gold leaf or silver leaf to it. When you eat this, you need to exercise a lot.

Dried Honey Carrot

A poor man's diet is made from carrots. You'll need one or more carrots (or apples), honey, glass jar, and cheesecloth. Steam a carrot (or an apple), peel the skin off and soak it in a glass jar filled with honey. Cover it with cheesecloth and leave it in the sun for 40 days to dry out. Serve it with gold or silver leaf. It is good for the heart.

Potato Peel and Pistachio Nuts

Here is another pure and simple poor man's food. The potato peels are steamed. Put the pistachio nuts with it. Blend the steamed skins with pistachio nuts and as little honey as you need.

Wheat Berry Day

Wheat berries prevent stomach cancer, intestinal tract cancer, or colorectal cancer. With them you will avoid pancreatic or kidney problems. Wheat berries are wonderful. You should eat wheat berries one day each week. Wheat berries are man's food and you guys make jokes about it because it is cheap, takes a long time to cook and doesn't taste good.

Q: Do you eat it plain?
Yogi Bhajan: You may add a little bit of honey. I don't take it with anything else, it is better that way. Train your children so that if there is any kind of difficulty in the world, your system has already adapted to eating wheat berries.

Q: We've been putting a little milk and honey on them, is that OK?
Yogi Bhajan: That is desirable. I don't want you to live poor and miserable lives. I cannot tolerate you doing things which in the long run make you old, senile and neurotic.

Q: Do you get the same effect by eating wheat berries with your other food every day?
Yogi Bhajan: No. No. No. Wheat Berry Day is wheat berry day. Your system has to be made accustomed to it.

Wheat Milk Powder Prasad Balls

Make wheat milk powder by boiling wheat berries until soft, grinding them and put it through a sieve. The liquid is wheat milk. Then evaporate the water and what is left is the wheat milk powder. Fry this in ghee. If you wish you may add pistachio nuts and raisins. Make it into a prasad ball and when it dries add raw brown sugar to your taste. Eat one prasad ball early in the morning with hot milk. It is very good for backache and for sexual stimulation. It is very good for feeling sexy, especially if you are feeling older and colder.

Q: How often should we eat it?
Yogi Bhajan: Once a day. It's very hot. If you have too much, it can bring blood out of your kidneys. You can have it every day, but just one ball, a muffin-sized ball.

Q: You let the milk evaporate?
Yogi Bhajan: No, you take the milk out, let it settle. The water evaporates; it dries up and becomes like a powder. It is called nakasta. Nakasta is a very old word. It is very good for you when you are over 54. It keeps you going. The best way to eat it is to soak it in milk at night, and early in the morning, eat it and go for a long walk, play football or hockey, or whatever physical exercise you want—very good. It keeps you going. It's the best use of wheat.

Q: How long do you boil the wheat?
Yogi Bhajan: Just boil it long enough that the skin becomes soft and the milk may be taken out. The best way is to just soak it for a few days, don't boil it at all. Just put it in water for four or five days, and then wash it out, grind the softened berries, etc.

Hypoglycemic Diet

People with hypoglycemia can take four spoons of mung beans and rice with yogurt every two hours.

Two Great Ways to Use Sesame Seeds

1. Use one or two pounds sesame butter (homemade preferred). Mix with a very sour sourdough bread. Make your bread adding apples or whatever appeals to you and bake. One toasted piece per serving.

2. Make a chapati dough using one-fourth whole sesame seeds and three-fourths dough. Use the dough to make stuffed chapatis.

Chawan Prash

Take one ounce of chawan prash every day, rolled in a silver leaf, with 8 ounces of milk as part of your breakfast. It must be taken in this fashion for a long time. This food falls under the category of Aryuvedic remedies, which is a slowly building system. It keeps you going, and it builds you gradually. Real chawan prash is the healthiest thing in the world produced by the human being.

Sex and **Longevity**

For men, sexual intercourse before the age of 25 can be very dangerous. This is because the timing of the testicles with the pituitary is only in synch, in rhythm, after the age of 24. If you stick to this law, then from the ages of 25 all the way up to 100, you will never get senile, weak or insane. Your propensity for creative consciousness and your psyche of projection will be very smart; you'll walk tall.

Usually, when you have not controlled yourself before the age of 25, (which includes masturbation and wet dreams), you pay a heavy price. After the age of 54 you start going downhill.

To correct this damage, there are two things which can be taken: One is chawan prash and the other is pistachio paranthas.

Pistachio Paranthas

This food can help take care of arthritis as well as help a man with building his potency. One day a week eat two paranthas; live on those two paranthas that day. In this way you can be resettled.

FLOUR:
- ½ cup Corn flour (not corn meal)
- ½ cup Garbanzo flour
- ½ cup Bhajara flour (available in Indian stores; if not on hand, use whole wheat flour)
- 3 cups Whole wheat flour

Mix the flours together until you have a dough consistency. You may want to use less of the garbanzo flour and more of the bhajara or whole wheat flour, as these latter two tend to make the dough stick together a little bit better.

STUFFING:
- 1 lb. pistachio nuts (unsalted, shelled)
- 1 cup minced cauliflower
- 1 onion chopped
- 2 teaspoons saffron
- 1 teaspoon red chiles
- 2 teaspoons salt
- 1 teaspoon pepper
- ¼ cup of milk
- ghee

To use the saffron, you must first take the saffron and soak it over night in milk. In the morning take all the above ingredients, and blend them together in a food processor until you have a fine mixture.

The pistachio nuts are the main ingredient in this stuffing mixture; use a smaller amount of cauliflower than you do pistachio nuts. All of the other ingredients can be used in any amount you wish as seasonings.

To prepare the parantha: Once you have the dough made and you have kneaded it for a while, place about a golf-ball sized ball in your hand. On a floured surface, roll the dough out with a rolling pin until you have it flattened to about 6 inches in diameter. Next take about ½ of the stuffing mixture, place it in the middle of the flattened dough. Next bring the sides of the dough up, and pinch them together at the top, completely sealing the stuffing mixture inside. Now roll it out again into a flattened 6" diameter. In a chapati pan or a frying pan, over a low-medium flame, place your stuffed parantha. Cook it on one side for about 10 to 15 minutes on this dry pan. After 10-15 minutes, turn it over and then take a lot of ghee, and pour it on top of the parantha. It will go through the bread to the other side. Cook this side for about 5 minutes on the same low-medium flame. Take a spoon and keep pressing down on it, until it is done. It is very delicious. It can be eaten with yogurt. It is a very pure food.

This is a very expensive diet because pistachio nuts and saffron are so costly. You don't need to eat any other food with it, since it is such a delicious and precious food.

This food was given to one person who had a very bad case of arthritis and was in a lot of pain. This person lived solely on it for about one month and was healed of this condition within this time period.

These paranthas help to remedy a particular situation which occurs in men. Most men, due to masturbation and overindulgence in sex, have bent organs. And about 50% of the men get a condition where their organs will not catch up from the base and then do not shrink back properly. The moment intercourse is finished, it just slumps down like a broken tree branch. This causes a very great irritation to the system. Its reaction comes back to you in 72 hours, at which time you will wake up feeling very heavy-headed, heavy-bodied, and you will have a feeling of sin. This pistachio parantha can put you back into gear.

Parsley Pilau

- 1 cup basmati rice (uncooked)
- 1 cup parsley leaves, dried
- 2 cups of unskinned chopped potatoes
- 2 chopped onions
- 2 teaspoons oregano or ajwan seeds
- 1 teaspoon ground red pepper or to taste
- 1 Tablespoon turmeric
- 1 teaspoon black pepper
- 2 bay leaves
- ½ cup ghee (clarified butter)

Sauté onions in ghee, adding spices to create a masala. Then add rice to that sautéed onion dish, add potatoes and parsley and then stir for a while. Add water to the dish (to steam the rice). Cook everything for 10-15 minutes.

Benefits: This is a very male, human food. It is good for when you get headaches and heaviness in the head, and you feel very dozy. It is very good for the brain.

Sometimes your skin feels very small and you feel very big. You feel you are out of your skin, like you are being suffocated and stitched in your skin. It is a combined irritation to the capillaries; the capillaries cannot hold their function of blood going through them. This happens to a lot of people who feel handicapped or inadequate. At this time, take this food as a monodiet, but be sure not to overeat it.

Try it sometime as a solo-food. It is very light when it is solely done. If you are a hard working fellow, you can use yogurt with it.

Eggplant with Saffron and Spices

Fry eggplant slices in pure ghee, with chopped onion, garlic, and ginger. Add cardamon, cloves, cinnamon sticks and bay leaves. When the dish is completed, pour saffron milk over it (2 Teaspoons of Saffron soaked in 1 cup of milk) and put silver leaf on top. Serve with flat bread.

Garlic Saffron Almond Rice

Enhances a man's creativity

- 1 cup milk
- 1 teaspoon saffron
- 1 ½ cups basmati rice
- 6 cloves garlic
- 2 cups homemade yogurt
- ½ teaspoon cinnamon
- 1 teaspoon salt
- ½ cup almonds
- 1 Tablespoon ghee

Soak saffron in milk overnight. In the morning, blend until smooth. Soak the almonds overnight or in boiling water to remove their skins. Then slice the almonds. Peel and slice the garlic into quarters. Sautee garlic and almonds in ghee. Rinse rice thoroughly. Boil basmati rice in saffron milk and 2 cups of water. Add garlic and almonds, Simmer for 20 minutes. (Add the saffron milk when dish is half-cooked.) It should be eaten with yogurt and the yogurt should always be homemade. To cleanse the internal organs, then eat this dish with Golden Yogurt, using turmeric. In that case, yogurt should be made from golden milk. Boil ½ teaspoon of turmeric in 1 quart of milk. Use this milk to make the yogurt.

Herbs for Men

1. Embellic Myrobolaus
2. Beleric Myrobolaus
3. Chebuic Myrobolaus

These three herbs provide a general tonic for the man. All three should be mixed together and powdered and a tablespoon taken in the morning. It's a tonic of all tonics. It is called the 'mother, father & child' of everything known or ever produced by God. (See page 360)

Rejuvenating Foods from Around the World

Presented by Soram Singh Khalsa, M.D.

In reviewing this list of rejuvenating foods, we will present the country of origin, the source, or foodstuff, and the qualities which make that food valuable.

■ ■ ■ Sweden

Rose Hips

The first item is from Sweden, and the rejuvenating source is rose hips. Rose hips provide Vitamin C. Vitamin C is necessary to the health of the body protein, collagen. For this reason rose hips keep the skin beautiful and youthful, preventing wrinkles, flabbiness and discoloration and the skin tight and smooth. Rose hips affect the adrenal glands which secrete hormones. Vitamin C has a rejuvenating effect on the glands.

Q: *Collagen, and its source, and how to take it?*
Dr. Soram Singh: Collagen is another aspect of rose hips which I don't know as much, about. It is the substance from which our skin is made and it helps keep the skin beautiful, youthful, prevents wrinkles, flabbiness, discoloration. This collagen is in rose hips. Some of the creams are now available in very natural forms, and they are rich, specifically in collagen, to help maintain that beauty and shine and glow of the skin.

Whey

The second item from Sweden is whey. Whey helps digestion and elimination of food. Whey helps us prevent the development of harmful bacteria by providing the proper nutrients for beneficial bacteria in the intestinal tract. (Acidophilus actually contains these beneficial bacteria.) It prevents constipation, is high in vitamin B and B2. Whey comes in tablets or powdered form.

Q: *The fact that Sweden's the country of origin, would you say that that would be the best place to get the food mentioned?*
Dr. Soram Singh: I don't think that that's necessary. I think that the procedure described is perfect for making whey (recipes) and in terms of convenience, it's available in powdered forms. You dissolve it in water and stir it up like powdered milk.

Q: *The separation that happens in homemade yogurt is that also whey?*
Dr. Soram Singh: No, that's acidophilus. It's different.

Q: *So the liquid part of homemade yogurt is acidophilus?*
Dr. Soram Singh: Not necessarily. However, acidophilus and whey are not equal.

Student: *To make acidophilus, Yogi Bhajan said to leave the yogurt out for several days and then the natural souring of the yogurt would create the acidophilus liquid.*

■ ■ ■ Finland

Sauna

Dr. Soram Singh: The next country is Finland. Its rejuvenating source is fever, as in a high body temperature. Fever is a defense against poisons, virus and stress factors. Healing high temperature speeds metabolism, inhibits growth of virus and bacteria. The Finnish people use saunas. However, you shouldn't take saunas often. It shouldn't be a daily activity. Once a month is fine, and never without a massage and a cold shower after. This is because the sauna routine is very powerful and can temporarily diminish the aura. Saunas and fevers also cause profuse perspiration using the skin to eliminate poisons. Also, I repeat that high temperatures help to kill off the invading organisms and speed up our metabolism which is necessary to fight infection. In other words, it gets the body running. Your heart's beating faster when you have a fever, pumping more blood, which lets you resist and fight bacteria.

Q: *Do you call that a curative measure or a preventative measure?*
Dr. Soram Singh: Sauna would be, as it's commonly used, preventative. There are countries, and I would imagine Finland might be one, where fever therapy is used. That is, intentionally raising your body temperature, whether it be through sauna or another form, such as hot baths that you soak in, as a curative technique. When you have a fever, we're suggesting that you let it go. The body is using the fever to help heal itself.

Rye

The rejuvenating source is rye as used in sourdough rye bread. Its qualities are beneficial to the health of the digestive and eliminative organs. That is, your intestines and colon. It is an anti-constipation food.

Germany

Fermented Foods

One rejuvenating source is fermented foods, including sauerkraut, sourdough bread, pickles, etc. The qualities of these fermented foods as listed here are: cures arthritis, scurvy, ulcers, colds, digestive disorders, and cancer.

This is an appropriate place to interject that in these qualities I don't think we should, any of us, get carried away and go out of here saying, "One of our friends has cancer and I heard at the course to give him pickle and he'll be cured." Similarly for ulcers or for any other thing. What we are saying is that these foods can be beneficial in those conditions.

Q: You said, "Cures arthritis." Do you want to say relieves it?
Dr. Soram Singh: I'm reading to you what's on this sheet as given to us by Yogi Bhajan, I think that it can cure arthritis in combination with other factors which would be contributing toward the cure.

Mineral Waters

Mineral waters have extensive beneficial effects. Mineral baths cure high blood pressure, arthritis, female disorders, cardiovascular diseases, skin disorders, nervous disorders, allergies, old age, and senility. Taken orally they can prevent heart disease, tooth decay, hardening of the arteries. That's quite an extensive statement for mineral water. But indeed, if you look through history, mineral baths in Germany, in Europe, the Bavarian hot springs, have been used for curing everything. Again I'll say that in times when we didn't have all the technology that we have available now, this is what they had and this is what they used. We have much more available today, so that something like mineral water can be used in a supportive way and one can take advantage of everything else to use along with it.

Juice Fasting

The next health tradition from Germany is juice fasting, mentioned earlier by Yogi Bhajan to be done with extreme caution and wisdom. Juice fasting increases the cleaning capacity of lungs, liver, kidney, bowels, and skin. It expels toxins, rejuvenates mental, glandular, hormonal and nervous systems. It can also expel decayed cells and stimulate new ones. Alkaline juices are the best.

Q: What are the alkaline juices? What generates alkalinity in the body?
Dr. Soram Singh: The juices that Yogi Bhajan typically suggests to people are carrot, beet, celery, quite often celery. For ulcers he recommends cabbage juice. He's also recommended cucumber juice.

Juice fasting, I would also emphasize, should be done with caution. Should be done by someone whose body is intrinsically strong enough to withstand the toxins that are going to be eliminated. The body should be prepared for fasting. It should be done in a program of building up and letting down following the fast, whether it's a juice or food fast.

Bulgaria

Soured Milk Products

It's known for the rejuvenating source of soured milk as in homemade yogurt and kefir. The qualities of these foods are that they prevent auto-toxemia and putrefaction in the colon. They prevent self-poisoning and improve health and long life.

Yogurt, as I think we all know, is a most beneficial food. It can be used in many, many ways. It can be used orally to replenish and rebalance the intestinal flora, those bacteria which normally grow in our intestines. It can be used as an enema to locally implant those same bacteria, to stimulate the friendly bacteria and to help knock off the unfriendly ones. It can be used by women as a douche.

Questions: Has Yogi Bhajan recommended enemas to anyone? Isn't he against them?
Dr. Soram Singh: I think in general that he doesn't recommend their use because they don't promote natural bowel functioning.

Q: What about colonics, would they be generally out of the question?
Dr. Soram Singh: If used for reasons of constipation, they would be in the same category as enemas, I would think.

Russia

Honey and Pollen

The next country is Russia which has given us honey. Mainly depending on the pollen content, honey induces longevity, is effective in treating asthma, hemorrhoids, allergies, digestive disorders, arthritis, hay fever, and multiple-sclerosis. It improves assimilation and elimination. Pollen is available in tablets (ten per day) or pure form. You can get the granules and you take about a tablespoon a day for a dose.

Sugar

What we'd like to talk about now is sugar. Sugar is not on the list of good things. It's on the bad list. We are mentioning sugar because so many people eat sugar and don't know it, for instance, in ketchup. Soft drinks are loaded with sugar. All colas are loaded with sugar. The best thing I think I can say to you is, whatever sugar you are eating, you should stop. Whatever honey you are eating, you should probably cut down. Honey, although it comes directly from a natural source, has been processed by the bees and it is a concentrated sweet. It can have the same detrimental effects on your body and mind as sugar.

I've traveled around the country from ashram to ashram, my observation is that people are eating too much honey, thinking that there is nothing wrong and that they are not hurting themselves. In the best of all worlds, in paradise, one could get along with eating honey as long as one were staying relaxed and didn't have much to do. But we're talking about living in cities and living under stress. An excess of honey in the diet is an enormous physical stress combined with the emotional and psychological stresses. All this precipitates an imbalance in the autonomic nervous system. You can call it hypoglycemia, which many people do call it. I'm increasingly getting away from calling it that name. It's the same syndrome. Basically it comes down to stress, and honey and sweets are a great stress on your bodies.

I've seen hyperactive children in ashrams. I don't mean necessarily in a pathological sense, but they weren't centered children. I made comments and the diet was altered. A few months later there was a whole different vibration to the children and to the people living in the ashram.

All day long, I teach people about what they are doing to their bodies. Almost all illness is self-induced, through self-abuse, and you can correct yourself by stopping that self-abuse. What we do at the clinic is speed that healing using therapeutic techniques. Even without these techniques, if you can stop abusing yourself, you'll get well. It's a question of being out of touch with how you are abusing yourself. Whether it's physically or mentally, it doesn't matter. It is not treating ourselves properly and our body reacts by getting what we call "sick." It's a way your body uses to heal itself, to attempt to heal itself through being sick.

Q: What about fructose?
Dr. Soram Singh: Fructose may be better because less is required to sweeten, but it is still a sugar and it still works as a stress.

Q: We're comparing it to honey?
Dr. Soram Singh: Yes, same category. Better than white sugar; white sugar should just definitely be out.

Student: *Honey is 75% fructose and fructose is more fat-forming than glucose (which is the sugar molecule in white sugar). In the chemical pathways, it can be fatted more easily. So if you tend to have a weight problem, fructose in honey is actually worse for you than sugar.*
Dr. Soram Singh: What you are saying is that honey will tend to make you more fat than white sugar. But white sugar has so many other negative things that I would definitely not tell you to eat it, for that reason.

Q: What is a tolerable amount of sweet?
Dr. Soram Singh: The tolerable amount is a very individual thing. I don't want to say one tablespoon and then everybody go home taking one tablespoon. Many of you may be able to eat two tablespoons, and some of you should have zero. But, by and large, you need to tune-in. From my experience of examining people, whatever you're doing now, it is probably too much, and start from there. I'm just saying this very realistically. It's just too much. You have to read the labels of things; sugar is just everywhere, in almost all canned foods. I think most of us are pretty conscious of that. Things like the so-called health food soft drinks are loaded with honey or fructose, and they really blow you out without you even realizing it, unless you're tuned-in to your own body.

Q: What about some of these fruit juices that are really, really sweet, like apple-boysenberry, but have no sugar or honey in them. Still the fructose can blow you out. Would you put that in the stimulating drink category?
Dr. Soram Singh: I definitely would. We're also talking about things like dates and raisins, which have natural sugar, yes, but in excess can really make you off-balance.

Now, why am I telling you these things? Is it because I want to make you suffer? Or that you shouldn't eat sugar because somebody told you not to? No, it's because as Sikhs and as Khalsa, we're making every effort to be able to focus our minds, to direct our consciousness, and to help support and uplift those around us. What I see in people who abuse themselves with sweets is that they are not able to do that—they get spaced out. Or even if they appear to be effective, they could be still more effective. For example, if they're tired in the morning when they wake up or too tired at night after they come home from work, often by decreasing the amount of sweets they eat, there can be a drastic change in how that person feels in terms of energy. The problem is that once you get into that cycle of sweets, your whole glandular system reacts to that over-stimulation. It begins to fatigue and you get what is called the adrenal-exhaustion syndrome, which subsequently affects the thyroid, and then the pituitary. What we're seeing increasingly these days, which I didn't see, say, two years ago, is that people come in not just with an imbalance in their adrenals, but now the vast majority of people who are blown out have also blown out their entire glandular system. These kinds of things are set off by stressors—of which sweets are one.

Student: *You said you wouldn't say it, but at one class, in a very general statement, Yogi Bhajan said, one tablespoon a day of honey and then only for medicinal use.*

Dr. Soram Singh: Yes, he said that about five years ago. Another thing he said in that same class was that if the skin and the hair were left on the meat nobody would ever eat it. Nobody would ever think of eating it. Likewise, if you were to sit down to a cupful of white sugar, you wouldn't even think of eating it. But, if you drink an eight ounce glass of a soft drink, that's exactly what you're taking in, a cupful of sugar.

Student: *I think some of the prasad[1] that I've eaten would fill the normal daily requirement.*

Dr. Soram Singh: I'm glad you brought that up. *Prasad* is indeed sweet, but there's a very, very interesting thing about *prasad*. We've done some measurements on equivalent types of situations. *Prasad* is not what it appears to be. The benefit that you get from *prasad*, is not from its nutritive value, "on the physical plane," but from the etheric vibration it is filled with through the blessings. I can tell you for sure that if you were to take the individual components of *prasad* before it's made, take a person who has a problem with stress, and muscle test them or measure them, they would definitely be blown out by the honey, and in many cases by the wheat. On the other hand, if you take the *prasad*, and take a person who's totally blown out on wheat on every muscle, and put that in their aura, everything will become strong. That is because of the etheric energy that is imparted to it through the prayers and all the energy that we direct into it.

[1] A sweet dish traditionally served after taking a hukam from the Guru Granth Sahib, made from flour, water, ghee and honey or sugar.

Student: *So throw away your Hershey bars.*

Dr. Soram Singh: I had a patient do that in my office one day. He came into my office with some kind of bread that he was very allergic to (he's been allergic all his life to wheat). I walked out of the room to get a phone call. I had just tested him and he had been totally blown out by the bread, and he was thinking he wasn't going to be able to eat it anymore. When I came back in, he said, "Test me for this just one more time." I said, "Sure." He was strong as a rock. I said, "What'd you do?" He said, "I said a blessing over it while you were gone." And we think when we bless our food for dinner, for breakfast, whatever, that this is just a ritual, this is a routine, we always do that, I'm in a habit. Very specifically, you're putting a great deal of energy into it, and that energy is what affects our consciousness.

Student: *Also eating with the fingers is part of that. Yogi Bhajan says that what you're doing is transfering prana into the food. The food, the nutritive value of food, is not so much in what it is made of, protein, carbohydrates, and so on, it is in the energy that we extract from that. That's why if you have a bad digestive system, you can eat all day long and still be very unhealthy because you're not getting the energy.*

Q: *How much **prasad** should one eat?*

Dr. Soram Singh: The questions here are coming out of the range of medical and into the range of spiritual and that's fine. The answer I think is you should eat what's given to you.

Garlic and Onions

Another one from Russia: garlic and onion. They reduce blood pressure, stimulate cell growth, and more. We have measured with some sophisticated, electronic acupuncture equipment, and found garlic to be wonderful for cleaning out all sorts of poisons that the body has accumulated, such as insecticides and pesticides, that we've gotten from our foods. We found that taking garlic every day, whether it's in the form of raw garlic or some of the other forms which are concentrated, like "Kyolic" (which we use a lot in the clinic), is very helpful in cleaning these things out. One reason many people are low in energy is that some of these toxins have accumulated in their body. Just by taking garlic and cleaning those things out, along with whatever else the garlic is doing to the glandular system, nervous system, a person can have a lot more energy.

Q: *Have you had any experience with garlic and radiation?*

Dr. Soram Singh: You mean garlic as a cleaning-out agent for radiation. There are better things than garlic for radiation. There are homeopathic medicines specifically for cleaning out radiation and that's what we generally use. I don't know that garlic would do it.

Q: *Can you comment on the conflict between garlic and homeopathic remedies?*
Dr. Soram Singh: Yes. I have heard Yogi Bhajan say that raw onion will neutralize homeopathic medicines and, in my experience, I definitely find that to be true. I'd like to speak to you today from my clinical experience, I feel that's the most I have to offer you, and, I can say, we have a lot of patients who are taking garlic in the form of Kyolic, who are getting homeopathic medicine simultaneously and between the two of them there seems to be no conflict. Now, with people eating raw garlic every day, in large quantities, it may fall more into that category of raw onions. I can't say anything specifically. Usually we advise people definitely not to eat raw onions, on the day that they take homeopathic medicines.

Q: *Raw garlic, is it as good as cooked garlic?*
Dr. Soram Singh: I would say that they would be similar and I couldn't tell the difference quantitatively.

Q: *Do you think powdered onion, garlic, and ginger are as effective as fresh?*
Dr. Soram Singh: I don't know. Kyolic is a therapeutic agent for people in the business community and people out in the world who don't want to eat raw garlic three times a day. Kyolic serves as a very excellent substitute; it comes in capsules, it leaves no odor, and it works, by the measurements that we've made. Now whether it works less effectively than raw garlic, I don't know, because I don't have that many patients taking raw garlic cloves three times a day as a medicine.

Buckwheat

Buckwheat is next. It is also from Russia. It supplies rutin and is beneficial in circulatory and cardiovascular system diseases. My experience with buckwheat is that it is a complete carbohydrate. As opposed to simple carbohydrate, it's a complex carbohydrate. It is balanced, and it can be handled well by the body. It is very good for people who have so-called hypoglycemia because it is a complex carbohydrate.

Sunflower Seeds

Sunflower seeds are rich in vitamin E and zinc which play an important role in the growth and maturity of the gonads (the male sex glands) and the prostate glands. Indeed, zinc is very important for male prostate function and male sexual functioning and vitamin E is also important for sexual functioning in men and women. Sunflower seeds are rich in these nutrients.

Zinc is very important for male sexual functioning. Older men with prostate problems definitely need zinc nutritionally.

Japan and Asia

Seaweed or Kelp

Nutritionally seaweed is rich in natural iodine and it helps the endocrine glands, especially the thyroid. Use kelp instead of salt.

Sesame Seed

Next from the orient is halva, sesame seeds. The qualities are extensive: increases virility; rejuvenates mental and physical capacities and endurance; has abundant potassium and magnesium; is an excellent source of lecithin; increases secretion of the pituitary, pineal and sex glands (one couldn't ask for much more than that); good for the brain and nerve tissues. What we've got here is a very solid food. Tahini is a common form of sesame seed butter. "Halva" I think is a popular form of candy.

Mexico

Papaya

Papaya is rich in papain, which is a digestive enzyme. It is also rich in vitamin C and an excellent cleansing food.

Lime

It aids digestion, is a powerful antiseptic, treats colds, liver complaints, scurvy, dysentery, and fever. Limes, of course, are rich in vitamin C.

Chile

Chile stimulates circulation, helps digestion (by stimulating enzymes and hydrochloric acid in stomach), is beneficial to the kidneys, spleen and pancreas.

Damiana

Damiana is an herb we use a lot at the clinic. It is a remedy for sexual impotence. It is also a tonic for nerves, and can be used for mental and physical exhaustion. Damiana also helps support the adrenal glands

Sarsaparilla

Its qualities are: blood purifier, helpful for chronic rheumatism, skin disorders, psoriasis, general weakness, sexual impotence, and as an antidote for toxic effects of strong poisons. It is a natural source of male and female sex hormones.

China

Ginseng

The healing qualities of ginseng: aphrodisiac; stimulates cell growth; increases hormone production; rejuvenates the nervous system; cures all ills (again temper this with modern knowledge); and, finally, strengthens the heart.

Gotu-kola

Its healing qualities are: keeping the endocrine and sex glands in peak working condition; energize nerve and brain functions.

Pitcairn Islands

Morning Cleansing Time

The tradition of eating only fruit in the morning, and a big meal at noon, because from 5:00 to 11:00 a.m. your body is cleansing. Eating at this time disrupts this process.

Two Magic Herbs from China

Li Chung Yen is said to have taken these two herbs (ginseng and gotu kola) daily and lived to be 265 years old. At 200 he looked like 50. He outlived 23 wives, and kept his own teeth and hair. He was also a vegetarian.

America

Vitamins

America discovered vitamins. There are no foods mentioned here, just vitamins.

Vitamin E

Aging is caused by oxidation. Vitamin E is a natural antioxidant and it increases fertility.

Vitamin C

We could talk about vitamin C all day really, as many of you probably know, and especially in view of the work of Linus Pauling and others, in megavitamin dosage of vitamin C. I can speak of my experience with it, which has been moderately extensive. We use vitamin C regularly for people who have infectious diseases, and for people who are under stress. (Stress will be mentioned many times as we review this list.) Stress can be in many forms. It can be the stress of physical labor, working very hard, lifting heavy things; it can be nutritional stress, that is, improper diet. Stress can also be pollutants around us such as smog or pollution from factories. Vitamin C basically helps to build our resistance and to maintain it. It offers specific anti-inflammatory and anti-infectious properties. We will often use 15,000 units of vitamin C intravenously for people who have an acute flu or cold. With that kind of dose taken intravenously, the flu can be completely eliminated in a few hours, if caught early enough.

If you can't use vitamin C intravenously, there are many, many oral forms. There's one particular powder which we have found to be very, very good. It's called "Emergen-C." This particular vitamin C is ascorbic acid in the ascorbate ion form combined with minerals such as potassium and calcium. It's prepared in a powder which you dissolve in water and drink. Because of the way these ions are combined, the ascorbic acid gets right into the cells and does the job. And so it's more effective than the tablet form.

Q: What about pure organic vitamin C, in very small quantities?

Dr. Soram Singh: Another company, Standard Process, puts out vitamin C tablets which contain only two-three milligrams of vitamin C. This vitamin C has been culled from a huge number of rose hips, the raw rose hips. It's my feeling, although I've never heard anyone speaking on this issue, that those two-three milligrams, because they are the pure essence of the vitamin C, are just as effective in the body as 2-3,000 of the kind I mentioned earlier. However, the Alacer "Emergen-C" is readily available in health food stores. The Standard Process type, which is very good, is available only through doctor's offices.

I want you to understand that the things that I tell you today are things that I feel very solid about based on extensive muscle testing, measuring with acupuncture instruments, and seeing clinical results.

Q: What about vitamin C poisoning?
Dr. Soram Singh: Vitamin C poisoning? People who are taking excess ascorbic acid may have side effects like diarrhea or nausea from the acid parts of ascorbic acid (usually that doesn't happen until dosages reach 10-15,000 milligrams a day). Again with the "Emergen-C." that is specifically avoided because the acid form of vitamin C is not used. The ascorbate is used.

Q: What about rebound scurvy?
Dr. Soram Singh: When you take a lot of vitamin C for a cold or infection, say you're taking 10,000 milligrams a day, and then you wake up one morning and you're well, don't drop your vitamin C down to zero, because you can get rebound scurvy. That is, scurvy is a vitamin C deficiency disease, and when your body is used to 10,000 milligrams a day and you suddenly withold the C, you have a relative deficiency. When you're taking those very high dosages, always taper off slowly over a few days or weeks depending on how long you've been using them.

Q: Have you had any trouble with the powdered form losing its activity when you store it?
Dr. Soram Singh: No, we haven't so far. In terms of survival needs, I don't know about long-range storing in terms of five to ten years. In terms of acute needs, six months to a year, there's been no problem.

Q: I've heard that if you have a cold, it's your body trying to get rid of the toxins or whatever, so if you take the vitamin C, it prevents this function?
Dr. Soram Singh: In my understanding it is not that way with vitamin C. A cold can be viewed as a way for your body to eliminate. You might say that with the use of vitamin C perhaps the body is eliminating in another way. There are many forms of elimination in the body. A cold is a way through the lungs or through the respiratory system, but it can also eliminate through the digestive system, through the skin, and so in my personal philosophy, vitamin C doesn't suppress, though there could be others who would disagree with what I've said.

Vitamin A
Vitamin A keeps skin youthful and gives healthy mucous linings.

B-Complex
Vitamin B complexes are good for the nervous system, especially when balanced with magnesium. Can also be used for long-term pain management.

Lecithin
There are quite a few qualities listed for brain and nerve tissue and the pituitary, pineal and sex glands, essential for semen production, and prevents hardening of the arteries. It is recommended to take two to three tablespoons of the liquid daily. When large dosages are taken daily, add calcium lactate to the diet to balance the excess phosphorous from the lecithin. Calcium lactate comes from dairy products or is available as a supplement.

Vitamin P
Vitamin P is rutin and the bioflavinoids. It is good for reducing blood pressure.

Brewer's Yeast
The last rejuvenating source from America is brewer's yeast. It is rich in vitamin B-complex and is a good source of zinc. Also it is the richest natural source of nucleic acids: DNA and RNA.

This list is meant to be a resource for rejuvenating yourself. I think that Yogi Bhajan felt that the way we take care of ourselves and our knowledge about what we are eating, wasn't adequate. He wanted me to go over the basics. As you go on, you can refine it according to your own bodily needs, but this is a good basic list.

Review of Rejuvenating Foods and **Recommendations**

Yogi Bhajan: Did you review the list of rejuvenating ideas from all over the world? Do you understand all of it?

Student: *There are a few questions.*
Dr. Soram Singh: The first one was about brown sugar.
Yogi Bhajan: Brown? Brown sugar is not a crystal sugar. Brown sugar is in a solid form. When you take white sugar, put molasses in it, and make it brown, that is not brown sugar. Any machine which makes white sugar contains lead, and lead is not good for the body. Period.

Dr. Soram Singh: Another question was about powdered garlic as opposed to raw.
Yogi Bhajan: Powdered garlic is 60% as potent as raw; but 60% is better than nothing.

Q: How about liquid garlic?
Yogi Bhajan: Liquid garlic is very powerful, 70%. I take it every day. Liquid garlic is good for circulatory pressures and that pump which is called the heart. It's far out. It's good for the liver, too.

Q: How about powdered onions and ginger?
Yogi Bhajan: Powdered garlic, ginger, and onion, the trinity roots, do maintain themselves, not much is lost except freshness. They lose about 30%.

Q: Rice bran syrup compared with brewer's yeast.
Yogi Bhajan: Brewer's yeast and rice bran syrup, both are okay. Brewer's yeast has a problem. Some people are called brewer's yeast freaks. I have seen a person taking scoops of cottage cheese with an equal amount of brewer's yeast. I asked him, "Can you do that?" He said, "Sir, what is wrong with it?" It is called too much.

Q: Does the antiseptic quality of honey destroy the flora of yogurt?
Yogi Bhajan: No. Honey has the quality to intermix immediately. Take the honey, mix it in the yogurt, and eat it.

Q: When you put the honey in, because honey is an antiseptic, it kills the lacto-bacilli.
Yogi Bhajan: Yes, but it takes time. What can it do when it is already in the stomach? It's okay. It's not affected that way.

Q: Liquid or powdered lecithin?
Yogi Bhajan: Lecithin in any form is wonderful. The problem is that it smells bad. There is a drink with cucumber juice, lecithin and water soluble liquid chlorophyll. It's the first drink I take in the morning. It has done me a lot of good. It takes away the fatigue.

Q: Sesame seeds, with or without the hulls?
Yogi Bhajan: Sesame seeds are a very unique thing. Sesame seeds are very difficult to blend. But there's a way to do it. Take two pounds of sesame seeds, and blend them at a low-frequency, not at a fast frequency, to make sesame butter. There are two types of blenders available. One is very fast: you put in the sesame seeds and hot butter comes out on the other side. The other blender works with pulleys and can work very slowly. The seeds come out as butter, too, but the temperature of the butter is the temperature of the seeds.

Q: Should children eat regular sesame butter?
Yogi Bhajan: It is good for them. They can handle a tablespoon, or two tablespoons, reasonably.

Q: In the chapatis, sesame seed or sesame butter?
Yogi Bhajan: Sesame seeds will do because you have to fry it.

Q: Hulled or raw? White or brown?
Yogi Bhajan: Both will work. Take your choice. Actually it is the inner ingredient of the sesame seed which is important. The husk is there just for elimination.

Q: Will it hurt the sesame seeds if we roast them before hand?
Yogi Bhajan: Sesame seeds should not be roasted, but when they are roasted they maintain themselves up to 40% and they are easily digestible. If you have more money you can roast them. We are paying for something and 60% we are roasting away.

Q: Sir, about tahini. We are wondering how long it keeps?
Yogi Bhajan: I think, within a reasonable time, it will be all right. It's not a big deal.

Q: There was a question about the banyan tree milk...
Yogi Bhajan: Folks, I owe it to my grandfather, the most saintly man I have ever met in my life. Take the banyan milk with yogurt and it works perfectly. There's nothing in the vegetable world equal to it. I think now that it's April—it's the right time to go on it for six days.

Q: Banyan and yogurt?

Yogi Bhajan: For the prostate: It regulates, it controls and it strengthens all the muscles. It's very good.

Q: You mentioned that there were three Aryuvedic remedies that the man should use. What were they?

Yogi Bhajan: Yes. We call those three triphala. The Aryuvedic names are *hardada, beda and amlaa*. Their Latin names are: Embellic myrobolaus, Beleric myrobolaus, and Chebuic myrobolaus. A beautiful medicine can be made using these three and the juice of a fourth called *glib*. A tablespoon of this in the morning with a glass of milk will be sufficient for any efficient man. It is a wonderful gift of God.

INDEX

3HO 81, 109, 181, 237

7-year itch 32, 54

Alcohol 320

Arcline (Arc Body) 77, 100, 105, 110, 133; wearing cotton 91

Arthritis 87, 348, 351, 352

Astrology 34, 285

Aura (Auric Body) 15, 24, 35, 47, 50, 77, 91; wearing white 14, 91, 105

Bana 51, 92, 105, 115, 153; and the woman 86; wearing white 14, 91, 135, 153

Blocks 71, 136, 162, 203, 209, 213, 216

Boredom 180

Breath of Fire 133, and the sexual urge 136-8

Chakras 7, 47, 75, 85, 219, 224, 326, 331

Charan Japa 298

Child rearing 5, 9, 18, 32, 46-8, 64, 67, 79, 90, 127, 132, 144-7, 211, 247, 268, 297-299; and birth control 296; and diet 353, 358; uncircumcised 18; circumcision 51; death 93; and divorce 262; and masturbation 17; and sex 62; and a spiritual teacher 20

Circumvent Force 79

Circumcision 17, 29, 51; female 62; and sex 295

Cocaine 133, 215

Commitment 46, 66, 77, 80, 86, 115, 117, 147, 214, 242, 267, 325; blocks and 210; duality and 205, 209

Communication 11, 21, 53, 58, 65, 71, 85, 94, 113, 186, 235, 256, 268, 324; arguing 8, 21, 53, 55, 84, 88, 119, 157, 235, 262, 284, 298; and the chakras 75, 85; criticism 9; direct 13, 65, 157; honesty 114; Kriya 189, 259, 265; as intercourse 304; silence 4, 7, 10-1, 113; 72-hour rule 84; time and space 6, 47

Cycles (see also Lifecycles): 238, 243, breath (nostril) 15; menstrual 3, 66, 88; man's 30/70 cycle, 66, 72;

Dating 83, 301

Dharma 32, 37, 46, 64, 76, 250, 271, 297

Dialogue Exercises (with the Master) 216, 261, 264, 269, 277

Divorce 5, 21, 24, 36, 54, 68, 77, 80, 89, 125, 211, 256, 262; rate of 33

Eating 71, 91, 105, 115, 218; meat 19, 56, 140, 354

Ego 3, 9, 29, 32, 34, 45, 51, 55, 66, 75, 81, 93, 100, 108, 127, 129, 144, 165, 182, 207, 214, 248, 260, 294, 303; as an asset 229; and children 6; and nudity 205; sexual ego 125; and the woman 325

Ejaculation 3, 29, 224, 235, 296, 30; and aging 317; alkaline, 129, 136; consistency of 29, 60; and father phobia 225; and indirect anger 141; kriya for 317; and masturbation 15; mental 60, 124; premature 74, 143, 320, 345; and the projection of the male 80, 124, 129, 211; suspension of 136-7

Emotions (commotions) 76, 86, 143, 154-9, 167, 179-180, 183, 192, 204-210, 213, 232, 242, 249, 256, kriya for 22; and rationality 220; and the woman 181, 293

Anger 141-144, 237, 242, 276, 293; exercise for 167, 235; and the woman 11, 88; as an outlet 124

Depression 65, 78, 124,183, 205, 216, 263; exercise for 313, meditation for 331, and testicles 322;

Fear 69, 74, 80, 102, 104, 144, 220, 232, 238, 247, 268-1, 304; about sex 136; kriya for 274, 280; of death 176, 183, 206; of intimacy 217; of failure 218, 225; of success 225; physical expression of 152;

Happiness 2, 34, 48, 78, 114, 119, 147, 164, 180, 183, 186, 242, 262, 285, 293, 304;

Jealousy 80, 119, 276;

Love 4-9, 24, 30-34, 76, 93, 101-4, 108, 112, 129, 145, 153, 199, 207, 209, 217, 237, 248, 256, 269, 285, 294; conditional 8, 107, 209, 304; and the woman 76, 92; kriya for 253

Failure 4, 48, 104, 110, 140, 151, 160, 216, 220, 225, 229, 242, 248, 298; dialogue exercises and 269; and the woman 76, 294

Finances 11, 16, 22, 31, 33, 75, 119, 125, 181, 192, 233, 249, 320; debt 217; temptation 198; and success 227, 262

God 30, 77, 90, 101, 110, 153, 180, 199, 205-6, 213, 224, 229, 238, 245, 249, 281, 300, 304; as consciousness 47, 110; and fear of death 104; Infinity 40, 4, 210; and meditation 80, and mistakes 79, 295; and security 10, 22; and the woman 48, 64, 80, 87, 94; as the Word 12, 77, 179, 315

Golden Milk 87, 339, 351; recipe 346

Guru Gobind Singh 28, 32, 51, 77, 110, 115, 152, 179, 214, 273, 300

Guru Ram Das 106, 153, 192, 300

Hair 78, 318

Health 40, 172, 179, 192, 195, 243, 292; and acidity 18; and diet 55; and ejaculate 60; and weight 19; slogan 238 (See also Appendix B); kriya 307

Homosexuality 94, 294

Horny 35, 53, 58, 119, 124, 132, 140, 160, 293, 318, 324, 339; meditation for 59

Hygiene 59, 293, 295

Impotency 51, 55, 58, 62, 84, 125, 136-40, 143, 172, 210, 285, 292, 306, 322; foods for 338; kriya for 128, 131, 174, 317; and money 11, 22

Initiation 233

Insecurity 45, 83, 181, 225, 237, 246, 268; and the woman 6, 11, 16, 20, 48, 58, 69, 83, 119, 305, 324

Intercourse (see also Sex): 56, 142, 216, 324; and depression 18; as communication 304; during pregnancy, 18; and impotency 144; post intercourse 59, 292, 343; sexual 3, 15, 23, 47, 48, 141, 267, 349

Intuition 78, 180, 193, 198, 284; and the woman 6, 77; kriya 333

Kachera 15, 18

Karma 23, 32, 36, 102, 238, 297; meditation for 239

Kidneys 87, 320, 346, 348

Kindness 101, 103, 106, 210, 272, 284, 300

Kirtan Kriya 22, 59, 103, 116, 133-4, 328, 334

Krishna 272; and Lila 29, 62, 141

Laws: compromise 46; fake it until you make it 70, 77; the law of approach 5; law of dharma/karma 23, 102, 238; the law of nature (wishing and wanting) 210; the law of one 110; the law of polarity 12, 46; law of projection 52, law of swing 54; law of rhythm 129; sun and moon 4, 6; yamas and niyamas 164

Leadership 88, 110, 257, 268, 304; and the woman 4, 34, 67

Lifecycles 11, 21, 30, 32, 45, 54, 89, 164

Magnetic Field 79, 119, 210

Male and female, differences in 76, 319; sun and moon 112

Man 284; appearance 151, Banana man 8, 9, 20, 87, 304; and child 204, 211; defensive 35; exercises for 131, 175, 309, 313-5; kriya for 307, 321; Nature of 15, 28, 52, 75, 88, 129, 164; needs 65, 76, 86; Nobility 8, 28, 324; as Sun 4, 36; social animal 147; weaknesses 72, 94, 232

Mantra 281, 315, 327; Ardas Bhaee 103, 106, 111, 121; Guru Mantra 103, 167, 327; Har Hare Hari 281; Maha Mantra 235; Mangala Charn 265; Narayan mantra 96; Panj Shabd (Sa-Ta-Na-Ma) 22, 59, 103, 116, 133; three and a half frequency 103

Marriage 24, 31, 34, 45, 48, 51, 54, 69, 86, 117, 198, 210, 262, 298, 325; to Self 207; in-laws 22; finances, 31; arranged 145; nagging 218

Masturbation 15, 17, 51, 63, 124, 140, 292; and circumcision 18, 29; healing foods 349; in women (tiding) 16, 29, 63; mental 124, 136

Money 11, 16, 22, 31, 33, 75, 119, 125, 181, 192, 233, 249, 320; debt 217; and temptation 198; and success 227, 262

Moon Centers 16

Nervous System 15, 59, 63, 70, 87, 91, 110, 124, 133, 235, 303; kriya 194, 331

Neuroses 2, 64, 71, 143, 208, 228, 249, 269, 320

Ojas 60, 293

OPI-OPM, (Other People's Intelligence) and (Other People's Money) 108, 183

Orgasm 16, tidings 61

Peacock Pose 126, 138

Penis 2, 74, 125, 160, 224, 292, 295, 305, 320; kriya 266

Personality 32, 62, 71, 74, 88, 107, 125, 129, 143, 154, 193, 305; and communication 113, 157, 180, 186, 192, 256; exercise for 89; and power 115; and sexuality 127; and sympathy 152

Phobias 20, 22, 74; intelligence 5, Mother phobia 4, 20, 68, 71, 225 Father phobia, 12, 21, 68, 71, 80, 87, 93

Pituitary, or master gland 56, 102, 108, 115, 125, 130, 152, 292, 320, 349; and the penis 2, 56, 119, 285; and masturbation 15, 292; and smell 126, 138

Polarity 84, 156

Potency 28, 125, exercises 38-44; foods, see Appendix B

Pranayam 133, 167; kriya 168

Pratyahar 167, 257

Prayer 179, 238, 258, 324, 354; and food 70, definition of 117

Prostate Gland 60, 130, 292, 322; foods for healing 296, 355

Prostitution 107, 144, 156, 199; and the story of Joga Singh 214

Relationship 51, 77; being single 71; man and woman 4, 12, 21, 30, 34-6, 50, 53; relating to a woman 2, 32, 86;

Relaxation 55, 65, 118, 129, 216, 272; and sex 23, 39, 130, 136, 302; and sleep 313, 345; and meditation 39, 104; and the woman 114; kriya 128, 314

Religion 32, 52, 117, 160, 183, 199, 206, 210, 250, 320; and dharma 32; and faith 271; definition of 285

Sadhana 2, 21, 23, 72, 77, 83, 89, 162, 192, 217, 258, 271; recuperative powers of 59

Security, and the woman 4, 6, 33, 48, 69, 112, 120

Self 2, 89, 117, 125, 217, 224; higher 85, 107-8, 117, 147, 159, 161, 192, 198, 208, 213, 218, 232, 238, 251, 261, 269, 299; in relationship 9, 186, 324; meditations for cultivating the Self 103, 128, 179, 226, 240, 244, 248, 249, 330, 331

Semen 12, 18, 29, 40, 60, 108, 219, 339, 347, 357

Service 23, 48, 50, 75, 107, 153, 308; and anger 141

Sex (see also Intercourse) 58, 92, 130, 132, 139, 141, 145; and creativity 124; on a full stomach 3, 16, 139; stimulating the woman 16, 48; maturation 35; multiple ejaculations 59; perversions 61; 72-hour rule 47, 58, 140, 172;

Shakti Pad 106

Sixth Sense 74, 92, 132, 219, 285, 292, 296, 305, 318, 325

Sleep 3, 39, 58, 80, 118, 161, 239, 257, 272, 309, 319; and sex 16, 23, 63, 108, 130; and food 139, 339, 345

Smell 29, 35, 120, 126, 138, 149, 155, 267, 292-5, 303; vaginal 17

Solstice (Summer and Winter) 25, 238

Spirituality 28, 35, 64, 70, 74, 100, 105, 115, 156, 160, 181, 186, 216, 224, 242, 248, 276, 292; and health 301

Stress 20, 92, 133, 193, 269, 284, 295, 304, 353, remedies 55, 356

Success, 53, 125-7, 150, 186, 225, 233, 242, 256; and work 129; and the art of nursing 140; meditation for 166, 245

Teacher (spiritual) 20, 36, 103, 107, 147, 158, 261

Ten Bodies 47, 77, 101, 110

Testicles 58, 132, 138, 219, 292; temperature of 15, 322

Trust 9, 22, 36, 46, 65, 75, 80, 102, 113, 151, 164, 186, 207, 216, 221, 232, 245, 293; and children 48

Turban 318; and the woman 81, 86

Wet dreams 60, 124, 132, 350

White Tantric Yoga 22, 162

Wife 20, 32, 64, 81, 86-9, 144, 211, 262, 298; and communication 9, 55, 65, 102, 152, 210, 218, 232, 267, 306, 326; and father phobia 68; and mother phobia 225; and sex 293; and work 297; 'why and if' 34, 93, 106, 298; kriya 233

Woman 31, and child 7, 18, 80, 86, 181; as moon 3, 61, 66, 112, 256, 293, 298, 319; fundamental nature 2, 5, 7, 33, 48, 52, 64, 69, 119, 305; questioning, 5, 7; the Mother Nature 7, 11, 181, 205, 225, 273, 296, being single 83; what a woman wants 4, 9, 33, 80, 82, 305; 'wow' of the woman 29-33, 46, 297;

Work 45, 55, 68, 87, 94, 109, 124, 181, 209, 216, 229, 232, 238, 242, 247-9, 248, 269, 286, 322; and identity 225; woman 33; and sexuality 130; story of Kabir 117; eating habits 91, 139, 356; and relationships 94; and wealth 325

Yogi, definition of 36

Yogi Tea 87, 322; recipe 344

Resources

This and other KRI products are available from the
Kundalini Research Institute (KRI):

www.kriteachings.org

Remember to always buy from 'The Source'!

For information regarding international events:

www.3HO.org

To find a teacher in your area or for more information
about becoming a Kundalini Yoga teacher:

www.kundaliniyoga.com

Of further interest:

www.sikhnet.org

Kundalini Yoga as taught by Yogi Bhajan®

Kundalini Research Institute